THE **STRONG** SYSTEM

TRANSFORM YOUR MINDSET AND BUILD YOUR BEST BODY AT ANY AGE

CORI LEFKOWITH
@REDEFININGSTRENGTH

I0110034

VB

VICTORY BELT PUBLISHING INC.

LAS VEGAS

First published in 2026 by Victory Belt Publishing Inc.

ISBN-13: 978-1-628606-60-7

Cover design by Kat Lannom

Interior design and Illustrations by Yordan Terziev and Boryana Yordanova

Photography by Duke Loren

Printed in Canada

TC 0126

CONTENTS

FOREWORD

When I joined Cori's program, I didn't know I was about to begin one of the most profound journeys of my life. I was at my heaviest weight physically, mentally, and emotionally. My confidence and self-worth were buried under years of disappointment, shame, and self-criticism. I had tried everything, chasing the next diet or workout plan, desperate to finally feel good in my own skin. But nothing worked. I was ready to give up. Cori's program was going to be my last-ditch effort.

What I didn't know then was that it would become a rebirth and total transformation.

From the very first lesson, I realized this program wasn't like anything I had ever experienced. It wasn't just about macros or workouts. Cori didn't hand me another rigid plan or impossible set of rules. Instead, she taught me to meet myself exactly where I was—not where I used to be, not where I thought I should be, but right there, in that vulnerable moment.

That shift of meeting myself where I was became the foundation for everything that followed. It allowed me to drop the judgment, release the "all-or-nothing" mindset, and start showing up for myself with compassion and patience. Cori's approach gave me permission to be human, to grow at my own pace, and to see progress not just in my body, but in my mind and spirit.

Her message that self-love is a choice hit me hard. I had spent years believing love for myself had to be earned by reaching a certain weight, looking a certain way, or achieving some version of enough. But Cori helped me see that self-love starts long before any number changes. It starts with a single decision to choose yourself, even when it feels uncomfortable or undeserved.

Through her method, I learned that transformation doesn't come from punishment or perfection; it comes from consistency, curiosity, and care. Making small, sustainable changes and letting them build on top of one another while adding a sprinkle of patience is truly the recipe for lasting change. And it works, because it's built on grace instead of guilt.

This journey has transformed every part of me. My body is stronger and more capable than I ever imagined, but the real transformation happened inside. I've learned to quiet the inner critic, celebrate small wins, trust myself and the process, and see setbacks not as failures but as lessons. For the first time in my life, I'm not chasing unrealistic goals; I'm practicing evolution.

The beautiful thing about Cori is her unmatched passion and her heart for every person she helps. She doesn't just teach fitness; she teaches freedom. She reminds you that strength isn't just measured in pounds lifted or inches lost but is in your ability to rise after every fall, keep showing up, and believe that you are worthy of feeling amazing right now, not "someday."

This book is your guide to transformation—to redefining your strength on every level. It's an invitation to meet yourself where you are, dig deeper than the surface, and build strength inside and out that will last a lifetime. Cori's words will challenge you, empower you, and inspire you to rediscover the best version of yourself.

If you're ready to break free from the old stories that have held you back, if you're ready to stop chasing quick fixes and start creating a life that feels aligned and sustainable, this is your moment.

I know, because I'm living it.

This isn't just a program. It's a journey home to the strongest, most authentic version of you.

I'm forever grateful, Cori.

—Lori Wrobleski

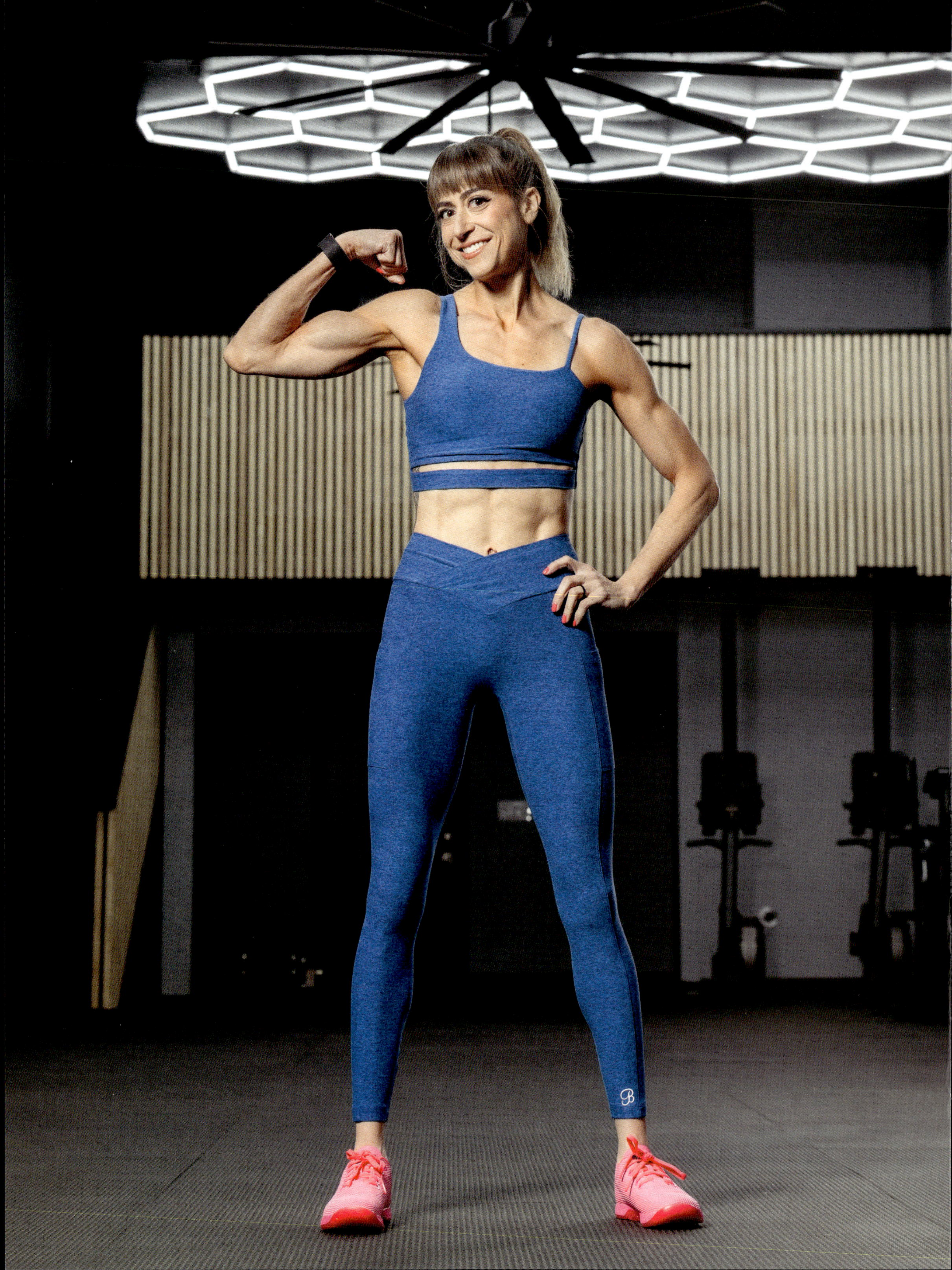

PREFACE

I know this part of the book is where the author is supposed to tell their own story, but this book isn't about me.

It's about you—creating the *you* that you want to be and seeing the results you deserve.

And while I will happily share more about why the heck you should trust a word I say, it's key I first highlight how important this focus on *you* really is.

This book helps you recognize that one size doesn't fit all and understand what you need to do to build the systems that will get you to your goals, even as your body, needs, goals, and lifestyle all change.

The systems and plans in this book aren't just about what I've found worked for me personally. They're also about what's worked for tens of thousands of clients just like you with the goal of conquering all the ups and downs that life can throw at you. My clients have been able to achieve things they would never have dreamed possible when they started out.

I could spend time on the certifications and training I have—from corrective exercise to performance enhancement, nutritional and macros certifications, menopause and pre- and postnatal certifications, classes and courses on kettlebells, battle ropes, lifting, functional fitness ...

I could spend time on all the publications, TV shows, and news shows I've been featured in, from *Women's Health*, Livestrong, *SELF*, *MindBodyGreen*, and *Well+Good* ...

This book not only utilizes my certifications and education and what's worked for me and the clients I've worked with for decades, but it also draws on the knowledge and experience of the coaches and dietitians on my team. Coaches and dietitians who have specialties and certifications that complement mine. They have their own experiences—overcoming different health concerns, pursuing sports challenges, reaching their goals, conquering different phases of their lives as they inspire our clients as well.

Too often, we get focused on what worked for someone else. Not on what will work for *us*. And that's why I don't want to focus on those things other than to show that this isn't a program based only on what worked for some influencer on your Instagram feed or some person who was willing to sacrifice by eating nothing but chicken and broccoli while doing two-a-day workouts. That's a lifestyle most of us can't sustain.

> **Too often, we get focused on what worked for someone else. Not on what will work for *us*.**

I only briefly want to mention all this because it's this diversity of knowledge, experience, and the fact that we've created systems and lifestyle wellness programs to help tens of thousands of individuals just like you around the world build their leanest, strongest bodies at any and every age—and break free of our fad diet, magic pill culture—that inspired me to write this.

When people focus too much on what other people have done (or are doing), I see them writing themselves off. They define themselves by an age. A health concern. A life situation. What they can't do.

But there is *always* a way to move forward. You simply have to recognize your unique path.

That's why this book isn't just another workout or diet plan.

Yes, I will give you those tools. But more than that, this book is a system and solution to meet you where you are so you can create lasting changes.

Over the years, you may have been drawn to the next "perfect thing." The *perfect* workout. A *perfect* diet. A *perfect* move. A perfect *perfect*.

When the goal is "perfect," it's common for results to fall short. There is no one "perfect" thing or habit. There is only creating a system that meets you where you are and leads you to your goals and lasting results.

In the pages of this book, you'll find the tools to help you act, including workouts and dietary changes that move you forward.

I can feel your burning desire to go right to that section. *Stop!* The plan is the reason you got this book, but skipping directly to that part won't make it work. Let me explain.

You've been searching for that single perfect program. However, to create lasting change, you instead need to do the most uncomfortable thing of all: embrace *building* a new you. That is what achieving results is all about.

That starts with truly recognizing who you are right now and the struggles you've had in the past. This recognition, self-awareness, and reflection are what will allow you to finally break free from the cycle of working hard to never truly achieve your goals in any lasting way. Because no matter how hard you work, if you're doing that work with the wrong system, you won't see the results you want. You might even be working in the wrong direction!

In this day and age of magic pills, quick fixes, restrictive diets, and intensive training programs that never really feel sustainable (and make you dream of going back to what you used to do), the STRONG system will help you meet yourself where you are, enjoy the foods you love, and train in a sustainable way. You will do *less* to achieve *more*, and it will help you find that balance that has you feeling, looking, and moving your most fabulous till your final day on this planet. The STRONG system will help you bridge that gap between knowing and doing so you can create the perfect system for *you*.

It's time to dive into what lies within the pages of this book, but remember, as tempting as it may be to skip right to the workouts and meal plans ...

Don't!

This is what most people do time and again, and it's why they've been stuck. If you've been one of those people, it's time to break the cycle.

INTRODUCTION

> **" A good farmer spends more time clearing the field than they do planting the seed. "**

People tend to want to jump to planting the seed before they've cleared the field when it comes to approaching weight loss, fat loss, gaining muscle, or health and wellness goals.

And this is why people often don't see results grow in the way they want. People jump to harvesting before they've planted because they want to get to doing the act they think will make the most difference—the part of the process they deem the most fun or important or exciting.

I see this comment daily on posts and videos: "This is too long. Stop telling me *about* it and just tell me what to do," or "Blah blah blah. Just get to the point of what I should actually do."

Everyone wants the "tactic":

» The macro ratio

» The food to cut out

» The workout to do

» The exercise to include

It's human nature to be less interested in learning *why* the changes would help or *why* they are key. People don't want to better understand why they're currently stuck. They don't even want to fully assess their current lifestyle to better understand what may or may not be right for them so they can see results truly build from the next thing they implement.

But this approach is like attempting to plant an apple seed in a field overgrown with weeds. Without understanding what's going on in general, there's no way you can grow that seed into anything, even if you want to!

You will never see the fruits of that labor (pun intended) even if you work super hard to plant it and take care of it.

I know you might not want to "waste" time planning and preparing and thinking through what you need to achieve results, but so much of why something leads to success is the prep work you do prior to getting started.

The more you have true clarity on what needs to be done and why it needs to be done, the more prepared you are to face any struggles. When you acknowledge potential pitfalls, you help yourself clear away struggles before they happen. You're truly addressing the weeds at the roots rather than pulling them out by the stems!

The more you do

» The boring mindset work
» The goal setting you feel is stupid
» The work to understand why macros are key
» The research to figure out why a specific workout design may or may not work

the more you create the perfect environment for *growth*, which yields the ripest, sweetest fruit.

You can't succeed if you aren't prepared to implement and sustain the new habits, no matter how amazing or perfect the habits are. You're not only fighting to create new habits but also fighting to clear away old ones. And those old habits are like weeds with very, *very* strong roots.

That's why it's worth your time to make the effort to understand where you are right now and *why* you need to do certain things to move forward. You need to recognize the old habits so you can prevent them from sabotaging new ones.

If you continue to skip to "doing" without learning and assessing, you'll stay trapped in the same cycle you have been (more on this change loop to come).

Look, I understand the desire to get right to planting something new. That's the reason fad diets are so tempting. They're just planting the seed. But that's also why you don't see results truly build and it gets harder month over month, year over year, to achieve your goals.

Stop sabotaging yourself by not pausing to clear the field first.

Set yourself up for success this time.

Do all the prep work. Learn the why. Embrace new mindsets. Then act.

You'll thank yourself for taking the time to really clear that field before you plant the seed.

THE UNSEXY TRUTH: BACK TO BASICS

There is no magic move in this book. No secret macro ratio. There are just the unsexy fundamentals you need to build off of—the basics you may think you're above. But you're not. They're fundamental for a reason. And the STRONG system is built off of them. That's why it works.

The truth of the matter is that you probably just need to be reminded what to do more than you need to be taught. You need to pull the right tool for the job out of your toolbox, not acquire a shiny new tool.

That's the reason I've laid out this book as a comprehensive system that builds. You figure out where you're starting from and begin there, not from some "ideal" point. Because there is no ideal. What's "ideal" is what fits your lifestyle, needs, goals, body, and mindset as they are right now. Knowing what you need takes some assessment, so that's where you will start. Honestly, although the assessment might not be all that much fun, it's the most important and most eye-opening part of the process. It is the part that will have you asking one very important question over and over again: *why?*

When you're starting a new diet and workout plan to lose fat, gain muscle, and be your strongest, fittest self, you're embarking on a process of behavior change. You'll be building self-awareness, and that happens through reflection.

For example, you'll ask yourself:

? Why you hold certain beliefs

? Why you repeat certain patterns

? Why you're resistant to certain changes or believe specific things to be the only "right" way

Often, people seek out the *what* and the *how* of making changes. They look for what they need to do, but they don't bother to understand the *why* behind it. Questioning why helps you dive into what has and hasn't worked so you can meet yourself where you are. And it helps you find the value in the new habits you're working to create.

You have to remember that you prioritize what you value. And understanding why something is important helps you prioritize it. It's why I frequently challenge you to reflect and ask *why*.

From this foundation, you can build the system you need, nerding out about the fun and exciting tactics and techniques you can use before you have to implement them.

Actually, that's another place where you may get stuck. It's easy to get excited about all the opportunities but then never take action. You might either hit a point of overwhelm or do something for a day or two and then let old habits creep back in. That's another effect of skipping the first stage of understanding the systems you need and jumping right to what you think is the "important stuff."

HOW TO USE THIS BOOK

So, to help you avoid repeating the same cycle again, I've set up this book in three sections:

» **Part 1: Understanding Your System**

» **Part 2: Building Your System**

» **Part 3: Implementing Your System**

In "Understanding Your System," you'll learn about the change loop that's been keeping you stuck, and you'll start to outline your origin story while truly assessing what your goals are. You'll break down everything you need to meet yourself where you are now to create a game plan for action by going through the STRONG system method.

In "Building Your System," you'll refine your plan and map out your habits so you're truly able to take action. I'm not talking about only your diet and workouts, the two habits most people focus on. You'll plan all the habits you need to create a system that will drive you forward.

To help you plan your system, I'll outline three different macros methods so you can choose the one that fits where you are. You'll be able to make eye-opening and sustainable dietary adjustments that don't require you to cut out the foods you love or label foods as "good" or "bad."

I'll break down how you can track without tracking with my hand-sized health method. There are fundamental principles you need to implement to see results, but that doesn't mean you can't be creative with your habit practice to match your lifestyle, mindset, and needs!

In Part 2, I'll also break down three different training methods so you can see results no matter what your current fitness level, needs, or goals are—even if you're short on time and training with limited equipment at home. If you've ever wondered how many reps and sets you should do, what types of moves are best, how much rest you should take, and what areas you should work, your questions will be answered.

I'll share training techniques you may have never seen before, such as the 6-12-25 method or compound burner sets. I'll teach you how to harness the power of interval workouts to build strength when all you have is your own body weight. I'll also help you assess how much cardio versus strength work you need and show you how you can use the cardio-strength continuum to your advantage to see fabulous muscle gains and fat loss no matter your age.

And if you're feeling doomed by your age or aches and pains, or if you're worried you won't be able to train the way you need to see results, I'm going to show you how you can feel and move better than you did even in your twenties and thirties with a three-step prehab process.

I'll go over all the unsexy stuff that is easy to ignore but also often the reason hard work in the gym and nutritional changes don't pay off. I'll cover the stuff that doesn't feel like it has benefits and makes you have to slow down but is ultimately what leads to better results faster—things like recovery, sleep, micronutrients (vitamins and minerals), and even taking breaks from the push to see results.

You read that last part right. *Breaks* in your training and diet can help you see results faster. In Part 2, I'll break down why. I'll even go over how to track progress, when to make changes, and how to know if something is or isn't working.

In the final section, "Implementing Your System," you'll grab the resources you need and start taking action. This is the section you'll find yourself returning to as your body, needs, and goals change.

Now, let's get to it! It's time to clear the field, plant those seeds, and put in the work to grow those apple trees so you can enjoy the delicious fruits of your hard work!

In Chapter 1, I'll begin with one of the most eye-opening realizations I personally had—the recognition of the change loop I was keeping myself stuck in. When you become conscious of a pattern you're repeating, you gain the power to change it and break free!

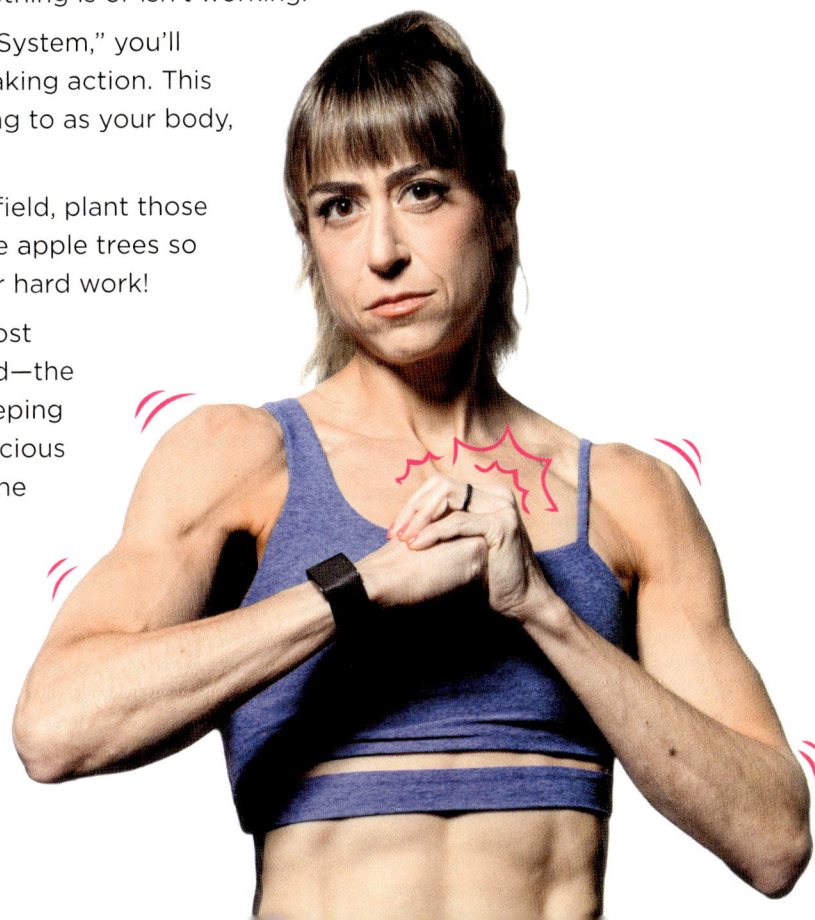

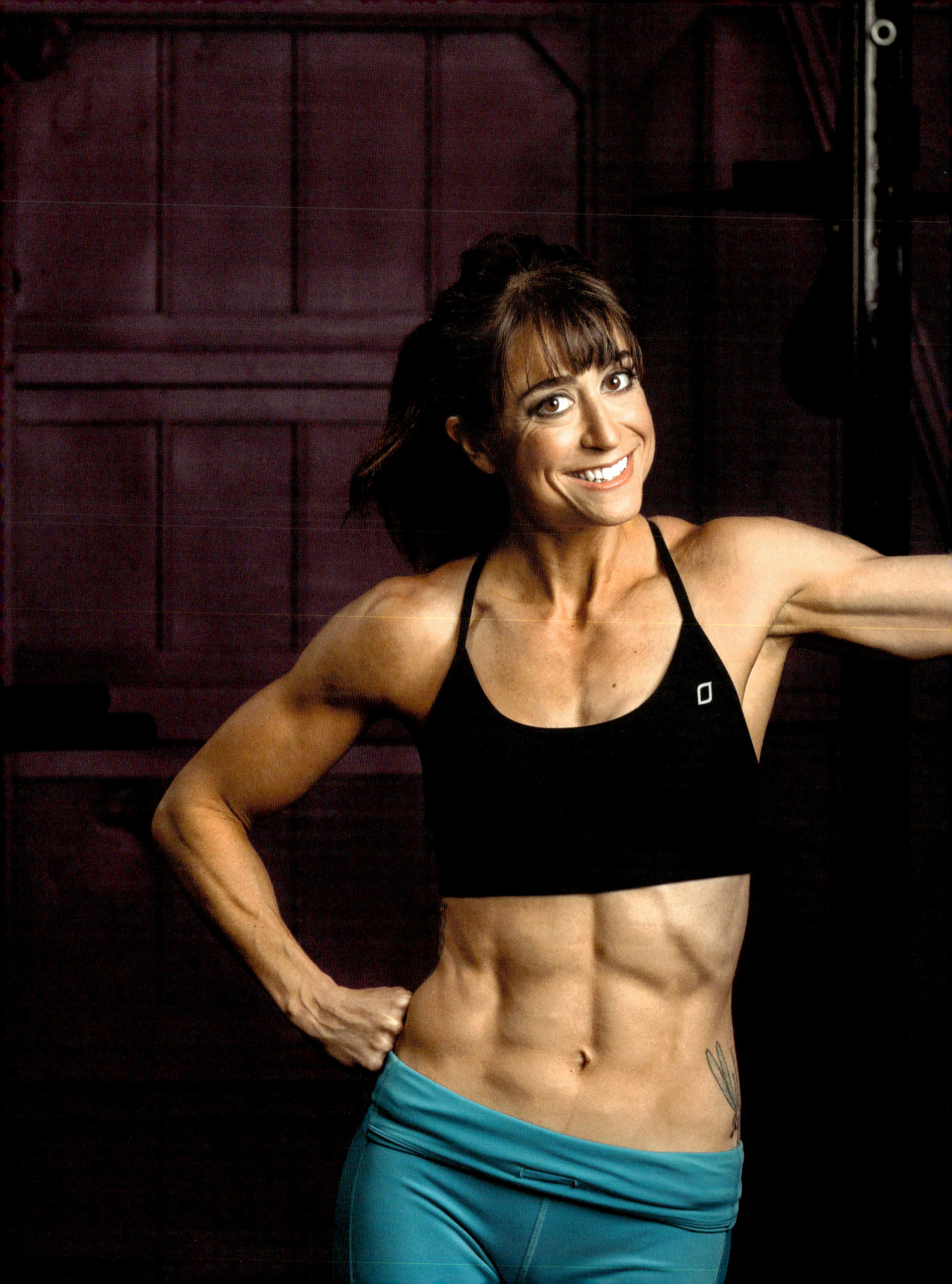

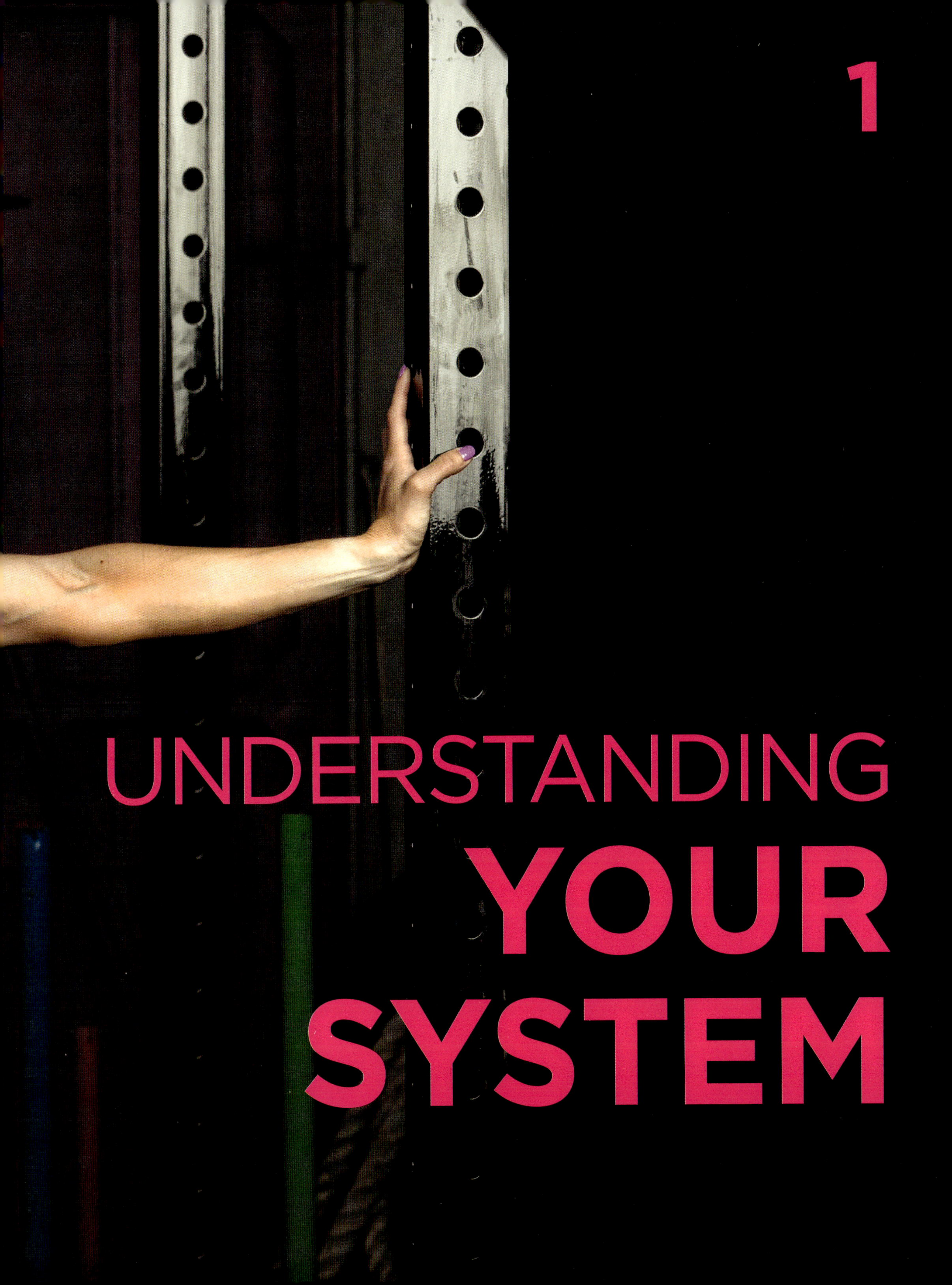

1

UNDERSTANDING YOUR SYSTEM

1 YOUR CHANGE LOOP

Right now, I just know you're itching to jump to the workouts and meal plans. You want to be told what to do so you can do it already.

But this attitude has kept you stuck in a loop of working really hard only to end up frustrated that results don't snowball. (And if you're confused by what I mean by "snowballing"—just wait!) If you're overwhelmed by all the conflicting information available and unsure of what to do, you probably don't do anything long enough to progress.

Your desire to skip straight to the action and work harder is holding you back.

You've been planting seeds in overgrown fields, and it hasn't worked. This time, you refuse to repeat that cycle.

You're reading this right now because you finally want to make a change. So, make it!

WHAT THE CHANGE LOOP IS

Slowing down and pausing to better understand what you need are the first steps of making a change because that "act-fast, do-more" approach can lead to worse results and a lot of frustration. In other words, you need to slow down to speed up.

I say this as a person who learned this lesson the hard way. I fell into this trap far more times than I'd like to admit. Taking action feels good! It makes you feel like you're moving forward even when you aren't.

Anytime I find myself trying to rush results by taking action, like I can out-exercise or out-diet time, I remind myself of the tale of two woodcutters. Let me explain, because you're probably now thinking, *What the heck does a story about woodcutters have to do with this?* (And don't worry, all my references aren't going to be garden and tree related.)

Two woodcutters were in a competition to see who could cut down more trees by the end of the day. The first woodcutter was older and more experienced; the second was a younger, stronger person eager to prove their ability and show up the seasoned foe.

Both set to chopping. After about an hour or so, the more experienced woodcutter paused, sat down to take a break, and invited the younger person to join in.

The second woodcutter replied, "No way! I'm going to keep chopping, and I'm going to beat you."

"Suit yourself," said the experienced woodcutter.

Throughout the day, the experienced woodcutter took breaks off and on, while the younger, stronger woodcutter kept chopping away.

At the end of the day, when the two woodcutters compared their results to see who had chopped more wood, the younger and stronger woodcutter, who never took a break, was astonished to find that the older woodcutter, who had taken breaks, had chopped piles and piles more wood.

The younger woodcutter was incredulous and said, "How is that possible? You spent far less time chopping than I did. I'm stronger and never once stopped chopping. What's your secret?"

The experienced woodcutter said, "Every time I sat down, I was sharpening my axe."

Hard work is key to results. But hard work without direction, focus, and intention is frequently energy wasted.

Too often, a person's tendency is to seek to do more in the gym. They restrict foods while searching for a magic fat-burning supplement. Instead, what they really should be doing is learning and dialing in the basics to focus on what they truly need right now.

It's not about effort. It's about efficiency.

Read that again. It's *not* about effort. It's about *efficiency.*

Trust me, if it was about effort, I'd know lots of people in far better shape than me. People who train twice a day for hours and eat only "clean foods," for example. Now, don't misunderstand me; I'm not the least bit lazy, but I do have my dessert. I love my Rice Krispies treats with buttercream frosting. And I'm going to train three days a week for thirty minutes if that's what my schedule needs.

Being consistent with what you need is what adds up. You don't want to work so hard that you ultimately burn out and end up bingeing on a whole pint of ice cream on the couch and saying "forget it" to your workouts for the next couple of weeks.

So, don't be afraid to pause, assess, and learn. Don't be afraid to take time to plan. Heck, purposefully make time for it. Often, considering the outcomes can save a ton of time going in the wrong direction.

This reflection helps you really assess what you need now. It helps you build the self-awareness that enables you to push through the ups and downs that life will throw your way (because no journey is ever without its challenges).

Before you start working, it's important that you have a focused direction. You need to understand what's driving you forward and what you need to be efficient in making changes—in other words, you need to "sharpen your axe." This is the different approach you need to take to help you push through hard situations that previously would have stopped you in your tracks and made you turn back.

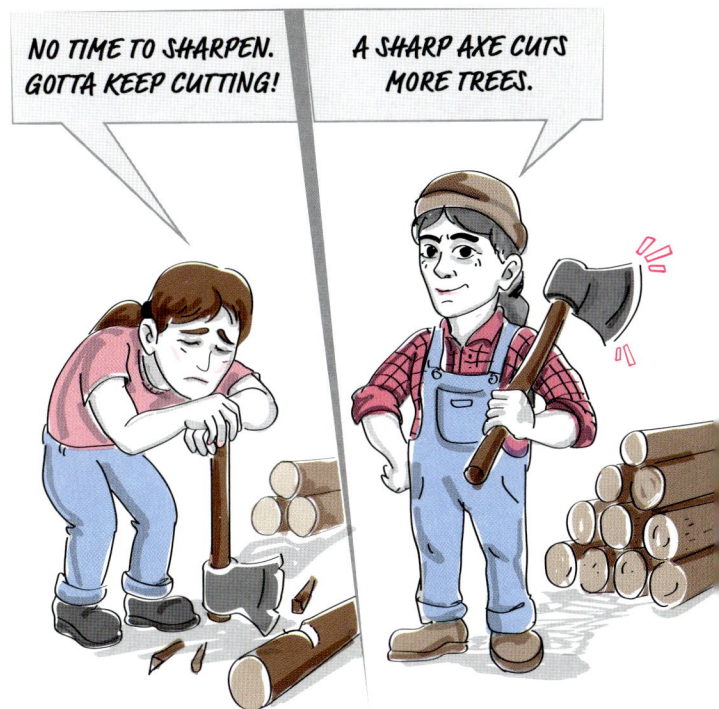

You're finally going to bust out of that change loop you've been stuck in. The change loop has made you feel like you don't have the willpower or self-control to see the results you deserve, and it might also make you feel like getting older means accepting weight gain and injuries and feeling ... well ... old.

But the amazing truth is that you can build your leanest, strongest body at any and every age. You just have to finally break free from repeating the same pattern you've always followed. It means embracing the hard stuff and doing things differently to see a new outcome.

THE END OF STARTING OVER

"No program will ever work. I've tried everything!" Lisa left this comment—complete with a crying face emoji—on my Facebook post about seeing results at any age.

Lisa and I first met when she commented about having struggled with trying to out-exercise her diet. After months of back and forth, wanting to reach her goal but being scared to fail at another thing, she officially started implementing the system. She started making hard changes. But her mental rebellion was palpable.

"What if this is yet another thing that doesn't work?" You could tell this question was running through her mind.

Inches began to shrink, but budging the scale was painfully slow. The fear and doubt began to add up.

The days ticked by as she slowly embraced the changes that went against everything she thought she needed. She was working to reverse decades of dieting culture build-up, metabolic adaptations, and lifestyle mindsets and habits she didn't even realize she had.

Nine weeks in, we were on a video call when she said, "I've been so consistent, and I've worked so hard, but results aren't happening fast enough! I quit."

I simply looked at her and said, "No."

She stared back at me. She totally hadn't expected that response. After a little bit of time—actually, it was a very awkward silence that felt like minutes—I added, "This is where you've always quit. You hit this locked door, and instead of trying to find the key, instead of even testing to see if it's really locked and not just stuck, you turn back. But if you don't this time, you'll finally achieve your goals. So, keep going."

I've been guilty of turning back too; everyone has. Along the way, you have challenges where the door may be open just a smidge, but you can see the light, so you keep going. Then you come to a point where you hit a door that's fully closed. It's your first real test.

Too often, when you hit that first sticky door, the one you have to put a little shoulder to, you turn back. You don't want to look like a butthead by continuing to try to push open a locked door. So, you give up.

Then you head back the way you came to try to find another way forward. But ultimately, you just keep repeating this cycle, always hitting another closed door that looks a little different. And each time, because you've taught yourself to turn back, you do.

Now, I want to show you how to finally unlock that closed door and keep moving forward. Because the key is right there—you just have to know how to look for it. It starts with recognizing the change loop you've caught yourself in.

IT ALL STARTS WITH A PROMISE

You're starting a change loop right now as you're reading this book. You're excited by this system. Hopeful. You feel like this could be *the thing.*

You're motivated and passionate about making a change, just as you have been every other time in the past. Think about the last time you started a new program. What had happened right before motivation hit you so hard that you had to act right then and there? Maybe it was one of these things:

» You tried on some pants that just didn't fit.

» You hit a number on the scale you'd thought you'd never see.

» You became tired and frustrated.

» You were in *pain*. Not necessarily physical pain, but you really didn't like where you were.

You were driven to make a change.

In those moments, the pain of staying stuck outweighs the pain of change. You're willing—even wanting—to make sacrifices if it means you hit your goals.

When you hit this stage, you go all in. You're an all-or-nothing person. It's like you just got a new, shiny, beautiful car, and you want to get in it and start driving as fast as you can! You want to be perfect with everything, so you put pressure on yourself to do the most you can. You make every change. You make sacrifices to get results faster. You read through everything, and you make all the changes recommended by the program:

» Cut out your favorite gooey, double-chocolate, fudgy brownie? No problem.

» Work out twice a day, hitting the gym morning and night to lift before logging endless miles on the treadmill? OK. You can manage that for a bit if it guarantees results!

» Convince yourself, *This isn't so bad. This could be a lifestyle.*

You don't like those delicious, salty tortilla chips and creamy guacamole or that large glass of wine you pour when you first get home and kick your shoes off to drink as you eat your bar of smooth, velvety dark chocolate on the couch *that* much, right?

You're doing everything you can all at once. You work harder and focus on every last detail. You see some progress, which motivates you to do even more.

But then you have a day when you forget your lunch at home. And, of course, your coworkers buy pizza from that local spot that has just the right amount of cheese and the crust with some crunch but a bit of doughiness, and it smells as good as it tastes, and you can feel the scent pulling you out of your office.

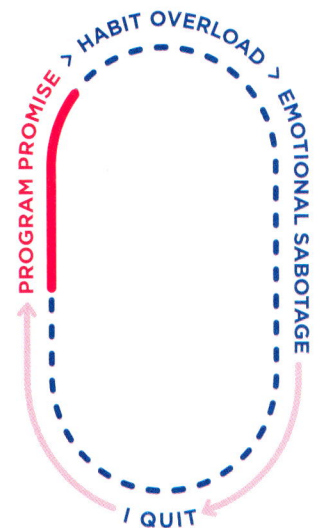

Then your friends want to meet up for dinner at the place with those amazing, freshly baked rolls with that light, flaky sea salt, and they're just screaming for butter. Skipping your workout isn't that big of a deal, right? You already ruined your diet today, so who cares?

No! you think. *I won't. I'll just go home. I'll work out.* But even though you're doing what you "should," you feel even more miserable. You remind yourself of the progress you've made. You tell yourself you just have to keep going to get to your goal. Progress has happened; you just have to trust the process, right? Wrong.

All these habit changes are starting to make you feel overloaded and overwhelmed. Your self-control gas tank is heading toward empty, and you're about to realize that while you've been driving fast, your car has run over a nail, and your tire pressure is slowly draining away.

WHEN HABIT OVERLOAD HAPPENS

Newton's Third Law states, "For every action, there is an equal and opposite reaction." This is especially true when it comes to your diet.

In your cabinet are these magically soft chocolate chip cookies your friend shipped to you from a shop near her house. You know they will come out of the microwave and melt in your hand with ooey-gooey goodness.

You put them in the cabinet because you couldn't bear to throw them out. But as time passes, the call of those cookies gets stronger and stronger. You can smell them through the wrapping. You've passed them by for days, and every time you think, *Would one bite be that bad?*

However, you know if you have just one, you'll eat them all. Then you'll just want to kick off your shoes, open that bottle of wine, and plop on the couch instead of going to the gym.

Your old habits call. And the call is getting stronger.

The more you force yourself to resist something, and the more you go against what you've always done, the more mental pushback you'll experience (Newton's Third Law at its finest!). People don't like change. The familiar is comforting.

The more you resist, the more you will want to give in.

But you want this time to be different! You think, *Do I just not have the willpower?* You keep trying to push through.

The burnout continues to build. Every habit feels like a chore. The workouts you enjoyed now have you dreading the gym. You're sick of watching everyone at work enjoy foods that you can't have. You feel the pressure mounting. Things don't feel sustainable. You're questioning how much longer you can do all these habits.

Still, you hold out. You're weighing in this weekend. If you see progress, it will all be worth it, right? You count the hours and white-knuckle your way through. Then you step on that scale.

Boom. You've just realized you have a flat tire, and you have to pull over.

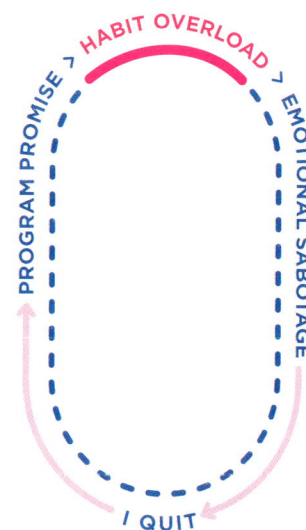

EMOTIONAL SABOTAGE: THE TIPPING POINT

*What the f***!* you think when you see you haven't even lost an ounce!

Frustration and disappointment hit at once, and you feel mentally drained. You want to throw the scale at a wall, cry, have a tantrum on the ground, and go eat every food you've wanted and passed up during the last few weeks.

You've hit the eff-it point. You're beyond caring. You give up. Emotional sabotage is about to kick in, and you're about to do everything you know you shouldn't.

You have a flat tire, and you've pulled over. But instead of calling roadside assistance or putting on the spare, you're about to take out a knife and slash the other three tires.

Does that choice make any logical sense as a way to fix the situation and get back on the road faster? Nope.

But emotional sabotage is illogical. It doesn't make any sense, but by the time you're at that point, you just don't care. It's that "I quit!" moment where rational decision-making is completely gone. Your self-control is on empty, and the effort you've given doesn't feel worth the outcome. You feel like you've wasted time, money, and energy—probably not for the first time.

You feel broken, so you completely self-sabotage. You want immediate comfort and couldn't give a flying fart in space about your long-term goals, so one cookie becomes ten. A bite of pizza becomes the whole thing.

And then you're starting over *again*.

But this is where you have a choice. The question you have to ask yourself at this point is, "Do I quit? Or do I double down?"

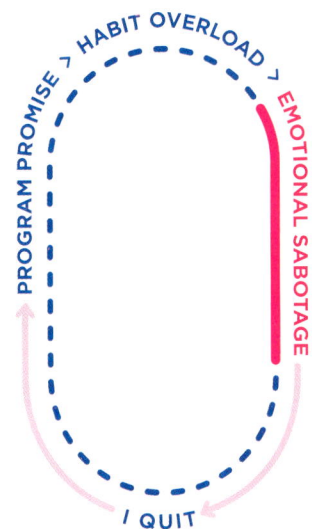

"I QUIT!"

One common reaction people have when they get frustrated is to give in to temptation, even though they know they shouldn't. You may grab a bag of chips, finish the whole thing, and lick the salt from your fingers when you're done. Now that you've satisfied that salty fix, maybe you need something sweet, so you go after those chocolate chip cookies with the extra-large chocolate chunks. You heat one up in the microwave and bite into it as the chocolate smears on your lips. You put two more in the microwave to heat up while you grab a pint of ice cream from the freezer.

Now, it's time to bust out the big, loose T-shirt and sweatpants. And you probably feel lethargic from the snacks, so maybe you not only skip your workout for one day but also for the whole week.

In these cases, every change you've made is *poof—gone!* It's immediately forgotten. Basically, you had one flat tire, and you not only slashed the other three tires, but you also decided to burn the car and leave it by the side of the road.

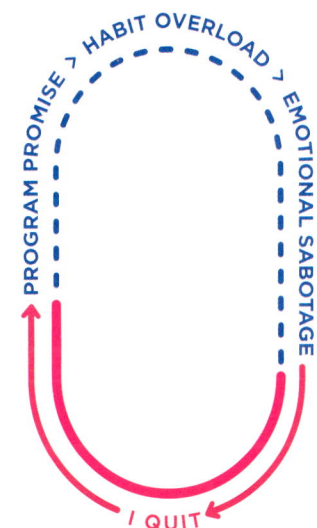

The tendency is to blame the program and try to think of all the reasons why something didn't work. You may question whether you have the willpower, the genetics, or the lifestyle to ever achieve your goals. You probably feel increasingly worse with time. The guilt mounts more and more as you get deeper into habits and routines you dislike.

Eventually, you realize you still need a car. So, you decide to make a change and go buy a new one. And this is where the change loop starts to repeat.

How far down the negativity spiral you go before you finally decide to stop the slide isn't always the same. But each time, you set yourself back a little more, so you aren't just starting over but also digging yourself out of a deeper hole.

The thing is, this pattern makes it feel harder and harder to see results as you get older. Being caught in the change loop can lead to feeling like you'll never achieve results—with good reason. Each setback means you now do have more you have to fight against. Going around the loop over and over again makes the journey harder. The good thing is that when you recognize a pattern repeating, you can gain the power to break it.

This is your chance to stop repeating this change loop. This time, when you hit a hard situation, feel that habit overload and emotional sabotage building, and want to slash the other three tires …

You won't. Instead, you'll …

DOUBLE DOWN

OK. I might have exaggerated earlier. In reality, when you get a literal flat tire, you don't slash the other three tires. Honestly, that concept is ridiculous when you think about it. But the spiral I described for overeating and giving up on exercise is what people often do with diet and workout habits. When a tire goes flat on a car, you'd find a solution to fix the problem and move forward.

That's what it means to double down, and that's what you need to do with your food and your workouts.

You need to step back and assess what is and isn't working. Where is the true problem, and what can you do to fix it? When you recognize the problem, you then need to tweak the stuff that doesn't work (note, I didn't say you need to completely stop doing it!) and do more of the things that are working. You double down on those habits.

Doubling down isn't necessarily about doing more or working harder. You can't out-exercise or out-diet time.

It's about *efficiency of work* (remember the woodcutter sharpening his axe!) and focusing on the habits that build progress. It's about building off of those habits to see changes snowball. It's about finding room for growth and improvement in what you're already doing to get even more consistent with it.

Doubling down isn't only about the actions you take. Doubling down also involves a huge shift in mindset, and, honestly, this is why the biggest payoff happens.

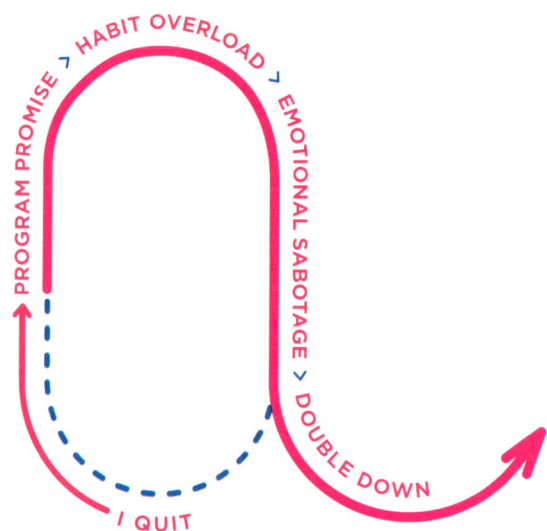

When you double down, you keep going. You look at that comfort zone and step past it.

When you double down, you realize that this is the point where you've stopped and fallen back into old patterns every other time. This time, you know the only way to break the loop is to do something different by not going back into the comfort of what you were doing prior. You know where those old habits lead—and it's not forward.

Doubling down means you recognize that even though progress won't be linear, you're still stepping forward. You've heard that pushing toward the hard and pushing outside your comfort zone is where the magic happens, and it truly is.

The ability to create workout routines and dietary habits that not only move you forward but also meet you where you are, allowing you to embrace building and pushing through the challenges to see results, is a big part of what you'll get out of this book. It also helps you reflect on those habits to own what is and isn't moving you forward as efficiently as possible so you can make changes without feeling like you need to start over.

Because there is no starting over. Instead, there is either repeating the change loop or breaking free of it by pushing through the "I quit" moments to keep going. By doing the hard work of not quitting when it would be so easy to do so, you show yourself how much you can overcome. You show yourself your true strength.

YOUR STRENGTH REVEALED

Strength is built through what you overcome.

The more you face, and the more you push through the challenges, the more you will be able to accomplish. Achieving your goals means revealing your strength as you push past that comfort zone and learn to get comfortable being uncomfortable in new ways.

With this book, you will try new habits. You will fail at new things. But most importantly, you will consistently reflect on what is and isn't working and keep circling back to doubling down on the successful habits that move you forward.

There will always be hard points and challenges on your path, but you don't have to make things extra hard on yourself by creating the habit overload that leads to emotional sabotage. So, in this book, I help you capitalize on your strength to make changes that fit with who and what you are. Because this is what most efficiently gets you from where you currently are to your destination and what leads to results snowballing.

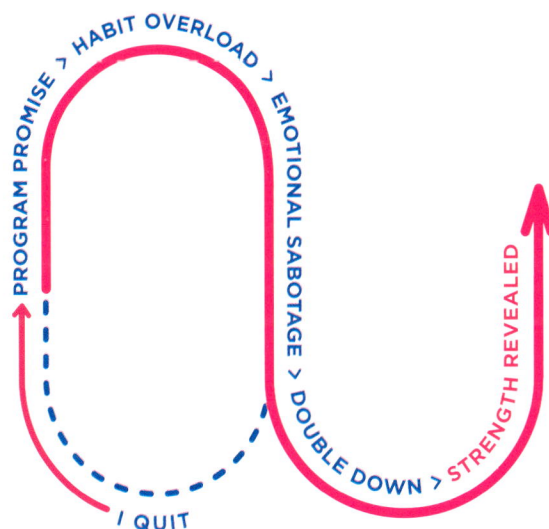

THE SNOWBALL

"I didn't get what Cori meant by results 'snowballing' until today, when I saw my progress photos. Holy cow! I didn't realize how much had changed just from looking in the mirror daily!"

Often, results happen slowly enough that we can't see the incremental changes until we take a bird's-eye view and step back to reflect. Moving an inch at a time doesn't feel like you're making progress, but even inch by inch, you can go a mile.

Through consistent hard work and consistent focus on habits that build, you move forward. That *consistency* is key. It's also what is often missing when you're constantly "starting over."

But remember what I said earlier: There is no starting over. Each time you repeat the change loop, you've actually dug yourself into a deeper and deeper hole.

Think of it this way: Success is never owned; it's rented. The daily, boring, basic habits you do to be successful are like paying rent. And rent is due. Every. Single. Freaking. Day.

Getting results means you have to put in the work *daily*. And you don't get to do sexy, fun, new things each day. You have to do the boring basics to get to your goal. And once you get to that goal? You have to *keep* putting in the work. Every. Single. Freaking. Day.

If you think you'll get to your goal and then be able to go back to life as it was before you made the changes, that's not how it works. You can *never* stop doing what made you "better."

If you've heard the phrase, "Fake it till you make it," I want you to learn this one instead: You've got to *act as if* until you're *acting as you are.*

You will never stop doing the healthy habits that got you results. You won't necessarily do them in the exact same form for the rest of your life, but you will do some version of them.

Because the simple fact is, you're never going to go back to what you used to do unless you want to lose all your hard-earned results and progress. Will you have some not "perfect" days? Of course! Will some days be easier than others? 100 percent! There will also be days you really don't want to do what you need to do. You'll have some days that stink.

But you've still got to stay focused on doing your habits day in and day out—paying that rent daily—if you want to move forward and maintain your results long term.

Now that you have a better understanding of the change loop and how you get stuck in it, I want to help you better understand how you can stop this loop from repeating.

It's time to set your GPS!

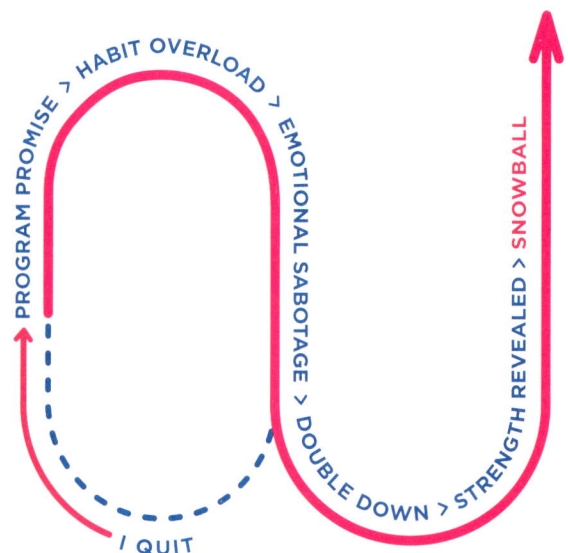

PROGRAM PROMISE > HABIT OVERLOAD > EMOTIONAL SABOTAGE > DOUBLE DOWN > STRENGTH REVEALED > SNOWBALL

I QUIT

2 SET YOUR GPS

A client named Deb emailed me to say that she wanted to lose weight but was struggling to make dietary changes. I asked what she was currently doing in terms of her nutrition.

"Well, I start my day with some oatmeal and a banana. For lunch, I may have a sandwich with chips or maybe a wrap and fries. Then for a snack, some crackers or maybe candy that's out at the office. And dinner is often, like, pizza or takeout if I'm feeling lazy. I don't really like to cook."

As I read about her average day, I made a note that it was carb heavy with lots of restaurant dishes and processed foods. Note: I wasn't making a judgment. I was just observing what changes may add up as I met her where she was in terms of macros and meal prep.

She wrapped up by saying she always struggled to find something sustainable and concluded with, "I think I'll just do keto."

My face looked like that emoji with the circle mouth as I read that last statement and reeled with shock. I emailed back: "Out of curiosity, with all that you just mentioned, why would you decide to start a keto diet?"

Her response: "I don't know. But it's super popular and seems to be getting results for lots of people."

Now my face turned into that half-blue emoji with the hands on both cheeks. I shook my head. I felt her frustration with repeating the change loop, and I could see the pattern was about to repeat itself—again. She was about to force herself into another fad-diet mold.

The loop ended for her that day when I said, "One size doesn't fit all."

Now it's your turn. Your loop can end today. Although you may see new diet and workout trends rising in popularity and enticing you with being the next magic quick fix, just being popular doesn't make it good or right for you. Even if it worked for your friend, who you perceive as being similar to you, that doesn't mean it will work for you. So today is the day you stop starting over. No more hoping the next thing will work.

You've probably been looking for a program based only on your goal—the end result you want. Instead, you need to pause and sharpen your axe by taking a good hard look at who and what you are. You need to build self-awareness of your habits, lifestyle, priorities, and excuses.

If you don't know who you are, you can't find what you truly need. While this may feel like a deeper exploration than you thought you'd have for "just some weight loss," I have news for you. It's your key for finally seeing the results you deserve and achieving more for yourself than you thought possible—not only in terms of your aesthetic goals but also in building strength to grow and conquer so much else you didn't think was possible in your life.

Right now, you're going to start to map out your route to results by fully owning who and what you are and the lifestyle you want to lead! And that all starts in this chapter with truly understanding your starting point.

WHERE ARE YOU STARTING FROM?

As Maya Angelou so perfectly put it, "You can't really know where you're going until you know where you've been."

Think about using your GPS in your car. When you set it to help you get to a destination you've never been to (or, if you're like me, a place you have been frequently but can't seem to remember what route to take), you set not only your destination but also your current location.

I love how the GPS almost always calculates *exactly* where I am. And when it doesn't pinpoint my exact location, I swear I always turn the opposite way I should. There's nothing worse than realizing you've gone the wrong way, can't make a U-turn until you've passed through seven lights, and have to spend extra time just to get back to where you started. But often, many of us do exactly that on our fitness journeys.

If you look only at your destination and not your starting point, you'll get caught up in a "perfect plan"—a plan that overwhelms you so you never get started because you're unsure of what to do. Or maybe you're trying a plan that you can't stick to long term because it leads to so many wrong turns you ultimately give up in frustration and feel worse than when you started. This is because you don't have clarity on what you need.

You need to slow down to speed up. When you barrel ahead without thought, your GPS can't calibrate to find your current location. And if your GPS can't find your location, you're likely to head in the wrong direction or feel overwhelmed by meaningless directions that don't address your point of origin. No one likes to feel overwhelmed and directionless.

So, your first step is assessing where you are *right now*. I'm not asking you where you used to be in your "prime" and where you'd like to get back to but where you are right this minute.

I know it's easy to want to be back where you were during your "glory days." You wouldn't be the first person I've heard say something like, "I used to be so in shape before having kids. I was running marathons without aches and pains. I just wish I could get back there," or, "I used to have abs; then menopause hit, and I look like I have this tire around my middle." You want to go back to where you were because you felt good at that time—not necessarily because of a number on the scale or a specific achievement but because you simply remember feeling your best then. That's what you're chasing now: a *feeling*.

Unfortunately, you can't go back. You can't change your age or the life events that have happened. Wishing you could only makes you feel more powerless to make a change. And honestly, how does where you were have any relevance to where you are now? Simply put, it doesn't.

If you want to move forward, you have to deal with the reality of all that's happened, including the injuries, less-than-ideal habits, and excuses. You also have to own that your priorities may have completely shifted. Continuing to focus on what "was" and what "used to be" will hold you back from moving forward because you're chasing something that will never exist in that form again. You're not the same person. Life has happened. Instead of chasing a feeling, you need to look at how you can move forward to feel your most fabulous now.

When I say you need to let go of where you used to be, I'm not asking you to ignore the importance of everything you've done to get to this point. In fact, when someone asks me, "How long did it take you to achieve *blank?*" (it doesn't matter what result they're asking about), I always say, "My entire life!"

Everything you've done to get where you currently are, good or bad, has an impact. It affects what you do and do not like and what changes you're open to. It affects your mindset about tools and influences how much pain you're willing to embrace. It determines how many unconscious habits you're going to fight against and how much your body will resist changes because it's become comfortable in its current state.

Part of owning where you are is assessing where you've been to help you find the clearest, most direct path forward. All your previous experiences shed light on what you need and even how long results will take to build.

> **OWNERSHIP**
>
> Note that I keep saying "own." Taking ownership is a key component to understanding your mindset and lifestyle. You need to realize the role you've played in getting into your current situation. Although life happens and things outside your control occur, you have to take back control of those things you have power over. This means being accountable for what your life looks like and the mindset you have right now so you can develop belief in your ability to move forward.

CONTROL WHAT YOU CAN CONTROL

Often, people don't realize how much they lack belief in their ability to make a change. People tend to think, "Well, nothing has ever worked for me before. So why should it now?" That's why this pause to build awareness of your priorities, needs, goals, and current lifestyle is so valuable. It enables you to create a solid foundation on which you'll build your future habits or plans.

As unfun as this reflection and focus on self-awareness can be, and as much as you want to skip it, doing so is like decorating your house when your foundation has a huge crack. You're not going to spend lots of time, money, and energy picking out furniture and paint colors if you know your foundation has a huge crack that would leak, are you? NOPE! You know that'd be wasting hard work and money.

That's why, right now, I want to help you start to create what I like to call your "Beastette (or Beast) origin story."

WRITING YOUR BEASTETTE/BEAST ORIGIN STORY

Pause for a second and close your eyes. Picture your favorite superhero. What does that person look like? Are they strong and attractive? Do they exude confidence and calm in the face of danger? Do they stand like a bada$$, challenging all foes to take them on? Are they unwavering, showing no fear as they go on the offensive?

This larger-than-life superhero who's the picture of perfection has an origin story—a beginning where they suffered setbacks and failures they had to fight to overcome. They saw success not despite struggle but because they used their strength to overcome it. They had to face obstacles that life and other people threw at them as well as challenges they made for themselves. Often, those internal doubts, fears, and struggles were the hardest to overcome.

Right now is your opportunity to own your origin story and let it become your superpower to achieve results. While you may not currently believe you can achieve your goals and doubt what's possible, you build confidence and strength through what you overcome.

You may not realize it yet, and it may sound cheesy, but you are your own superhero or, as I like to call it, your own Beastette (or Beast). Own this fact!

Your current struggles and your current situation aren't bad things, but they are things that make you unique. They give you strength and empower you to achieve more than you realize is possible right now. The key is learning to harness these powers!

You may be thinking something like, "But I just want to lose 5 pounds and see some ab definition. It's just a vain and unimportant goal." However, it's more than that. It's about you feeling as fabulous as you've always dreamed you could feel. It's about proving to yourself you can be leaner and stronger than you thought possible. It's about conquering your doubts and fears and loving how you look in photos.

Often, people are afraid to own how important their goals are because they're worried others may label them as "silly" or "vain," but you shouldn't feel that way. Stop judging yourself. Instead, recognize that life is about seeing how far you can go and growing constantly. As New York Times bestselling author and empowerment and self-love advocate Mandy Hale said, "Growth is painful. Change is painful. But nothing is as painful as staying stuck somewhere you don't belong."

You have one life and body to pursue the greatness you're capable of, so pursue it. When you pursue greatness, even in a small part of your life like your fitness goals and body composition, you may also see great success in other ways, and you may inspire others to pursue more for themselves.

If it feels awkward writing your origin story, think about the story of your superhero. Think about how much knowing where they started inspires you because you also know the powerhouse they became. And think about how your story can not only become something to move you forward but also inspiration for others in your life who need a change.

As you write, remember your story needs more than the dry details. Don't just write down your weight or make a list of habits you do every day. Include what your

Beastette/Beast is going to overcome. Recognize the struggles you'll face, both internally and externally.

Draw on the power of pain. Although you probably often run from the negative, in this case, I want you to embrace it. Heroes draw on their pain to help themselves find the motivation to keep going through the ups and downs. They've embraced pain to help them find their superpower. Greatness is born out of struggle!

Something motivated you to get this book. Maybe it was seeing a photo of yourself at a party where you had a lot of fun, but now, when you look at that photo, you're so embarrassed you wore that outfit. Maybe you're tired of seeing the number on the scale creep up. Maybe you felt out of shape when you recently tried to hike a route that was fine last year. Maybe you tried on jeans and realized you can't button the top button, or you have shelves of clothes collecting dust because they don't fit.

Those things have something in common. There is some pain in them, and it makes you want a change. You can harness pain and convert it to motivation and passion to drive you toward your goals if you take ownership (yup, there's that word again) instead of letting it drag you down.

As you write your origin story, connect this pain to your current lifestyle, the struggles you've had in the past, and the reasons why you want to move forward. The more the pain of staying stuck outweighs the pain of change, the easier it will be to start to build new habits and take on new challenges so you can move forward even through setbacks. The more you feel the pain of where you are now, the more "sacrifices" you'll be willing to make. Think about other times you've felt great motivation. You've really wanted not to be where you were at that time, and you were willing to do anything needed to move forward. You need that kind of motivation now.

You're willing to eat boiled chicken and steamed broccoli. You're willing to shovel in uncooked, dry spinach. You're willing to hit the gym at 4 a.m. and again at 9 p.m. if needed. You're willing to do everything.

And while you need to capitalize on this motivation to help you get started, you also need to recognize this motivation and passion to make a change will fade. So, before it does, it's important to have an accurate picture of your current lifestyle and the changes you need to make to let passion shape your purpose.

Passion alone is fleeting, so it must transform to purpose if you want to create sustainable changes and new habits. When the passion fades and you feel like you're running out of motivation, the new habits you've created that didn't feel so bad at first start to feel super overwhelming, and you become overloaded. You start to shudder at the thought of having to weigh out chicken again, eat salad for yet another meal, and do the same cardio session over and over.

By drawing on pain to map out your origin story, you can use your passion to plan, prepare, and create a process that keeps you focused on your purpose and implementing habits through the ups and downs. Having that purpose is what creates discipline.

So when you're mapping out your origin story, draw on the pain. Play it up. Don't run from it.

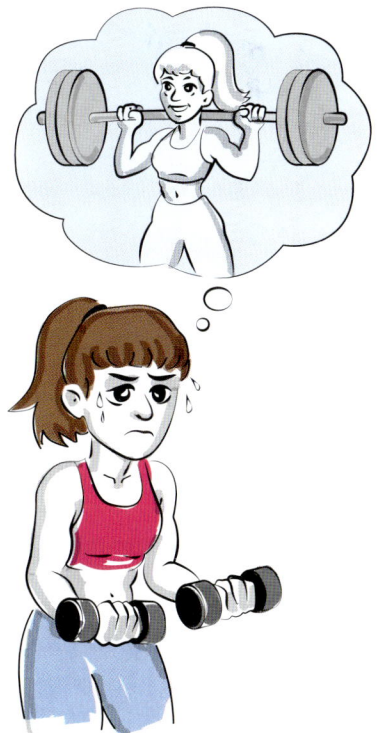

DOING THE WORK

In addition to embracing your pain, your struggles, and your feelings, you need to tie them to your current habits. The more you tie emotion to what you're currently doing, the more it will help you shed your current habits and embrace the "unlearning of them" while being willing to sacrifice and embrace the discomfort of the new.

In the past, you probably haven't created this "pain" association. Consequently, it's been easy to fall back into the change loop when new habits feel uncomfortable or hard.

I know creating this pain association can feel awkward, and I know you probably want to skip it. You're here for the workouts and dietary changes, not some mindset, learn-about-yourself, self-help stuff. But before you're tempted to skip ahead, my client Melissa said something you need to read.

Melissa was wrapping up her program and posted the following in the Facebook group: "We start programs like this because we know we need change. Half of that change is food and exercise. The other half is learning about and loving yourself. That is always a bigger challenge than anything else."

It's easy to get caught up in the quest for a perfect macro ratio, a perfect move, or the best workout routine. You want some earth-shattering new diet or workout design to make everything happen magically. Unfortunately, there's no "perfect" food or exercise plan that will work if your mindset doesn't also shift.

Honestly, I've seen people with "perfect" plans who don't achieve results, but those who commit to the learning process, truly embrace change, and seek to better understand themselves succeed even with not-so-perfect macros or workouts. I think the reason is that there really is no "perfect" lifestyle.

Ultimately, what works comes from finding your personal balance and embracing your personal quirks. As I like to say, you embrace your little inner freaks. You also have to realize that your personality, needs, goals, and lifestyle are constantly evolving. You need to be in a continuous state of reassessing what holds you back and what moves you forward. You need to embrace tracking so you can constantly adjust as you learn and grow.

Success doesn't happen overnight. It happens as a result of the 1 percent improvements you make a little at a time and having a better understanding of yourself. Learning to love yourself while always wanting to improve is a process of constant evolution, but by embracing who you are right now and what you need, you can figure out how to keep moving forward!

The workbook at redefiningstrength.com/extras includes guidance for writing your origin story, so make sure to check out the worksheet and reflection sheets included there. Here's some other food for thought to help you start jotting down some notes:

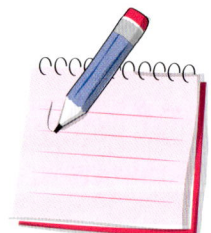

? What does your current day look like? Don't just write what you do in a day. Make notes about how things feel. Assess *why* you do the things you do. Think about how those things contribute to your current situation.

? What is the reality of your current situation? Fully face where you are now: weight, size, performance achievements, injuries, and energy levels.

? **What routines in your lifestyle do you love and can't imagine living without?** What parts of your life would you struggle to give up?

? **How are your current habits, things you may enjoy, impacting your life and keeping you stuck?** What habits do you think could help you move forward? What habits do you have that hold you back? Are there habits you aren't willing to adjust or think could be part of the problem? Step back and really try to see your current habits in a negative light. If you try to justify why things are good or work or shouldn't be let go of, it can hold you back!

? **What routines and habits do you find yourself repeating that make you feel bad?** What things do you wish you hadn't done that you keep doing even though you don't like them?

? **Why do you want a change?** Go deeper

than just "losing a few pounds" to get to the real reason. What would these changes bring for you mentally and physically?

? **What setbacks have you recently had that made you want to see a new and better result?** What is your reason for feeling the pain right now?

? **What struggles have you had in the past?** When have you always quit in the past? What has led to you being in your current situation? What may have created this origin story?

? **Why is the pain of staying stuck worse than the pain of change? What pain will lead to your purpose?** As the hero of your own story, what is driving you to go from victim to victor?

Make notes as you reflect on these questions. As you progress through the book, you will want to return to your origin story and add to it.

As you face new challenges and set new goals, you want to return again and again to this assessment, building your self-awareness as you create clarity on where you are and how you need to move forward. Your current situation (or location, in GPS terminology) is constantly changing. You periodically need to reassess where you are because the destination you're shooting for may need to change.

The simple fact is that you don't truly know what's possible until you prove it possible. I touch on this more in the next section as I talk about where you want to go and what you want to achieve.

WHERE ARE YOU GOING?

Now you have a better idea of where you are. You've dug into your pain, so you may be more than ready to get on your way to reaching your goals. You might even be tempted to jump to the workouts and get down to business. However, you can't know what steps forward you need to take if you don't know what direction to head in. You need to create a clear goal to get from where you are to where you want to be. The question is, what is a realistic goal?

Direction drives people. You need a clear vision of where you're going if you want to map out your plan to get there. But sometimes, it's hard to know what goal to set.

You may be wondering *How do I know what's truly possible?*

The simple fact is that you don't know what's possible until you prove it possible. Given that, if you don't set a goal that pushes you, you don't go nearly as far as you could. In striving for less, you achieve less.

It's important to recognize that you may often hold yourself back when you say something isn't possible. This is a defense mechanism to protect you from failure because no one likes to fail! But you need to take the risk if you want to get the reward!

As you consider where you want to go, I don't want you to set a "realistic" goal right now. I want you to dream big.

Try considering people you admire who are living the life you'd like to live. As you look at what they've achieved, don't just look at what they have; examine their whole lifestyle. What are their mindsets, attitudes, and actions? Consider what it would take for you to get there.

When people shoot for a big goal, they tend to immediately go into a mode of self-doom because of doubt. You may think of all the reasons why it can't happen, why it won't happen, or why it isn't possible for you. You might bog yourself down in all the potential roadblocks rather than allowing yourself to find solutions. You may see yourself as the *victim*, not the *victor.*

To combat this, don't see this situation as what you can achieve; see it as what your Beastette or Beast can conquer as they break free from that origin story you wrote.

> **You need a clear vision of where you're going if you want to map out your plan to get there.**

ARE YOU THE VICTIM OR THE VICTOR?

If you have the mindset that "nothing's ever worked before so nothing will work now," you write off your potential and give away your power and agency to make a change. One reason for this is that you've never assessed what it looks like to be a victor—to become your Beastette or Beast version. You've only ever looked at how far you have to go and all the changes that need to happen. You may even have tried to force the end lifestyle on yourself without realizing you have to *grow* into it. But that's what this journey is—steps and stages and phases of growth.

Think about a road trip. You don't arrive there after the first turn. As you're driving, you can't see the full route or even the next turn. There will be pauses and setbacks along the way. Forty-five minutes into the drive, you may need a bathroom break because you drank your water too fast as you listened to a podcast. Or in two hours, you might spill your trail mix all over your car and have to stop to clean it up. Or perhaps there will be an accident on the highway from a butthead driver texting on their phone and not paying attention to construction, so now you either have to find another route or be delayed for hours. You may have known you'd need to stop for the night, but you couldn't foresee that the hotel where you'd planned to stay would be full.

You also can't know exactly the experience you'll have once you get where you're going. The vacation could end up being the best experience ever, including a chocolate lava cake you'll never forget and the most beautiful, picturesque hike. Or it could rain every single day so that you're trapped in your hotel room with a TV that won't play a movie without the sound cutting out while the people in the room next to you fight constantly.

You can never fully know all that will happen on a journey, but by planning to the best of your abilities and in recognizing the reality of where you are *and* where you're going, you can give yourself the power to adjust and adapt along the way.

This is the reason you need to have a clear picture of not only what you want your goal to be but what is required to be the person that maintains that goal long term. By examining every aspect of your goal and being creative in how you implement habits, you can find small changes that progress you forward. It helps you to realize that everything doesn't have to be changed or fixed or adjusted right away—potentially even at all.

This knowledge also shifts your mindset by giving you clarity about what you want and helps you form the belief that you can achieve your goal. Lack of clarity is often what makes you feel most overwhelmed, uncomfortable, and unsure. You may think you give yourself clarity through specific, measurable, numeric goals—like weight-loss numbers or personal record race times—but these specific numbers are useless because they don't help you understand the habits or mindsets that go into achieving the results.

Often, people visualize the end score on the scoreboard but make no attempt to understand what it takes to get there. What plays are necessary? What skills are required? What mindsets are needed? What does winning actually look like? These details of where you want to go and what success really means give you the clarity to drive forward.

You aren't just "going on a diet." You're *adjusting your diet.* You aren't doing a plan or program. You're evolving your habits and lifestyle. You're *acting as if* until you're *acting as you are.*

As you build your system, you'll learn to embrace this mindset shift—going from "faking it till you make it," to "acting as if." When you fake a habit or action, it means you don't truly believe in or value it. You'll never prioritize or consistently do things you don't value. They'll just be habits you overload yourself with until you hit emotional sabotage and fall back into the cycle of the change loop.

The only way out is to change yourself and your identity to reach your destination and goals. Again, I know I'm asking you to dive deeper than you may have thought you were going to go to make some diet and workout changes, but this exploration is what makes this program different. It's what helps you become that lean, strong Beastette/Beast you want to be 'til your final day on this planet!

FORGET "FAKE IT 'TIL YOU MAKE IT"

Faking habits and actions won't move you forward in any lasting way. That fake-it-'til-you-make-it attitude is what keeps people constantly doing twenty-one-day challenges and six-week programs. They get stuck in a loop of seeing results only to fall back into old patterns—repeating that change loop over and over and over again. Being stuck in that rut is what makes you feel like diet and workout changes need to be a full-time job to create results rather than being a component that fits into your lifestyle and priorities.

> **You're *acting as if* until you're *acting as you are.***

DESTINATION BEASTETTE/BEAST

You've probably been limiting yourself by what you've done in the past and the knowledge you currently have. You don't see potential and possibility. You let that negative little voice in your head constantly sabotage you and hold you back from seeing opportunity in options and obstacles. However, when you outline your true goal, you aren't just telling yourself what you believe you can achieve; you're dictating the changes you can make and the person you can become.

I call it "Destination Beastette" (or Beast) because you create a kind of alter ego. You're creating the person who you know can have the goals you want to have. The person who can repeat the necessary habits. The person who is the version of you that you want to be. You aren't limited by what you see as your strengths and weaknesses. Instead, you're outlining what's possible and what you need for this goal.

Through the STRONG system, I'm going to show you how you can assume this alter ego. Embrace the opportunity to step outside yourself; otherwise, you will limit yourself by your current perceptions and beliefs. You don't want your current boundaries to limit your future potential.

You can't stop thoughts and emotions from happening, but you can change the impact they have on your actions. You may still be thinking, *Look, Cori. I want to drop a few pounds and have people compliment my guns in my sleeveless black dress. I don't want to go this deep!*

Guess what I'm going to tell you. Suck it up, Buttercup, and do this work!

Avoiding this mindset stuff (gosh, I personally hated it for the longest time) is what has sabotaged your habit changes in the past. You haven't been able to use many tools and form many habits because of your self-doubts. Your little negative voice tends to speak up and question you or say, "You can't," at the worst of times. You know that constant annoying chatter that seems to overwhelm your thoughts every time you look to make a hard change? The chatter that you find yourself giving in to because you consider it to be your true problem and something you can't change about yourself or your reality?

» *You can't ever stick with your diet. You just don't have the willpower. Let's just pour that glass of wine and relax on the couch.*

» *Are you really going to eat that? You're ruining the day. Oh well, you may as well have the rest of the cookies now.*

» *Do you really want to do that? I mean, you can't do that move. You're not an athlete.*

» *Tracking is so restrictive. You'll be miserable. You don't want to do that.*

Well, that chatter—the little voice—isn't you. And those doubts aren't a problem that can't be solved. You just have to gain distance from those thoughts to make a change. You can create distance by thinking of that annoying little hater voice as a bad roommate who's trying to take over the place.

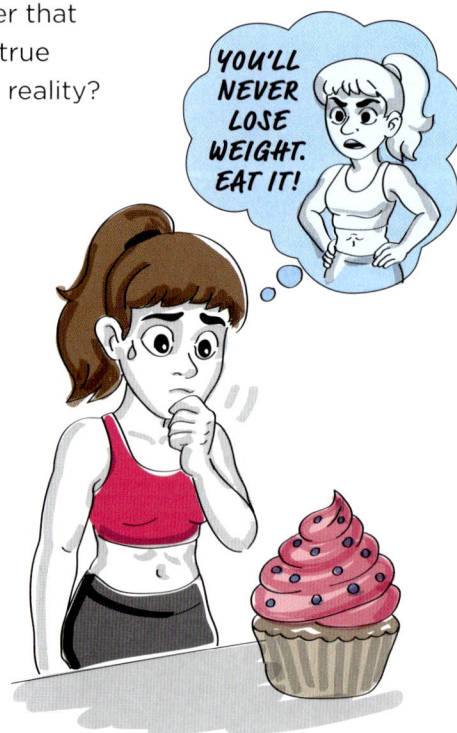

You don't have to let that voice take control, and I used the word *let* for a reason. Once you recognize those thoughts aren't irrefutable truths or valid problems—they're just doubts—you can stop letting them dictate your actions. You can gain perspective on how you want to act by regarding those thoughts as a separate entity (like a roommate) that you can ultimately kick out. The key is not to let that roommate's negativity continue. When you *let* them take up more and more space, it drags you back to old habits. When you *let* them take over, your thoughts go into a negative spiral. Instead, you can give them the boot.

Start to recognize the questions and criticisms and push back against them. Reflect on why you have those doubts and show yourself how you can overcome them. Remind yourself you aren't that person anymore.

Reflect on the doubts to understand where they're coming from. Don't feel like that voice has to have control. Stop letting it rent space in your brain by recognizing that it isn't who you are or who you have to be. It's simply an unpleasant roommate with bad opinions. Now, let's give the boot to that annoying roommate by focusing on the mindsets and actions of your alter ego Beastette or Beast.

For help writing out your vision for your goal, check out the worksheet and reflection sheets at redefiningstrength.com/extras. You may also find it helpful to jot down some notes by asking yourself these questions:

? What goal do you want to achieve? What other goals and wins would come by achieving this? Don't just list a weight or performance goal. Really think about other aspects of the goal. What other signs would you see when you've reached your goal? What other impact would this goal have on your life? Would you sleep better? Take on new hobbies? Travel more?

? Who embodies this goal and what does their lifestyle look like? Have you ever had this goal in the past? One size doesn't fit all. You can learn so much from the journeys of others or even by reflecting back on times you've had the success you wanted. Look at the lifestyles, habits, and mindsets of those with the goals you want to achieve. Use these models to help you better understand what your life and habits may need to look like and what changes you may need to make so you can assess what adjustments are realistic for you. But also use this comparison to help you avoid making some of the same mistakes!

? How would it feel to be at this goal? People are driven by *emotion*. Own this! Use it to your advantage and really think about how you'd feel at this goal because feeling is what honestly makes you attached to a specific outcome in the first place. Really show yourself why achieving this goal is worth the ups and downs along the way to return to this motivation when you need it!

? What would a "day in the life" look like? Begin to understand the habits you need to reach your goal because it will help guide you in the plan you create and how you break down changes that will occur over time. Picturing it can also help you avoid being distracted by changes that don't matter or wasting effort by working hard at things that aren't necessary in the long run. It can also help you realize that what you sometimes need to do to reach a goal is not what you will do to maintain it. Understanding this can help you embrace some short-term pain on the journey!

? How would you feel doing these habits? You're not going to like everything you have to do to reach a goal, but the upsides have to be worth the downsides. So, you have to evaluate whether they are. If not, how can you help yourself value any necessary habits more, or how can you get creative in finding a way to the same outcome without using those habits?

? What mindsets would you have? What beliefs about yourself and your life would you have? As you're working to reach a new goal, you're building a new identity, and you can't fake a new identity. Your actions and your mindset have to evolve, and you have to believe in who you're becoming. What beliefs will you hold as you reach your goals? What beliefs will you need to have along the way? And how will your goal change how you view yourself and life? Strength and confidence are built through what you overcome, but you have to embrace the mindset shifts with the actions!

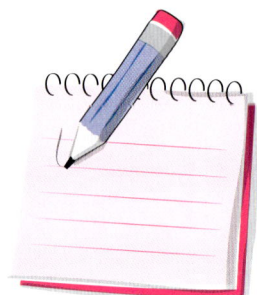

? How would other people view you? What would your community look like? As you change and create new habits, your relationships with others will change. You have to watch that the people you have relationships with don't push back against your changes and ultimately sabotage you. The more you recognize the people who support you and move you forward and those who may push back against your changes, the more you can see what type of community you need and even plan for how to handle any peer pressure. This can even help you find new support systems based on the lifestyle you want to lead while helping you make sure you've communicated your goals with your loved ones so they're also on board!

? What changes may occur along the way? What habits would you no longer have? What habits would you have built? What you do to reach a goal isn't the same thing as what you do to maintain it, but you also won't return to your old habits. Recognizing what may need to change and what may be constantly evolving is key. Think about things that may seem important to you right now. Are they holding you back? Are they truly important? If so, why? How could they continue to be part of your new life, or how can you slowly evolve past them? What new habits may come out of these changes to support your new life?

Take time to reflect on and assess not only your current lifestyle but the one you want to build. Don't hold yourself back with what you've accomplished only so far. Don't doom yourself with doubt. Remember, the Beastette or Beast is coming out. Your alter ego has kicked out the bad roommate instead of letting them take over the place! It's time to stop being the victim and start being the victor!

This will help you really break down the habit changes and 1 percent tweaks you need that will help you use the STRONG system not only to reach your goals but create lasting changes to keep growing until your final day on this planet!

3 STRONG

Here's a cold, hard truth: You're here because nothing's working the way you want. You believe more is possible, but doubt and struggles have crept in, and you feel doomed to be a hamster running on a wheel—working really hard to get absolutely nowhere.

I've been there. In fact, it's how the STRONG system came into being. I was sick of trying to force a square peg into a round hole. If you're like me, you've tried program after program—all of which are touted for amazing results—only to have each ultimately fail.

I've personally gone on countless diets, including the potato diet. (Trust me, it's not french fries, which would have been delicious.) I've seen some "fast" results that seemed like I dropped pounds overnight. Unfortunately, those fast results led to an even faster rebound. If you're like me, the rebounds make you feel even angrier and more frustrated and like you're carrying more weight than when you started.

Some programs work in the short term, but ultimately, these fast fixes that seem like they'll help you avoid pain now lead to suffering a lot more pain later. These diets are why so many people start blaming age and feel doomed to never see the results they want. But age isn't the problem. It's all the poopy dieting and training practices that rush the process.

That sucks, but it's true. Hopefully, you've seen them as learning experiences that help you grow. It's tempting to quickly seek out the next thing without assessing why things did or didn't work, and that's probably what you've done in the past. When you do this, the doom of nothing ever working continues to build.

I saw a change in my personal results and in the results of my clients when I had us all sit down, think, and assess. Asking yourself, "Who am I?" is important. While I do mean this in a slightly existential way, I don't need you to assess your existence on this planet right now, but I do need you to assess what truly is realistic based on who you are at this time, considering your lifestyle, the goals you have, and the mindsets and habits you've built.

The best results—the changes that actually work—come from a plan that takes who you are into account. It's why keto or intermittent fasting or Weight Watchers or whatever the heck else has worked for a friend in a similar situation ultimately has not worked for you.

Because you aren't that other person.

The STRONG system always works because it's not some magic pill or a diet or workout "ideal." It's not a plan made for someone else. The STRONG system is a plan you create for yourself based on where you are right now. When you follow a plan made for you, it's impossible not to see results! The best results come from making small changes based on your personal needs, goals, and lifestyle. But I realize how hard this actually is to do.

I was working through this whole process in my head when I woke up at 2:35 a.m. on November 13, 2022. I had what I thought was probably my most brilliant idea ever. I typed it in my phone's note app and tried to go back to sleep, but I couldn't. I knew the idea was amazing, and my brain just wouldn't shut off. Finally, at around 5:30 a.m., I did sort of fall asleep.

When my alarm went off about thirty minutes later, I barely let Ryan, my supportive husband, open his eyes before I began brain vomiting everything at him. Usually, he kind of stares at me when I wake up talking at him, and he waits to respond until after he's had his morning coffee. This time, though, his immediate response was, "Holy crap! This idea is really as good as you think it is!"

Ryan was so excited about it! We talked about it during the entire two-hour car trip to our little Palm Springs staycation. I filled my phone with notes of what were the beginnings of what I've now refined into this book.

I'm pretty sure I barely got more than an hour of straight sleep during the next few weeks after my middle-of-the-night brainstorm. I kept waking up to type more jumbled notes on my phone. I was trying to get down each thought before it disappeared!

Today, I'm still excited every time I get to share this knowledge with someone new because I truly believe this is the secret to the success we've all always wanted but never believed was possible!

WHAT DOES STRONG MEAN?

Strong can mean many different things to different people. That's part of the magic in the word. Heck, if you look up *strong* in the *Merriam-Webster Dictionary*, you'll find more than ten definitions.

For me, this word is *everything.*

I want to help everyone I come in contact with recognize how strong they are—both physically and mentally. That's why I felt making the word strong into the acronym for our system for success seemed so appropriate: We're helping people build their strongest, fittest, healthiest selves!

The letters in STRONG stand for ...

S IGNIFICANT

T ARGETED

R EPEATABLE

O PTIMIZED

N ONNEGOTIABLE

G O

The idea behind it is basically goal setting for people who think goal setting is BS. I'm one of those people because setting SMART (specific, measurable, achievable, relevant, and time-bound) goals never worked for me. However, I do realize that direction drives people, including me. Without a way to measure progress, keep myself accountable, and have a game plan in place to take action, I would never achieve the success I wanted.

Goals without actions are wishes and dreams that never materialize. That's why I saw failed attempt after failed attempt. I had to find a way to get over my personal hang-up that goal setting was ... well ... stupid (being 100 percent honest) because the fact was that I knew everyone who was wildly successful did some form of it. So, I began to research the evidence in favor of goal setting. Because the changes people resist the hardest are the ones they need the most—for example, goal setting. But you can't really force yourself to do something. If you're mentally still saying, "Well, this is dumb," you're not actually embracing the changes. You're *faking* it, which doesn't create lasting change. That's the reason I research all the evidence in favor of the habit I'm fighting against. This doesn't mean I then just blindly do the action. Nope. Instead, it often leads me to realize how I need to tweak the habit to fit my unique freak!

People know, but often forget, that one size doesn't fit all. By researching all the benefits of goal setting while I worked out the STRONG system, I was able to pull the benefits and morph them into a system that addressed everything I found wrong with SMART goals and goal setting in general.

I learned that most goal-setting approaches ignored five key things. Too often with goal setting, we don't do the following:

1. Stop and assess current habits.
2. Connect to our *why*.
3. Assess obstacles.
4. Create a roadmap or system to move forward.
5. Start with action.

With the STRONG system, I was able to address all these components and make my little action-taker, do-er heart very happy, and you'll be able to do the same. So, if you've ever thought, *Goal setting is pointless*, you're going to hate to love the STRONG system. It will give you that roadmap to take action and work efficiently (yup, that woodcutter story from Chapter 1 will haunt your dreams when I'm done with you), but you'll also know when it's time to adjust, because when you build a lifestyle, you don't do one thing forever.

However, people often "go on a diet" and think, *This is a lifestyle! This is what I will do from now on!* They deceive themselves into thinking they've found a solution and that they'll do this exact thing forever without thinking about the fact that there is no area of life in which everything stays the same without end.

Over the course of a year, our habits shift with the seasons. For example, I find it way easier to get up in the summer, when the light peeks around the shades early and the dogs start trying to play with the covers and wake me up by scratching at my back. In the winter, when it's cold, even the dogs want to roll over and bury themselves under the covers when my alarm goes off.

Life doesn't stand still. Your body, needs, and goals are constantly evolving, and so are your priorities and lifestyle. The more you accept this need to adjust, the less you'll find yourself hitting that plateau, feeling broken, and placing blame on your age, hormones, or schedule as the reason why you can't see results.

Your system isn't stagnant. Embracing the reflection and assessment will help you have that power to adjust so you're never wasting time or energy on another New Year's resolution that doesn't pan out.

But no system works, no matter how much it's designed to shift with you, if you don't truly embrace the changes and take action with them. You need to act as if with the habit changes instead of going through the motions and faking them, ultimately dooming yourself with doubt. You can't be thinking, *Yeah, yeah, yeah ... I'll give this a "try,"* because that thought isn't you committing; it's really just you feeling like you'll go back to old habits at some point. And creating a system that evolves is never about going back—it's about moving forward to match where you're going, not where you've been.

A system only works if you embrace stepping into the mindset and actions needed to get to the destination you outlined in Chapter 2. You're just about to create that true roadmap to get there with the STRONG system outline!

ACT AS IF

The smallest of small tweaks in phrasing, perspective, and actions are ultimately what dictate your success or failure. Although "Fake it 'til you make it" may seem like the exact same thing as "act as if," it's not. Not in the slightest. Don't believe me?

Imagine begrudgingly going to a family gathering—a party you just really don't want to go to. During the whole car ride, you complain about different family members and annoying conversations you're going to have. How one aunt always pushes food on you and how you don't feel like having to explain your macro goals to her again.

You walk up to the door and put on a fake smile. Minutes feel like hours as you make small talk with person after person. You keep declining the food people force on you and the drinks being handed to you.

Then your aunt walks out with your favorite cheesecake from that place you have to order from months in advance. It's a cheesecake you order only once every year because you just want to devour the whole thing the second it lands on your doorstep. You can't believe your aunt got it this year. She turns to you and cuts you a piece and says, "Your favorite!"

She wins! You can't *fake* it any longer. You're tired and grumpy from all the questions, and you not only devour your piece before everyone has gotten one, but you're also going back for seconds and grabbing some wine and those rolls you've been eyeing all night.

You aren't having fun, and things spin out of your control. You end up groaning in the car because you're so full. You put on sweatpants as soon as you get home, and you dread getting on the scale the next day.

You repeated a common pattern because you were trying to fake being what you thought you "should" be. You went to that party telling yourself you weren't going to have a good time—maybe even that you weren't going to have any of the food. You felt restricted and probably a bit bitter about having to pretend to be this way. So, of course, the first sign of overwhelm was the final straw that broke the camel's back, and you caved!

You can't force new habits you don't believe in. You can't just pretend to be a new person or that you don't have old routines. Instead, you have to "act as if" until you're "acting as you are." You have to embrace the changes truly and honestly because they define who you're becoming. You have to find value in them and understand why you're doing them.

Now, imagine that you go to the party and recognize that, yes, it isn't your ideal event, but you've chosen to go because you value family and know it means a lot to them. You know that you're going to embrace the questions and conversation because you know others care about it. You know that you're going to "act as if" you value these things too because you want to be there for others. And when your aunt pushes food on you, you're going to say, "No, thank you," and even ask her how her routines are going because you know she always struggles around this time of year.

Then when that cheesecake comes out, you're going to have a piece and *not feel bad about it* because part of having balance is owning that sometimes you want something and plans change. But *choosing* to make a change doesn't mean the day is ruined or that you now have to grab the rolls too. (Wink wink...fix that flat; don't slash the other three tires!) Heck, you can even plan to eat lower calorie and higher protein earlier in the day in preparation for your aunt the food pusher and the surprise treats she's always showing up with that can throw you off your game plan.

You do all this because you're embracing the person you're growing into. You believe in the habits you need. You also aren't trying to force actions; you're shifting your mindsets. You value your choices and recognize that all your actions are just that ...

Your choice.

That's the difference between the two phrases. One is forced, pretend, and something you don't believe in. The other is your choice, a change you want, and something you believe in.

You're shifting from "I have to" to "I get to." You're owning that your mindset really impacts your actions and how consistently you keep doing those actions to achieve the results you want. Results are built off those consistent, daily actions, and you get good at things you consistently do, but you won't consistently do things you don't value, prioritize, and believe in.

> **You're shifting from 'I have to' to 'I get to.'**

So as *bleh* as mindset work can be, nothing truly changes in your actions and routines until you shift your mindsets about those habits.

It's cliché, but it's spot on: "We are what we believe we are."

It's why going back to that destination you outlined is so important. You want to truly understand the person, your destination, who has the goals you want to have. Because only by knowing the mindsets, actions, and habits you'll need can you start to build the system to get there.

You don't grow into this new version of yourself overnight. Like a seed that's been planted, your identity needs to be nurtured and grown. If you aren't careful, your identity can suffocate, or its growth can be stunted. But the STRONG system gives you the tools to nurture and grow healthy so you thrive through every season because you know how to adapt based on the evolutions in your life.

Here's the thing, though: "Acting as if" is sometimes easier said than done. Wanting that new identity and being willing to do everything needed to make the changes to grow into that person isn't always easy. (They don't call them growing pains for nothing.) Change is hard! But nothing changes if nothing changes.

The change process will take time because you aren't just learning new habits. You're also letting go and *unlearning* old ones. That takes time, conscious reflection, and often a lot more willpower than you may recognize.

LET GO!

Who you were two years ago, a decade ago, in college and high school, is not who you are now. Yet, for some reason, after a certain age, many people resist change. They even see it as a bad thing. Some people cling to their identity even when it doesn't serve them. This is why people often achieve results only to fall back into old habits and then see success slide.

Achieving a goal and embracing new routines means truly shifting who you are and how you see yourself and the world. That sounds super deep—again, probably more existential than you expected from a book on fat loss—but it's true. And you need to *own* it if you want results.

Unlearning old habits as you learn new ones takes time because unlearning requires you do these things:

1. Recognize that a pattern or habit exists and reflect on it.

2. Break down the mindsets that lead to it and make it "valuable."

3. Recognize and shift your perspective to see how the habit is not serving you.

4. Catch yourself in the act of repeating the behavior and start to address it.

5. Stop the habit or pattern before it happens.

6. Find a new habit that's in line with your goals to replace the current, comfortable routine.

7. Learn the new habit while making yourself conscious of not repeating the old one.

8. Correct setbacks when you fall back into old patterns.

9. Shift the new habits little by little until they stick.

10. Build upon the new habits to fully create the shift.

That's ten steps. Ten freaking steps to unlearn and learn one—probably small—habit. And none of these steps are super simple or quickly accomplished. It's why habit change isn't the clean twenty-one days people often say it is. Changing habits actually takes an average of about sixty-six days.

I love hanging this quote on my fridge and having clients write it out to see it daily when they first start their journey. I also tell them to remind themselves of the following things each time they hit the hard part, where they feel like they've been at it long enough and things *should* have happened faster or *should* be easier:

» Changes take time, and there are lots of ups and downs along the way!

» It takes three to four months to build a habit. You're practicing until you get it right.

» Then it takes sixteen to eighteen months to build a lifestyle. You're practicing until you can't get it wrong.

» Finally, it takes three to four years to transform your identity. You're practicing until it's part of who you are!

The time frames aren't the only thing that make this quote significant. It's the emphasis on *action.* "Practice" means taking consistent action day in and day out as you move forward through the ups and downs.

As you move through the stages of unlearning and learning, practice makes it so you can do things without thinking. You shift from "acting as if" to "acting as you are." It's a process that takes years, but people often give themselves only to the end of a twenty-one-day challenge or a six-week cut. No wonder changes don't stick!

The STRONG system is different because you're recognizing *right now* that you not only have to learn the new strategies in this book, but you also have to *unlearn* and let go of many habits and mindsets you have.

You started to see the habits and mindsets as you wrote your origin story in Chapter 2. You'll break down these habits and mindsets as you get deeper into the STRONG system, especially as you start to optimize things. Right now, I'm not asking you to know all the patterns you're repeating or to start listing them. I'm just asking you to be open to reflecting on them because your innate response is going to be to fight against the changes.

The more uncomfortable the changes you feel you have to make, the more your brain is going to want to retreat from the discomfort. As I've said, the changes you fight against the hardest are the ones you need the most.

One reason you may fight changes is because you feel bad and think you were wrong or dumb for doing those habits in the first place. No one likes to feel dumb or wrong. It's hard to own up to the idea that your comfortable habits aren't serving you. It can feel like admitting guilt or that you aren't right. And you probably want to be right. I know I like to be.

Also, you may have some valid habits that worked in the past. They may be based on solid practices and research. You know their value. It's hard to let go of what used to work, especially if the habits have become a part of your identity.

Everyone ties their identity to habits sometimes. Ever thought of yourself as a runner? The hardest worker in the room? A low-carber? A plant-based eater? An athlete? The person who could push through anything? The person who didn't need to track?

When something is part of your identity, it's extra hard to let go of it, but you have to if you want a new and better result. You have to recognize the dieting and training practices that may have worked at one point but aren't working now. You have to recognize that they may even be holding you back.

Instead of finding all the reasons to cling to and validate these habits while you also find reasons to doubt the new habits you're confronted with, you have to be open to questioning and finding all the reasons why you need to make these changes. At this point, I'm not asking you to know what needs to be changed. I'm only asking you to recognize when you feel that wall come up in response to something new and to question *why*.

Why do you want to fight this change? What in your current identity is the change pushing against? The more you question, the more you can help yourself embrace change.

This time, instead of fighting change, you're going to own that change means you're open to growth. You're ready and willing to see the results you deserve. You believe you can achieve more and that constant evolution is a good thing, and you're controlling the direction you're growing.

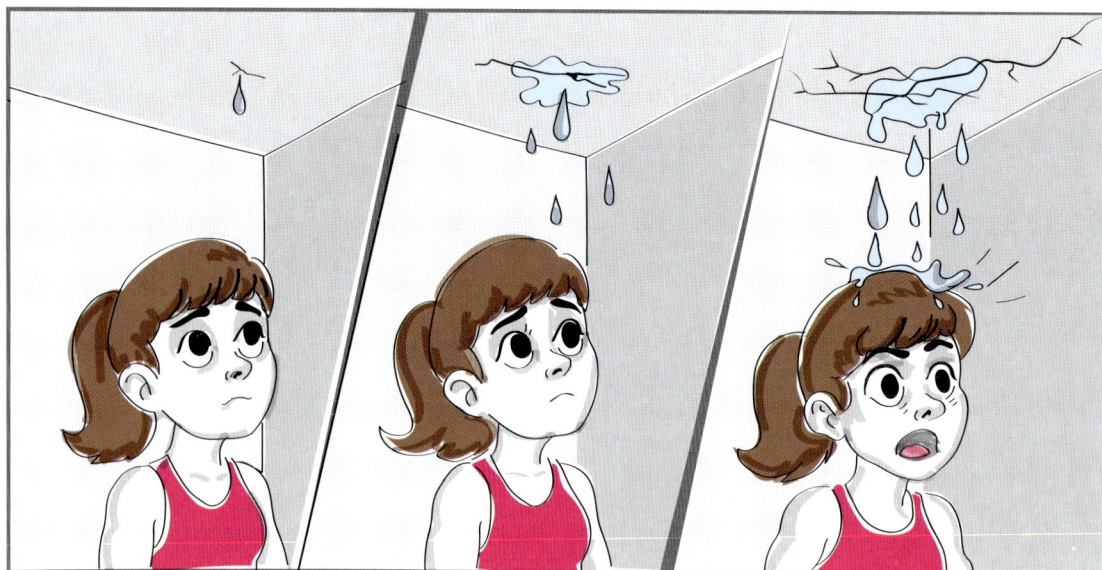

THE LEAKY CEILING EFFECT

Picture this scenario: The ceiling tiles collapse. Buckets of water start spilling from overhead. Where the heck is it all coming from!? That slow drip drip drip of water from the leaky pipe has finally added up, and the leak can't be ignored any longer.

This is usually what happens when you finally seek to make a change. Your pants no longer fit. You feel so disgustingly out of shape that you can't stand it. Your lab numbers come back, and your doctor tells you it's time to make a change. Symptoms of menopause are making you go crazy, and the lack of sleep is making you so irritated that the next person to look at you wrong is going to get punched in the face (not really ... but maybe).

Basically, you've ignored the problem until you can't any longer. And then you make a change. However, you're less than happy to have to address the problem, which makes the changes seem even worse.

This time, you aren't going to just set habits and forget them. You're going to create systems that have checkpoints and reflection points. The idea is to pause to sharpen your axe so you can keep it from getting too dull and slowing you down. The same thing goes for the leak. If you had stopped to assess the situation when you first noticed some slight dampness or discoloration on the tile, you could have caught the problem before it built up.

I've already asked you to do quite a bit of reflection work, so you might be itching more and more to get to taking action. *Don't*. Now you're getting to the hard stuff, but it's the stuff that will keep that leak from becoming a massive problem.

Remember: Don't run from the problems you see popping up. The sooner you address them, the less they add up. Having a problem isn't a flaw. Problems are a part of the process. It's only when you ignore them that they add up and ultimately sabotage you!

NOT JUST SETTING GOALS, SETTING SYSTEMS

"I always achieve my resolutions," she commented on my post about goals around the New Year.

"That's awesome. How do you do it?" I asked because I'm always curious about what drives others.

"I don't set any," she wrote back.

Ba dum tss!

This is a pretty common thought process. There have been times I've not set resolutions or goals myself, believing they were a waste of time. I took action anyway, so did it really matter whether I had a specific goal? That's when I realized there's a difference between setting goals and setting systems.

What you need to do—and what the most successful people do—is create a *system*. In other words, you need a vision that drives *action*.

In the rest of the chapters in Part 1, I break down each component of the STRONG system:

S IGNIFICANT

S
T
R
O
N
G

Why is your goal significant? The thought of diving into your why might make you want to run for the hills, roll your eyes, or both, but as I've said before, digging deeper than "I want to lose a few 'vanity' pounds" to get into what this journey will truly mean to you and your life is key. Your why may not feel that deep, but the shifts in your habits and mindsets are often that far-reaching. So, get specific. Own what you truly want out of life and what your destination will look like. Force yourself to honestly step into the discomfort of owning what you want without shame or filtering!

Conquering even seemingly small goals builds confidence and shows you your physical and mental strength. You build strength and confidence through what you overcome. The more you understand why you want something, the more you will prioritize it. And prioritizing your goals isn't selfish. It's leading by example to encourage those around you to also work toward the goals and life they deserve.

S
TARGETED
R
O
N
G

I will set out ways to measure success, not only through short-term or mini goals but also through complementary targets. Complementary goals work alongside your main goal to give you other ways to measure success and see your habits paying off. Complementary goals, like performance goals, help you do the habits that pay off for weight loss while seeing progress even when the scale doesn't budge. I'll go over ways to set complementary targets to keep you on track in Chapter 5. The more ways you have to be successful, the more likely you are to succeed.

If you've ever made changes and wondered, *Is this really working?* Chapter 5 will help you not have to guess. When you make habit changes, you may not see immediate progress toward your main goal, but you *will* have other signs showing you that you're on the right track. You just have to know what to look for so you don't miss them.

It's like knowing the exit to look for on the highway. If you aren't paying attention and looking for it, you can miss it. Then you either end up turning around before you hit it or driving far out of your way before getting back on track.

S
T
REPEATABLE
O
N
G

After setting your targets, you have to focus on habits to get there and actions that move you forward—specifically, habits that are repeatable. You will create a habit stack to build lasting habits you can do consistently.

People are the sum of their habits and actions, but when they set habits, they often set ideals rather than habits that line up with where they are at the start. The habit roadmap you'll create will help you build lasting changes and create true discipline, which isn't something you're born with. You have to build it.

S
T
R
OPTIMIZED
N
G

You're going to go where you don't want to go. You're going to embrace the negative and take a hard look at every single failure you can. You're going to wipe that makeup off and see all the pimples and blemishes. Because as hard as it is to step back and really own where you've messed up in the past and why program after program hasn't worked, the more you can reflect on those experiences to learn and optimize, and the more your next changes will truly be based on who you are and the lifestyle you lead.

Failures are just learning experiences with frustration. Learning experiences that can help you avoid future speed bumps. Be ready to own the negative and oversell future struggles to plan for them. This optimization is so often missing but can help you conquer the hard while thinking, *Wow, that really wasn't that bad!*

STRONG: NONNEGOTIABLES

As you work through the process and face challenges, you don't want to make things harder than they need to be. That's where nonnegotiables come into play. You're going to do something you've never done before. Instead of restricting things you love and fighting against your priorities, you're going to embrace them and plan for them.

People often don't embrace who they are and what they value. They stuff it down and force a mold over themselves until they come oozing out of it, breaking the mold. The nonnegotiables are truly the biggest *secret* to success. And it doesn't have to be hard work. It's about the efficiency of work.

STRONG: GO

This is the section that people often want to skip to, but they do it without understanding how it connects back to their starting point. With each of the preceding parts of the process, you've put in place the steps toward your goal. You're giving yourself small steps to climb your way up rather than being faced with a box to jump onto that's as tall as you are. One is ultimately not only easier but also a much less intimidating or risky approach. So, don't skip this step and don't stop short. While it feels good to dream and think about what you will do, you need to actually do it. I'll help you make taking action easier and less overwhelming through this system.

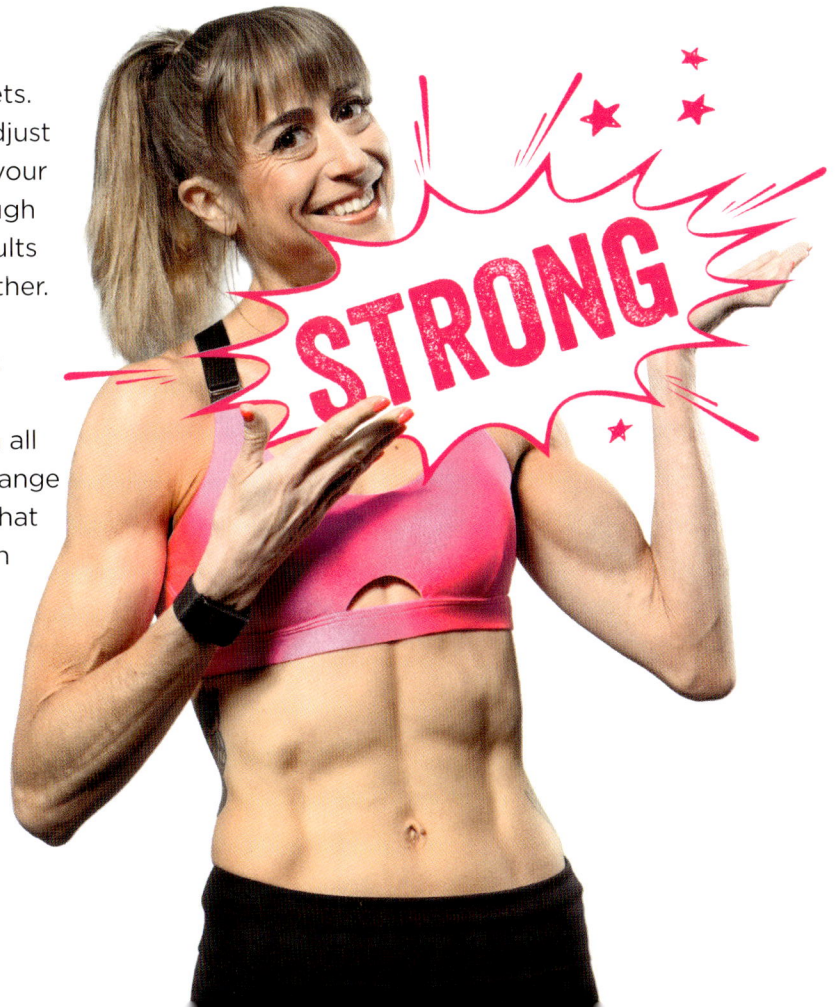

With each of these steps in the STRONG system, you'll do more than assess mindsets. You'll be outlining habits and actions to adjust not only your diet and workouts but also your entire lifestyle. Results don't happen through just one perfect move or macro ratio. Results happen through all systems working together. That means assessing sleep, recovery, micronutrients, outside stressors, changes in schedule, priorities, and so many other components. So, don't forget to reflect on all these other factors. Some are easier to change than others, but the more you recognize that each part has an impact, the more you can control as many aspects as possible.

So, let's get started setting the system in place and taking action to clear the field for reaping the sweetest fruits as a reward!

STRONG

4 WHY IS IT SIGNIFICANT?

"Well, since Sharon joined Redefining Strength, the sex is way better," her husband said in a testimonial video.

And while he was joking, he also wasn't.

People often don't see the far-reaching effects their goals will have on their lives and the lives of those around them. Too often, they downplay the importance of their goals, especially when society labels the goals "vain" or small because they're seemingly not a priority in the grand scheme of life. The question is, why should you have to?

Why can't these goals have a huge impact on you? Why don't people validate their significance and importance? Why do you let yourself feel guilty or silly for having these goals in the first place? Honestly, we should *value* these goals. These seemingly small, "insignificant" goals can actually have the most life-changing, farthest-reaching impact. Yup. You read that right. A vain or "small"

goal—a goal you push off and put behind everything else in your life—can have the most life-changing effect. I mean, consider what Sharon's husband said. She came into the program for weight loss and is leaving with a deeper connection with her husband!

This is why the STRONG system starts with you owning why your goals are significant to you: You prioritize what you value.

In this chapter, you'll focus on understanding the significance of your goals to help yourself prioritize and value new habits and changes even when life throws you curveballs that threaten to sabotage you.

Now, before you start to think your goals just aren't that significant, I want to share a huge lesson that changed my life: It isn't just in the destination, but in the journey that we realize how important and life-changing even small goals can be.

WHAT MATTERS TO YOU?

I've seen the massive transformation and impact a "silly and vain" weight-loss goal can have, because it affected my own life. It's why I'm here right now writing this book. Heck, it's why my company Redefining Strength exists, and it's helped hundreds of thousands of people around the world. My original goal was a super vain one. It was super unimportant and something I totally could have lived without. It was a goal that many people don't want and many think is stupid or ugly, especially for women. That goal was that I wanted to have … six-pack abs.

I'd downplayed this goal for years. I told myself it was stupid. Vain. I'd written off achieving this goal many, many, many (did I say many?) times before. I'd given up on all previous attempts, throwing the laundry list of excuses at myself. I told myself I liked food too much. That it just didn't matter. That I didn't have the willpower or the discipline. That it wasn't my body type to have abs. I blamed everything and tried to ignore the fact that I really, really wanted it! I made myself feel bad for caring about it.

But then I realized something. Why shouldn't it be important to me if I wanted it? I have this one body, this one life, to see what challenges I can conquer and to pursue the ones that matter to me. Why did I give a flying fart in space what anyone else thought about my goals? And why shouldn't this be significant to me? Why shouldn't I find out what I was capable of and believe I could achieve more?

I also began to realize that the more I made up excuses, the more I needed to conquer this challenge. It represented something I needed to prove to myself. And that was why this goal was so significant to me.

So, I took on the challenge. And I got freaking abs!

Here's the interesting part: Having abs didn't really change anything for me other than I was more willing to take half-nakey photos with weird faces to post on social media than I had been before. Yes, that was partly because I was proud of the lessons I'd learned to get abs. But really, the journey led to so much more than I'd expected because the process was far from easy, and there were many times I wanted to give up.

When you pursue any goal you think you can't achieve or that you tell yourself isn't important, you often do that to protect yourself and your ego from failure. Sometimes, the "smaller" the goal, and the less "important" it is to your survival, the easier it is to give up and let other priorities get in the way. You probably feel you don't deserve to prioritize yourself in that way because doing so would be selfish. You don't realize the huge impact that valuing yourself, even in these seemingly insignificant ways, can really have.

Getting abs showed me how much resilience and fortitude I have. It demonstrated my ability to overcome obstacles, stick with things, and evolve. It challenged me to slow down to speed up. It taught me life lessons that I needed to learn. Yup. Losing some stubborn belly fat taught me things about myself I didn't know.

All those things are true because, although this goal may have seemed small or unimportant, it was still a challenge I hadn't conquered and had even given up on before. It made me question myself and my limitations to build strength, confidence, and discipline. No matter what challenge you're

49

overcoming, those things are built through the struggle. The goal itself doesn't matter. It's the mental fortitude and physical strength to keep going that's important.

Through achieving this goal, I realized how much I could now help others in their fitness journeys. I could inspire them to pursue the goals that mattered to them while ignoring the judgments of others. I could inspire other people to believe that age, injury, schedules, and other obstacles or previous attempts didn't have to define them. They could create the person they wanted to be and inspire others to do the same.

My mental shift created a snowball. Now that snowball helps improve the health of thousands of people worldwide daily. No, I'm not being conceited. This is a fact. You may be thinking, *Great, Cori. But I'm not some half-nakey influencer posing on social media.* Well, I'm not an influencer either, even though I will pose half-nakey on social media. But seriously, it doesn't matter. Committing to a change helps you value this one life and body you're given and pursue other changes. You also lead by example. Show, don't tell. That's the way to change the world. (I know. So deep.)

You need to stop downplaying the importance of your goals and instead realize the web of impact that your goals can have. You have to really understand your why because that is the significance of your goals and will help you keep going and value the changes you're making.

You'll need to do an assessment like I did to determine what makes your goals significant to you. You can't worry about what other people will think. Ultimately, you have to be happy with you. You have this one life to lead. What do you want out of it? Why do these goals matter to you? Don't worry about what you "should" do. What do you want to pursue? What would help you feel you've accomplished something meaningful?

WHAT'S YOUR WHY?

Natalie came into the gym smiling from ear to ear like the Cheshire Cat. She was still grinning as she sat down to foam roll, and I was impatiently waiting to hear what she was going to say.

"Well?!" I finally said as she just sat there rolling her calf and smiling.

"I got the promotion!"

The previous week, Natalie had been crying and cursing me out as I told her she couldn't leave the gym until she did the monkey bars. She told me she couldn't. We battled back and forth. I held her legs as she went across. I *knew* she could do it, so I told her she couldn't leave the gym until she did. Halfway through the next class, after tears and multiple fake attempts at the monkey bars, guess what happened.

Natalie did the monkey bars! Not only did she do them, but she went all the way across and probably could have crossed them a few more times. Did she smile or thank me or even throw a kind word my way? Nope. Did she even give herself credit for achieving the goal? Nope.

But the confidence she gained in overcoming those monkey bars led to her asking for a promotion she'd been holding off on asking for—one she was sure she'd be passed over for. She not only asked for it, but she also got it!

Originally, she'd just wanted to do the monkey bars, something she hadn't been able to do even as a child, but the significance of the goal was far greater. Often, health and fitness achievements reveal a strength, resilience, dedication, fortitude, and willpower that you might not know you have. The confidence and strength to achieve those goals ultimately makes you ask for more of what you need and deserve in other areas of your life.

That's why a goal of wanting to lose 5 pounds isn't just a goal of wanting to lose 5 pounds. You need to pause and consider the importance if you want to succeed and make lasting habit changes.

No matter how much you prepare, set systems in place, and try to break down changes to accommodate where you currently are, there *will* be pushback. And at those times, you will be willing to keep going only if the pain of staying stuck outweighs the pain of change.

THE PAIN PUSHBACK

You prioritize what matters most to you.

If you value a goal, you will do what you need to do to achieve it on the worst of days. You may not do it perfectly. Things may not go exactly as planned. But you won't say, "F*** it!" to skip your workout and grab a box of cookies to devour as you sit on the couch while crumbs accumulate on your sweatpants.

Instead, you'll find a way to still do something. Don't get me wrong; those "forget everything!" days will still happen, but they'll become fewer and farther between because you'll know what you truly want and prioritize the habits and actions that get you there.

The hard part is making sure you remember why your goals matter and why they should be priorities to you even when life tries to get in the way. The pain pushback won't hit just once. It will hit throughout your journey, often when you least expect it. It will hit as your priorities shift over the course of the year.

You've probably had the pain pushback sabotage you before. Most people have. It's that point in the change loop where habit overload slides into all-out emotional sabotage, and you hear your inner voice utter the phrase, "This just isn't worth it!"

It's the point where the effort doesn't feel worth the outcome, and the pain of change starts to feel so great that the pain of staying stuck no longer drives you forward. It's that point where motivation fades, and you begin to believe you won't ever have the willpower to be able to keep going long enough for results to build.

I mentioned Newton's Third Law earlier in the book: "For every action, there is an equal and opposite reaction." Well, this is where it comes in with an emotional vengeance! That's why, before you jump right to making changes, I want you to really recognize the web of change and success this goal could create in your life. However, I do want to recognize that no matter how much you create a strong why, there will be times you still can't out-why the effort.

For example, even though I want to help others get lean, stay lean, and feel their most fabulous and strongest until their final day on this planet, there are days I don't do what I "should." Some days, the "shoulds" and "have-tos" don't feel like things I "get" to do. Some days, I know better and want better but don't do better. I'm human—a weird one, but human nonetheless—which means that no matter how strong my why is, there will be times I don't act in alignment with my goals, and that will happen to you too. However, little mistakes and the times you don't do what you "should" aren't the opposite of progress as much as they seem to be. They're a part of the process. When you recognize this, you can keep moving forward through the pain pushback. You can prevent yourself from cycling through the change loop again.

Recognizing that little blips are to be expected means you can address the other side of the pain scale. You determine which changes feel worth the discomfort and where the pain of staying stuck outweighs the pain of changing to move forward.

The idea is to make the pain of the changes feel worth the effort. You have to step back and ask yourself questions like these:

? Why do the habits feel too hard?

? Why doesn't this feel "worth it" to do when I really want my goal?

? What habits and actions would I be willing to do?

Your answers can help you better understand the cost involved in reaping the rewards you want. They can help so you don't have to rely on motivation to move forward, and you can set realistic timelines and repeatable habits that evolve as you progress.

DON'T RELY ON MOTIVATION

People crave motivation—yearn for motivation even. People rely on motivation and think it's the secret to success. People tend to blame all their struggles on a lack of motivation. But motivation actually is what holds people back. It's a passion bomb that usually explodes right in their faces and sabotages them.

Close your eyes and think about the last time you started a program. You went through all the resources. You were super excited about the promise of new things. You probably thought, *I've got this. I'm going to do everything exactly as it's laid out. This is going to be the best thing ever! I need a change, like, yesterday. All these changes are perfect, and I hate where I am right now.*

Many people experience that excitement right before they start something and before the reality of change, hard work, and nonlinear progress hits. They feel hope and motivation about the new thing, and the pain of the current situation makes them feel willing to do *anything.*

I used to get excited when someone would tell me they'd do anything. But now, I think, *Uh oh. We've got a ticking passion bomb.*

I know. I'm being a buzzkill. But I'm here to tell you that if you don't recognize the power of this built-up passion, it's going to blow up right in your face. The passion and motivation you feel driving you forward makes your brain ignore the hard changes you will face. You think, *Oh, it won't be that bad! I can live without [insert thing you most definitely can't live without that will come back to bite you in the butt...hard].*

Now, I tell myself or anyone else with a passion bomb that's ticking down to zero, "Pause." Otherwise, you get caught up in action that explodes. So, I say, "Pause. This is going to be hard. As tough as it is to take a step back and pause right now, and as passionate as you are about getting started with all the changes, you have to slow down before you speed up."

Womp womp. You know that sound effect? I told you I was going to be a buzzkill.

When you feel that kind of excitement, you're relying on motivation to help you make a change. It drives you to do over-the-top things like two-a-day workout sessions, eating plain spinach leaves and boiled chicken, and telling yourself that you *enjoy it.* Motivation makes you feel like any change is worth it, but then you hit that pain pushback before results have a chance to build. It's why you repeat the change loop over and over and over again.

The change loop stops for you today. Instead of relying on passion and motivation and making a million and one changes today, you're going to recognize that the all-or-nothing attitude has always led to burnout. Stop cleaning out your cabinets and treating today like it's your death row last meal. Recognize that passion must shift to *purpose* with a *plan* if you want to see lasting changes and reach your goals.

Pause in your passion and excitement and truly lay out a clear plan. Earlier, I asked you not to jump ahead in this book to get to the workouts and nutritional changes; now, I'm asking you to pause in wanting to do everything at once. You can use your passion to prepare, plan, and create the process. Take time for reflection. That is the first step.

Reflection helps you understand the process that will help you reach your goals. As you plan, prepare, and process, passion will shift to purpose. You will go from thinking about all the things you want to all the actions you need to take to get there. You shift from focusing on things outside of your control to those things within your control. You stop staring at the scoreboard hoping it will change and instead start playing well on the field and scoring the goals you need.

As you do this, you face reality and consider the actions and mindsets you need. You step into who you want to be and act as if. These are the things that will carry you to the finish line because passion will fizzle as it has before. Fizzling passion is why you think, *I just don't have the willpower or motivation. I'm not disciplined*, every time you fail to reach your goals

You actually do have enough willpower. What you don't have are clear steps for moving forward from where you are to be able to build discipline—because discipline is built from consistency.

You become good at what you consistently and repeatedly do, and to repeat habits and actions consistently, you have to believe in their purpose. This process will include

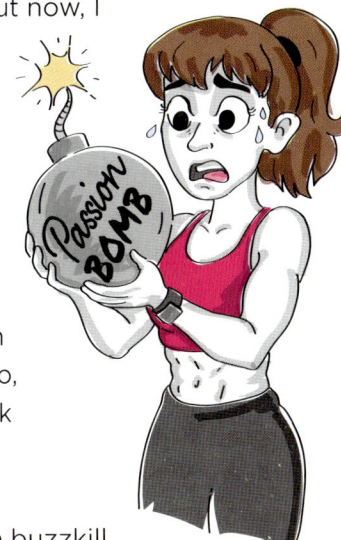

things that you won't like, but when you know their purpose, you will continue to push through.

Understanding why you want to meet this goal and what uncomfortable habits and actions are worth it prepares you for the ups and downs to come. Recognize that you may be willing to sacrifice more in the immediate future to see better results faster and that how you implement habits may have to shift as the pain driving you forward from your initial motivation wears off.

I keep reminding you to pause because I know how excited people get to jump ahead. Defuse that passion bomb and instead focus your energy on creating a deeper purpose for your goals to drive you forward with a clear plan in place.

REFLECTING ON YOUR WHY

Now comes the inward look and self-awareness building that kinda stinks but is truly what makes for a strong foundation for lasting results.

I want you to write out the most basic version of your goal—a one-sentence summary of your destination from Chapter 2. Think about that Beastette or Beast and how fabulous they feel and also think about their origin story.

As the author of your own story, why do you want to end up at your goal? Consider the following questions:

? Why are you sick of being stuck where you are? Really consider why your current situation is painful. What do you dislike most about it?

? Where will making changes have an impact on your life?

? Where can achieving this goal lead? Could it help you get a promotion? Could it inspire other family members who have grave health concerns but won't take action? Will you be able to travel? Will you want to pursue new relationships? Think about the far-reaching effects this new identity could lead to and the new lifestyle it could bring.

? What will be the more subtle effects? What changes will this create that will improve other areas of your life? How could this mentally create a change, making you more confident, open, adventurous, and so on?

? Who else will this potentially impact in your life? Who will you need to connect with to achieve your goals? Who may not stick with you on your journey? Consider the community you will need and even who in your current life may give you a bit of "hate."

Remember that strength and confidence aren't built by achieving your goal, and the result alone doesn't bring happiness. Everything that occurs along the way contributes to who you want to be. Your new identity will be able to achieve things you may not dream are possible right now. So, realize you aren't just losing a few pounds and starting a new workout routine; you're growing into who you want to become!

CHANGING YOUR ENVIRONMENT

Now that you've reflected on your why, I want you to do something that may feel a bit silly. I want you to create a visual reminder. This visual reminder will help you connect back to your why when you feel the pain pushback. It will also help you recognize when the pain of staying stuck doesn't outweigh the pain of change, which means your habits need to shift. Lastly, it will help you stay focused on the habits and mindsets you need because a visual reminder is a shift in your environment.

Shifting your environment is one of the best ways to become more disciplined almost instantly. (You're welcome!) It's a constant reminder to maintain the habits you want to implement and not to default back to habits you're trying to unlearn. You need to be reminded far more than you need to be taught, yet the tendency is often to look for new things to learn over better ways to remember all that we already know.

When you write your why on a piece of paper, you create a visual reminder so every time you see it, you feel an instant pick-me-up. It's an instant cue. It's like putting out your workout clothes at night so you feel a push when you wake up to go to the gym or putting your foam roller in front of your TV so you feel extra guilty when you walk past it without doing your mobility work. It's like the opposite of having all the foods you love sitting in your cabinet with a "Do not eat" sign on them.

I mean, really, you'd never do that, right? You'd throw out things you don't want to eat, or you'd just not buy them. At the very least, you'd hide them on a high shelf or put them in the freezer. These are all shifts in your environment to remind you of the habits you want or even to help not remind you of the habits you're trying to move away from.

Pick a picture, write out a quote, draw a symbol, find an object that represents where you want to travel to, buy a plane ticket, put out a piggy bank and some coins to drop in as you go—something that gives you a visual reminder of your why that you see every single day and inspires you to keep moving forward while taking time to pause and reflect.

Heck, maybe you can even get a mini toy axe. Whatever you pick, make it something that will give you an extra boost on the days that you don't want to do what you should to *keep on going*!

5 MAKE IT TARGETED

I want you to consider something for a second: How are you defining success?

Your answer is probably why you haven't reached your goals in the past or maintained your results long term. Your lack of success isn't because your plan hasn't been good, you haven't worked hard enough, or you're just broken and genetically doomed. There's also no secret out there that you just don't know yet.

Here's an example. A client messaged me and said, "I'm losing inches but not losing weight! *<grrr>*"

As I read the comment, my face (with its very thick, expressive eyebrows) cycled through expressions of shock, amusement, and confusion—just about every emotion possible. I wanted to shake sense into her. I'm sure she saw my message bubbles pop up seventeen different times over the next minute as I tried to type a reply.

Finally, I said, "Out of curiosity, why do you say that as if it's a bad thing?"

She replied quickly with five sobbing emojis, "Because I need to lose 50 pounds, and the scale isn't budging!"

First, the scale had been changing—slowly, as defined by the client, but let's face it: Everything is slow compared to what we want. Second, why did she consider the scale the *only* measure of progress? Why was she ignoring a key sign that she was losing fat without losing muscle? Why didn't the inches she lost count?

I realized something right there and then, but instead of trying to point out the progress she had been making, which would only have resulted in her focusing on how slow her progress was or how much further she had to go, I asked, "So, what now? You give up?"

Now, it was her turn to make message bubbles pop up and disappear. I could tell she wasn't sure how to reply. Finally, the bubbles stopped. I waited. Eventually, she replied, "No. I just really want to see progress."

So, I asked, "What would count as progress if these inches you've lost don't count?"

Your expectations can make or break your success. Manage your expectations.

I want to repeat something I just said: Your expectations can make or break your success.

When I asked you to reflect on the question of how you are defining success, you may have had thoughts like these:

• Losing *x* pounds.

• Fitting back into my skinny jeans.

• Hiking a trail with my family.

• Lowering my blood pressure.

All these goals are fabulous.

But if your only measurement of success is direct progress toward reaching a singular goal, you're probably going to give up before you get there. Progress is never linear. The bigger the goal, the longer it will take to get there, which

> **Your expectations can make or break your success. Manage your expectations.**

makes it easy to get caught up in only seeing how much further you have to go. And, boy, can that "further to go" seem to stretch on forever the harder you're working, the more effort you're giving, and the more you really want it!

To complicate things even more, you can't control how long results take to manifest. Although you don't have control over time frames, you do have control over your consistent, daily actions.

Think about planting an apple seed in a field you cleared. Just because you want to eat an apple tomorrow and did all that work to plant the seed doesn't mean that *poof*—the tree will grow faster magically, and the apples will be ripe right away. If you try to water the seed more to make it grow faster, you could ultimately kill it. Your extra effort would sabotage you.

Yet people often approach habit changes this way when there aren't obvious signs of growth or progress. In the end, that extra effort only sabotages the whole plan. The sucky thing is that results take time.

The push to out-exercise and out-diet time as you measure progress in only one way makes it harder to embrace the ups and downs and causes you to struggle to find ways to stay consistent during the weeks you go backward. When you have one singular focus or one singular definition of success, any steps backward feel like stabs to the heart. They make it hard to stick with it and push on even when you know that you have to keep going to leap forward.

Maybe you know the story of the two miners. Both were told they'd find diamonds if they just dug deep enough. So, both started mining down into the dirt. Dirt above them. Dirt below them. Dirt all freaking around them. They dug for days. On the fourth day, little did they know they were both inches from breaking through to the diamonds. The first miner, who saw only dirt all around, threw up their hands and said, "Forget this! I'm not making any progress. I'll never get there!" That miner gave up and turned back.

The second miner stayed focused on chipping away at it. This miner's goal was to dig a certain number of inches every single day. Through dirt. Through stone. The miner wanted those diamonds and expected to *just keep digging* until they got there. Because this miner set the expectation of digging a certain number of inches every single day and focused on the action of digging and seeing it as a win—*boom*! The miner struck diamonds.

Honestly, this story is exactly how it feels to achieve goals. You have to do hard stuff every single day, and it often isn't fun. It isn't sexy or cool or exciting. It's dirt. Digging in freaking dirt. And so often, when your sole focus is on just "being there already," you give up right before results snowball. You don't see all the progress you've made and let that fuel you to keep moving forward.

Don't let the dirt all around you distract you. Don't let how you're defining success sabotage you.

Now, let's talk about how you want to be able to answer so your expectations don't break you the next time I ask, "How are you defining success?"

THE UNSEXY EXPECTATION EVERYONE SHOULD HAVE

You're in a rush and running late, so you're driving a bit above the speed limit. You're trying to go around the slowpoke in the outside lane and don't see a piece of plastic in the middle of the street until it's too late. Pop! You hear the unmistakable sound of a flat tire. Ugh!

You pull over to the side of the road and get out to take a look. It's completely flat. You need to put on the spare or call roadside assistance to get going as quickly as possible. Instead of doing either, you go back to your car and grab the knife you've brought for the cake you baked. You'll never make it to the event in time, so you may as well slash the other three tires. Wait. *What?* You'd never do that, right? *Right.*

Doing so would make absolutely no sense. The thought is laughable and ridiculous. Why would you want to repair more damage and take longer to get back on the road? You wouldn't.

Yet this is exactly what people do when a "setback" happens with their diet or workout plan. One cookie becomes the whole box. A missed workout becomes a week without training. One thing becomes a bigger problem to fix. But you can change this approach to stop the change loop from repeating. What makes this time different isn't a new macro ratio or workout plan; it's a shift in your perspective and your expectations.

Instead of seeing the failure, the off-plan eating, or the progress toward your goal that wasn't exactly what you wanted to see as an excuse to say, "Forget everything," see it as your first chance to fix the flat and get back on the road. Every time you can rapidly fix the problem to get back to your trip, the progress happens faster. Don't add to your mistake. Move forward from it!

Now, the question is, how do you do that? How can you avoid compounding the problem? How can you avoid seeing every mistake, failure, or setback as a reason to give up? It all comes back to managing your expectations and how you define success.

There's one unsexy expectation you need to set for yourself every time you start working toward a new goal if you don't want to end up moping by the side of the road with all four tires deflated: expect to *learn* from everything you do.

Learning should always be your goal. I know that isn't what you want to hear. Learning is boring, and the process often *sucks.* But the simple fact is, failures are just learning with frustration. Success doesn't happen despite failures; it happens because of them. But only if you realize what the failures are teaching you.

> **Success doesn't happen despite failures; it happens because of them.**

"We learn more in the reflection than in the doing." I'm not sure where I first heard that, but man, oh man—it was a lightbulb moment. If you reflect on each experience and expect to learn from everything you do, you'll ultimately move forward faster toward your goals. Nothing—I repeat, *nothing*—you do will be wasted effort because reflecting on it means you'll always get something out of it. You won't always make the direct forward progress you hoped for, but if you learn something, even if it's what not to do, you will grow. You'll gain knowledge that will move you forward, and that makes the experience valuable. That's why, as you read through this book right now, I want you to focus on the learning.

If you already know something, good! What more can you learn from reading it said in a new way? How have you not reflected on or truly implemented this tactic or perspective in the past?

If you mess up with the macros or skip a workout, good! How can you see this as an opportunity to reassess your priorities and schedule? How can you see this as that opportunity to fix the flat faster and move forward?

When you set your expectations to be to learn from anything new you start, you always hit your goal, not only because the goal is to learn but also because you don't give up at the slightest setback or failure. You don't sit moping by the side of the road. Managing your expectations and seeking to always learn is just part of it.

WHAT DOES SUCCESS TRULY MEAN?

The more ways you have to measure success, the more successful you will be.

Remember the last time you stepped on the scale after a week of hard work expecting to see fabulous progress only to ... well ... *not*? You spent all week feeling hungry every night as you went to bed, getting up at the crack of dawn to do your workout, meal prepping for hours on a Sunday when you really wanted to be out at brunch with friends, and then you stepped on the scale, and you hadn't lost any weight. Maybe the number even went *up*. Sure, maybe the increase was only 0.2 pound, and you hadn't yet pooped that morning. But gosh darn it, you *deserved* results for all that work, right?

Instead, you feel like a horrible failure after working so hard, and you just want to say, "Screw it," and go out to breakfast to eat everything you know you "shouldn't." This constant feeling of failing isn't going to keep you wanting to move forward with your new habits. It definitely isn't putting you in a positive mindset to embrace the changes.

The more you feel like a failure, the more you're going to see yourself start to fail. That's why you have to manage your expectations and give yourself more than one way to measure success.

Success can't mean only one thing (achieving your ultimate goal) because the bigger or harder the goal, the longer it will take. The more you're pursuing a goal you've never had or haven't had in a long time, the longer it will take. You have to remember that the longer you haven't been at your goal, the more your body is used to its current state and habits, so the more you resist the process of change. You've "built up" a stronger resistance to the change becoming more entrenched in your current lifestyle. Any way you look at it, progress won't be quick. Because progress is never linear, you're looking at a lot of days and weeks you simply don't and won't feel successful if you define success only as reaching your goal.

No wonder people often want to give up along the way!

Consequently, you need to manage your expectations and not only set your ultimate goal but also *mini* targets within that big goal and *complementary targets.* Mini targets are little progress markers or benchmarks. If you want to lose 50 pounds, your first target may be losing 10 pounds. Mini targets can help you celebrate wins along the way.

Complementary targets are goals you set that you know will help you repeat the habits and maintain the mindsets you need to reach your ultimate goal. They're basically other ways to keep you doing what you should and feeling successful.

I love to call them nonscale victories, or NSVs. They're ways to measure progress outside of the scale, and that's especially important when your goal is weight loss. The scale is a fickle frenemy that fluctuates all the time; it would change hourly if you were to step on it. NSVs occur more frequently along your weight-loss journey than the scale wins do, even when you're making fabulous progress. Yet people often don't bother to pause to appreciate and recognize them.

That's why you need to consciously set complementary goals. Consider the habits you need to succeed at your ultimate goal. How can you measure progress in those habits? How can you know success is snowballing even if you can't see it yet? Could you set a performance goal in the gym? Could you set a meal prep focus for hitting your daily fiber? Could you enter a race? Can you get a health test or blood drawn to watch markers? Can you try on a pair of jeans to see if they're closer to fitting?

Find as many ways as possible to celebrate progress and know you're on the right track with your habits, even setting celebrating consistency in those habits as a goal itself! Take some time right now to write out a few goals that will support doing the habits you need to reach your ultimate goal. How will you measure progress toward them? Also, consider little benchmarks within those goals and your ultimate goal so you can measure progress along the way. You might even consider having some complementary targets that are super simple habit consistency wins you can celebrate daily!

SUCCESS BREEDS MORE SUCCESS

While I was getting out of the car, I was juggling coffees in one hand while I reached into the back seat to grab my dog Kiwi's leash with the other. My husband, Ryan, saw my struggle and asked, "Do you want some help?" Because I was in a horrible, no good, very bad mood—one of those cut off your nose to spite your face moods—I said, "No. I've got it."

Famous last words. Kiwi leapt from the car, yanking the leash as I closed the door. I felt a cup of coffee start to drop, so in a panic, I squeezed it, and coffee began spurting out from under the lid. The coffee spewed across my jacket, all over my feet, and onto the driveway. I tried to stop the spillage, and I let go of Kiwi's leash as she sprinted to the door. I felt like throwing myself on the driveway to have a temper tantrum right then and there, but my neighbor was out washing his car, so I trudged inside, tossed my jacket in the washer, and sat down at my computer to pout.

Honestly, it wasn't really that big a deal. Very little coffee even spilled, but I was in a horrible mood, and that was simply the last straw. As a result, I didn't care about doing anything I should. Eat well and hit my macros? Meh! Work out? Who cares! I "ruined" the day—all because a little bit of coffee spilled.

That's the power of mindset.

Feeling unsuccessful and like everything is going wrong often leads to more going wrong as you spiral down into the pit of negativity from the slightest prompt. You start to doubt yourself, call yourself stupid, and believe you aren't worth the effort.

The flip side is that when everything goes right, you want to do more and feel better about every change you're making. Success makes you feel more confident, empowered, stronger, and more capable, leading you to do more.

Owning the power of mindset and momentum can help you use this perspective to your advantage. It can help you use success to create more success. And it can help you recognize when your momentum is starting to carry you the other way.

It's important to control the direction your momentum is carrying you. You can do this in the way you set your expectations and goals and by how you break down the habits you implement. It's why even the small habit goals that are daily wins are so important. As I've said, there will be weeks you step on the scale, test your pull strength, or have a pace on a run that doesn't improve and maybe even goes backward, but that doesn't mean you aren't moving forward. It can be hard to remember that, though. It can make you feel like you're failing if you don't have other measurements of success to keep you motivated and moving forward. It's so important that you're able to measure success in many ways and break down your targets into repeatable habits (which is the subject of Chapter 6).

As you set your complementary targets, think of goals that will give you some quick and frequent wins. You want to set your mini targets so the victories add up rapidly, which will build the progress and make you want to do more. It's also why you need to set targets based on where you are now rather than based on where you want to go. Finally, focused deadlines and end dates that are realistic hold you accountable.

That raises an important question you're probably wondering about.

HOW LONG WILL IT TAKE?

The annoying and most honest answer to this question is this: It depends. With any goal you set, you don't really know exactly how long it will take to achieve it. When I post a picture of a "before" and "after" photo, I often get asked, "How long between these two photos? How long did it take?" The answer I always give is, "My entire life."

Everything you've done up until this point will have an impact. How long you've had the weight on, how inactive or active you've been, any pain and discomfort you feel, and the sacrifices you're willing to make all play into the changes you can embrace and how your body responds.

You know that show *Fit to Fat to Fit*, where the trainer would gain the weight to be able to lose it with the client? I hated that show. It wasn't fair. The trainer knew the pain that came with changes. They knew exactly what changes to make. They had the discipline of habits already in place before they gained the weight. Besides, they hadn't had the weight on for very long. All that made it easier—mentally and physically—for them. It's also why you can never compare yourself to another person, even if that someone is about your height and age with the same amount to lose. Your journey will be different.

Even though you don't know exactly how long results will take, you need to set an end date or deadline to hold yourself accountable.

Think about the last time you were truly motivated to get started right away and were able to stay focused the entire time. Was it before your wedding? Before a big reunion or birthday? Before a beach vacation where you wanted to rock a bikini? End dates and big events create motivation and "urgency." They make you more focused and intentional. When you haven't had a deadline, you may have found yourself thinking, *I'll start tomorrow*, only to have tomorrow end up being months later.

Deadlines and end dates, especially ones tied to big events, help motivate you to get going and stick with things to push through the hard parts. They add emotion or "pain" to your why, as well as a sense of urgency. It's why you want to set deadlines for your targets, especially the main goal. You want this deadline to have some pressure on it as well. Maybe you plan a vacation to hike a challenging trail or even schedule a photo shoot in celebration of your body recomposition. Maybe you plan a race or a very special party. But make your deadline meaningful to hold you to it and even try to involve others.

Now, while you do need deadlines, too much pressure can backfire. Success and failure are dependent on the mindset you create. When you feel like you're constantly failing at hitting deadlines, you'll want to give up. If you feel like you're hitting every end date, you'll want to keep going. Part of how you view success and failure is baked right into the word we use to define these dates, especially for the mini targets within the main and complementary targets. I like to change the term *end date* or *deadline* to *checkpoints* because that's what they really are—points to check on your progress and reassess what you need to keep moving forward.

Some checkpoints you want to hit easily and even know you will likely surpass. Those checkpoints help you feel successful and wanting to do more. Others may be lofty goals to hit in the time frame you outlined, but that pressing date may be motivation for you to get started immediately and stay more focused and intentional with the plan. You can use a combination of both to create motivation and focus, as well as success momentum.

Viewing these dates as checkpoints rather than deadlines also contributes more to your success mindset. It isn't a failure not to hit that target by that time. That

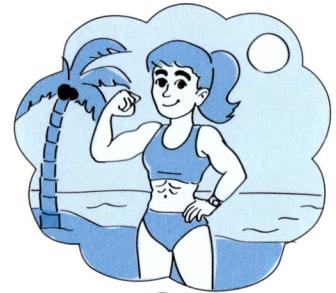

checkpoint is just a time for reassessment to adjust future targets and even make sure your habits and routines are still in line with your goals and where you currently are. When you don't pause after hitting, or missing, a goal deadline to see what else may be going on, you miss the chance to reflect, which holds you back from creating lasting change and continuing to move forward.

BUT I HAVE MORE THAN ONE MAIN GOAL!

You might not want to hear this, but you can't have more than one primary focus at a time. Where your attention goes, your energy flows. The less energy, dedication, and focus you give one thing, the less likely you are to be successful.

That doesn't mean multiple things can't work together. That's the beauty of the complementary goals. So, if you have multiple things you want to achieve, you need to recognize that sometimes a goal has to take a back seat if it's pulling you even slightly in another direction.

By prioritizing one thing at a time, you can often achieve all your goals faster. Even slightly conflicting goals can help propel you forward when you place them in the correct order. Like a weight-loss goal and a performance goal. You may choose to value performance over losing weight faster, but in training hard for your performance goal, you set yourself up for success later when you prioritize the weight-loss goal. Or by prioritizing losing weight first, you may then set yourself up to be fit for your performance goal.

Your budget and the goals themselves will dictate how many can work together and in what ways. So, as you set your main target and complementary targets, consider whether they're all pulling in the same direction. It's like walking a pack of dogs; if they're pulling in every direction, it's going to be a battle to go anywhere. But if they're all pulling in the same direction, you'll be propelled forward even faster!

CAN I LOSE FAT *AND* GAIN MUSCLE AT THE SAME TIME?

This is a question that often comes up. My answer is yup, you can. Honestly, it should be your goal: body recomposition (recomp).

Saying, "I want to lose fat and gain muscle," is different from saying, "I want to gain muscle and lose fat."

These may seem like the same thing, but they aren't. While both are body recomp, each has a different main focus. Which one you pick affects how you design your weekly strength and cardio schedule as well as how you adjust your diet.

So, what is your goal? And don't say weight loss. As much as you may think you care about what the scale says, what you ultimately want is to feel and look a certain way. Those things can often happen at very different weights on the scale if you let go of the power that number has.

You want to look more defined and feel stronger. You want to see your hard work in the gym pay off so you look like a freaking rockstar in your bathing suit or an outfit that makes everyone compliment you.

This is body recomp at its finest. If you want to lose fat and gain muscle, you will want to have that primary fat-loss focus in mind as you dial in your workouts and diet to match. If you want to gain muscle as your primary focus while losing fat, you want to set your systems in place to match.

If you aren't sure which is your primary goal because you really want both, here's a good rule to follow:

» If you're basically at your desired weight (maybe you would like to lose 10 to 15 pounds) and near the leanness level you want, then you want to focus on building muscle while losing fat.

» If you have more weight to lose (16 or more pounds) and want to look lean and defined while adding muscle to stay functionally fit as you get older, you may start by focusing on fat loss while building muscle.

Having this clear goal in mind can also help with complementary targets. When you want to lose fat as you build muscle, your gym goal might be to maintain your lifts rather than seeing huge increases. Maybe you even focus more on improving push-ups or pull-ups. If you want to build muscle while losing fat, you should focus a bit more on seeing bigger gains in your lifts and numbers.

Remember, you want everything to have a purpose. The more clarity you have about your goals, the better off you will be. (More on the impact this has, and even stepping off the scale to measure your results, in Chapter 14.)

Take some time now to write out your goals, assess how they work together, and consider how you'll measure progress toward them. Really think about what those measurement tools are telling you!

REFLECTION

Brainstorm ideas for your targets and keep in mind how you're managing your expectations and giving yourself more ways to feel successful and see progress. By setting these complementary targets, you can help yourself focus on creating and maintaining the daily habits you need to reach your ultimate goal.

So, consider things like this:

? What related goals can you set that will mean you're doing the habits you need to achieve success?

? How can you break down these goals into mini targets to track improvements in these other areas?

? What mini targets can you set to keep you on track toward your ultimate goal?

As you list out these targets, create a firm end date for your ultimate goal. Make it meaningful. Then set checkpoints for each of your mini targets and complementary goals. And don't worry right now about whether they're "realistic." You're setting assessment and reflection dates.

First, create short-term checkpoints for your primary target. State something you can measure at that time. Set a firm date for that checkpoint so you know when you're checking in on your progress (and how you'll measure it).

Being able to evolve your workout and diet systems and habits means having accurate data. Will you use progress pictures? Will you do weekly food log overviews to see consistency? Will you watch your weights, reps, and sets on specific moves? Will you enter a few races and track your times? Will you take body measurements or use an item of clothing? Outline how you're measuring progress toward each goal so you have some form of data rather than just feelings. (Feelings often sabotage you!)

Then name two other goals that will complement your main goal with their own mini targets to keep you accountable. Give yourself checkpoints to keep you motivated, hold yourself accountable, and prevent you from waiting until tomorrow to get started! The whole thing will be structured like this:

MAIN TARGET:.. checkpoint date:
....
1. SHORT-TERM TARGET:.. checkpoint date:
....
2. SHORT-TERM TARGET:.. checkpoint date:
....
3. SHORT-TERM TARGET:.. checkpoint date:
....
How will you measure progress for each?...
....
....

COMPLEMENTARY TARGET #1:... checkpoint date:
....
1. SHORT-TERM TARGET:.. checkpoint date:
....
2. SHORT-TERM TARGET:.. checkpoint date:
....
3. SHORT-TERM TARGET:.. checkpoint date:
....
How will you measure progress for each?...
....
....

COMPLEMENTARY TARGET #2:... checkpoint date:
....
1. SHORT-TERM TARGET:.. checkpoint date:
....
2. SHORT-TERM TARGET:.. checkpoint date:
....
3. SHORT-TERM TARGET:.. checkpoint date:
....
How will you measure progress for each?...
....

Habits are the *how* to get what you want. You need to plan them strategically and assign clear action items to them. It's easy to identify a habit, like "drink more water," but people often don't outline how they're going to implement the habit, so they stay stuck where they are. So, in this chapter, you're going to really dive into the actions and daily routines you need and decide how you're going to do them.

THE HABIT ROCK PILE

I have a question for you: How many stones can you carry?

Are you wondering whether I've lost my mind? There's a point. Just stay with me here.

Your answer is probably, "It depends." The bigger the rocks, the fewer you can move at once, right? With smaller pebbles, you can easily grab and move a bunch in one swoop.

You need to think about changing your habits in the same way. Not all habits are the same magnitude, so how you go about changing habits depends on what the habit is, just like how many rocks you can pick up depends on their size.

Your habits are like different-sized rocks. You have a pile of big rocks, medium stones, small stones, and little pebbles. You need to get these rocks from one side of a field to the other using only one bag that can accommodate up to 100 pounds.

You realize you can fit only so many big rocks into it at once. Try to stuff in too many, and you either can't carry the weight, you run out of space, or you risk the bag ripping as you travel across the field. Wouldn't that be fun? Not!

More of the medium and small stones fit into the bag. But as they shift around in the bag, you feel there is wasted space you could fill. The pebbles are so tiny that you could almost carry the whole load across in one go, but then you'd still have to make many more trips if you moved only those first.

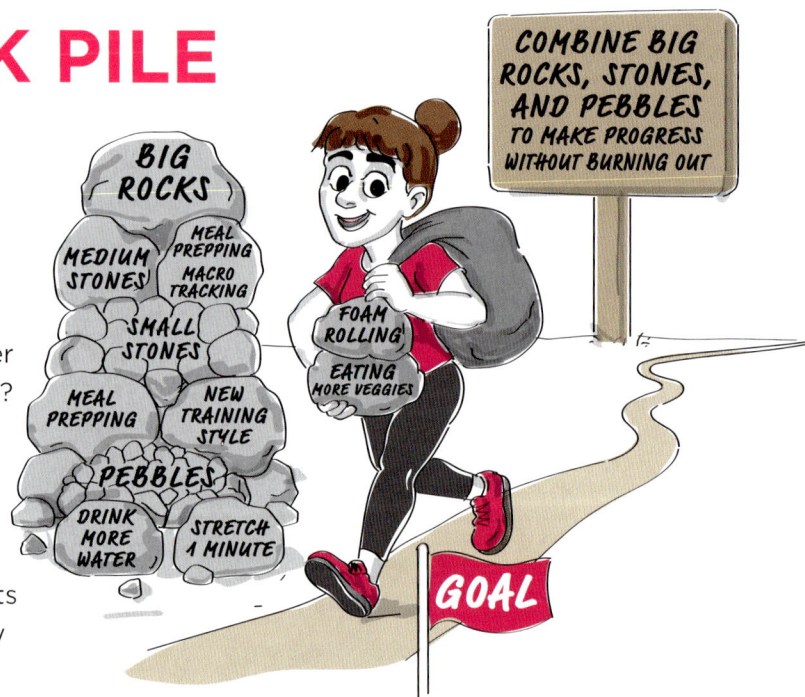

How do you make the fewest trips and not waste time or effort or cause yourself to fail so you ultimately can't reach your goal? You combine different sizes to fill your bag to the max weight it can carry! That way, you're optimizing each trip. You can put in one big rock, then fill the space around it with medium and small stones before packing the extra space with pebbles. Doing this allows you to make it across the field efficiently without tiring or the bag ripping. Yay!

The big rocks represent those habits that feel like big changes from your current routine. They're far outside your comfort zone, don't necessarily feel sustainable or realistic in the long term, and require energy and focus to implement. These are the habits that really make you embrace being a beginner.

The big rocks are often overwhelming and awkward, and your brain doesn't especially like them. These are the habits you feel like you really have to power your way through. They challenge the identity you've found in your current diet and workout practices, and they're the changes you need the most but probably push back against the hardest. The big habits vary from person to person, but they tend to be things like these:

» Tracking macros. A lot of people think about doing it, but because it seems daunting, they don't start.

» Becoming a morning workout person if you've always trained at night. It just seems impossible to get up that early!

» Lifting if you've always been a runner. Maybe you just love cardio and believe you need it to see results. And it feels so good. You know you "should" lift, but you don't want to. It's so hard!

The medium stones are changes that are more in line with your current lifestyle and values. They're habits you may be interested in, somewhat like the idea of, or are even comfortable being uncomfortable with. While they take some effort to do, you're OK with that. These things are just slightly outside your comfort zone but close enough that you can see the steps forward. They're the changes you don't really have a mental block against, but they still fall by the wayside because they require some planning or effort. Here are some examples:

» A new style of training that will really challenge you to lift heavier and do uncomfortable new moves. But you like training, so you're up for the challenge.

» Meal prepping weekly. You're comfortable planning out meals and enjoy cooking, but it's hard to find that set time to bulk prep!

The small stones are the habits that don't take a ton of effort, but you just don't feel comfortable doing them, or you don't enjoy them, especially the first few times. They may be unfamiliar or awkward, so you hesitate even though you can easily do them. They fall off your to-do list, not because they're hard, but because you don't value them, especially when other priorities get in the way. They are habits such as these:

» Foam rolling or doing your mobility work. You know you "should" do it, and it doesn't really take much time or energy, but you don't like it, so you don't make time for it.

» Eating more fruits and vegetables. It's not a hard thing to do, but if you don't like fruits and veggies, it can be an uncomfortable change to make.

Finally, you have the small pebbles. These are tweaks to what you're currently doing. They don't require much effort, and they're comfortable to make. They even feel natural right from the start. Honestly, these are the habit changes you probably don't often make because they don't feel like they add up fast enough! They are the changes you could get up right now and implement without much thought, like these:

» Drinking another glass of water daily.

» Doing one minute of stretching at your desk.

These habits are the most unsexy, boring basics, but they're still important.

THE HABIT ROCK PILE

BIG ROCKS

1. TRACKING MACROS.
2. BECOMING A MORNING WORKOUT PERSON AND GETTING UP EARLY!
3. LIFTING.

MEDIUM STONES

1. A NEW STYLE OF TRAINING THAT WILL REALLY CHALLENGE ME TO LIFT HEAVIER AND DO UNCOMFORTABLE NEW MOVES.
2. MEAL PREPPING WEEKLY.

SMALL STONES

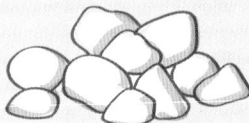

1. FOAM ROLLING OR DOING MOBILITY WORK.
2. EATING MORE FRUITS AND VEGETABLES.

LITTLE PEBBLES

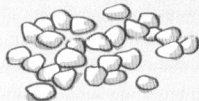

1. DRINKING MORE WATER DAILY.
2. DOING ONE MINUTE OF STRETCHING AT MY DESK.

Looking at your rock pile, what combination can you carry this week?

Now, the efficient way to carry the rocks across the field is to combine a variety of sizes in the bag. You need to do the same thing with your habits.

The different kinds of habit changes have different values and need to be combined for the best results. When you don't take this approach of combining different types of habits—those more or less comfortable and more or less effort—you ultimately don't see the results you want and quit.

If you combine too many big rocks and medium stones at once, you'll overwhelm yourself. Your bag will rip halfway across the field, or you'll go to lift what you just stuffed in and not be able to carry it even a foot. It's just too much effort. You can't rely on willpower to take you through for long. Something will give before you've reached your goals, and you'll feel worse off than when you started.

But if you focus only on carrying small pebbles or stones, you may feel like the process is taking *forever* because you aren't really seeing that pile get smaller, even though it's dwindling a bit at a time. So, you give up out of frustration. You need to make big enough changes that progress is more obvious. As I mentioned in Chapter 5 in the discussion about targets, success breeds more success!

By combining habits of different magnitudes, you can be more efficient. You can help yourself see results in the fastest possible way while not burning yourself out. Also, each trip across that field does not mean you have to carry the same habits each and every time. As you go through your fitness journey, your habits will evolve. Sometimes, you may be able to fit in a few more big rocks and medium stones. At other times, you may be tired and need to lighten the load. Heck, at some point, you may even find a sledgehammer to break those big rocks down into smaller stones!

The key is recognizing that habits come with different costs and that the cost can change. By recognizing the difficulty, or ease, of making different habit changes, you can meet yourself where you are to move forward.

WHAT WILL IT COST ME?

There is a cost to every reward. A downside to every upside.

Success is never owned. It's rented, and rent is due every single day in the form of your habits. The exact cost depends on the habit. The question you have to ask is, "Can I pay this price, and am I also *willing* to pay it?" In Chapter 5, when you worked on outlining your target, I mentioned that the pain of staying stuck has to outweigh the pain of change. You can't change the pain of staying stuck, but you *can* alter the pain of change.

That's where the different sizes of rocks come into play; each comes with a different cost and reward. With more effort, discomfort, and sacrifice comes faster progress toward your goal, but the mental cost is greater. Smaller pebbles cost less both physically and mentally, but progress is often slower. It's especially true if we've chosen to break down big habits into smaller pieces.

For example, making a big diet change is often what yields sexy, quick changes on the scale. But it comes at the cost of people not being able to maintain the restriction for long and ultimately seeing their weight rebound or gaining even more. Instead, if you break down some of the big diet changes into one small change of drinking more water, you may find yourself able to more easily build on those healthy habits, but you may also find that the scale takes longer to change. The fewer big changes you make at once, the less immediate progress you may see, but the more you can mentally handle the changes and stack the habits to see results snowball long term.

For the cost of a habit to be worthwhile, the reward has to have significant value. If the cost doesn't feel worth the reward, you won't do the habit in the long term.

When you're motivated, you're strong enough to carry all the big rocks across the field. The problem is that motivation and energy don't last. Basically, you lift more than you can carry and end up "injured" and unable to implement any of the habits you've built. This habit overload from motivation is the passion bomb exploding in your face, and you fall back into the change loop. Passion must turn to purpose if you want to see results, and motivation can make you take on *faaaaar* too much all at once. That's why you have to take a sledgehammer to some of the big rocks.

You have to recognize the power of the 1 percent.

TEAM 1%: DROP THE ALL-OR-NOTHING MINDSET

You might have heard that a habit takes twenty-one days to build. If that's the case, why do people do so many twenty-one-day or thirty-day challenges only to sabotage their results by falling back into old habits and routines? Wouldn't all these challenges pay off?

The thing is, they could. The way people go about making changes during the challenges is what holds them back from long-lasting results.

Researcher Dr. Phillippa Lally and her team at University College London found that it takes an average of 66 days to form a true habit, but the time frame for habit formation can range anywhere from 18 to 254 days. The amount of time required to create a new habit depends on the complexity of the habit, the individual, and consistency in practice. People get good at what they consistently do.

This is one reason I say my results are based on my entire life. Many of the habit changes I'm comfortable being uncomfortable with, or am unwilling to make, are based on previous experiences and current mindsets. This also contributes to why you have to recognize that it's sometimes best to break down a few of the big rocks into smaller pebbles.

The bigger and harder the habit, the more willpower and focus it will take to keep repeating it day after day. There is only so much mental energy you can expend on habits like this, especially as life priorities shift. Have you ever had a habit that didn't seem "that bad" at first but became almost intolerable as stress mounted in other areas of your life? The reason is that the effort of habits can change based on other priorities and motivation.

It's why you have to recognize that you can carry only so many big rocks at once, but you can break those rocks down to make them more manageable. When you break things down for yourself, you can find it easier to keep moving forward even though your lifestyle has shifted. The effort is less, and the cost feels worth the reward.

Breaking things down so they feel manageable is the power of the 1 percent. It allows you to do what you can be successful with. Seeing a small success builds motivation for you to keep pushing for the 1 percent changes that lead to a snowball of wins.

However, it's hard to embrace this attitude of less is more. You may get caught up in the all-or-nothing mentality and think, *If I can't do everything and do it perfectly, why do anything at all?*

But you need to join Team 1%, a loving name a client gave to my program because of how much I push these small changes that fit where you currently are. When you do this, you will find that you do the minimum even when life gets in the way.

This ability to maintain a minimum of your habits through even tough or stressful times builds because habits need to be repeatable.

ONE SIZE DOESN'T FIT ALL

One reason you may struggle to make a change (or end up making too much of one) is that you see habits as very set, definitive, one-size-fits-all things. When you view habits this way, you end up forcing yourself into a habit mold that doesn't fit.

You may also let habits get attached to feelings, and that can hold you back from making the changes you need. You need to recognize that you'll break down habits and implement them in different ways based on your lifestyle as it changes over time. Habits have many different variations and implementations, so you can adapt them to what you need at any given time.

You need to assess why you have certain attitudes toward habits. Do you hate the scale because the only time you focus on your weight is when you feel fat and want to lose weight? Do you hate tracking because every time you've logged your food, you've felt hangry and deprived? Often, people associate tools and habits with specific feelings based on how and when they've used them. The scale itself is not evil, even though most people hate it. And your tracker isn't restrictive; it's just data. You're the one being judgmental about it.

This is why one person can love weighing to track their trends, while other people would love to smash the scale to bits. This is why one person can see tracking macros as a fun game of Tetris, while another feels like the math is going to cause their head to explode. You might get tired of reading this, but one size doesn't fit all.

This is the reason I've included different training methods and schedules as well as different nutritional macros methods in this book. You may even use more than one method over the year as you adjust based on progress toward your goal. That's habit evolution! You constantly adjust things in your life, whether you realize it or not. The key is recognizing when you need to do it consciously.

Your holiday habits will be different from your "New Year, New You" habits, and you need to recognize that. There's no one way to build a habit or one form of a habit that's right for everyone or right for you all the time. If I put it in terms of cost again, your so-called "budget" may change based on what other priorities you have going on in your life. I'll talk more about this in Chapter 7 when I cover how to optimize.

Emotions are powerful, and they can make what is a small pebble to someone else look like a boulder to you. So, you also have to remember that you might push back the hardest against the changes you need the most. You have to recognize the association you've created between habits and emotions in the past so you can adjust your habit implementation to control the pain of change.

To draw on the power of the 1 percent, you have to recognize when the boulder is immovable for the time being and break off the smallest pieces to get yourself started. As long as you don't burn yourself out by trying to push or lift something you can't budge, little by little, you will move that boulder.

Are you starting to remember some habit boulders you've tried to lift in the past? Maybe it was two-a-day workout programs, making yourself get up at 4 a.m. to train, meal prepping the same chicken and broccoli to eat for every meal, or slashing your calories down to 800 per day to lose weight.

Now, I'm asking you to do a bit more self-reflection. (Go ahead and groan. I'll wait.) Ask yourself these questions:

? What habits have I really struggled with in the past?

? What habits do I do now that I really love?

? What habits do I easily repeat right now?

? What habits do I have right now that I know really aren't serving me?

? What habits are moving me forward?

? What habits would I like to change?

There's one more question you need to ask yourself with all the preceding questions: Why?

? Why have I struggled with these habits in the past?

? Why do I love the habits that I do?

? Why are habits easier or harder for me to repeat?

? Why are habits not serving me?

? Why am I still doing them?

? Why are these habits moving me forward?

? Why do I want to change these other habits?

Why, why, why?

The more you not only list the things you're doing but also dive into *why* you're doing them, the more you see how you can tweak things to make those 1 percent changes add up. You can also assess what you need to move forward.

You are the sum of your habits.

You are what you repeatedly do. You can repeat the same old habits and get the same old results, or you can implement new habits to work toward a new goal! Each habit is like a grain of sand on a beach. Alone, it's just a grain of sand, but put them together, and they're a beautiful beach. Each habit alone isn't who you are, but together, they shape your identity.

YOU ARE WHAT YOU REPEATEDLY DO

Your current situation is a result of your past hustle. If you don't like where you are now, you'd better take a good hard look at the habits you've been repeating—not only for the last few days but also for the past weeks, months, and even years. You're the sum of these habits. Are you simply repeating habits because they're comfortable? Because they worked in the past? Or are you repeating habits specifically focused on your goals and the lifestyle you want to lead?

Humans are creatures of comfort and convenience. We all create habits and routines so that we can repeat things unconsciously and without effort. The downside is that these habits, routines, and patterns become instinctive, which means they can become a part of our identity, so they can be incredibly hard to break. That's the reason understanding them to find ways to make them less unconscious and harder to repeat is so important.

You can't simply disown your old habits and—*poof*—magically be comfortable with new ones. You have to unlearn old habits, and that often needs to happen before you can implement and learn new ones. The more natural and comfortable a current habit feels, the more it's tied to your identity and the harder it will be to unlearn. In addition, the more uncomfortable, unnatural, or complicated a new habit feels, or the more the habit feels like something a person like you wouldn't do, the longer it will take to learn the new habit.

This whole process of unlearning to learn is one reason why habit change can be so hard. If you're lucky and there aren't old habits that conflict with and fight against new habits, change sometimes happens faster. You can simply add the new ones. But when you have current habits that are big rocks and so tied to your lifestyle and identity that they're as valuable as gold to you, you're going to be less willing to let go of them. You're also not necessarily going to embrace putting other big rocks on top of them. In these cases, you need to join Team 1% and carry over some pebbles as you push back on what you see as a valuable habit you're unwilling to let go of—maybe even helping yourself realize that what you think is gold is actually fool's gold.

It's also why you need to step back and ask, "Who am I?" and reflect on the way your habits contribute to your answer. You answered this question when you wrote your origin story. Get it out now. Don't just read through what you wrote; also recognize that you don't want to be there anymore. As you feel the pain, realize the situation is a result of your past hustle and your current habits—the ones that "feel good." Those are the habits that created the pain. They don't feel so good anymore, huh?

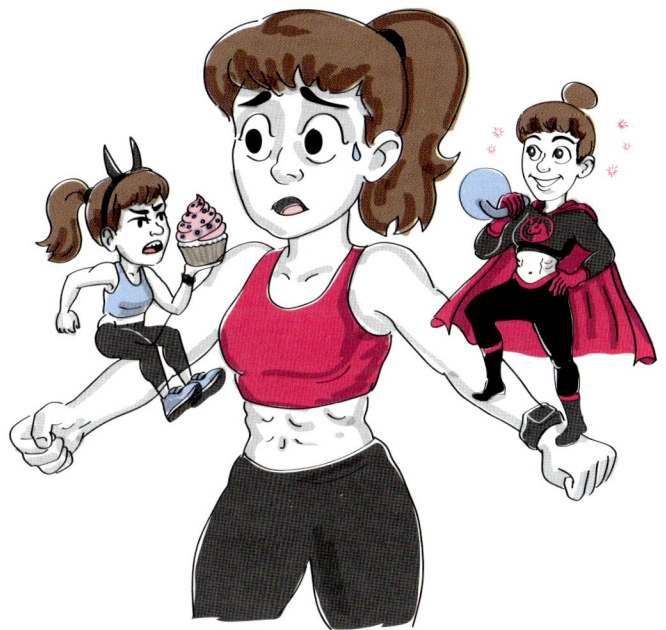

"Good habits are hard to form but easy to live with. Bad habits are easy to form but hard to live with." I find this quote to be such a good reminder, and it may be something that can help you embrace the cost and pain of change even more. It can remind you that the changes you need the most are the ones you often fight the hardest; you need to push through that pushback. But it can also remind you to give yourself grace when you do fall back into some old habit patterns.

So, it's time to take action. Take a good hard look at some of the habits that make you who you are and an even harder look at the mindsets behind those habits. Regardless of whether you want to recognize it, your actions are a reflection of your attitudes and beliefs, so if you don't change how you view your current habits and the ones you want to build, you're never going to make a change. You'll ultimately hit habit overload again and tear your bag as you try to carry those big rocks across the field.

HAVE TO VERSUS GET TO

One thing you want to note as you list the habits you're doing currently that don't serve you as well as the ones you want to implement is how they make you *feel*. Think about how many you feel you'll *have to* do. This language and feeling is what leads to habit overload that builds toward emotional sabotage, when you ultimately say, "I quit!" The more you feel you have to do something, the more important it is to assess how you can make it feel more like something you *get to* do.

One way to do this is to embrace those 1 percent tweaks and remind yourself that habits don't look the same for everyone. So, if your habit list includes "macro tracking" and you can't help but feel the *have to* wave looming, make note of that. It could be a reason to start with the minimalist macros or the hand-sized health approach I'll go over with the macros methods in Chapter 12. While you won't always feel like you *get to* do the habits you need and should do, the more you can feel the value, the more the cost of the change will be within your "budget" to make.

THE UNLEARNING

Part of assessing your current habits is recognizing the habits you should double down on to keep moving forward out of the change loop. You also have to recognize the resistance you're going to face as you make changes. This helps you assess how you're going to implement new habits and whether it's realistic to add certain big-rock habits to the bag or if it's better to carry them as pebbles. It can even help you assess how you'll implement specific habits.

Think about the statement, "Track your macros." What comes to mind? An annoying app? Obsessively weighing and measuring every crumb that goes in your mouth? Struggling to hit specific numbers and feeling like you can't enjoy any of the foods you love? Pay attention to the adjectives you use and the tone of your thoughts about that habit.

While tracking your macros may be key, you're never going to do it, especially not in the form you're envisioning, if you have a negative attitude about it. What may actually be an easily movable rock can become a huge boulder you can't lift based on your mindset. But this is also a boulder you've created. You're seeing it as immovable when the reality is that it's some big rocks stacked together. It's crucial to know what habits feel like boulders so you can take a sledgehammer to them and break them down into manageable pieces, or maybe you even leave them to be carried across when you feel more ready to handle them.

For example, although you may see tracking your macros as ideal, it can take different forms. Tracking can be taking pictures or using your hand and visual guides to measure. It can even be focusing on one specific macro. You'll become open to these other options when you realize that one size doesn't fit all and you don't have to have an all-or-nothing approach.

In assessing your current habits, you can also see what routines have become so natural and comfortable that you may cling to them. They sometimes include habits you don't even really like or habits you know aren't valuable, but they're now so set that you struggle to let go of them. Recognizing this can help you focus on the unlearning process as you start by implementing easier 1 percent changes in other areas. It's like recognizing you're tired, so you start with what you can to get the momentum going instead of forcing yourself to carry big rocks right away.

So, take a look at your origin story, consider other habits and patterns you've realized you're repeating as you've read through this section, and reflect on the following questions:

? What current lifestyle habits and repeatable actions are you doing that will work against the changes you want to make?

? Why do you like some of these habits? Why are they comfortable, convenient, or easy? What are they attached to in your life and environment?

? Why do you feel they aren't serving you?

? Why do you feel like they're key but against what you feel you may need? (We've often done a lot of research to fight the habit changes we need the most, and some of our current habits may be tied to this!)

? What can you do to help break some of these habits? How can you help yourself start to unlearn these behaviors as you learn how to repeat the new ones?

YOUR NEW HABIT SYSTEM

You're the sum of your habits, and in reflecting on your current habits, you can start to see how you've gotten to where you are now. Yeouch! Your habits shape your identity, and that includes not only actions but also mindsets. It's cliché, but it's true: You are who you believe you are!

When everything works together as a system, results build. Daily, weekly, and monthly actions create the system you need to reach your goals. It's not a habit done in isolation every once in a while. You get good at something only because you consistently do it, and you consistently implement habits and changes only when you truly believe in them. What you value, you prioritize and do!

Do some reflection on the habits you need to reach your destination. Consider your main target, complementary targets, and mini targets. What actions do you need to get there? What you write will help you determine the workouts you do, the nutritional changes you make, and even the other lifestyle changes you need (some often-ignored factors like mobility and sleep because you need to think beyond your plate and the gym if you want to see the best results as fast as possible). Here are some questions to guide you:

? What daily habits (food tracking, 2,000 more steps, workouts, drinking water, doing mobility work) will you need? Don't worry right now if you aren't sure of the form but make note of whether it's a rock (R), medium stone (MS), small stone (SS), or pebble (P). This can help you assess what habits you start with.

? What weekly habits (meal prepping, workout scheduling, grocery shopping, weighing in, measuring) will you need? How will these help with the daily habits and planning? How will these help you see progress and assess consistency to reach your targets?

? What monthly habits (reflection, planning workout progressions, switching macro ratios) will you need? How will these help and be built off of your daily and weekly habits? How will these help you measure your progress toward your mini targets and targets? Don't forget your complementary goals!

As you map these habits, consider what the struggles may be in repeating them. Have you tried some of these and failed in the past? If you have, which habits did you struggle with? Are you confused about how to do some of these things? Are you worried you won't be consistent?

Ask yourself why you're concerned. Reflecting now helps you meet yourself where you are as you build your complete system and then get to the fun stuff of implementing new workouts and nutritional changes. As you take a look at the habits you'll need to unlearn and learn, consider how you're going to make these changes easier.

THE HOW BEHIND HABITS

"I always hesitated since I've spent a fair penny in the past and end up pretty much back where I began. I'm sixty-eight, and I guess it's taken me a while to internalize the truth that you can't pay someone to do this work for you."

Ultimately, whether you succeed or fail, it's your fault. No one can want it or do it for you. It sucks, but it's true. However, knowing that it's up to you means you can take control of what you can and do everything in your power to reflect on what you need to meet yourself where you are. You need to recognize that it isn't enough to know what habits you "should" do; you need to find the connections to make them something you can actually act on.

This is why your mindset about the changes is key. You need to recognize when you're mentally resisting what you "should" do. You need to make a conscious effort to not only flip your language but also find other ways to lower your mental resistance.

Here are some things you can do to help yourself create habits faster:

» Break them down and make them simpler—for example, focus on 5 more grams of protein at a meal rather than trying to hit 150 grams when you're currently at 60.

» Do the habits first thing in your day as often as possible to make consistency easier. Doing your workout first thing in the morning when you know you have a busy day and are likely to skip it is one way you might do this.

» Pair new habits with habits you already have and enjoy so you remember to do them—for example, meal prep and listen to your favorite podcast.

» Celebrate and track your consistency in doing the new habits to "reward" yourself. You might set a complementary target to be doing every workout in your progression with a mini target of hitting all four workouts that week.

» Change your environment to create reminders and reinforce new habits, such as by setting your water bottle by your coffee machine so you remember to stay hydrated or even putting a quote that reminds you of what you're driving toward where you can see it frequently.

» Learn the value of the habits and remind yourself that you get to make these changes to reach your goals! For example, foam roll and remember how achy your shoulder used to feel and now doesn't.

The easier and more comfortable you make habits you want to create, and the harder and less comfortable you make habits you want to break, the more you'll find your lifestyle evolving and your results building! Just remember, habits take longer to build than you think they should. How long it takes to create them varies, so you need to be vigilant in your changes for as long as it takes.

Take the list of daily, weekly, and monthly habits you've written and start to list how you're going to help yourself repeat them. Also, consider using the opposite of those "hows" to list ways you're going to help yourself unlearn those old habits.

7 IS YOUR PLAN OPTIMIZED?

"I can't believe you eat that. It's such crap."

Someone made that comment on a picture I posted of my oh-so-freaking delicious Vanilla Bean Supreme Freeze from Koffi. Had they made that comment in person, I probably would have taken a huge, loud, slurping sip and said, "Yum!" That drink is legit a milkshake barely pretending to be a coffee. And it's *delicious.*

I literally dream about it before a summer trip to Palm Springs. And I get at least one every trip. Thankfully, I drink it on the balcony of our hotel room, so I can lick the whipped cream and leftover blended chocolate-covered espresso beans off the inside of the cup. If my tongue can't reach it all, I'm not above licking my fingers to get what my tongue misses.

I'm telling you this story not to make you really want one right now but because I believe comments like these can often sabotage people's success in finding their own lifestyle balance. Critical statements create guilt and often cause us to struggle to create the changes we need to move forward.

I have an unpopular opinion to share: I believe that not everything people do in life is 100 percent "good" for them, and that's OK. Heck, I'd even argue it can be beneficial to do some "bad" things. Sometimes, you might do something that has no direct value but a ton of indirect value.

My Palm Springs Koffi routine is an example. Getting the coffee, walking back to my hotel when it is already scorching hot at 8 a.m., and then sitting on the balcony and looking up at the mountain gives me so much enjoyment. It's something Ryan and I have done together for more than a decade. I truly do not feel one smidge guilty in having my coffee drink.

I believe it honestly helps me be healthier overall. The mental payoff is so great that I feel it is worth any cost. And no, I'm not excusing the sugar and processed "who the heck knows what makes it taste that good" ingredients, but I believe this "crap" promotes a better lifestyle balance for me that allows me to be more consistent on other days. It encourages me to do what I need for long-term results. It contributes to the long-term consistency that pays off. It doesn't create a feeling of restriction that could add a big boulder in my path. And it's that recharge I need to more consistently carry the big rocks across the field at other times. Making those hard habit changes would wear me out otherwise!

Don't let someone else's judgments hold you back from finding your lifestyle balance. As a human, you need to find what feels right for you. You need to do things that provide enjoyment while helping you move, feel, and look your best! This whole "good and bad" attitude honestly only keeps you stuck in the change loop. You try to be perfect and eat clean only to ultimately fall off your "diet" and feel guilty until you again force yourself into giving up all the things you want to enjoy. And then you repeat the loop again and again and again and again. Instead, embrace your balance.

You'll be surprised by how much allowing that 20 percent flexibility, instead of trying to pressure yourself to be perfect, creates an even better 80 percent, leading to overall better health and well-being.

In this chapter, I talk about creating a plan optimized for your lifestyle with repeatable habits that evolve as your body, needs, goals, and lifestyle change. Optimizing your habits and programming isn't just about looking at who you are and all you want out of life; it's also about taking a hard look at why things haven't worked in the past, taking ownership of your failures, and learning from them. Remember, failures are just learning experiences with a nice side of frustration!

EXAMINING WHY YOU HAVE FAILED

Lucille Ball. Michael Jordan. J. K. Rowling. Steve Jobs. Oprah Winfrey. Walt Disney.

When you read these names, you probably think of their greatness and successes. But all failed before they succeeded. They often even credit their success to their failures. Failures, if viewed correctly, can be the experiences that drive you forward the most. The key is in your perspective. Do you see opportunity or obstacle? A learning experience to grow from or a roadblock to turn away from?

I actually had a very funny example of this occur when my friend and assistant to the regional manager (bonus points if you get that joke) Ashley sent me a video of Kiwi and Sushi, my two mischievous and loving Bichons. Ashley was housesitting while Ryan and I were gone. The video shows Kiwi and Sushi standing at the sliding glass door, begging and whining to get in. Kiwi keeps pawing at the door as Ashley keeps saying, "Well ... come on in!"

As the video goes on, Kiwi and Sushi become more frustrated that they couldn't reach Ashley, who gradually zooms out on the video to show me that the door is 100 percent *wide open*. The dogs could easily walk 2 feet over to go through the

The boneheads

door. Instead, they stand in place for minutes, feeling frustrated and depressed, before Ashley *finally* gets them to walk where they need to.

That door was a "failure" to the dogs, but it wasn't actually blocking them from anything. They only needed to shift their perspective.

That's also what you need to do. You need to realize that the door hasn't been closed on you when a mistake or setback happens. You can choose to let it block you, or you can see it as an opportunity to learn and keep moving toward what you want!

The best inventors often arrive at amazing ideas precisely because their original plans failed.

Success is struggle. The more you own those struggles, the more you succeed. That's why you need to recognize why you've failed; then you can create your perfect system to see the best results as fast as possible.

Failures for sure show you what *not* to do, but they also show you what could have worked if you pause to assess what the opposite action could have been. To be able to dive into your past habits and why things did or didn't work out, you have to shift your mindset first about what failure is.

Something isn't a failure unless you give up. Sometimes, you have to try something and bumble through it to move forward. It's like the idea of crawling before you walk. It's why you need to constantly remind yourself that failures are essential to success. Every time you hit a speed bump, you need to reflect on the following things:

? Why did that happen?

? Are there triggers I can note to avoid it happening again?

? What can I learn to move forward from it?

? What did this teach me about myself?

The last question is the most important because roadblocks and speed bumps often relate back to previous mindsets or patterns. Sometimes, they relate to priorities and beliefs. The more you recognize why the stumble may have happened and what you need to do to make a change to move forward, the more you can meet yourself where you are now.

On any journey, your location shifts, and this one is no different. Where you started, your origin story, shouldn't be where you are halfway through. That change in location may mean that a reassessment of your priorities, lifestyle, and goals is necessary. Your body may need something different than it did before, and you want to optimize for that.

Part of this journey means facing the fact that you will fail. The more you own that failure will happen and realize that your strength, resilience, and confidence are built through what you overcome, the more you can push into the hard stuff and keep going.

One of my favorite phrases to help myself keep going is, "Suck it up, buttercup." I recommend finding a saying that speaks to you and reminds you that success comes from the learning and growth you get out of failures. You have to pick yourself back up, reflect, and keep going. And I include *reflect* for a reason. A failure you just move on from is one you're bound to repeat if you don't learn from it!

While you can control only what you can control, you have to recognize that the more you take the blame for something, the more you gain the power to change it.

FAULT VERSUS RESPONSIBILITY

"Ah! It's raining. Guess I can't get my run in today! Now, my whole week is thrown off. Maybe I'll just have a glass of wine and chill on the couch watching some Netflix."

It's easy to blame outside forces for sabotaging you— people, weather, *life*. And while things outside your control do happen, like rain, you can control your reaction to the event.

Do you see obstacle or opportunity? Do you place fault on the outside thing or take responsibility? One moves you forward; the other keeps you stuck. No matter what happens, and no matter how bad it is, even though it's not your fault and you may not have chosen this situation, you are responsible for what happens next.

The easy response is to say things were out of your control, but that doesn't change the fact that you have to take responsibility for your actions and mindset. Dwelling on what happened, or blaming what happened, doesn't change it. Nothing will.

How you choose to react to something and then take action is 100 percent your responsibility and within your control. No, it may not be your ideal situation. Sure, you may have to take massive steps back and handle things you never wanted to handle, but ultimately, you're responsible for yourself. You're in control!

Being in control is a good thing. Is it easy? Oh, heck no! It often stinks worse than a dog fart not to be where you want to be and have to shoulder the "blame" even when something isn't your fault. However, by accepting responsibility for yourself, you can move forward to achieve even more than you thought possible. You have a choice anytime something happens.

Choose to take responsibility and focus on moving forward! That includes owning your struggles and your priorities; otherwise, they become your excuses.

OWN YOUR STRUGGLES

I'm bringing up *ownership* again because that's what everything comes back to— taking back your own agency and power to make a change. Take a hard look at your life and priorities to assess what you need to move forward. This good hard look at what you need means reflecting on why you've failed, and the reason you fail usually relates back to your priorities.

When you don't own your priorities, they become your excuses. Chapter 8 focuses on those priorities (nonnegotiables) in your life so you can plan around them. For now, it's important you recognize that when you've failed in the past, it's been because your habit changes haven't been in line with your identity. While this may sound sort of silly, part of my "identity" had always been that I was a dessert person. (I will dive even deeper into this nonnegotiable in the next chapter!) I wanted dessert every night. Every time I tried to lose fat to get a six-pack, I'd cut out dessert to cut my

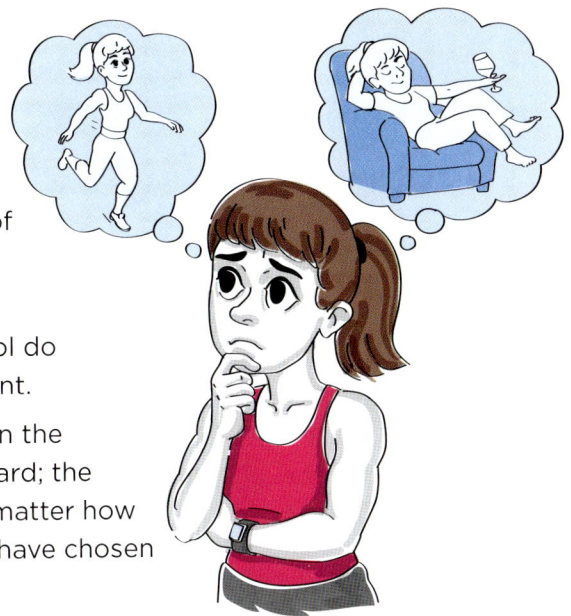

calories. It makes sense, right? Dessert isn't the healthiest thing, and it's calorically dense. But in cutting it out, I felt instant mental rebellion hit, and I'd want dessert even more. When I instead made it a nonnegotiable and planned my dessert as part of hitting my macros, I felt things shift instantly. And getting ab definition finally became achievable! I owned my priorities so I could plan around them, and you need to too.

It comes back to doing that reflection people so often skip. Before starting to read this book, you may not have assessed which habits are serving you well right now and which ones aren't. You may not have assessed which habits would have been easy in the past had you not been bearing the weight of other things. And you may not have really looked at which habits weighed you down so much that you can't keep carrying anything else because of them.

You may not have owned the reality of your work-life balance and what it means for a realistic workout schedule. Or why certain habit changes are hard or feel awkward. Or why old, unhealthy habits feel so comfortable. You may not have owned what you truly enjoy in life and don't want to miss out on.

If you haven't owned that change is hard (which is 100 percent OK for you to admit), you're going to struggle. Not to mention, results are going to take a whole heck of a lot longer than you'd like!

OVERSELLING THE NEGATIVE

Think back to the last time you started a program (or maybe even to when you picked up this book). You may have thought, *Yes! This is going to be amazing, and I'm going to see fabulous results! Yay!* That feeling comes from the program promise I mentioned in Chapter 1 when I talked about the change loop. The excitement of something new is the passion bomb building.

You rarely pause at that point, with your excitement and motivation bubbling over, to reflect on the changes you want to make and how hard they're going to be. You may even try to make things seem easier. You justify all the reasons so many of the changes won't be "so bad" because you want immediate results. You keep reviewing all the other people the plan or program worked for and tell yourself, "If they can do it, so can I!"

Then, when you don't feel like your results are as good as other people's, habit overload occurs quickly. It's followed by the scale sending you into a downward spiral of emotional sabotage until you finally give up—again.

Not this time!

This time, you're going to assess what will be hard so you can break down those challenging habits into smaller changes. You have to find *all* the reasons why a certain habit or change may be even harder than you're realizing, especially if you've struggled the teeniest bit with it in the past, and break it down to little pebbles. This is overselling the negative.

Find as many big rocks buried in the pile in a way that makes them look like small stones as you can and bring them to light. Then take a sledgehammer to them—or at least be prepared for when you have to carry those heavy rocks.

This is part of planning ahead. You're not just mapping out what you need to do or why you need to do it. You're also understanding the cost so you can plan your budget. Otherwise, you'll go into habit debt, which leads to emotional bankruptcy and putting on the sweatpants so you can plop on the couch with a pint of cookie dough ice cream.

So, take some time to make a list of some habit changes you've tried in the past. Why did you not feel prepared for them? How did they not fit with where you were at the time? Would they work now? Why or why not? Now, assess what you could do differently this time.

What habits will be the big rocks you'll struggle with and why? What habits may seem like small pebbles but may end up being harder to carry than you think, especially when you combine them with other things? The more you assess the challenges and what may conflict with your current mindsets, routines, environment, or priorities, the more you can not only outline Plans X, Y, and Z but also be mentally prepared to face the hard and conquer it.

You want to face the difficult stuff and be able to think, *That wasn't that bad!* even if it wasn't something hard you had anticipated. You want to be able to get that flat tire and not only have a spare but also have snacks, blankets, and extra things just in case any other issues pop up as you're fixing it.

The more you can optimize your plan for the struggles and mentally prepare yourself, the more you will be open to evolving. Learn why these habits are important so you prioritize them and build your new identity to maintain your results long term.

PRIORITIZE YOU

"But I need to …" You can insert any number of priorities or life situations that will pop up—usually at the worst time—here. Life is going to happen. The question you have to ask yourself is, "How can I still find a way to prioritize *me*?"

Self-care isn't selfish.

I mentioned this in Chapter 4 when I outlined the significance of what you want. While you may want to "just lose 5 pounds," the ramifications of your goals are often further reaching than you realize, especially when your health and fitness goals and the lifestyle changes you make have a huge impact on so many other things.

While it can be hard to prioritize your needs and goals, and it can maybe feel selfish, you can't pour from an empty cup. Basically, I'm giving you the same instructions you hear every time you get on an airplane: Put your own oxygen mask on first!

Prioritizing yourself is the key to seeing the results you want. You will make time for those things you prioritize. You will choose to do it. You will find a way—no matter what. There is a cost to every reward, but you have to believe you deserve this and are worth these changes.

If you're struggling with this, think about what you'd tell a friend who's trying to make healthy changes. You'd tell them to take care of themselves because they deserve to prioritize their health, and you'd try to help them. You'd tell them they should make time for their workouts and meal prep.

Be your own best friend. Or, heck, get your best friend involved so you can support each other. Write out who you can inspire to make a change themselves—who you'd like to see value themselves and their goals more. Then lead by example. Show, don't tell.

Now, I want you to consider when the last time was that you gave yourself permission to assess what you want out of life. Yes, I say *permission* because I think we often don't really allow ourselves to dream big (or even dream at all). We limit ourselves. We put boundaries on what we can do.

Think back to the destination you started imagining and writing down. Now, I want to ask a question: Is your dream big enough? Did fear of failing hold you back, or were you ashamed to want to admit you craved more? By owning there will be difficulties, recognizing that failure is a part of the process, and planning for it, can you make changes so that you get what you want out of life? Should your destination be loftier? Give yourself permission to ask for more of yourself and your goals. Give yourself permission to focus on yourself and consider what you *personally* want out of life. Embrace dreaming big.

This attention to what you want is self-care and self-love. It's what will help you embrace your choices as you make changes.

Consider these two questions as you reflect:

? What do I want *more* of in my life?

? What do I want *less* of?

When you consider these questions, think about how your habits may need to adjust as life gets in your way. Reflect on the habits you wrote down. How could you break down those big rocks you want more of in your life into habits that you can prioritize even when everything is going wrong?

You can't control the rain, but you can control whether you sit on the couch on a rainy day or switch your workouts so you still do something at home before completing your mileage the next day.

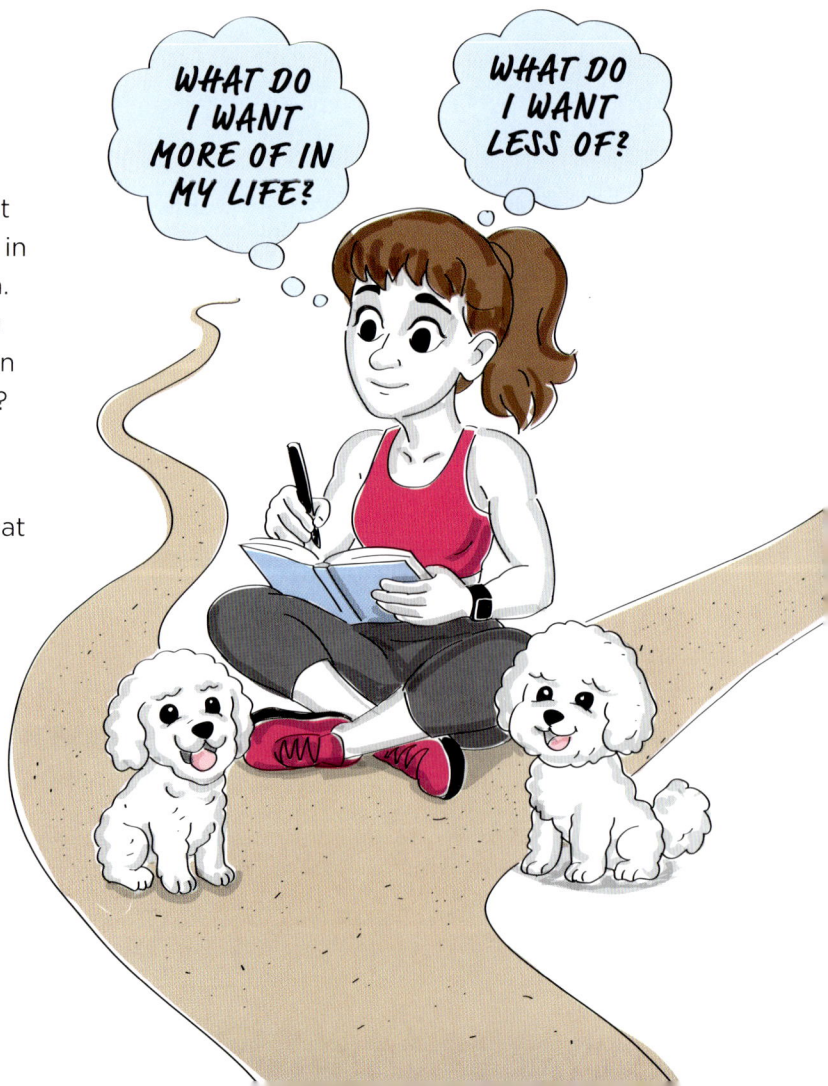

REFLECTION

What have you struggled with in the past that's prevented you from reaching your goals? What failures have you had, and why do you feel they occurred?

While it stinks to relive negative things, the more you can reflect on past issues and setbacks, the more you can learn and avoid repeating the same mistakes. Reflecting also helps you go in mentally prepared for the challenges that are ahead of you. You know there will be challenges; ignoring them ultimately makes things worse. Struggling with things you could have been prepared for can make you feel like there's something wrong with you.

What will your mantra be to remind yourself that you knew it would be hard and that you need to push through? I shared one of mine earlier: "Suck it up, buttercup!" Mantras or affirmations don't have to be flowery or directly positive. If that's not your style, pick something a little more tough love.

For a final reflection exercise to help you own and recognize challenges you'll face, consider what struggles may come up with the new changes you're making. List them based on the repeatable habits you outlined while reading the previous chapter and think about what you're worried you may struggle with:

? Which rocks may become bigger if priorities in your life shift? What if you get busy at work? What if you're traveling more? What about the holidays when cookies and parties are popping up?

? Which small pebbles may end up being combined into more than you can handle?

Now, list things in your lifestyle that will push back as you move forward (yes, this includes people):

? What old patterns have pushed back when you've tried to make changes in the past?

? What priorities have always made certain things hard?

? Who in your life may resist or question your changes? Do you have a "food pusher" who tries to get you to eat all kinds of things as soon as they find out you want to make diet changes?

Finally, write down strategies to overcome obstacles from both lists:

? How can you include more foods you love and own your nonnegotiables? (More on this in the next chapter.)

? What is the minimum you can do for the habits you outlined so you still do *something* when things get tough because something is better than nothing?

? How can you do less and achieve more to avoid setting off the passion bomb?

Take time to write your reflections and own your struggles because you'll return to this after you assess your nonnegotiables in Chapter 8. If you've realized some of the habits you created aren't as repeatable as you originally thought, go back and break them down into smaller habits that are more easily repeatable.

8 OWN WHAT'S NONNEGOTIABLE

You don't want a cookie, do you? Mmmm ... a warm, ooey-gooey chocolate chip cookie fresh out of the oven. Nope, you don't want to eat it. Don't look at that melty chocolate. Don't even think about how soft and doughy it looks. Cookies. Cookies. Cookies ...

Have you ever had that happen where you weren't even thinking about or wanting something, and then someone tells you that you can't have it, and suddenly, you can't live without it? Perhaps you also know you "shouldn't" have it because you're on a diet. It's bad for you. It's not a "clean" food. It's off-limits.

You want it even more, right?

Then you think, *It can't hurt to have just one.* Famous last words. Remember the flat tire incident I described in Chapter 1—the one where one tire went flat, and then you ended up slashing the other three tires? This is like that. One cookie leads to eating seven, lying on the couch with a food baby, skipping your workout, and starting over on Monday. Change loop repeated.

You blame your lack of self-control. Your lack of willpower. Life, priorities, and stress. Heck, you even blame hormones. All these reasons have some validity, but they are symptoms of the true problem. The true problem is your approach to change.

You're restricting things you really have no desire to cut out. You're eliminating habits that you want to do. You're also trying to make these changes first, which is like trying to carry all the big rocks across while telling yourself they're small pebbles.

So, I'm going to ask you to take a step back from what you've heard is ideal. That probably means going against the way you've always made changes in the past. I'm arguing *against* clean eating, restriction, and making foods or habits "off-limits" or "bad."

IT'S NOT A DIET; IT'S AN ADJUSTMENT

Just think about the word *diet*. What comes to mind? Restriction? Deprivation? Misery? Hanger (you know, when you get so hungry that you get angry)? None of those terms are in the true definition of *diet*, which is "the foods we habitually eat."

I don't see anything there about cutting out the foods you love, feeling hungry all the time, or restriction. Heck, I don't see judgment of any kind. *Anywhere.* People have created that miserable association with changing the way someone eats. *Diet* has become a dirty word because people are always "going on a diet" rather than adjusting their diet and lifestyle.

If this is your attitude toward how you're making changes, it's keeping you stuck. Food is no longer just fuel, and you have to recognize and account for things like the annual Thanksgiving meal with family where you all sit around reminiscing as you take a third serving of the sausage stuffing you look forward to each year. It's the pumpkin pie you savor as you tell embarrassing stories about each other and catch up in a way you only do once a year.

It's a hot dog at a baseball game, which honestly isn't even all that good, but you crave having it because it brings back fun childhood memories of super hot summer days.

It's a piña colada on the beach as you relax and read your book while you soak up the sun and think life couldn't be better.

Diet isn't about food alone; it involves habits too. It's taking time to listen to your favorite podcast while you drink coffee on a Saturday morning rather than rushing out of the house to get in a workout.

> **Diet isn't about food alone; it involves habits too.**

It's attending your kids' sporting events and being at every game. It's being the embarrassing parent who cheers inappropriately loudly. Most importantly, it's spending quality time with them and letting them know you're in their corner, not just in the game but also in life. You don't want to miss a second of anything with them.

Diet encompasses a lot of things you *value* in life—your nonnegotiables. What you value, you will prioritize.

Now, think about how hard it is to cut out something you value or something you prioritize. Often, it doesn't happen. Instead, your priorities become your excuses. But what if, instead of focusing on cutting these things out first, you owned them and their value to you?

WHAT DO YOU VALUE?

The last time you started making changes to your diet and workout routine, what did you do? Did you cut out your beloved dessert because you knew it wasn't good for you? Did you avoid girls' night out and restaurant meals with friends because you were on a diet? Did you prioritize workouts and extra sessions over other hobbies and events you love?

And then you burned out.

This approach sabotages you each and every time because you aren't embracing what you value. You aren't owning what you consider nonnegotiable—at least right now. Your identity is shaped by what you value, and you find a way to prioritize those things so they gain your full attention and focus.

When you try to avoid prioritizing things you truly value, it eventually comes back to bite you in the butt. That's what happens with the whole "going on a diet" versus *adjusting* your diet approach. When you fall off the diet wagon, you believe you don't have the willpower you need. In truth, you're defaulting to prioritizing what you value.

You consistently repeat the habits that support what you value, and you seek to return to them. You know what that means? You need to find ways to value the new habits, but you also need to own the value in your current habits to create a balance. In this case, "balance" is more of an act of constantly balancing; you constantly have to reassess what you value and why. The reason I'm writing this book now is because I've done this exact assessment myself.

You may have noticed I talk about food—a lot. I consider myself a foodie and a cocktail girl. When I travel, literally the first things I look for are the good restaurants and cocktail bars. Trying new places and craft cocktails is an experience I value more than anything. It's a nonnegotiable for me. So was dessert for the longest time (more on this shift in a bit).

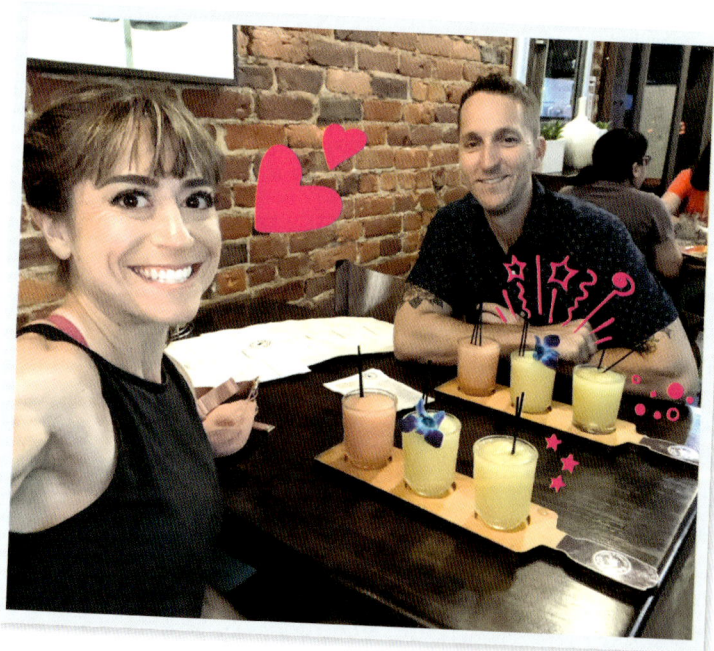

I valued food experiences so much that I'd told myself I "loved food too much" to ever get abs. I'd told myself I couldn't maintain the restriction for long enough for my results to snowball. When I got my first job at a gym, a coworker asked me to do a figure competition with her. I told her, "I don't have the discipline to do that." At that time, I would have loved to achieve body recomp more than anything. It was a huge dream of mine, but I felt the habits went against what I valued too completely, and there was no balancing of the two.

Even just a hint of ab definition would have made me ecstatic. It wasn't that I didn't like the idea of the goal; I really did want it. And it wasn't an issue of not being motivated to achieve the goal; I would get motivated enough to restrict—for a bit. I just thought I wasn't a person who could eat "clean" enough to get amazing muscle definition.

Let me repeat that: I thought I wasn't a person who could achieve that goal. I wasn't limiting myself because I didn't have enough discipline. I'd trained hard and sacrificed for many other things in my life. It wasn't that I didn't have enough willpower. I'd trained plenty to get a Division I tennis scholarship.

The simple fact was that I wasn't ready to embrace that *identity.* I wasn't ready to own my priorities and values and find ways this goal could also fit. I would say this is the case for most people.

Embracing a new identity isn't easy to do. You can't just be like, "Welp, I'm a new person!" and expect results to happen. You have to create a new identity through habit changes. You have to *act as if* you're the person you want to be.

In earlier chapters, I mentioned the difference between "acting as if" and "faking it 'til you make it." Remember that? "Acting as if" isn't just about forcing new habits and pushing yourself into a mold. You can't just say you should do certain things and "should" all over yourself. You have to truly create your balance and shift your values and priorities.

It's a slow process. You're changing your mindset, routines, and habits. You're becoming a person who can achieve those things. You have to assess the actions you need to take to reach your goal and then connect who you are currently to the person who would do these things. It goes back to you owning your origin story and understanding what the destination looks like for you.

Your ability to change comes back to the fact that you are what you believe you are. At any point, you can evolve and grow as a person by changing your beliefs. So, if you've believed you're a person who can't do something, that's who you are—*right now.*

However, your current identity isn't unchangeable. Will the evolution happen overnight? Heck no! But if you focus on becoming the person you want to be and create habit changes, it will happen.

Earlier, I said I believed I didn't have the discipline to get abs. Now, I'm leaner year-round than I'd ever come close to before. I'm leaner than I thought I could possibly be and have the ab definition I claimed I couldn't get because I liked food too much, didn't have the genetics, and didn't have the willpower or discipline to get it.

I was able to get abs because my habits fit my new identity. My habits are in line with my priorities and values, which have shifted over time.

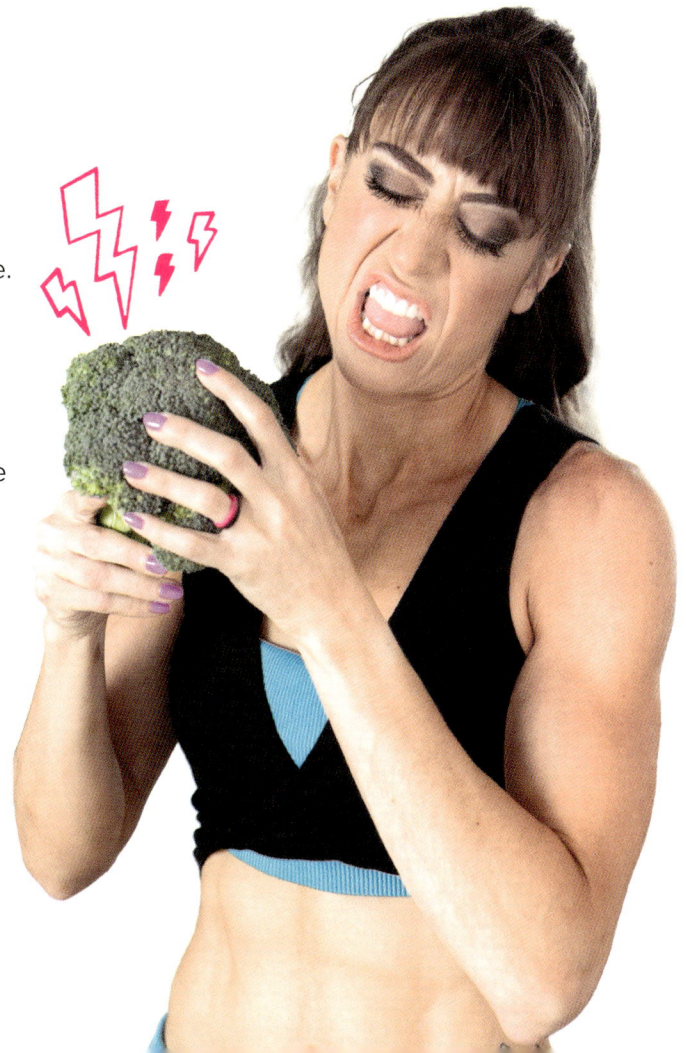

Nonnegotiables are things you deem important and that reinforce your identity, but they can shift as your identity evolves. They shifted for me because I gave them time to change and owned them when they weren't something I wanted to change. That's right. I said, "wanted to change," not "couldn't change," because you can make any change you *want*.

Your approach to change is what matters. It's why a key component of the STRONG system is owning what's nonnegotiable.

In the hierarchy of habit rocks, values and priorities are boulders. When you try to make habit changes, you often start by trying to push them instead of going around them. Pushing them gets you nowhere. If you do happen to budge them, you ultimately burn yourself out after working very hard to make very little progress. Sometimes, you've probably felt like you've made progress only for them to roll backward.

Stop trying to push the boulders! Instead, make habit changes *around* them. Recognize that the boulders are there and find the easiest path around them so you can move the other rocks in the pile first. You can always revisit those value and priority nonnegotiable boulders. You will often find they aren't as nonnegotiable as you once thought!

For now, consider the things you value and prioritize. Consider the things that feel important and that you don't really want to give up. Consider what things always become your excuses and make you fall off your plan. Consider what things require a ton of self-control, focus, and discipline to avoid doing. You usually can identify your nonnegotiables by looking at the habits you feel like you have to white-knuckle your way through. They're often the things that seem to go against what you *want* to do.

By determining what you truly want and what feels nonnegotiable *right now*, you can see why changes become harder and harder and why you start to dislike certain habits and tools more and more. They are things you're constantly feeling forced into, things that often eliminate what you love. And the more you feel forced into doing something, the less you want to do it.

As you look at your nonnegotiables further, realize the pushback you've created for yourself. You can feel this pushback when you've eliminated your nonnegotiables or avoided them. Realize how hard you're working to try to push a boulder that you can't push right now. This constant effort isn't helping you create a repeatable habit that falls in line with your current lifestyle or moves you forward toward your goals. It's you basically wasting energy you could be using to move forward and make a change.

Now, I'm not saying all habit changes will feel easy, but the more you *own* who you are and your nonnegotiables, the more you give yourself control and power to make a change. And the more you recognize your power of *choice*.

EMBRACE YOUR CHOICE

"Yesterday, my favorite cupcake place was featuring two of my favorite cupcakes: almond raspberry and one called the Irish triplet. I was seriously considering heading there to buy one of each to sample. But I just had a feeling the scale was gonna budge. I have been bouncing back and forth for a while, and I just felt I was close to good news. So, I skipped the cupcake. They will have the flavor next Saturday, so I told myself to wait! And yep!! The scale budged!! I'm down 7 pounds since starting the program, and no cupcake would be worth missing this feeling. Not at this point anyway! Next week, if I feel good about it, I can work that cupcake into my day. So tempting!!!"

That would not be the last cupcake she would ever have the opportunity to eat. She recognized that, weighed her options, and decided based on what she truly valued most at that moment.

But how often do you instead act like you're being *forced* into a decision you don't want to make?

After saying, "I'll start my diet Monday," have you ever acted like you have to cram in all the foods you love like you're on death row and about to have your last meal? I know I have. I've acted like that cupcake is the last cupcake I'll ever have the chance to eat.

That's the kind of attitude that keeps you feeling like healthy changes have to be miserable and restrictive. You probably act like success means sacrificing so much that you have to be super strong with unwavering motivation and discipline to achieve your goals. It makes you feel like people who do achieve success have some quality you don't.

And they do, but it's not what you think. They don't have extra motivation or willpower. What's different is that they realize they have a *choice*. A choice to eat something or skip it. A choice to do the workout or not. No one is forcing you to do either. No one is judging you, either, except yourself.

The more you recognize this and embrace it, the more you gain control of the changes you make and realize the balance you can strike. Eventually, the things that *seemed* nonnegotiable become—surprisingly—negotiable!

Part of what makes something nonnegotiable isn't just that you value or enjoy it but also that it's a habit or thing you've prioritized in your life that has good feelings associated with it. You feel like you can't have it if you're doing what you "should." Things become more nonnegotiable when you're already weighed down with the habit rocks you're carrying. You can't exert any more control or feel like your identity is changing even more.

When you aren't being forced to do something, you suddenly care far less about it. This is why you want to plan around the things you enjoy and the things that feel nonnegotiable. When you choose to include them, you give power back to yourself.

This control frees you to make a different choice at another time. The power you feel makes you feel strong enough at another point to make more sacrifices. With this freedom to choose, you may even cut something out that once seemed impossible to change.

Your perspective shifts. If you're stuck below a rock, it's going to look a lot bigger than if you're standing above it. The rock hasn't changed size. Your perspective has shifted.

If you acknowledge your "budget" and weigh the costs of everything to start, you can spend wisely on more habit changes while striking a balance. Later on, you may have enough left in your balance to spare so you can implement more changes to see results faster!

The flip side is that you can blow through your budget trying to eliminate nonnegotiables only to go into debt and fall back into old patterns. So, as you assess what has caused you to fall off habit changes in the past or has made certain habits feel like big rocks, consider what you value. What habits do you enjoy? What things do you often try to cut out first despite the fact that they're nonnegotiable for you? The more you own these things instead of making yourself feel guilty for them, the more you can start reducing the resistance against making changes.

Too often, people create negativity and overwhelm instead of finding ways to make themselves happier about the changes. As time goes on, you can reassess what you thought you couldn't live without. Ask yourself, "Is this worth it? Do I really want this?" If the answer isn't a resounding affirmative, then ask, "Am I willing to *choose* not to have this right now because my goal is more important?"

CLIENT STORY

"One of the things I have noticed these past sixteen weeks is that I've had a complete mindset shift. They had all kinds of free food at work today (donuts, cookies, mac and cheese, you name it), and before this program, I would have decided not to grab anything because I wanted to be 'healthy,' but then I would cave in, eat a bite, and feel completely guilty. Today, I actually thought to myself, 'Do I want to eat it or not?' It really threw me off because the mindset shift happened so gradually, and I didn't even realize that I don't really label foods as healthy and unhealthy anymore. I decided that I really didn't want to eat anything today, but I did grab a to-go box of some food so I can fit it into my macros tomorrow!"

You are in control of how you balance things. There is no right or wrong. When you recognize your nonnegotiables, you meet yourself where you are so you can move forward rather than becoming stuck. You clear a path rather than putting hurdles in front of yourself.

Remember, you are choosing what is important to you *right now.* You can always adjust how you spend your habit budget. No one is forcing you to do it one way or another. Stop "shoulding" all over yourself. Embrace your balancing act.

Note that even as you include things you love and try to meet yourself where you are, you aren't going to like *everything* you do in pursuit of your goals. No one ever does. The key is recognizing that you have the power of choice regarding the sacrifices you make and the sucky hard things you're willing to face.

HOW TO CARE WHEN YOU DON'T CARE

You might have heard the phrase, "If you do what you love, you'll never work a day in your life." Eh ... wrong! While I get the sentiment and have even repeated this phrase myself, well, it isn't true. It should say, "If you pursue what you love, the suffering will be worth it."

This idea goes back to the habit budget I talked about earlier. The more pain you feel by staying stuck, the more pain of change you're willing to embrace.

In Chapter 7, I talked about overselling the negative—breaking down the things that cause you problems into the tiniest habits. This idea is key to getting through the sucky things you don't like. It mentally prepares you for those times you don't feel motivated so you can still find a way to do the minimum. Minimums you can fall back on are what keep you going when you don't care. They're the habits that feel almost so silly and simple that you could do them in your sleep. They're habits so small, you can do them without needing a lot of motivation.

Because motivation is a little bit mythical. Motivation is a feeling that can help you build momentum, but you can also build momentum when you're not motivated. When you see the benefits of your effort, you're more willing to care about doing it even when you're unmotivated.

A big part of learning how to care when you don't care is to stop restricting the things you do care about first. This is why hanging on to your nonnegotiables is important. You first cut out or change the things that aren't tightly tied to your current lifestyle and identity. When you maintain the things you care about, you don't hit habit overload or emotional sabotage nearly as quickly or as hard.

Consequently, sufficient results build that things feel sustainable enough for you to keep going. You find your habit budget increases, so you can double down on what's working. You might even feel more confident in your ability to overcome!

You'll be more willing to carry more medium stones because you'll know that although they're heavy, they'll help you get that rock pile moved faster. And in the times when you aren't as willing to carry them, you can still create momentum by doing *something*, even if it means carrying across half-filled bags of pebbles.

Now, think about the repeatable habits you wrote down. Which ones conflict with your nonnegotiables? How can you adjust them? How can your plan include things you love so you make habit changes that address other things first? Think about *why* you value each and every one of the habit changes you're making, especially if they do push against your nonnegotiables. What would make you care about them on days when you want to do absolutely nothing or when the call of old patterns beckons you back?

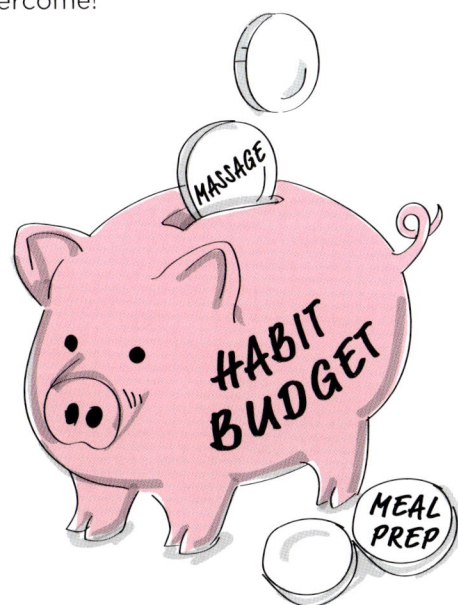

How can you make them priorities in your day? Can you do them first? Can you connect them with habits you value or enjoy? Assess those habit changes, recognize you are *choosing* to do them, and then really think about their value and whether they fit your habit budget.

Don't forget to own that you won't like everything you have to do all the time. Oversell that negative. Think of what you can do on your worst of worst days so that you're prepared for the times you don't care, don't feel like doing anything, and *do it anyway!*

REFLECTION

In addition to the questions in the previous section, think about things you feel you've cut out or not prioritized in the past that truly are essential to your lifestyle now:

? What do you love in your life that brings you enjoyment?

? What do you miss in your day when you don't get to do it?

? What do you do for yourself even if it isn't healthy or ideal?

? What have you cut out in the past and then regretted and thought, *I can't wait to have X again?*

Based on your answers to those questions, list your nonnegotiables. What things would make habit changes and your lifestyle feel more balanced if you could keep them in? Your coffee with creamer every morning? Your dessert at night? Runs on the weekends even though you know you need to weight train for body recomp? Pizza night with the family? Wine on Friday nights?

As you list your habits, routines, and priorities, make note of why these things are so significant. This can help you better plan out how to act and determine where you have some wiggle room to tweak these things to strike a better balance. Remember, habits don't have to be done in one form, and the more you recognize why you value something, the more you also gain the power to choose whether to include it based on your true priorities right now.

Knowing isn't doing!

Earlier in the book, I mentioned that the STRONG system isn't only about setting goals. You're also creating a roadmap for action because achieving results is very much like a road trip.

Think about the last road trip you took. You set your GPS with your current location and destination. You may have recognized where you might run into traffic or issues on the road. You may have planned your pit stops as targets or checkpoints where you could reassess and possibly adjust course. You may have had to evaluate changing routes to make better time or look for side streets that would keep you moving toward your destination even if you weren't traveling as quickly.

If it was winter, you may have oversold the negative to yourself, knowing the weather might slow you down. You may have even allowed yourself some detours to see things you felt you couldn't live without, like the world's largest mailbox.

The point is, the planning you do for a smooth trip is exactly the same type of planning you've done for your STRONG system. The planning helps you reach your destination quickly while still enjoying the ride.

If you've rushed through the chapters up to this point, pause, take time to sharpen your axe, and prepare for your trip. This preparation gives you as smooth of a ride as possible so you can look back at the challenges you thought you'd face and think, *That wasn't that bad!*

Use this preparation to be ready to embrace the specific techniques and methods I'll go over in Part 2. Those are the details of the exact turns and speed limits you'll encounter along the way.

If you feel good about the reflections you've done and the aha moments you've had so far, don't stop reading now. While this mindset work can feel good at times, you still need to put it into practice because knowing isn't doing! You implement and take action—not tomorrow, Monday, or next month, but now.

BYE-BYE, SOMEDAY SYNDROME

You've said it before: "I'll start _____ *someday*." This "someday syndrome" is why you never see results snowball.

"But Cori, I've read through everything. I'm just going to pause to sharpen my axe and start on Monday! Today isn't the right time."

First off, touché to using my words against me, but no. Pausing to sharpen your axe is still taking action. And in pausing to sharpen your axe right now, you should see something you can do *today*.

When you say, "Now isn't the 'right time,'" you wait … and wait … and wait. But I'm about to smack you in the face with some tough love: No time is the right time. And the wrong time to start is actually the right time you've been waiting for. Wait. How is the wrong time actually the right time? Let me tell you:

A. Waiting for the "right time" means you may never start, and nothing changes if nothing changes.

B. Making changes at the "right time" never shows you what is maintainable at the "wrong time," so you ultimately work really, really hard to create new habits and routines that simply aren't sustainable.

Waiting to start at the "perfect time" is what keeps you stuck in the change loop. You sabotage yourself with habits and routines that you ultimately let go of the second life gets in the way. You won't always care or feel motivated, so you have to prepare for that! What leads to results is creating habits you can do on your worst—yes, *worst*—days, not just your best.

STOP THE CYCLE!

If you're thinking that now is the wrong time to start, good. Start today. Jump into those small-pebble habit changes and start reading through Part 2. Don't wait. Don't let yourself reflect on all of the work you've already done. *Act*. This will finally bust you out of that change loop and help you build habits in a lasting way so your results can snowball.

If someday is going to be the right day, make "someday" today.

You've owned your struggles. You've recognized what's nonnegotiable. You've optimized your habits. So, what can you take action on *right now* (even as you read this) to build some momentum and create that success mindset to make you want to do more?

> **If someday is going to be the right day, make 'someday' today.**

As you start taking action, read through everything in Part 2. (Hint, hint: Reading Part 2 is taking action.) I still don't want you to skip to the workouts and meal plans in

Part 3 because you think you've "done enough" reflecting and learning. Learning the why behind *everything* is what will help you value the changes and repeat them even on horrible, no good, very bad days.

Make sure to take time to write out the reflections in each section in Part 2. This action will help you select the correct path and accurately map out the exact route for your road trip. There are multiple routes you could take, so you want to plan the one that's best for you (and know that what's most efficient may change).

The more you outline your STRONG system, the easier it will be to combine the correct macro method and training technique to see those results happen faster than you ever thought possible.

YOU CAN DO HARD THINGS

Strength is built through what you overcome. The nutritional changes, workout techniques, and 1 percent tweaks you're going to make to many lifestyle habits will challenge you.

What challenges you will change you.

Muscles adapt and grow stronger through challenge. You're basically like one big muscle (isn't that a fun way to think about yourself?) because you adapt due to what you are given. You will make mistakes and falter. You will mess up, and you will get stronger from pushing through until you conquer what you're faced with.

As you make changes, embrace the learner's mindset. Give yourself grace but also remember that your strength can only be revealed if you keep going.

> **Remind yourself that you can do hard things. What challenges you, changes you.**

Remind yourself that you can do hard things. What challenges you, changes you. Heck, tell yourself to *suck it up, buttercup*, and *do it anyway*!

As a final action before the diet and workout fun, write some reminders to help yourself push through challenges and encourage yourself to care when you don't care. Because learning to see the hard as a good thing is the final secret to success!

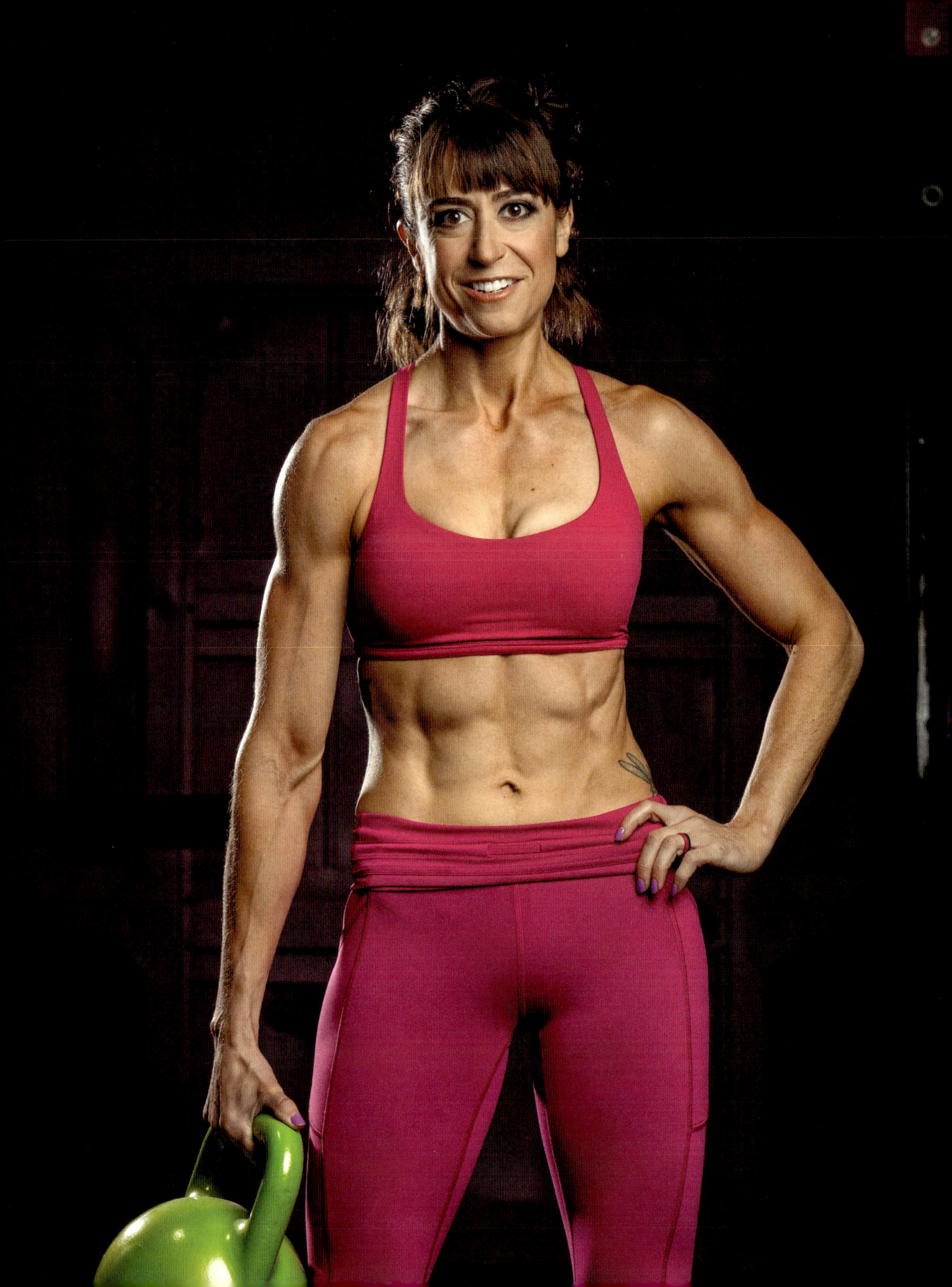

2

BUILDING YOUR SYSTEM

10 TAKING ACTION

Alright! Now we're getting to all of the nerdy stuff that makes my trainer's heart happy. I love geeking out about nutrition and workout changes that can be oh-so-fun in that torturously, amazingly miserable way.

I know you're still itching to get to what to *do*, but you should *not* skip this. What I cover in this chapter connects the dots of the habits you need while avoiding the struggles you've had in the past by having a clear system and roadmap in place. You'll also understand *why* certain changes you may have resisted the most are so important, and that can help you budget for them.

After reading through the different methods, pause and sharpen your axe by reflecting on your STRONG system. Then get to chopping!

First, I'll give you an overview of the different training techniques. I'll share why emphasizing strength work and building muscle is important even if your goal includes fat loss. I review the workouts first because your activity and training will impact how you adjust your diet. One perfect move or food won't fix a broken process. The pieces have to work together.

After I go over the three different training protocols, I'll dive into how to adjust your diet. The focus is on macros.

For many, tracking macros is far harder than the workout changes. I used to think, *I'll work out all day if I need to, but adjusting my diet feels next to impossible!* Like me, many people are more comfortable being uncomfortable in the gym than they are when making dietary changes.

You can't out-exercise your diet, though. Trust me; I've tried and seen *faaaar* too many other people try as well. Now, if you're thinking, *I hate tracking macros. It doesn't work for me. It's overwhelming. Too complicated,* and are considering closing this book right now, don't.

Remember how I said one size doesn't fit all and habits can be done in so many forms? So can tracking macros. I outline three different methods to adjust your portions and dial in your nutrition to match. And while you may not start out with tracking because it may be a big habit rock you're not willing to embrace or something nonnegotiable for you right now, that's fine, but I will ask you to pause and circle back to the STRONG system reflection from Part 1. Assess *why* you're resistant to this habit change. Separate out how you've used it in the past and the feelings it's created from how you can use it now.

These reflections may open you up to the opportunity of tracking in the future. I'll help you see how you can achieve the mental shift to take back control even if you still decide not to track in one specific way.

As you review the training protocols and diet adjustments, assess which meet you where you are at right now but also consider the opportunities and obstacles that you find in the other options. This can help you evolve as you need to implement different strategies and take different routes as needed.

Remember, nothing changes if nothing changes. I honestly hope I repeat this phrase enough that you get sick of reading it and it permeates your being so much that you can't help but take consistent daily action toward your goals. There isn't just one "ideal" plan for making changes. Each person is different, and I'm giving you the resources to create your uniquely perfect plan based on where you are right now.

METABOLIC MUSCLE-BUILDING PROTOCOLS

Have you ever added more cardio to try to lose weight faster? Have you ever thought to yourself that you need to sweat more, suffer more, and burn more calories in your training? I know I have.

Many people turn to cardio for weight loss and fat loss because they've heard it burns more calories. And if it burns more calories and a person needs a calorie deficit to lose weight, cardio must be great, right?

What if I told you that turning to cardio actually sabotages your results despite it seeming to work at the start? Yup. "Do more cardio for fat loss" is the big fitness industry lie. You need to stop believing it. (Calories in versus calories out also isn't the whole truth—but more on that later.) So, if you feel like your metabolism is broken, that your age has doomed you to weight gain, or like you have to do more and more to see results, your previous cardio practices have finally caught up with you.

Your workouts are so much more valuable than just the calories you burn. Being intentional with your training and keeping the focus on building muscle is … well … magical. Often, less is more. Feeling destroyed from your sessions doesn't mean they were better. It doesn't mean you'll see results faster. Often, it just means you worked hard, but you can work hard running on a hamster wheel and get absolutely nowhere.

It may feel satisfying at times to see the sweat dripping on the ground as you think about collapsing, struggle to catch your breath, and feel shaky and destroyed. (No? Is that just me?) However, that feeling doesn't mean you moved toward your goals. You may have just used up gas in your tank to drive in circles or even go completely the wrong way. Unfortunately, training hard and training smart with intention and focus on your goals aren't always the same!

If you're about to close this book because you *love* your cardio training and refuse to give it up, just hold on a second. I'm not telling you to make that sacrifice. But you do need to know the cost and reward of everything you include in your STRONG system so you can budget for different training practices and strategically plan for things you love.

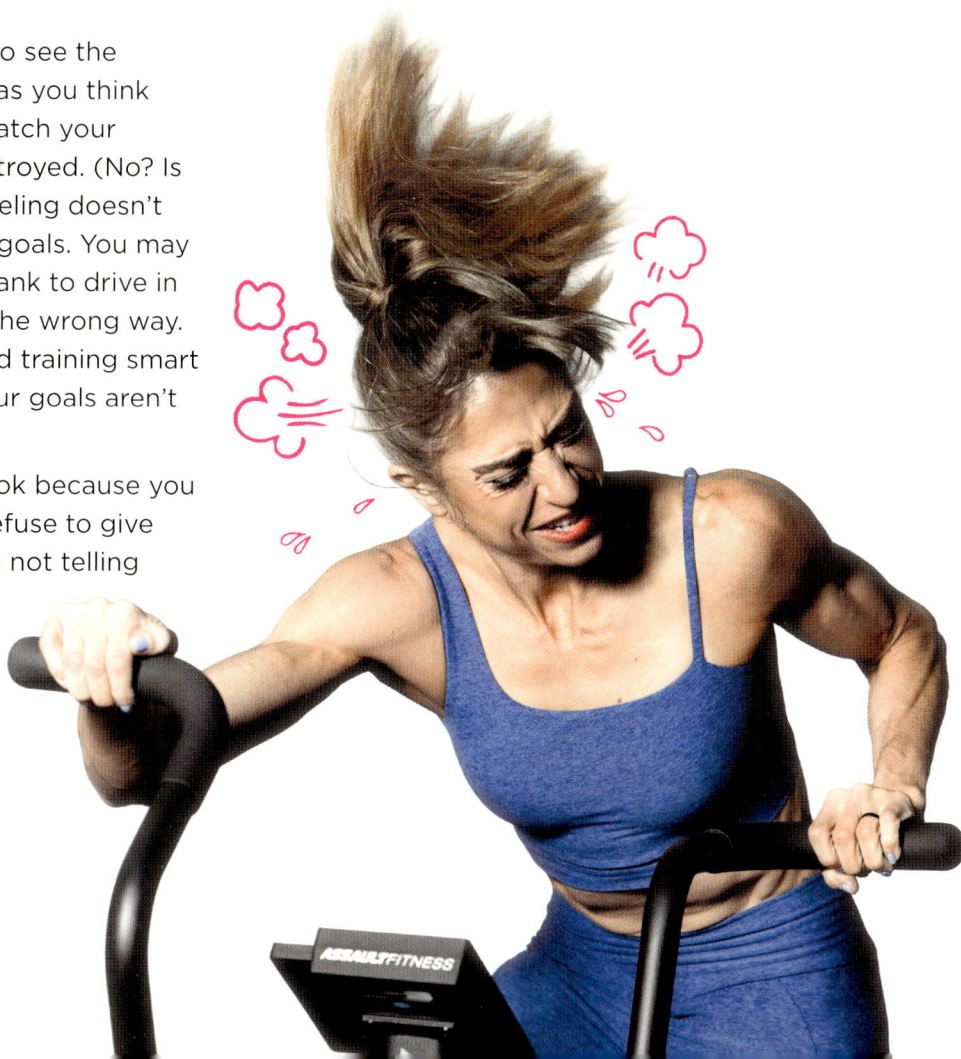

It's also key that you understand what may not be within your budget if you want results as fast as possible. As you work to reach your goal, you can't always just do what you like. You will make some sacrifices, and this is where you need to refer back to your STRONG system to assess what you want and what your nonnegotiables are. You may discover you have some nonnegotiables that you didn't consider previously, so you need to account for them now.

Here's an example: You're a fan of steady-state cardio but want to work on body recomp, so you might be willing to sacrifice the cardio temporarily because it will fight against your muscle-building efforts. You have to make a choice and embrace that your training practices need to evolve based on how your priorities and goals shift over time. Owning your goals and acknowledging what you enjoy in your training is why you outline your workout routine *before* you tweak your nutrition.

Honestly, exercise and nutrition are connected in a loop you keep cycling through. You have to constantly assess, adjust, and take care that all systems are working together!

You're not trying to look good for just a day. You're here to build your leanest, strongest body ever, no matter how old you are.

MUSCLE IS MAGICAL

Even if your goal is weight loss right now, you have to focus on building muscle. Muscle is magical and truly the answer to looking and feeling your most fabulous (and even seeing your health improve!).

If the idea of muscle makes you imagine the Hulk or bro bodybuilders whose arms can't hang flat by their sides because their lats are too big, and you're about to tell me you don't want to get bulky, rest assured that's not what I mean. However, if you want to bulk up, I'm happy to share tips for that as well.

I'm actually talking about building the lean muscle that makes you look toned and keeps you functionally fit and independent. Lean muscle is the key to definition and metabolic health. If you need an extra push to focus on muscle, here are fifteen reasons why muscle and strength work are important:

1. Muscle helps you look leaner.
2. Muscle helps you keep the fat off by improving your metabolic health.
3. Strength training protects and strengthens your skin.
4. Muscle powers your movements so you can remain strong and independent. (Sarcopenia, or loss of muscle mass and strength, is a leading risk factor in all-cause mortality in older adults.)
5. Muscle keeps your joints healthy.
6. More muscle means stronger bones.
7. Muscle improves your blood sugar levels.

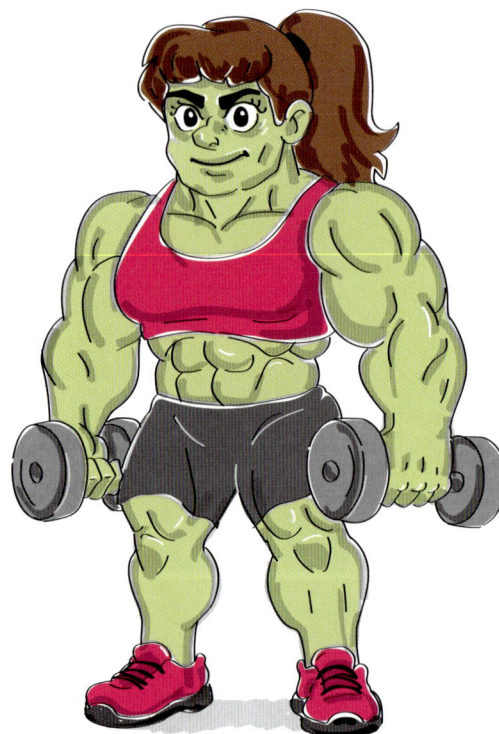

8. Muscle helps keep your heart healthy.

9. Muscle improves your immune system.

10. Muscle aids in better recovery from injury and disease.

11. Strength training improves mood and anxiety.

12. Muscle helps you feel more energized.

13. Building muscle improves your sleep.

14. Muscle helps keep your brain healthy.

15. More muscle means a longer, healthier, better life!

Achieving these things comes back to using your workouts strategically and being purposeful about what you include, from the exact reps and sets to the moves and types of equipment you use. You may even find you have to check your ego and regress to progress to see better results. I'll dive into this more when I discuss how to customize the workouts to what you need.

When I say that you don't have to feel destroyed by your workouts, I don't necessarily mean that your workouts will feel easy. You need a challenge to create a change, and pushing hard to create progression in your training to build lean muscle and lose fat is often both physically and mentally taxing. It's why prehab work (page 110) and a balance of intensities are key.

In this process, you're going to have to let go of many of your beliefs about training because many are probably built off of quick fixes and *only* losing weight with little regard for maintaining your results. That's why I'm harping on shifting your view of the goal for working out from burning calories to building muscle.

You may find it hard to shift that mindset because you may have been a cardio bunny who's been chasing that killer sweat for decades. You may also have viewed workouts as cardio *or* strength, and that's really not the case.

THE STRENGTH-CARDIO CONTINUUM

Seeing workouts as only strength or only cardio limits your opportunities. It also doesn't allow you to make small tweaks to how you include cardio or strength training to see better results faster. Not only is there a whole strength-cardio continuum you can use to your advantage, but there are also different ways to include even "nonideal" forms of training that you simply love to better fit your budget.

In Chapter 11, I'm going to break down this continuum to explain how you can include more metabolic forms of lifting with a realistic time frame and schedule so you can get the best of both worlds. While these training protocols are essential, how you use them needs to be based on what is a repeatable schedule for you.

Too often, "I don't have enough time" becomes an excuse not to train, so I designed the protocols to make them fit into your life. You can do them whether you have access to a full gym or train at home. There's an option whether you have three days and thirty minutes or six days and one hour. Results happen because you design for the time you have!

If you fall in love with one particular protocol, keep in mind it may not work for you year round because your lifestyle, needs, and goals may change. Recognize the opportunity in all three training protocols as your schedule shifts over the year.

With both the training protocols and the macros methods, you shouldn't try to make things fit a mold. Instead, understand that the right answer to the question, "What is best?" is often, "All." At the same time, the answer could also be, "None."

Remember, one size doesn't fit all—and the same plan won't even fit you forever!

THE THREE TRAINING PROTOCOLS

Chapter 11 gets into the why, what, and how of the training protocols, as well as who each one works best for. The three training methods are

» **The 6-12-25 method**

» **Compound burner sets**

» **Time strength series**

As you read through Chapter 11, take time to understand the upsides and downsides of each protocol to determine which is best based on the reflection you've done so far. And in determining what is best, consider not only what is best for you now but also what may be best for you at another point in your journey. What about when you travel? Or are busy during the holiday season? Seeing opportunities in each will help you plan.

These protocols all use what I consider to be the strength-cardio continuum sweet spot for body recomp—gaining muscle as you lose fat or losing fat as you gain muscle. All of the protocols help you build and retain lean muscle as you get older and your hormone levels aren't as ideal as they once were.

While getting older doesn't doom you to feeling old, you do want to use strategies that help you feel your best when your body isn't as primed to lose weight or gain muscle as it may have been when your hormone levels were optimal in your twenties. You also want to do forms of training that help you move better than ever so you can see results whether you're just starting back to working out or have been working out for decades.

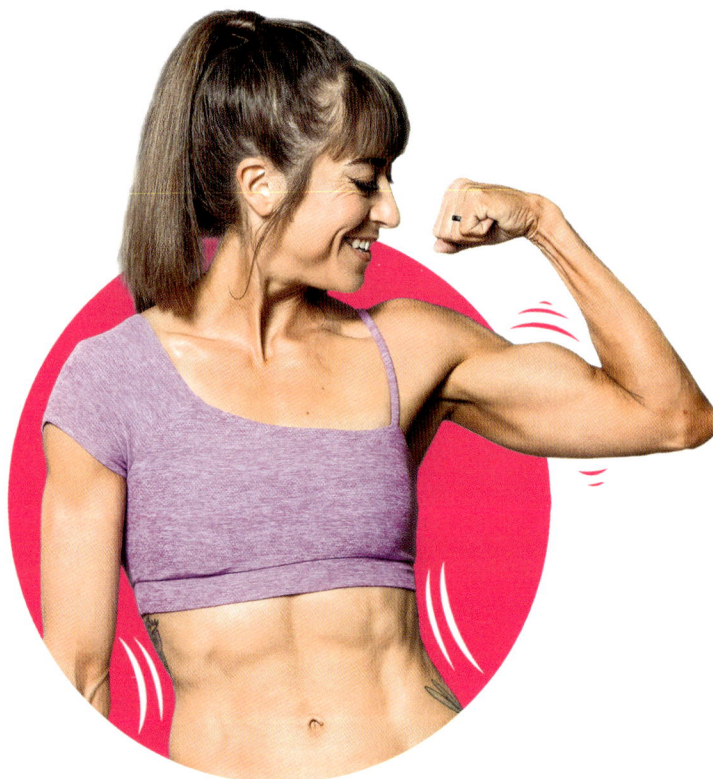

THE MACROS METHODS

Have you ever tried tracking macros and felt like you were staring at a board of math equations that go right over your head? Like you were the opposite of Matt Damon's character in *Good Will Hunting*?

Right now, you may be thinking that this program isn't right for you just because I mentioned the word macros. Or maybe you're saying, "What the heck are macros?!" (See the next section for the answer to that.) Don't worry. I'll break down the basics and outline some options to help you adjust macros without feeling like you're back in math class.

On the other hand, if you're saying, "Yay! Macros are like Tetris!" you're in luck too. There's a method for every person because a habit doesn't have to be done in just one form. Embracing the variation you need right now, even if you ultimately want to do another, might be the ticket to finally seeing the results you not only desire but also deserve.

Whether tracking macros is a big rock or a small pebble to you, doing it makes a difference in how fueled you feel and the results you achieve.

WHAT THE HECK ARE MACROS?

Even if you're raising your hand because you know the answer, take a second to pause and read through this section. If you take yourself back to that learner's mindset and refocus on the fundamentals, you may read something in a new way that makes other things really click.

Macros is short for *macronutrients*, which are the nutrients you need in large quantities from the foods you consume: proteins, carbs, and fats. Each has a different purpose in your body, and how you adjust the portion of each you consume can have a huge impact on the results you get.

That's the reason you may feel frustrated when you eat "healthy" but don't see results. Not only may your calories not be in line with what you need, but you also may not be getting the right amount of protein, carbs, or fats to match your body, needs, and goals, especially because your needs can shift over time.

When you track macros, you figure out how foods impact you and your results. Whether you realize it or not, every diet out there ultimately boils down to how it makes you adjust your macros. Keto, low-fat, Mediterranean, WeightWatchers, Atkins, Paleo—all of these diets are ultimately about adjusting your macros.

One of the issues with these eating plans is that they can keep you stuck because they hide the exact portions they are helping you create by eliminating specific foods or food groups. Then you go on diet after diet because you don't see the "secret" ratio behind the food restrictions. You ultimately fail when you're no longer willing to restrict the food you love. This is why assessing your lifestyle and owning your nonnegotiables before you begin is so key to the STRONG system.

STOP THE RESTRICTION

If you love bread, maybe you can do keto in the short term or go Paleo for a bit, but you can't permanently restrict something you love. If you don't learn how to work that thing you love into your life, it will become your downfall.

If you've tried some of these diets in the past, you might not have understood *why* they worked (temporarily). That's where learning about macros and how they relate to these methods comes in. You can optimize your nutrition based on *your* lifestyle and goals (rather than a generic formula), and you can then learn how to adjust based on your progress.

Sure, you may decide a low-carb ratio is right for you at this phase in your weight-loss process. You may *choose* to cut out the amazingly delicious, warm rolls that your friend bakes (and that you love), but you'll also know you can work them in at some point. They aren't demonized and off-limits forever.

That's the key. You can fuel according to your goals while creating a balance and enjoying the foods you love! It's also why all of the macros methods I share focus on nutrition by addition rather than only cutting out. Even if weight loss is your goal, it helps to focus first on adding certain things before you cut out other things.

Macros can work no matter your dietary preference: vegan, vegetarian, pescatarian, omnivore, gluten-free, dairy-free, or low-FODMAP. You can adjust your portions and eat foods that not only make you feel best but that you also enjoy.

THE THREE MACROS METHODS

People often fall into one of several camps when it comes to tracking macros:

» Some love mapping out meals to hit specific amounts of protein, carbs, and fats. They feel like they're a macros master and food tracking is a fun game of Tetris. Well, if you're one of those people, you're kind of weird, and I like it! I have a macros method for you: the macro cycling method (page 169).

» Other people have found that tracking macros has worked in the past, but they give up the second life gets busy. They feel like it's unsustainable even though it works. Or, in some cases, they just don't enjoy it or feel overwhelmed by the idea of fully doing it. The macros method for people in this camp is the minimalist macros method (page 159).

» Then there's the group that says, "Nope, nope, nope." No food apps. No weighing and measuring everything. If you feel this way, I may try to get you to reconsider your mindset in Chapter 12 because what gets measured, gets managed. However, I understand where you're coming from 100 percent. I resisted tracking macros for a very long time. Because one size doesn't fit all, tracking in one form isn't right for everyone, and some of us have some not-so-fond memories of tracking and restricting while feeling obsessed and deprived. There's still a macros method for you that helps you separate the tool from the feeling. It's the hand-sized health method (page 151).

You may switch among the methods as your lifestyle evolves or as you reach your goals. You may even find that even though you love tracking, the other methods come in handy during the holidays or when you travel.

So, don't skip reading through each method in Chapter 12 to see the opportunity in the options!

LOVE YOUR FAILURES

By going through this program and not skipping *anything*, you're setting yourself up for success. Consistently returning to and tweaking your STRONG system will help you meet yourself where you are with the changes you are going to make.

As excited as you may get after having read through the 6-12-25 method or the hand-sized health method, don't jump to acting without assessing the other methods first. This is key to helping you see little tweaks you can make in how you're using each technique to completely tailor it to what you need, even as your needs and goals evolve because nothing in life stands still.

No matter how much you plan, prepare, think through your past struggles, and do all of the STRONG system reflection, you will still encounter bumps along the way. *Life* is going to happen.

> **You're human and flawsome. Instead of seeing mistakes, setbacks, or failures as a bad thing, you need to learn to love them.**

Let's face it: You're human and flawsome. Instead of seeing mistakes, setbacks, or failures as a bad thing, you need to learn to love them.

Failing is not failure unless you give up. Progress is never linear. And if you consider every mistake an opportunity to learn and accept responsibility instead of placing fault, you'll end up failing forward. Each failure will be a learning experience that teaches you something new and allows you to better optimize your plan. It can also help you reflect on the habits you need and the way you're breaking them down.

Failures can help you reassess what you want and what sacrifices you're willing to make. They can help you see the road to take as well as the road to avoid.

Success is struggle. So, take consistent action and reflect on those actions. Use the mini targets and complementary targets you established in Chapter 5 to help you set checkpoints where you can reflect and assess. Consider not only your successes but also your opportunities for growth. Take a look at your consistency in your workouts or your macros and identify places you could make some 1 percent improvements to be better.

Be excited to recognize your areas for improvement and growth. Those little areas of optimization are what will take you to the next level. As I talked about in Chapter 7, failures are how you succeed, so reframe failure for yourself into a good thing. Sara Blakely, the founder of Spanx, has shared how her father helped her do this when she was growing up. Sara's father would ask, "What did you fail at today?" If Sara didn't report any mishaps or mistakes, her father would be disappointed. Take time to ask yourself, "What did I fail at today?" and take pride that you took a risk and pushed yourself outside your comfort zone to grow.

Be excited by the challenge that lies ahead with new workouts and nutritional tweaks. And return to your STRONG system often to help you meet yourself where you are to drive forward!

11 THE METABOLIC MUSCLE-BUILDING PROTOCOLS

Now it's time for the fun stuff—the stuff that makes my nerd heart especially happy. We're getting into the stuff you get to *do* to make exciting changes.

As you go through this chapter, remember *one size doesn't fit all*! A small tweak in a move, a slight change in schedule, cycling through only one of these designs (or all of them)—how you use these protocols is based on the STRONG system outline you've put together.

Don't get caught up in what you think is ideal. Focus on yourself and what *you* need. That's why I call the first section, "*Your* Perfect Protocol," not "A Perfect Protocol"!

YOUR PERFECT PROTOCOL

Everything you do should have a purpose. You need to design with intention.

Right now, reflect on your origin story: What are you currently doing for your workouts? Three days a week? Thirty minutes? An hour six days a week? Zero days a week and barely getting off the couch? Where you start affects what you can realistically do as a first step forward.

If you don't move carefully from where you are into your first step, you're going to get caught in the change loop. Remember that from Part 1? What do people often jump to that leads to the passion bomb exploding? The "ideal"! In their excitement to get started, they determine that six days of exercise must be best, and it must be an hour a day. Sure, some of the protocols have that option, but that doesn't mean you have to do it that way. Each of the protocols and progressions are designed for different schedules, needs, and goals.

I designed them that way with the purpose of fitting your lifestyle as you work to reach your goals. You need to own your current lifestyle and schedule first, so assess what you're doing now. Then consider what's repeatable. What seems so doable you know you can be consistent with it immediately—and maybe even crave more?

If timed strength work for 15-minute sessions three days a week is what you can do consistently, great! If the 6-12-25 option on six days a week for an hour in the gym works with your lifestyle and schedule, terrific! Instead of focusing on what you think may be best, remember that sustainability and results are about meeting yourself where you are by doing something you can build off of.

Take some time to reflect on your lifestyle and write down how many days a week are realistic for you and the time you have available. From there, you'll adjust based on your goals and how your schedule evolves.

Also consider other times of year as you're reflecting now. Is there a busy season where you may need to adjust your training? Or is it busy now and you may have more time soon? Do you have a vision of the schedule you'd eventually like to grow into on your way to your destination? These reflections can help you not only lay out what you need now but help you stay open to other options as you go along!

As you're creating your perfect protocol, you may feel a little bit like you're building Frankenstein's monster. You may have to piece together different components of the protocols. (I'll explain how.) However, you don't get to do only the things you like best.

For example, take something like including the three-part prehab process in every single warm-up. Have you ever skipped your warm-up to get to the "good stuff" because you're short on time? I have. Then years later, I felt aches and pains cropping up. During a workout, my back would get achy or I would have to stop because little pains started to add up. So as much as mobility work may not "feel" beneficial in the moment, doing it helps you optimize a routine to get better results faster.

Cherry-picking the things you like or ignoring components of the system leads to feeling like you're working really hard without seeing progress build. Recognize the underlying mindsets you've had about some of these systems to find ways to value them and see the opportunity in them now. Assess your mental hang-ups against them.

You also might have to let go of what used to work or something that was effective to get you to one specific goal. What helped you reach one goal may hold you back from taking things to the next level.

Refer to the notes you made when you read Chapter 7. They'll be helpful when you feel yourself pushing back against new things—like routines that go against what you've always done, higher or lower rep ranges than you've normally lifted, or even the way you measure progress.

As you read through the protocols in this chapter, keep your main target and your complementary targets front of mind to help you have direction. You aren't just picking a workout because it looks fun (although all of these are!). You always want to have a clear purpose to your plan and a definitive way of measuring progress. In Chapter 14, I'll break down multiple ways to measure progress.

Another thing to remember is to be targeted in your approach—something I talked about in Chapter 5. In that chapter, I compared it to walking a pack of dogs that pull in every direction. You can have more than one goal at a time, but you'll see results quickest in the goal you put first—what you prioritize. Otherwise, you're just going to end up tripping over tangled leashes and working really hard only to make no progress, no matter how fabulous these protocols are.

Also, balancing multiple goals may affect how quickly you see results. So consider your budget and what will keep you motivated. Assess what is most significant to you right now. If you want to improve your performance *and* lose weight, you want to figure out which you value most and prioritize that thing. If weight loss is your priority, you may be more aggressive in the short term, even if you see a dip in training. If performance is your top priority because you have a race around the corner, you may need to embrace slower changes on the scale.

Everything you're designing has purpose. You want everything you do to have a big bang for your buck. That's why you have to let go of doing only what you like.

Embrace the protocols and processes in this chapter and value each component in them because the way those components work together as a system is significant. Things won't turn out the same if you choose only some pieces of a system.

Before you worry too much, I'm not telling you that you can't tweak or customize the protocols. I'm only saying that you can't decide to do only the things you're comfortable with. For example, you need the rest that's built into the protocol, and you need to do reps that are more volume than you're used to. You need the stuff that sometimes doesn't lead to an immediate payoff.

So let's get to it. First, I discuss what's probably the most important—and most underutilized—training tool.

THE PREHAB PROCESS

Have you ever walked into the gym, hopped on the treadmill for about five minutes or done a few casual arm swings, and then rushed to your killer HIIT or lifting workout? And then have you wondered why you feel like you're never getting more flexible or why your back always hurts after your workouts even though you have good form?

If you're thinking, "Well, I'm getting older. It's my age," I have one thing to say: Yeah, that's not it.

So much of what you're blaming on age is actually the accumulation of missed mobility sessions that are finally catching up with you. Those pains are from the ankle sprain you never rehabbed and rested or the elbow injury you ignored that flares up right when you feel like you get in a groove. You need to *stop* skipping or slacking on your prehab and warm-up.

It's a simple but sucky answer. Every workout you do should start with the three-part prehab process. Honestly, if you take only one thing from this program, I hope it's that you give prehab a chance so you can move better than you ever have before.

This prehab process was born out of my own ego and subsequent stupidity. It's led to me now being able to train the way I want year-round. It's also what my clients have said is the biggest difference maker in their results, and it's the reason countless Redefining Strength members text me things like, "I feel like I'm moving better than I did in my twenties and thirties!"

Because you might have some mental resistance and warming up may be a big-rock habit right now, I want to explain the value so you can break down how you can start including it in your routine. Who knows. Maybe it'll become the single biggest workout game changer for you.

WHAT IS "PREHAB"?

Prehab isn't just any old warm-up. It's not just about warming up your body, although that's important. Prehab is about addressing daily postures so you can perform movements correctly in your workout to get the most benefit from every rep.

Prehab is *preventative rehab* that addresses mobility restrictions, muscle imbalances, postural distortions—all the little irritations and aches and pains—*before* they add up. People are often reactive and sabotage their consistency and success by training hard; then they hit a point where they have to back off or train through pain, only to see diminishing returns.

Prehab is a three-part process of foam rolling, stretching, and activation. One component alone doesn't have the benefit as the full system.

Do any of these situations seem familiar?

» You feel like you warm up only after a few rounds of your workout.

» You joke you need oil for your joints after waking up in the morning.

» Your hips are achy from sitting all day.

» Your neck and shoulders constantly get tweaked from sleeping wrong.

» Your joints sound like Rice Krispies cereal—snap, crackle, pop—when you move around.

» You feel frustrated because it seems like your abs just aren't getting stronger and more defined, and you constantly feel your back when you're doing core work.

If you agree with any of those statements (or others like them), you need prehab!

In the next sections, I break down the three components and cover how you can design your own prehab routines to use as five- to ten-minute warm-ups or as full recovery days. If you're feeling like even five minutes is too much, let's sledgehammer that rock to a pebble you can start today!

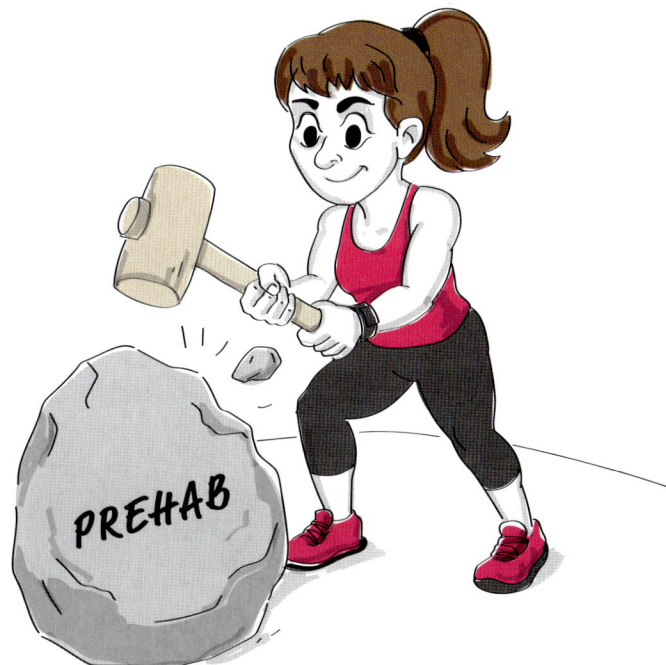

FOAM ROLLING

Foam rolling is a slightly "controversial" protocol. The rehab sectors of health and wellness give it some love, but other people (in more old-school powerlifting or bodybuilding spheres) often say, "Meh," and write it off as not valuable. However, that dismissiveness is probably because it's often used in isolation instead of being combined with stretching and activation to capitalize on its value.

If you're not sure what I'm even talking about when I say, "foam rolling," don't worry. I'm about to break down what it is, its benefits, and how to do it as the first part in the prehab process.

What Is Foam Rolling?

Foam rolling, or self-myofascial release (SMR), is one of the cheapest and easiest ways to give yourself a massage. Although it's called "foam rolling," you can do it with a variety of tools—a ball, a true foam roller, or some other trigger point tool. The goal is to help relax and release tight and overactive muscles and knots.

The Benefits

Here's a quick list of the benefits of SMR:

» Relaxes tight and overactive muscles

» Corrects muscle imbalances

» Improves joint range of motion

» Maintains optimal length-tension relationships of muscles

» Increases extensibility (the ability to be stretched) of the musculotendinous junction

» Improves neuromuscular efficiency (aka the mind-body connection)

Foam rolling helps relax muscles so that you can engage the correct muscles at the correct times during exercises and work through a full range of motion.

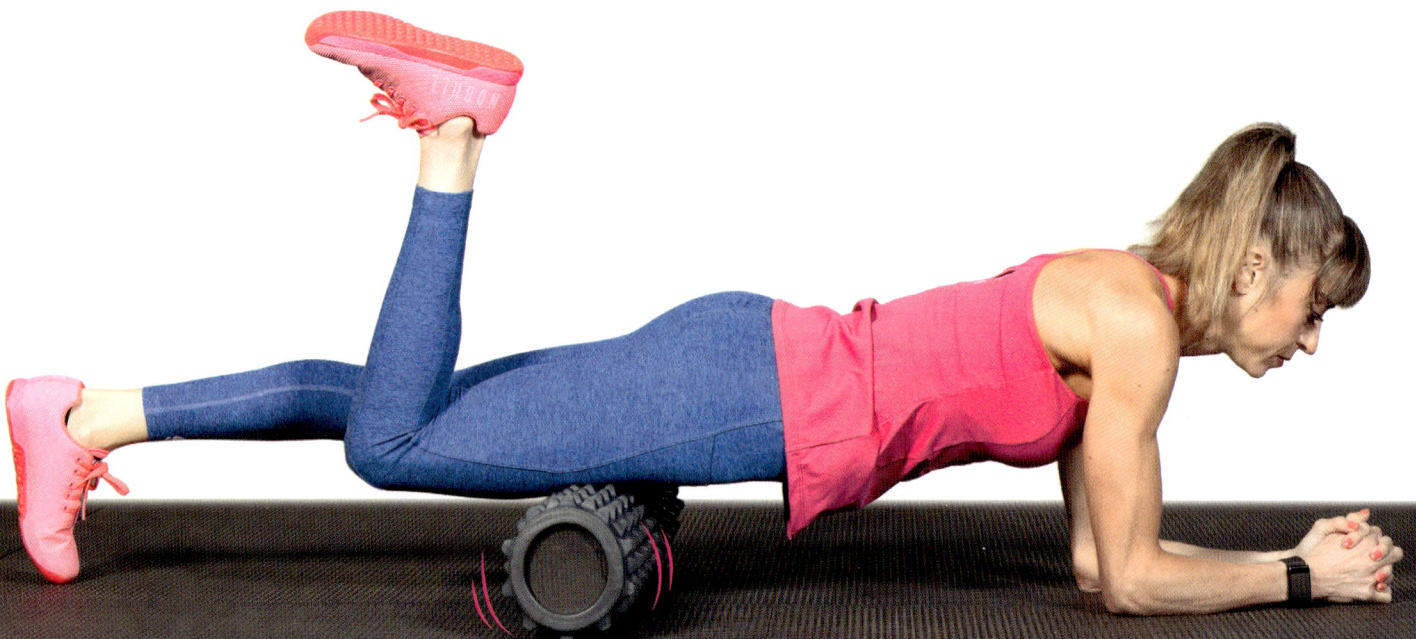

Trigger points (muscle knots) can restrict or alter joint range of motion, which can result in a change of neural feedback to your central nervous system. This can cause your neuromuscular system to become less efficient, which can lead to premature fatigue, chronic pain and injury, and less efficient performance over time. In other words, foam rolling is the first step to feeling ready to work hard in your workouts.

You want to use foam rolling before a workout to prime your body to work correctly, which will enable you to get the most out of your workout and lower your risk for injury! When you do this step first in the prehab process, you're better able to stretch and activate your muscles without interference.

If you don't do the foam rolling step first, it's like you're stretching a shoelace with a knot in it. Stretching can make things worse. Also, jumping into the activation moves means you continue to overuse muscles that aren't meant to carry the load you're asking them to carry. That perpetuates muscles and joints being overloaded and injured.

So while there may be some validity to the belief that foam rolling isn't "worthwhile" because the direct effects are technically short-lived and have an acute impact for only about 15 minutes, those issues aren't concerns here because it's just the first step in the prehab process. You follow it up with the other two components to maintain the relaxation and optimize engagement of the correct muscles.

If you're thinking,

But a warm-up should warm up your body. I've heard that static stretching is bad because it relaxes tight muscles and can hurt strength and power output. Wouldn't foam rolling have the same impact?

rest assured that the answer is, "No!"

That's why you use foam rolling rather than static stretching; it won't diminish power output or strength as it improves muscle flexibility. You're using foam rolling to relax overactive muscles that *would* negatively impact your strength and want to compensate and work when they shouldn't, making your training less efficient and effective!

You do foam rolling before stretching or activation because foam rolling can improve your tissues' ability to lengthen during stretching, which allows you to use stretching not only to improve your flexibility but also to improve your mobility.

By relaxing overactive muscles, you allow your body to more easily establish the mind-body connection with the muscles you struggle to feel working during your exercises. Foam rolling primes your muscles to be able to contract properly and help your body move well!

> **Foam rolling primes your muscles to be able to contract properly and help your body move well!**

How Foam Rolling Works

I want to nerd out a bit more and help you appreciate all that foam rolling does. Understanding the basics of how foam rolling works will help you better see the value in what may seem like a boring change!

Foam rolling (or SMR), works through autogenic inhibition. Put more simply, the muscle relaxes itself because of the pressure applied by a trigger point tool.

When you apply and sustain pressure to a trigger point with a foam roller, you can cause the Golgi tendon organs to "turn off" muscle spindle activity, allowing the muscle fibers to unknot, stretch, and realign.

When you reduce the soft-tissue tension, you decrease pain, restore muscles to their proper length-tension relationships, and improve their function, which means you help them contract better so you can perform better!

There is very limited research on foam rolling helping improve recovery and reduce delayed onset muscle soreness (DOMS), which is also why you include it with some static stretching in your cooldown. It helps prep your body for work the next day!

How to Foam Roll

You can foam roll to relieve discomfort or tight muscles at any time, but the purpose of rolling during the prehab is to focus on the tight muscles that may affect your workout. Rolling out other areas, such as those that may be tight from sitting, can be done at another time, especially if you're short on time.

When you use foam rolling as part of your warm-up, focus on any muscles that may alter the movement patterns you want to perform or inhibit the correct muscles from working. For example, if you're struggling with your hamstrings taking over during glute moves, you will want to roll out your hamstrings in your warm-up to relax them to better activate your glutes and improve your hip mobility.

I suggest you target one to three areas, depending on the type of workout you're doing. A full-body workout may demand a couple more areas than a hemisphere (upper or lower) split workout will.

Recovery workouts are the best time to address commonly overactive muscles caused by sitting or hunching during the day. If you're not certain what's tight, do a little "search and destroy" mission to find new areas that you may need to address.

When you roll out a muscle, use a trigger point tool to find a tight spot. Hold on that point as you breathe to help the muscle relax and release. The smaller and harder the tool, the more it will dig in to the muscle. If you find yourself tensing against the tool, you may need to switch to a softer tool, or you can try rolling off a wall or bench. If you're tensing against the pressure, you aren't going to allow the muscle to relax.

The only time to tense as you hold is if you contract the muscle deliberately against the tool and then consciously relax over it. This tense-and-release action can help you truly relax the area as you exhale as you release. People often tend to roll back and forth over an area quickly, but if you want to help the muscle relax, you need to hold on the trigger point. Hold and breathe for up to thirty seconds and then move on. You can spend up to one minute on a spot, but holding for any longer won't necessarily give you added benefit.

The next step after foam rolling is to use mainly dynamic stretches to improve your range of motion, warm up your body, and help maintain the mobility and flexibility you've started creating through foam rolling.

STRETCHING

"I need to stretch more." How many times have you said that?

When I would think about flexibility and injury prevention, I always thought *stretching*. But stretching is just one component of the full prehab process, and there are multiple forms of stretching that can be used at different times for different benefits.

If you're using stretching in your warm-up after foam rolling, you will want to use dynamic stretches to increase your range of motion, improve your flexibility, and get your blood pumping to prepare your body to work. This helps you make sure your muscles and joints are ready to engage efficiently.

What's the Difference Between Dynamic and Static Stretching

Dynamic stretching involves movement rather than just holding a position. You move a joint through a range of motion as you stretch your muscles. Many of these stretches address more than one muscle. They warm up your body as you work on flexibility and joint mobility. The dynamic stretches also begin the activation process as you focus on the muscle driving the stretch. Really focus; don't just go through the motions.

Static stretches are stretches that you hold and relax and breathe into. You often try to stretch further as you relax and hold, but you're not doing any truly active movement. The focus is on muscle tissue length rather than joint movement.

Both types of stretches are beneficial; however, you should use them at different times.

Knowing When to Use Dynamic or Static Stretches

A general rule of thumb for stretching is to use dynamic stretches as part of your warm-up and static stretches as part of your cooldown.

Because of the movement involved in dynamic stretches, they warm up your body and help you restore proper joint mobility while loosening tight muscles. They prime your body for movement, so it's a good idea to use dynamic stretches that mimic the movement patterns or exercises you plan to include that day. While they don't have to be the exact movements you'll be doing, you want to prep the body to be able to do the movement patterns required in your workout. For example, you may use a dynamic squat stretch before a lower body day, especially one in which you're doing back squats. Using dynamic stretches prior to your workouts helps ensure you get the most out of the very first rep you do in your training instead of needing multiple rounds to really get over any prefatigue and loosen up.

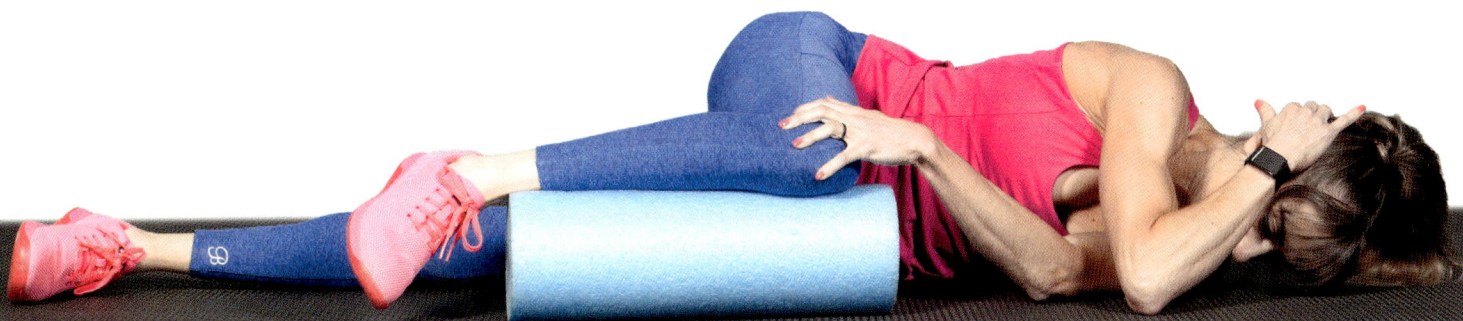

Using dynamic stretching as this second step in the prehab process also provides a transition between relaxing overactive muscles and activating underactive ones. When most people stretch, they think they should be focused only on elongating a muscle. They don't focus on what is driving that stretch. But when you shift your focus to engaging the muscle that's driving the stretch, not only do you often stretch the muscle more effectively and move the joint through a more stable range of motion, but you begin to activate muscles that tend not to work when they should.

An example of this is your hip flexors. Have you ever done a hip stretch and felt like your hips are still so tight and you can't squat any deeper? Maybe you've even felt like your lower back is constantly hurting no matter how much you work on your tight hips? The reason may be that you're not actually stretching your hip flexors. You're compensating and seeking out flexibility, stability, or even mobility from other muscles and joints. Instead, you may be arching your lower back or letting your pelvis move into what is known as anterior pelvic tilt.

If you shift your focus from doing the movement to driving the stretch with your glutes, you may suddenly realize how much you now feel the stretch not only in your hip flexors but also your glutes. Win-win! This is what will truly improve your flexibility and mobility, not to mention start to work on the stability and activation you'll address with the third part of the prehab process.

Dynamic stretching, when done correctly, helps prevent injury because you've prepped your body to handle the loads and range of motion required to help prevent compensations, imbalances, and overuse. A 2008 study found that a proper dynamic warm-up decreased overall injury risk by 35 percent and serious injuries by almost half![*]

Static stretching doesn't have this same preparation benefit. In some cases, it's been shown to impact strength and power output negatively. A 2006 study found it created neuromuscular inhibition (altered muscle stiffness), leading to reduced power.[**] That doesn't mean you shouldn't include it in your workout routines at all. It just means you won't often use it for the prehab in your warm-up.

Of course, there's always a "but" or "maybe" to every situation. If you've had a previous injury or issue, and mobility and flexibility are things that need your primary focus, then you may occasionally include a static stretch in your warm-up. In these situations, you aren't going to be focused on lifting your max anyway, so a reduction in performance isn't important; your primary concern needs to be on moving well while building back. A 2019 study also found that shorter static stretches done in combination with other warm-up techniques, even when paired with dynamic stretches, may then not impact performance.[***] The way you include things matter. And as I like to say, sometimes you need to "Regress to progress!"

Part of what makes static stretching good and beneficial for your cooldowns and prehab work on recovery days is that static stretches relax muscles, improve flexibility and even relax your central nervous system. Relaxing your central nervous system

[*]Torbjørn Soligard et al., "Comprehensive Warm-Up Programme to Prevent Injuries in Your Female Footballers: Cluster Randomised Controlled Trial," *BMJ* 337 (2008), https://www.bmj.com/content/337/bmj.a2469.

[**]Taichi Yamaguchi, Kojiro Ishii, Masanori Yamanaka, and Kazunori Yasuda, "Acute Effect of Static Stretching on Power Output During Concentric Dynamic External Resistance Leg Extension," *Journal of Strength and Conditioning Research* 20, no. 4 (2006): 804–10, https://pubmed.ncbi.nlm.nih.gov/17194246/.

[***]Helmi Chaabene, David G. Behm, Yassine Negra, and Urs Granacher, "Acute Effects of Static Stretching on Muscle Strength and Power: An Attempt to Clarify Previous Caveats," *Frontiers in Physiology* 10 (2019):1468, https://pmc.ncbi.nlm.nih.gov/articles/PMC6895680/.

can help optimize hormone levels, improve recovery, and keep your body healthy and happy so you can go hard during your next workout. So as easy as it is to finish your workout, pick up your stuff, and head home without a thought about a cooldown, taking time for some static stretching may be just what you need to get more out of your next session!

The key to stretching is to use each type in the proper way for the best possible results. Love stretching or hate it, it's essential. But as important as it is, you don't have to spend hours doing it. You want to make sure you're creating a stretching plan that works with your schedule.

How to Use Dynamic Stretching

The idea in creating your warm-up is to try to keep your routine to no more than six stretches. How many you plan to do depends on the number of reps you do per move and how many areas you're working at a time. Remember to select moves that fit your schedule. It's better to do one full body stretch than to program six you have to rush through!

Focus on the muscles and movement patterns you plan to use in your workout. The more a joint is restricted or a muscle is tight, the more you may need an extra move that isolates an area. You also want to make sure to address any overactive muscles or mobility restrictions so you don't compensate or perpetuate imbalances when you lift. This can mean addressing daily postures that could impact your workout as well as areas of tightness from previous workouts.

The warm-up should get your blood pumping but not make you tired. It should get you over that little prefatigue hump you may feel as you first get moving. After you've stretched to mobilize your joints, improve your flexibility, and get your blood pumping, you're ready to include a few activation exercises.

ACTIVATION

This is the step most often ignored and underutilized, but it's invaluable for staying free from aches and pains because what you feel working in an exercise is what is benefiting from the movement. If you're using the incorrect muscles, no amount of stretching or foam rolling is going to help. It'll seem like you're constantly foam rolling and stretching only to feel like you're never making any progress.

If you're wondering how to know if you're compensating, consider these questions:

? Do you feel your lower back working rather than your abs during core work?

? Do you always feel your hamstrings during glute bridges and never your glutes?

? Do you feel your traps and neck instead of your shoulders when you press overhead?

? Do you feel your biceps when you do a back row?

? Have you ever had a muscle that's constantly sore or tired and achy during a move and assumed it's "weak" and needs more strength work even though those aches and pains continue to add up over time?

If you answered yes to any of these questions, or questions like them, this means you have an activation problem. You have muscles doing work they shouldn't be doing while muscles that should be working aren't! That's why this activation step of the prehab process is so crucial.

Activation helps you improve the mind-body connection so you can properly engage the appropriate muscles to the correct extent at the correct times to power a movement. This helps you avoid overload and injury and ultimately be stronger, more powerful, more efficient, and faster.

Strength, speed, power, and even endurance are about moving by using the correct muscles efficiently and not overusing or underusing anything. Even coordination and agility—your ability to react and catch yourself—relates to that mind-body connection and the efficiency of that connection.

The more easily you can engage the correct muscles, the more quickly you can do this process without thought, and the better you will move! This means you'll see more benefit from those workouts where you've been putting in a lot of effort!

What Are Activation Exercises?

Activation exercises are those boring fundamental moves that seem too basic to be worth the effort. In some cases, they're slightly silly-looking moves you may have written off as being something only people clad in bright leotards did in old workout programs on VHS tapes. Fire Hydrant is a good example. It's aptly named because that's exactly what it looks like you're doing—lifting your leg like a dog does on a fire hydrant.

Even if these moves look silly, they have a lot of value. They're basic isolation exercises that allow you to focus on the muscles that should be working. The isolation and small range of motion often involved with these moves make it easier to really focus on the muscles that are working, and it's harder for other muscles to compensate, especially when you've already rolled out tight areas and done your stretching to mobilize your joints.

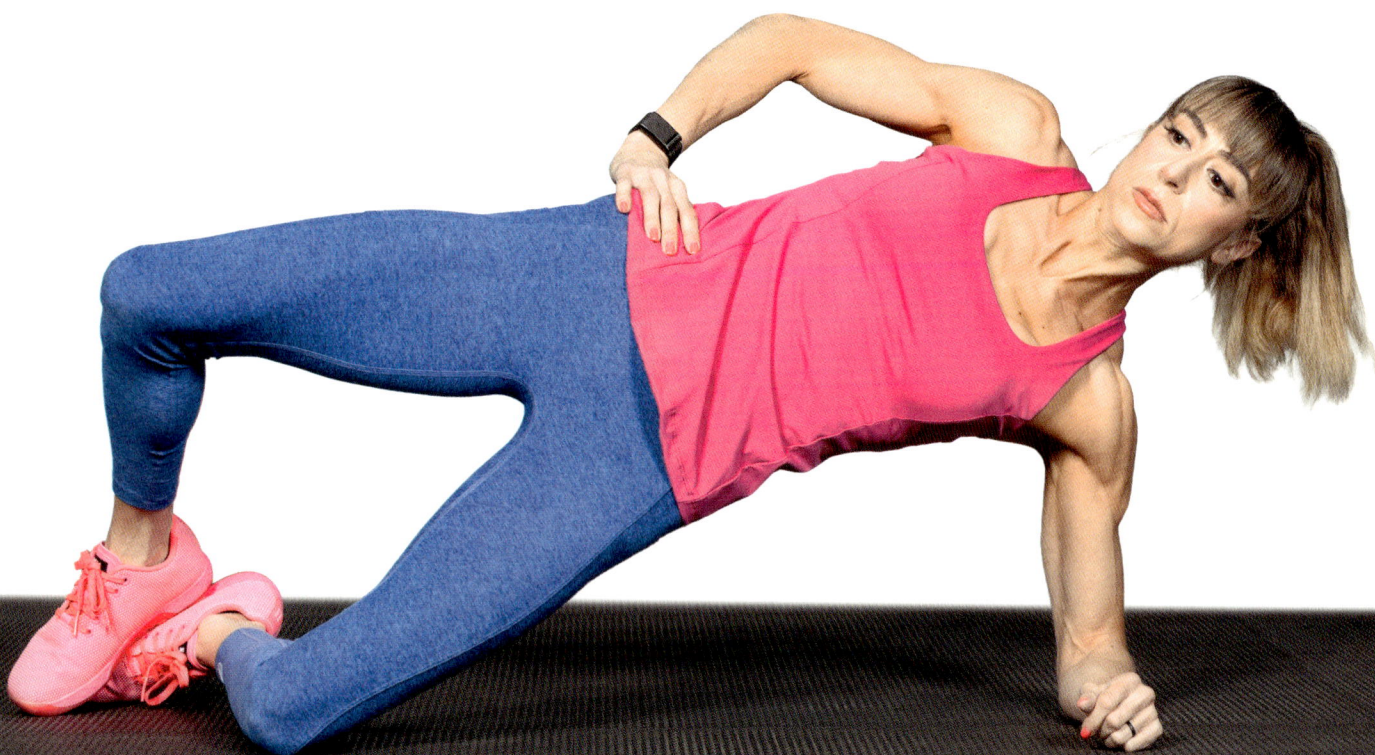

They're also done with little to no weight or resistance. Resistance isn't used so much to build strength or make you feel so tired you hit failure as it is to make sure you get a little "pump" in the muscle that should be working.

Although these moves are called activation exercises, many of them can also be great dynamic stretches. Dynamic stretches start the activation process, and activation moves continue the mobility and flexibility process. As you focus on engaging the correct muscle, you move through a range of motion that automatically "stretches" the muscle on the opposite side of the joint. For example, activation exercises can help you focus on hip extension. You stretch your hips by activating your glutes to drive the extension.

When you're short on time, you can pick moves that double as both stretches and activation exercises. With activation exercises, you're basically alerting your mind to the fact that a particular muscle is there and ready to work. You're helping the muscle to "wake up" so it can pull its weight during compound movements. These moves help correct dysfunctions due to poor posture and muscles that have become overactive because of your posture issues.

The better your mind-body connection, the more quickly you'll feel the muscle working without having to add weight or make the move more challenging technically. If you're just starting out, you may need more reps of a move before you feel a muscle fully engage, and you may find it helpful to place your hand on the muscle you want to work so you know it's contracting. Slowing down the tempo can help.

There's more to activation than just finding the "right" moves. In fact, you may already be doing many of the moves without seeing the benefit.

That's why I want to explain the difference between *movement* and *recruitment* patterns to help you get the most out of your activation work and be more intentional with your strength training.

Movement Patterns Versus Recruitment Patterns

Getting results is about more than doing the "right" moves. As I mentioned earlier in the book, there is no "best move" or "magic move." Even if you do moves that are beneficial or in line with your needs and goals, you may not be reaping the full value. That's because repeating proper form doesn't always mean you're using the correct muscles to power the movement. Honestly, many people are really good cheaters!

The more advanced and experienced you are with specific moves, the more you can cheat and mimic proper form to make the movement pattern look good. This ability to "cheat" is what leads to overload and injury. Your body finds the path of least resistance to do what you're asking it to do.

If you don't have proper spinal mobility of your upper back, your body will seek extra extension from your lower back to mimic the flat back position you want for your bent-over row. And that's why your lower back always hurts.

So if you've thought, *I have great form! I don't understand why I have certain aches and pains*, it may be your recruitment pattern.

Your recruitment patterns are the muscles being used to power the movement and the joints providing the range of motion for the movement. You want the correct muscles to be working at the correct times to only the extent they need to work—no more and no less.

This is easier said than done, especially if you sit at a desk all day or have had injuries in the past. The more you've created mobility issues or compensations, and the longer you've had them, the more you've trained new "natural" recruitment patterns.

These patterns are hard to break, and the bad patterns are what the prehab process addresses. It's why it's worth taking the time to do silly activation moves.

It can help you realize why your hamstrings always feel tight, you don't feel your glutes in moves, and your lower back is constantly achy despite your good form. Sometimes you have to step back to move forward. As I like to say, regress to progress!

> **Sometimes you have to step back to move forward.**

If your form looks good, don't stop there. When you're doing your activation work and during your strength routines, ask yourself, "What do I feel working?" This question will change everything. You will not only see strength and muscle gains but also avoid aches and pains because you're able to maximize each and every rep!

How to Use Activation Exercises

In your prehab routine, there are two places you'll use activation exercises: your warm-ups and your recovery days. I'll touch on my favorite type for a full recovery day (hint: they're isometrics!). Generally, in a cooldown, activation exercises aren't needed.

Use activation exercises to focus on underactive muscles and the muscles you will be working in your workout. Often, you'll be targeting muscles on the *opposite* side of a joint from the muscle groups that are tight. There are of course "buts" to this—or literally butts; however, it's a good rule of thumb.

You can also use activation exercises to address imbalances. For instance, if you've had an injury on one side or one side is weaker, you may do more reps of the activation move to help correct the imbalance and make sure both sides are working.

Select isolated movements and do them for higher reps—for example, 15 to 30 reps for about 1 or 2 rounds. Timed intervals are a good way to go so your brain doesn't have to focus on counting reps. Instead, you can focus on what you feel working as the timer ticks down. Some isometrics, such as plank holds, can also be good. They give you a chance to focus on engaging muscles that are hard to activate.

Simple isolation movements are best because they allow you to focus on the muscles that should be working. The more joints and muscles that have to work at once, the more you will be "distracted" by form. Keep in mind that you aren't trying to fatigue the muscles you're working; you just want to wake them up. Focus and think about the muscles that should be working. Because you're using light loads, a bit of volume can be helpful, but don't go crazy.

Once you've done your activation exercises, go right into your workout so your body is primed to move well and recruit the right muscles for the job. This doesn't mean you skip doing a few warm-up sets before a super heavy lift, but you should feel like your warm-up rounds are easier than ever before!

You'll find warm-up templates and workouts in Chapter 17. I designed them to address the joints and muscles you'll be working in the workouts. I've also provided recovery sessions, but I'll dive more into those in Chapter 13!

When you're doing your prehab routines, remember to address previous injuries. Don't ignore an elbow issue that's no longer giving you problems right now. Injuries never really go away, so even if something isn't bothering you at present, you can never stop doing what made you better. Simply resting an area doesn't correct the movement compensation or imbalance. It's one reason you do prehab—to prevent problems from resurfacing!

THE STRENGTH-CARDIO CONTINUUM

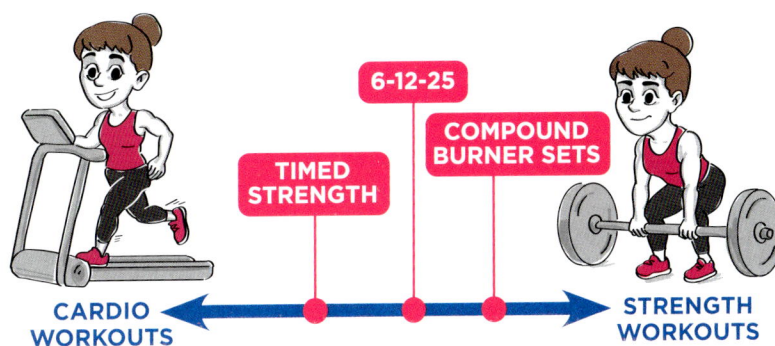

Cardio or strength? Which is better? You may guess I'm going to say strength. Strength work is crucial because muscle is magical, and too often, people turn to being cardio machines when they want to lose weight.

However, the honest and true answer to which is better is *both* (even if I'm annoyed to admit that)! It doesn't have to be an either-or situation. When people aren't training for a specific sport, they should program their workouts in that amazing space between "true strength" and "true cardio."

In that magical middle, where metabolic strength workouts thrive, you can often optimize for body recomp—which is especially helpful for people with crazy busy schedules. In this section, I break down the continuum to explain how you can use it to your advantage!

WHAT IS *CARDIO*?

When people think "pure cardio," they often think of steady-state, long-distance endurance-type training. Long runs and long bike rides. But that type of steady-state cardio works one energy system: the aerobic system.

In general, sprint intervals and interval training have become more popular, but these forms of training aren't fully on that "cardio" or aerobic end of the spectrum. You may even find you're currently using a beneficial form of power or sprint training that technically, in terms of energy systems and work-to-rest intervals, falls on the "strength" side of the energy continuum.

Too often, people end up not reaping the full benefit of interval work because they try to make themselves feel more tired by eliminating the rest periods. This constant desire to feel worked means the workout is just an aerobic session, it holds you back from working other energy systems, and it can also prevent you from building speed or power or improving your recovery. The rest isn't there just for fun. It has a purpose!

Although burpees, jump squats, and other such moves may come to mind when you think about interval work and conditioning, even lifting sessions can get your blood pumping and work on your "cardio." You can also use them to address a variety of energy systems and move you along that continuum from aerobic to anaerobic.

Next, I want to clarify what is often called *strength* work to highlight how different workout designs and training techniques can use all the space in the middle of the continuum.

WHAT IS *STRENGTH*?

When people think of pure strength work, they think about those powerlifting, 1-rep max workouts with 3- to 5-minute rest periods between sets. That's definitely one way to build maximal strength. The rest time is necessary so you can lift your heaviest every time. This work uses the ATP-PC or anaerobic lactic energy system, whereas "pure cardio" uses the oxidative or aerobic energy system.

When lifting heavy, you may wonder why you need so much rest between sets when you don't feel like you're gasping-for-breath fatigued. Just because you don't feel out of breath doesn't mean your muscles didn't expend effort and don't need a chance to recover. You have to recognize that "pushing hard" and "working at 100 percent intensity" doesn't always mean you're going at a true 100 percent.

Have you ever noticed that the number of reps you can get done in an interval workout often decreases over the rounds? You may still *feel* like you're working as hard as you were at the beginning, but your body isn't able to give the same effort. This isn't a bad thing, but it does change the energy system you're working—and even what you're training.

It's also the reason you may feel like you're doing a ton of strength training right now but struggling to see the muscle gains you want. Are you actually giving yourself enough rest to lift as heavy as possible and push that progression with moves? Or do your workouts "feel" hard because you're out of breath and a little bit shaky because you always cut out rest?

During your lifting sessions, if you're using loads that allow you to move quickly and eliminate rest, you're turning your strength training into a cardio workout. Although it can feel hard, and lifting weights as conditioning can be useful, you won't gain muscle and strength, improve your metabolic health, and see the fabulous definition you want.

To use the strength-cardio continuum, you have to assess what type of output you want and determine how you want to push fatigue and failure based on your fitness level, goals, and schedule.

USING THE CONTINUUM

Workouts can work in multiple energy systems over the course of the session when you work along the continuum, including the glycolytic or anaerobic lactic energy system. This energy system is where a lot of interval training and hypertrophy (muscle-building) work happens.

It's not only that you're working in different energy systems along this continuum. You're also taking muscles to fatigue in different ways and increasing your calorie burn based on which muscles you're working and how you're working them in sessions.

If you think about this continuum from a time-efficiency standpoint, it's no wonder people often use the "I don't have enough time!" excuse. If you feel you need to do pure cardio and pure strength, you'd have to spend hours in the gym every day!

The "pure" ends of the continuum are often longer training sessions. If you're logging a lot of miles or doing maximum lifts, you need extra time because of the rest periods. I think it's important we note *why* these sessions are long so you don't fall victim to trying to make your sessions longer just because you've heard you need an hour or more in the gym. You don't.

If your workouts with the training protocols included in this program are long, it should only be because of set-up or prehab work. Not because you're adding *more*! The muscle-building protocols in this program live in the middle sweet spot of the continuum because they combine different variables to be efficient. I call the workout progressions "muscle-building" while labeling the bonus cardio session as "cardio" because of their primary focus. For example, the 6-12-25 method and compound burner sets live more fully on the strength side of that continuum, whereas the timed strength work can slide a little toward one side or the other a bit, which I'll cover.

Interval Work

High-intensity interval training (HIIT) and Tabata training have become very popular over the years. Some elitist trainers get a bit mad at how the use of these terms has evolved. People often use them to mean general hard interval work, or in the case of Tabata, any workout with 20 seconds of work and 10 seconds of rest. But Tabata and HIIT are two different things. Tabata, in its true form, is more what we would call sprint interval training, or SIT. HIIT has different meanings; it can be anything from power work to timed strength work. I'll discuss both methods for building muscle.

The muddying of definitions can be why people don't see the opportunity or value in the different interval designs. Not all interval work benefits you in the same way. The moves you choose to include and how you set up your work-to-rest intervals can affect the results you get—not only because of the workouts themselves but because of the effect they have when combined with other sessions.

So for creating effective routines to build strength and muscle to get and stay lean, I want to focus on SIT and power interval protocols in terms of interval work. These are more intense, more explosive, and shorter intervals than HIIT sessions.

When I cover timed strength work, I discuss some benefits of HIIT. HIIT sessions like these SIT and power protocols should be short. Sessions designed that way can be super efficient for muscle-building and fat loss when you have only 15 minutes to train. If they stretch to longer than 20 minutes of work, you're no longer doing the true protocols!

Because my muscle-building protocols are more metabolic and not as close to the pure strength end of the spectrum, you need to be conscious not to overdo the intensive cardio because it can fight against your muscle gains.

The steady-state cardio people often turn to for losing weight catabolizes muscle mass. Again, I'm not telling you *not* to include steady-state cardio, but you should consider the cost it has on the speed of achieving your goals. If you're going to include it, it may be worthwhile to consider including more strength workouts closer to that other end of the continuum to balance things out.

For now, I want to explain a little about SIT and power protocols and why they're beneficial. When you get to Part 3, you can select the sessions that match what you need!

NOTE: *Too often, people get caught up in a short-term focus rather than seeing the long-term value. Even if you're in love with an endurance sport and want to focus on performance, consider the value of strength and these protocols that can help with speed, power, and recovery for your long-term training goals. While focusing on fat loss and building muscle may have you cutting back on mileage in the short term, what you do to reach a goal isn't what you do to maintain it. The improvements you see over this time can have a long-term payoff!*

SIT/Power Protocols

Want to improve your body composition, speed, power, reaction times, recovery, heart health, insulin sensitivity, and so much more? Don't sleep on SIT and power work! This type of training becomes even more valuable as you get older, but it's often the training people back off of because it's "too intense."

However, this explosive, short, and intense quick training helps keep your body healthy, functionally fit, and leaner while retaining that amazingly magical muscle. These quick and dirty intervals are often what you need to age well and look your most fabulous. They're especially helpful for women who have to navigate the hormonal changes of menopause.

Defining SIT and Power Work

SIT and power work are short intervals of high-intensity work during which you exert max effort. It can be anything: sprinting by running, all-out effort on a bike, some explosive lifts, or medicine ball drills and burpees. Select an exercise you can go all-out on and work for no more than 30 seconds. If you can go longer than 30 seconds, then your intensity isn't high enough.

Your work intervals with this type of training are eight to 30 seconds depending on exactly which protocol or type of work you're doing. Rest intervals vary based on your goals. You might rest for half of your work time up to five times the time you work. With both SIT and power work, you're trying to work at maximal effort. Both types of training are done in short sessions because of this intensity.

If you're training pure speed and explosive power, you do power work intervals with shorter work periods (8 to 12 seconds) and longer rest periods (40 to 60 seconds). At the end of the rest, you need to be itching to go again to truly be training explosiveness. If you're slowing down because you're not resting long enough, you're training ... well ... slowness. A huge benefit of this work is to improve your mind-body connection and reaction times. All of this helps you not only recover better and be functionally fit but also lift more! Being able to lift more in your sessions and improve your maximal strength will help you see amazing body recomp!

If you're using the SIT protocols, your intervals of work may be a bit longer than with the power work (from 8 to 30 seconds), but your rest may be shorter. You want to keep that true 100 percent intensity while almost pushing your body past failure. You're resting just long enough to keep the pace during each interval but not really long enough to feel recovered. This means you may rest for half the work interval to up to two or three times longer than the work interval. This is what creates amazing metabolic and conditioning benefits.

Knowing Why to Include These Protocols

Honestly, everyone should be including these protocols in some form as appropriate for their fitness level. If you're rebuilding from injury, you may be more limited in how you can use the protocols.

But as soon as you can, you want to include power work and SIT training because they truly make you metabolically healthier, stronger, and leaner. They're the perfect complement to your muscle-building protocols for feeling and looking your most fabulous at any age. They're also amazingly efficient! Even just 5 minutes can go a long way!

These protocols help you balance your hormone levels, something that's especially important as you get older and your body isn't as able to use protein as efficiently or recover as quickly. These protocols help address changes in insulin sensitivity during perimenopause, menopause, and postmenopause, which may help you avoid gaining the dreaded "menopot" or middle-age spread. For real, you can stop blaming your age and writing this off as inevitable! These protocols—but especially SIT—help, and a big reason is that they work in that energy system between pure strength or pure cardio. Even though they're often labeled "cardio," they can assist in building muscle, unlike steady-state cardio, which is often catabolic.

Power work helps with reaction times and neuromuscular efficiency (aka a stronger mind-body connection). SIT protocols have been shown to decrease fat mass and increase muscle mass and even aerobic capacity. They've also been shown to help with a reduction in fat—specifically in abdominal/visceral fat. Furthermore, these improvements were enhanced by doing muscle-building protocols in combination with the power work. YAY!

Another incredible feature of these protocols is that they benefit you beyond the time you're doing them. The workouts aren't just about the calories burned *during* a session. They can improve your fat-burning after your workout, and they keep your metabolism healthier so it burns more calories overall during the day.

NOTE: *Some of the SIT/power protocols, which are essential if you're entering those perimenopausal, menopausal, and postmenopausal years, technically fall on the strength side of the continuum, and you'll be tempted to cut out rest. Don't do it! These protocols can also help you improve your speed for the steady-state cardio you may love!*

Using These Protocols

Part 3 includes some different SIT and power work protocols. These sessions should be short: usually 5 to 8 rounds, and never more than 10 rounds. Just two or three sessions done weekly can pay off. They don't have to be sessions on their own. However, if your focus is on power and speed, doing a power work session before you lift may be key.

SIT can be great to include after workouts that target your more "stubborn" areas of fat. You mobilize more fatty acids from tissues surrounding the muscles you worked. Then you utilize these mobilized fatty acids with these high-intensity conditioning intervals. Win-win! However, if you include a SIT session after your strength work, you will be more fatigued going into it, especially if you're running after a lower body day.

Keep these sessions short and start with just one per week. When you first start, you might find it helpful to do these protocols on a recovery day. Because they're short and intensive, they shouldn't negatively impact your training session the day after.

However, if you're using the timed strength work, you might not include any SIT or power work sessions to start because those strength workouts are already more metabolic, and some implement HIIT.

With all of the protocols I talk about, remember three things: Design with intention. Design with purpose. Design for the time you have.

There are many ways to use all of these techniques to match what you need, so refer back to your STRONG systems from Part 1 to assess what you're doing now and where your biggest (but also the easiest) opportunities for change are!

The Fat-Burning Cardio Everyone Should Do

There's one form of cardio that everyone should be doing. It's not sexy, but it's essential, and it's probably the best kept body recomp maintenance secret out there. The best fat-burning cardio is ...

WALKING!

As amazing and necessary as SIT and power protocols are to body recomp and overall health, walking is the perfect recovery cardio to complement them. It's a tool everyone has in their toolbox, and it's a form of cardio you can do no matter your fitness level or age, yet most people ignore it as an option!

Walking is a great form of cardio for a variety of reasons:

» It works in the fat-burning zone.

» It doesn't stress your body.

» It helps you maintain hormonal balance while allowing you to be more active and burn more calories to maintain your body composition without the stress of a full training session.

» It's amazing for destressing your mind.

You've probably heard that you should move more throughout the day, and walking is the perfect form of movement you need. It's truly good for not only your physical but mental health.

You can't just add more and more intensive exercise without reaching a point of diminishing returns. Also, although more intensive forms of training may burn more calories during the session, they raise cortisol levels and take longer to recover from. This constant stress can backfire.

With walking, you burn fewer calories than with steady-state running, but more of the calories you're burning are from fat. This can help you stay leaner without any negative impact on your muscle mass. It can also improve hormone regulation and production and help you prevent insulin resistance, especially if you're going through menopause.

Walking after a session where you've mobilized more fatty acids from stubborn areas can help with fat loss. You might even choose to use walking after a session where you want to lose fat but also have struggled to build muscle in that same area. The reduced level of strain and greater percentage of calories burned coming from fat can be beneficial.

Trying to hit about 7,000 to 10,000 steps a day is a great way to maintain your lean physique and stay functionally fit and healthy. However, when you're first starting out, even 10 to 15 minutes per day of walking can go a long way!

The 6-12-25 Method

Diversity yields the best results. This training technique helps you use diversity to your advantage as you combine different rep ranges and different types of movements to help you zero in on stubborn areas and work muscles fully to fatigue.

This method requires you to let go of a lot of the common "fears" of working out that people can fall victim to, including these:

» Higher reps and lighter loads
» Heavy weights and low reps
» Isolation moves
» Rest
» Not doing one exercise at a time
» Not sticking to just body part splits

This workout design goes against what I call "bro splits" that you often see in mainstream bodybuilding magazines. But that is exactly why it works. You may not believe it, but this method actually *is* a more traditional, although advanced, lifting technique popularized by Charles Poliquin, although it never fully made it mainstream—until now.

First, let me break down what the 6-12-25 method is and how it works; then I'll discuss how to use it in your weekly schedule and explain why you may want to include it based on your needs and goals.

What Is the 6-12-25 Method?

The name of this method states exactly the reps you'll be performing during the workout: 6 reps, 12 reps, and 25 reps. With this method, not only do the reps change over the series but so do the types of moves and loads/weights you're using. You do a different move for each of those rep counts, and you do the moves back to back before you rest. You want each move to work the same muscle group, and you progress from 6 reps of a more compound move to 25 reps of an isolation exercise.

An example is a series with 6 reps of front squat, 12 reps (on each side) of front lunges, and then 25 reps on each side of a quad or leg extension. Your main focus is your legs, especially your quads. Over the course of the series, you go from a heavier compound lift near that maximal strength rep range to a still compound but accessory lift at the top of the hypertrophy rep range to end with an isolation exercise in the strength endurance rep range that targets the prime mover you worked in the first two exercises (your quads).

While no weights should ever feel light, your loads will get lighter as the reps go up. You'll feel your legs, especially your quads, fatiguing more and more with each move, making each weight at each set rep number feel harder than it may when done alone.

Do all three moves without resting; then you need to rest at least 90 seconds and up to 3 minutes between rounds. The variation in rest may be based on how experienced a lifter you are. Especially with the 25-rep exercise, you may find a little rest-pause technique pushes you past failure, so you need those full 3 minutes to maintain the same weight, if not go heavier on the 6 reps in your next round.

If your primary focus is on muscle, you want to push the weights enough that you crave the full 3 minutes of rest. If your primary focus is on fat loss, you may push the weights but embrace a little fatigue as long as your form doesn't falter by resting for only 2 minutes.

You'll do 2 to 4 rounds of the series before resting for up to 3 minutes and performing a second 6-12-25 series for another muscle group depending on how you design your weekly schedule.

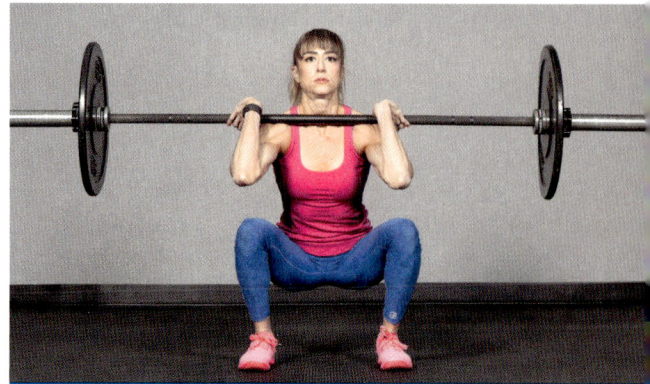

6 reps FRONT SQUATS

12 reps FRONT LUNGES

25 reps QUAD EXTENSIONS

NOTE: *Rest-pause technique is where you do as many of the 25 reps as you can, say 15, then pause for 15 to 20 seconds to finish out the full 25 reps with the weight. This can be a great way to push past failure with quality reps. But this will create extra fatigue, so make sure your form is good and you can maintain quality work in the following rounds!*

How and Why Does It Work So Well?

This method is so effective because of the combination of three traditional rep ranges, compound and isolation movements, and the targeting of specific muscle groups to create full fatigue in an area.

Combining many training techniques into one design results in a greater training density, which leads to massive lactate spikes and increased growth hormone production. That's why it's thought to work so well. As a result, this method can not only lead to amazing muscle gains but better fat loss.

With the heavy compound exercise done for 6 reps, you're working at that maximal strength range. Over time, you help yourself be able to lift more quality loads, resulting in more strength and muscle gained. These moves also create more muscle tissue damage, which can be a driver of muscle growth. As you progress with this design, consider selecting a move that forces you to pause after the fifth rep for a few seconds to complete the final rep. You want to err on the side of being able to do only 5 reps rather than being able to complete 7.

When you're doing the 12-rep exercise, you select a compound move that's a great accessory exercise to target the same muscle groups. This will allow you to really utilize that hypertrophy rep range and continue to fatigue the muscles you worked in the first move. The perfect moves to use are more unilateral (one sided) or those you just can't go as heavy with because you would struggle to max out at 6 reps.

NOTE: *You never want to stop at a rep number just because it's what the workout said. You want to feel that it's all you can do.*

The higher reps and slightly lower, albeit challenging, loads allow you to recruit more muscle fibers as you fatigue, but you're still using heavy loads. It's another way to push past failure and recruit more muscle fibers. Many of these moves create more mechanical tension to drive muscle growth.

Then, with the final move, you isolate a muscle group to work it fully to fatigue. This helps build that strength endurance, which will ultimately help you recover faster and do more quality work in future workouts and progressions.

This isolation move combined with an increased volume of work is a great way to help you build muscle in stubborn muscle groups. Make sure this move really isolates the muscle you want to target. You want to feel that pump or burn add up at 15 to 20 reps so you have to pause for a second to complete all 25. This ensures you're recruiting more muscle fibers as the fatigue adds up to stimulate better muscle growth in those stubborn areas. With this move, you're often creating more metabolic stress, which is that third driver of muscle growth.

Don't cut out rest! Honestly, you should crave rest for longer than the 3 minutes if you're truly seeing each drop in load and increase in reps and isolation as a way to push past failure. However, if you aren't used to lifting near that maximal strength range or have injuries that dictate you can't go as heavy, you may find that ninety seconds of rest allows you to push hard but feel the fatigue build.

The way you design the series going from more compound to more isolated can be used to your advantage to focus on your specific stubborn areas. You can also use it to really target those big muscles that may not get fatigued during your heavy compound lifts.

For example, you could design a 6-12-25 series to be bench press, chest flys, and triceps extensions if you really want to zero in on your triceps, but you could also do bench press, dips, and then chest flys if you find you struggle to fully fatigue your chest during the other moves as your shoulders or triceps limit you.

The rest only between sets allows for fatigue to build over the moves but then allows you to rest long enough to be able to lift heavy again starting with 6 reps. How you adjust your rest between sets and resting for longer can move you toward the strength side of the continuum. You can also choose to include a single heavy compound lift before any 6-12-25 series if you want to gain muscle while losing fat. Alternatively, you could do a SIT protocol after your two 6-12-25 series if your goal is fat loss while retaining muscle.

This combination of different movements and drivers of muscle growth while working an area to fatigue is what makes this series so challenging and leads to such amazingly efficient muscle and strength gains, but the back-to-back movements also mean this workout has metabolic benefits for fat loss.

How Should I Set Up My Weekly Schedule?

If you have only 15 to 20 minutes to train, I recommend you not start with this method. Instead, check out the "Timed Strength Work Techniques" section later in this chapter. If three days per week is your ideal, the compound burner sets method may be slightly better, but you can also make three days per week work with the anterior/posterior split (see Part 3). The 6-12-25 method is ideal if you have about 45 to 60 minutes and four to six days a week to train.

You want to design for the time you have because if you miss a session, you aren't going to get the full value of the workout progression. Everything is designed to work together to strategically create training density and frequency not only in individual workouts but over the weeks! Too often, people get caught up in looking at workouts in isolation, but how the sessions work together over a three- to six-week progression is what matters.

Part 3 includes not only a workout builder to design your own 6-12-25 but two different weekly splits: anterior/posterior (more frontside and backside muscles targeted) and hemisphere (upper/lower). The 6-12-25 method is best done when two or three muscle groups are being worked in a session; more than one 6-12-25 per muscle group is often far too much volume.

Of course, there is always a "but," and that "but" is that if you're short on time and doing six days a week, you may choose to do one compound lift for an area and then a single series of 6-12-25 for the same muscle group on that day. However, a hemisphere split is my recommendation, just with a more anterior/posterior focus based on the day.

Using a single lift at the start of one of your workouts can be great if your primary focus is on building muscle. If your primary goal is fat loss, you may choose to include a SIT session after your 6-12-25 series are complete.

The SIT may be better implemented with the hemisphere design than with the anterior/posterior option because it's working upper and lower in one session. It may surprise you how much it gets your heart rate up already, and the SIT is overkill!

You'll find in the progressions laid out, there are also details on how to include SIT, walking, power work, and even recovery sessions based on your schedule. But don't jump to Part 3 already, as much as you want to; because while this design may sound amazing, you need to know if it's truly best for you right now.

Who's This Method Best For?

I mentioned 6-12-25 was designed and popular for bodybuilding, but based on how and why this training works, it may be even better for all of us "normal people" who are struggling to see recomp. The more advanced an exerciser you are (the longer you've been training and the more types of training and volume you've done over the years), the more you've adapted to. That makes it harder to keep creating progression to drive changes.

Muscle gains slow the more advanced you are. You'd think it would be easier, but it's not because you can simply handle more! Your ability to handle more stresses and physical challenges is a good thing for life … just not when it comes to your aesthetic goals. But that's why this method helps. It uses a combination of techniques you may not have used in this way before. And the way it creates that hormonal response and uses multiple drivers of muscle growth is where the magic is!

So if you're struggling to build muscle, this needs to be your go-to method, especially with the hormonal changes of perimenopause and menopause or if you're finding yourself struggling to retain lean muscle postmenopause. When your hormone levels are simply no longer optimal, you need something that optimizes your body's response. This protocol does just that.

Don't fear the heavy weights. Don't fear the isolation moves or lighter loads. Don't fear pushing that intensity and your body to failure. This technique helps you do it in a safe way to drive growth!

Even if you're just starting back to training, don't fear this design. It can be a great way to create volume as you safely challenge yourself with harder moves for 6 reps. However, I will say that the compound burner sets or even the interval strength/density intervals in the timed strength work may be better. The more you can push that weight and those harder variations on those heavy compound 6-rep lifts, the better your results will be.

Regress to progress! Remember just because you did lift heavy or you feel like you "can" lift a weight doesn't mean your body is ready to. Your muscles may still be strong enough, but your connective tissues can become deconditioned. So rebuilding and meeting yourself where you are now is crucial!

One last thing: This method can also be great if you're still logging the miles, especially if you go with more of a hemisphere split. It can be great to build your strength and endurance if you want to help yourself PR in an endurance sport.

Should I Use This Method?

Now, go back to the R in your STRONG system and consider what is a repeatable habit for you. What is a design that works with the time you have? Not the time you'd like to have but the schedule you know you can easily hit? If you know you can do three or four days, maybe you use this design but with an anterior/posterior split to make sure everything is covered if you fall one day short. Or if you know you can do four days easily but you want to include that SIT or your other runs, you do more of a hemisphere split. On the other hand, maybe after reflecting, you decide that as amazing as this design sounds, you're ready to check out the other options, and you see opportunity in this for another time.

Do more than assess your schedule. Assess where you're starting from. Are you rebuilding after an injury? Maybe you aren't yet ready to try to test a 6-rep heavy lift. But if you've been lifting super heavy without seeing gains, maybe you jump in.

Is this design something that you feel would complement your targets or even other performance goals you set, like pull-up or push-up improvements? (This can help with that!) Or is this design something so outside your comfort zone that you aren't yet ready to embrace it, and you need to try one of the other designs closer to what you're doing now (while optimizing and owning your past struggles)?

NOTE: Go back through your STRONG system and don't get caught up in how awesome this protocol is on its own.

All of them are fabulous and made even better when you use them based on what you need.

Compound Burner Sets

If you've ever struggled to build muscle in a specific muscle group, this workout design leaves those muscles nowhere to hide! Over the course of the year, as you cycle between these different protocols and techniques, the 6-12-25 and compound burner sets build especially well together.

What Are Compound Burner Sets?

You may have heard of compound sets—which are sometimes labeled as supersets—but the "burner" in this name is there for a reason.

First, compound sets traditionally are two moves done back to back for the same muscle group—think barbell back rows and inverted rows. Supersets are technically two moves done back to back but for different muscle groups—think bench press and bent-over row or even bench press and squats.

With compound burner sets, you're not only working the same muscle group with back-to-back moves, but you're making that second move more of an isolation exercise to zero in on one muscle worked with the first move. You also change the rep range on each move. While the first move for an area may be in that 6- to 12-rep range and is a compound exercise done with heavier loads, the second move done right after is in that 15- to 25-rep range and more of an isolation move to fully fatigue a muscle worked in the first move.

There is no rest between the two moves, which leads to "burning out" a muscle group then resting 90 seconds to 2 minutes between sets. This rest doesn't feel like enough, and each round you may find it harder and

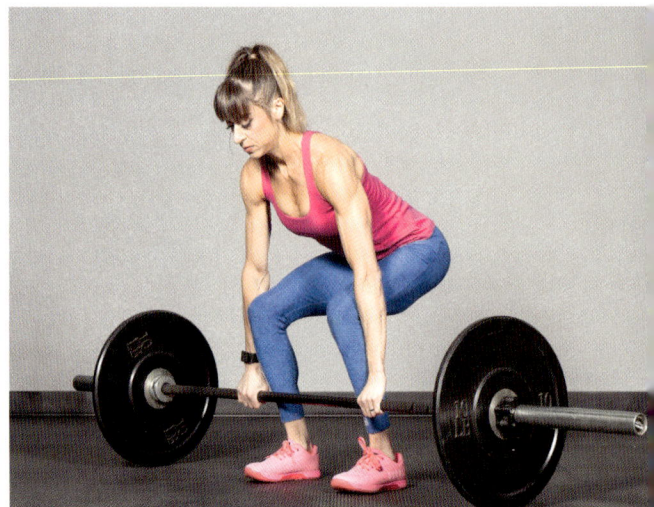

6 to 12 reps DEADLIFTS

15 to 25 reps GLUTE BRIDGES AND CURLS

harder to maintain the same weights; you might slightly lower the reps to maintain the loads you used in previous rounds or use the rest-pause technique (see page 128 in the 6-12-25 method) to complete the same number of reps.

You will do 2 to 4 rounds through the compound burner set. How many rounds you do is partly based on how you split up your weekly training schedule and partly based on how advanced you are and the training volume you're used to.

The back-to-back moves combine compound sets with post-exhaust technique. This means you're fully fatiguing an area worked during the first move.

How and Why Does It Work So Well?

With compound burner sets, you're taking a muscle past fatigue and failure to recruit more muscle fibers and create metabolic stress and mechanical tension to drive growth—just as you do with the 6-12-25 method. You're able to lift heavier loads while creating a great volume of work for a muscle. The slightly shorter rest periods also help create a greater training density, meaning you're doing more work in less time. These things combined are what drive your gains!

While normal post-exhaust technique doesn't have to be implemented as a set with another move, it does help you more fully exhaust the area. It creates that beneficial training density (how much work you're doing in a set amount of time). It's not only more work that leads to results but also the timeframe in which that work is happening. That's the benefit of timed strength work, which we'll get into in the next protocol!

The simplicity of the two moves done back to back with rest periods can also help you work in that middle space on the strength-cardio continuum, where you can technically tap into your glycolytic or anaerobic lactic energy system—specifically, slow glycolysis. This can be great for improving hormone levels and insulin sensitivity to build muscle. It can also improve your recovery time and work capacity to bust through any plateaus you may be seeing or push that progression your body needs as your hormone levels aren't as optimal as you get older.

Unlike 6-12-25, which involves performing two compound lifts back to back, compound burner sets include only one compound lift. This design helps you to push closer to your maximum effort within the hypertrophy rep range rather than entering that rep range already fatigued from the initial lift. This design is also a bit less volume per set than the 6-12-25, which can allow you to cover more areas in your workout over a few different compound burner sets.

If fat loss is your goal, and you're limited on how many days you can train, consider more full-body workouts using this technique. These full-body routines can help you get better results in fewer sessions by burning more calories per session while targeting stubborn areas more frequently over the week.

Also, unlike the 6-12-25 protocol in which there are set numbers to hit and a bit more precision in selecting your weights, with this design, you have the ability to use double progression to your advantage, which can be significant if you've hit a plateau in your lifts. For your first move, you can start with a weight you can do 12 reps with. If you fatigue, you can use rest-pause to stick at 12 reps if your form is good, but you can also go down in reps to 10 to maintain the same weight rather than reducing your loads.

The next week, you can stick with that weight to see if you can get 12 reps for all the rounds. This double form of progression can be helpful because people do hit ceilings with weights. Another way it can work is to increase to the next weight by dropping from doing 12 reps to 6. You can then stick at that weight as you work back up to 12 reps with that compound move. This double form of progression is so beneficial if you're feeling stuck!

This design is also easier if you use unilateral, or one-sided, exercises on both moves in the set; this enables you to correct imbalances if you have any. However, if you're short on time, doing bilateral moves back to back will be quicker because doing two unilateral moves back to back can make a workout longer, and cutting out rest isn't always an option. In moves like lunges, both legs often need the full rest time between sets; however, if you're doing a unilateral move like a single-arm press and the other arm does get to fully rest, you may use that active rest to shorten your workout duration while not seeing a detriment in your strength and output.

How Should I Set Up My Weekly Schedule?

The compound burner sets design plays well with 6-12-25 but isn't ideal if you're super limited on time, although it can work well if you only have three days to train. You can make the workouts full body, use an anterior/posterior split, or even do a hemisphere split. However, I *don't* recommend you use the hemisphere version if you aren't super advanced and haven't already been doing high training volume.

And now for the "but": Unless you do want more frequent but shorter workouts or you plan to do fewer rounds to target a few more areas more frequently, compound burner sets mean a lot of volume per workout. You can include two or three compound burner sets in a program. Like with the 6-12-25 protocol, you can also do a single heavy lift to start the workout if strength and muscle are your primary focus. Or you can include a SIT protocol to end your session if fat loss is your goal.

Because of the strength endurance work with this method, it can be great for an off-season cycle if you're an endurance athlete. You may include the power work interval session before you do the compound burner sets. There are so many options and opportunities with this protocol!

Part 3 includes the workout builder to design your own workouts. I've also included a three-day-a-week full-body split and four-day-a-week anterior/posterior split. With straight lifting, the schedule is often only three or four days a week, but you're still hitting areas two or three times a week. This configuration allows for some flexibility in your schedule but also allows you not to skip the necessary prehab and recovery work.

In Part 3, I include one five-day-a-week lifting hemisphere option for those advanced trainees who really need volume to bust through a plateau. But that progression is a ton of volume that requires a recovery week and a shorter duration on that progression. The body part splits often dictate lifting five days a week no matter what, but you're often hitting areas less frequently even though you're lifting on a fifth day.

Remember, you're going to have to do some things that feel awkward and different than what you've always done. Because of the intensity of these sessions, you should crave the lower intensity training sessions between.

Another thing to bear in mind when selecting your workouts is that you will also want to stick with the same progression for at least three to six weeks.

Who's This Method Best For?

If you're an advanced lifter who's hit a plateau, if you're struggling with a number of stubborn muscle groups that just don't seem to grow (especially postmenopause), or if you're an endurance athlete who wants to focus on building strength to improve your endurance training, this protocol is for you.

Although this technique doesn't require the lifting experience of the 6-12-25, you want to be conscious of truly maxing out on the reps listed rather than stopping at 12 reps for the first move because that's the top end of the range.

Also, you might be tempted to cut back on rest because you won't feel as out of breath as often. *Do not do that*. It'll backfire and lead to you not seeing the full muscle-gaining benefits you should.

If you're currently doing a ton of volume, really want to focus on muscle gains, and have more days to train, consider the hemisphere split. However, if you're an endurance athlete and still logging high mileage, consider only the three-day-a-week full-body option. This leads to less fatigue of muscles on a single day but still offers enough volume over the week.

Should I Use This Protocol?

I'm going to ask you again to go back to your STRONG system and consider what is a repeatable habit for you. Really assess where you're starting from and the different targets you've set. What design works for the time you have? Don't think about what you'd like to do; consider the schedule you know you can easily hit. If you know you can do three to four days, maybe you use this design but with a full-body or anterior/posterior split to make sure everything is covered if you fall one day short. Or do three days because your runs require longer distances on other days and you really don't want to cut them out; they're a nonnegotiable right now!

Or maybe after reflecting, as amazing as this design sounds, you're ready to check out the other options. You might see the opportunity in this for another time because you really need something that allows you to get your workout done in less than 30 minutes right now!

Just remember to assess your STRONG system honestly:

? Where are you starting from?

? What's a realistic schedule?

? Would this design help you hit your complementary targets?

? Is this design too far outside your comfort zone or just the push you need?

? Does this allow you to own your nonnegotiables and optimize your plan?

Remember you're designing based on what you need now—not just the goals you want to reach!

Timed Strength Work Techniques

When you think about intervals, or timed workouts, your brain probably instantly thinks cardio. When HIIT workouts became all the rage, people started to see timed training only as a way to get the blood pumping. I know when I used to think about strength workouts, my question was always, "How many reps and sets?" not "How long should I work?"

But intervals and timed sets are amazing techniques to use to build strength. In this section, I break down three different variations of timed strength work you can implement to use training density to your advantage.

This approach to training density is different from the usual approach of adding more reps and sets, which means more time spent in the gym to try to achieve results. Instead of adding volume and causing the length of the workouts to get longer, timed strength work forces you to create a great volume of work or move more loads in a set time frame to increase training density.

The focus for this timed strength work is on building muscle because muscle is magical for ... well ... everything you want to achieve in life, especially being functionally fit and independent for all the days you're on this planet. However, I want to touch on how implementing this type of training strategically can also benefit you for metabolic cardio purposes.

I mentioned earlier that HIIT has had many different definitions. Now, it's often used to mean any interval workout. Honestly, if you do an internet search for definitions, you'll find a ton. Originally, HIIT was a short all-out sprint burst of 8 to 12 seconds with long rest periods of three to five times the rest to work. Then Tabata became one of the most popular HIIT strategies in its original form of 20 seconds on, 10 seconds off for just 8 rounds of sprinting all-out. This was supposed to be done at 170 percent of your VO2 max.

However, over time, Tabata training has become any 20/10 interval workout, and the intensity of those 20 seconds of work has really changed. HIIT morphed in definition as well. SIT became a better term for short sprint work and all-out 100 percent max-out effort. HIIT is now interval work that's greater than 80 percent effort but not max-out intensity done for intervals of work at about that minute or longer time frame with variable rest to keep that intensity high.

NOTE: *VO2 max refers to the maximum amount of oxygen that you can utilize during intense or maximal exercise. It's your maximal aerobic capacity, and in general, the higher your VO2 max, the better your aerobic conditioning.*

I bring this up because if you're short on time, timed strength work can double as some of your important conditioning work based on how you tweak reps and sets, the moves you include, and even how you load movements. Things aren't set in being used in just one way! There are many options and opportunities.

I'll start by highlighting the three different timed strength work techniques that can help you see amazing muscle and metabolic improvements, especially if your excuse for not seeing results has often been, "But I don't have enough time!"

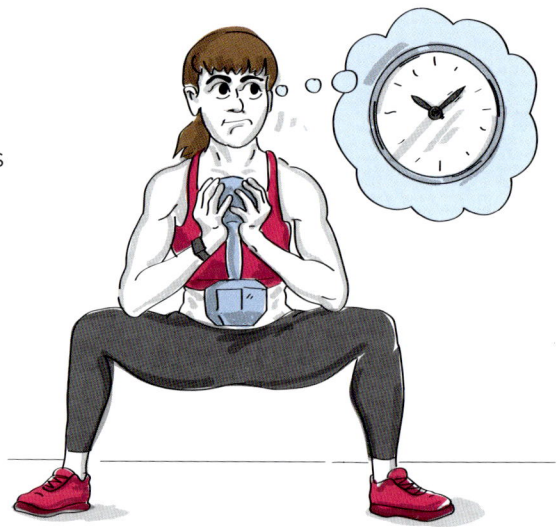

What Are the Three Types of Timed Strength Work?

The three techniques are

- » **Density training/density sets**
- » **Strength intervals**
- » **Density intervals**

All three of these techniques are great ways to help you fit in a workout even if you have only 5 minutes to work out. While 15 to 30 minutes is ideal, part of why these techniques are so fabulous as shorter sessions is that they're timed. You know exactly how long your workout will take, and you can't really rush through. You have to work for the set time!

Not only are you guaranteed to be done when you need to be, but you can also help yourself stay focused on the quality of your work and be intentional with your movements because you can't really get done any faster.

With these designs, the devil is in the details. (Honestly, as I've said before, nuance and seeing opportunity in tweaks are everything with all of these systems.) One small change can have an impact.

I mention this because strength intervals and density intervals especially have overlap, although strength intervals are often slightly longer than density intervals. Both use intervals ranging from 20 seconds to 1 minute on a move and cycle areas worked in supersets, compound sets, or even circuits (honestly, even trisets or quad sets—lots of options!).

Strength Intervals

With strength intervals, you want to cycle the areas you work back to back so that one area can rest as another is working. This allows areas to recover while still "saving time." So, think about alternating upper and lower or front and back muscles. The intervals also push you to do more reps than you would have done otherwise had you just had a rep range of 8 to 12 reps in a shorter time frame.

When you use these intervals to focus on building strength and muscle, don't go light just to make it through the time you've set to work. You want to almost force yourself to have to pause for a very brief couple of seconds to keep going with the weight or exercise variation. (Again implementing the rest-pause technique I've brought up before! YAY! So many uses!) You don't want to turn this into cardio with weights.

You will want to include an interval of rest after completing the moves outlined. Supersets, trisets, and quad sets or circuits work best in intervals of 30 seconds to 1 minute.

Density Intervals

With density intervals, you're creating more volume of work for an area in a shorter amount of time, and you'll need a full rest. But you aren't just working longer on one move for the same body part; you're using back-to-back moves to target the same area in different ways.

This may mean the same move with different tools, ranges of motion, or tempos, or you might make slight tweaks to position and posture. An example of this may be a goblet squat for one interval followed by a goblet squat pulse for a second interval and then a slow eccentric goblet squat for a third interval. These changes in tempos and ranges of motion may require different weights as you do them back to back, but they drive growth in different ways and create the training volume with quality work. They can also help you work past failure for a muscle group.

You can also use different types of moves for the same muscle group in back-to-back intervals, whether you use two compound moves, use a compound move and isolation move, or go from more compound to more isolated over the moves in the series as you would with the 6-12-25 method.

The key with this specific tweak to the density intervals is that you're focused on that back-to-back work for the same area. You must plan for full rest between rounds because you aren't cycling the areas you work.

Compound sets, compound burner sets, or trisets work well for this design, with intervals of work from 20 seconds to 1 minute, depending also on how many moves you're doing back to back. You can use multiple work intervals as you cycle through the moves based on the difficulty of moves just like you use multiple rep ranges in back-to-back exercises.

Density Training/Density Sets

Density training or density sets are longer timed series of work. Instead of intervals for each move, you're setting a time frame of 5 to 15 minutes to work to complete as many reps and rounds of a series as you can.

CrossFit has called these AMRAPs (as many rounds as possible) because you're trying to complete a series as many times as possible in a set time frame. But density training and density sets don't have the same focus as AMRAP, which is more metabolic. The emphasis with AMRAPs is on HIIT and metabolic conditioning *instead* of maintaining a focus on strength. And the rep ranges and types of moves you may include would differ between both. You may use a slightly higher rep range with the HIIT version with moves that push to get your blood pumping.

However, this also shows the benefit and diversity of options with these designs. You could include a combination of density sets and AMRAPs based on your goals to really embrace that middle space on the strength-cardio continuum!

With density training for strength, you will set your time frame, ideally about 10 minutes. Pick one to three moves. It's best to alternate the areas of the body you're working so one area can rest while the other works to maximize the volume (number of reps and rounds) as well as the total loads lifted in a session.

You will work most often in that 5- to 10-rep range to build muscle and strength with a focus on mainly compound moves. Select a weight or exercise variation for a move that you max out at about 10 reps. You may do only 5 to 8 reps with this weight or move, keeping a few reps in reserve so you aren't too tired to keep moving through the series.

Over the rounds, you will end up completing a lot of reps with a heavier weight than you may have been able to use for that volume had you done higher reps. As you fatigue, don't be afraid to do 3 or 4 reps in a row if needed to be able to keep moving without reducing weight! You may include the occasional isolation exercise, especially in the third set. If you do, you may increase to 15 reps and use that slightly to create a pump in another muscle being worked. Include 2 or 3 different timed sets in your routine, although even one 15-minute set is where this design can come in handy when you're short on time!

How and Why Do They Work So Well?

The more quality weight you lift, the stronger you're going to get. Intervals or timed sets help you get in more high-quality work in a condensed time. This training density is what yields amazing results.

With the strength and density intervals, you create a greater training volume to push past failure. And you can do so in multiple ways, such as the two moves back to back for the same muscle group with the density intervals. You also allow yourself to truly stay intentional and not just stop because you hit the top of the rep range. This can be a great way to really make sure you're training to push that progression.

With density sets, you're often able to lift more weight in the set session because with low reps that build volume, you get in more working rounds. When done right, this is deceptively brutal but often easier to optimize as you become more advanced and comfortable in that maximal strength rep range. You need to be able to max out at about 5 to 10 reps; you may even fatigue enough to be able to do only 4 reps toward the final rounds. This requires experience with lifting heavy.

You won't hit failure with this design, but you will be surprised, after totaling your reps and sets and weights, how much more weight you moved in the workout than you would have with your standard reps and sets. This is what makes this design brutal and makes it work so well for building strength and muscle.

With these three techniques, you're going against the "extend your workout to do more" attitude and approach, and instead "forcing" more work to be done in a set amount of time, which is what positively impacts the training density you're able to do. So, if you've blamed a lack of time for not being able to see results, you haven't tried these amazing workouts!

Creating Your Weekly Schedule

All of these timed strength work designs are super efficient, especially when you're short on time. You can use them whether you have three days a week to train or six. One of the best parts about timed workouts is that you know exactly how long the session will take, especially if you also do intervals for your prehab work. (And that's super easy to do; I offer a layout for it in Part 3.)

The more certain you can be that your workout will wrap up in the time you have, the less you rush through, and the more likely you are to do it!

With strength and density intervals, you can do full-body, hemisphere, anterior/posterior, or even body part splits based on your schedule. I gravitate toward the full-body or anterior/posterior options because those create a greater training frequency and volume over the week, especially since these designs are ideal even when you have minimal equipment. If you have just 5 minutes on five or six days a week, you may decide a density interval workout that focuses on one area each day is best. Opportunity in the options! Remember there is no right or wrong unless it doesn't meet you where you are. So optimize your repeatable routine around yourself. (That's what the O and R in STRONG are for!)

With density sets, I recommend a schedule of three to four days a week because this design is deceptively brutal when done for 2 to 3 sets of 10 minutes each and you really max out on weight. You may choose to do five or six days if you're doing more of a hemisphere design with some metabolic circuits. But if you do a full-body or anterior/posterior design, you'll be amazed at how much you need the recovery between days. This is where that walking cardio and those recovery sessions in Part 3 can be great to stay active between lifts!

Because these techniques sit a bit more toward that cardio end of the strength-cardio continuum, I suggest walking as the bonus cardio. However, you could add SIT a couple of times a week to the strength or density intervals or one of your density training sets could easily be turned into a HIIT series. You could also include just a bit of power work on a recovery day for a few rounds with long rest to recover, but note you may be fatigued the first couple of weeks going into that work.

Who's This Method Best For?

Short on time? Training at home? Are you an advanced lifter who's struggling to build strength and muscle? Timed strength work can be amazing for all of these situations. These techniques are diverse in their use and implementation.

Because these techniques use volume to help you see amazing results, they can be great to use when training at home. You do need to progress bodyweight moves through variations, tempos, and the ranges of motion you use, but a slightly greater amount of work or volume to your sessions helps create that challenge and progression. With intervals, you'll often push yourself to do more reps than you would have if you were just counting reps.

The density sets are a kick in the butt if you're working to build strength to drive better muscle gains, but you have to have experience lifting heavy to optimize these unless you're going the bodyweight route. That low-rep range of 5 to 10 reps for heavy loads is what keeps this design toward the strength end of the continuum rather than making it purely cardio.

Because these techniques are more metabolic or super intensive due to the loads and pushing work capacity, they're not something I'd recommend if you're already logging a ton of miles with your endurance sport. However, short, timed strength work may be something you could use as you wean off the lifting and focus more on maintenance as you near your race. You may just shift it to more of an activation focus.

And if you're worried about form or short on time, these timed designs help you make sure your workout fits the time you have available. You focus not on counting reps but on what you feel working as the timer ticks down. Of course, counting reps to see if you can do one more rep the next week can be helpful for creating progression, but focus on what you need most to start!

Should I Use This Protocol?

Once again, I'm going to ask you to go back to your STRONG system and consider what a repeatable habit is for you. Assess where you are now and the different targets you've set. Also consider what has caused you to struggle in the past and own your nonnegotiables.

These timed strength techniques can help you design for the time you have with so much flexibility to create options for home on those days you can't make it to the gym. Honestly, if you're planning to do the compound burner sets or 6-12-25, you may have a few timed strength workouts in your back pocket when things don't go as planned. That's what I do. The more prepared you are with a plan B in place, even if it's not your ideal, the more you still do *something* and keep the momentum building!

With regard to where you're starting from, have you been lifting super heavy but not seeing gains? Are you stuck with those traditional reps-and-sets bodybuilding designs? Take a risk! Often the change people are most hesitant to make and the thing they don't want to let go of is the thing they need to change! The density sets are especially good for taking your gainzzz up to a level you didn't think possible. (They're so good that I have to write it with Z's to make it more gnarly!)

Really consider which of the techniques is right for you: Is the design something that you feel would complement your targets and let you get more quality work done? Perhaps one of your targets is to be consistent with a routine four days a week, so timed strength work may be perfect. Or maybe you've really struggled to see muscle gains and want your strength to improve with heavy compound lifts like deadlift, squat, and bench; try density sets.

Go back through your STRONG system and don't get caught up in how awesome each of these protocols is on its own. All of them are fabulous and made even better when you use them based on what you need.

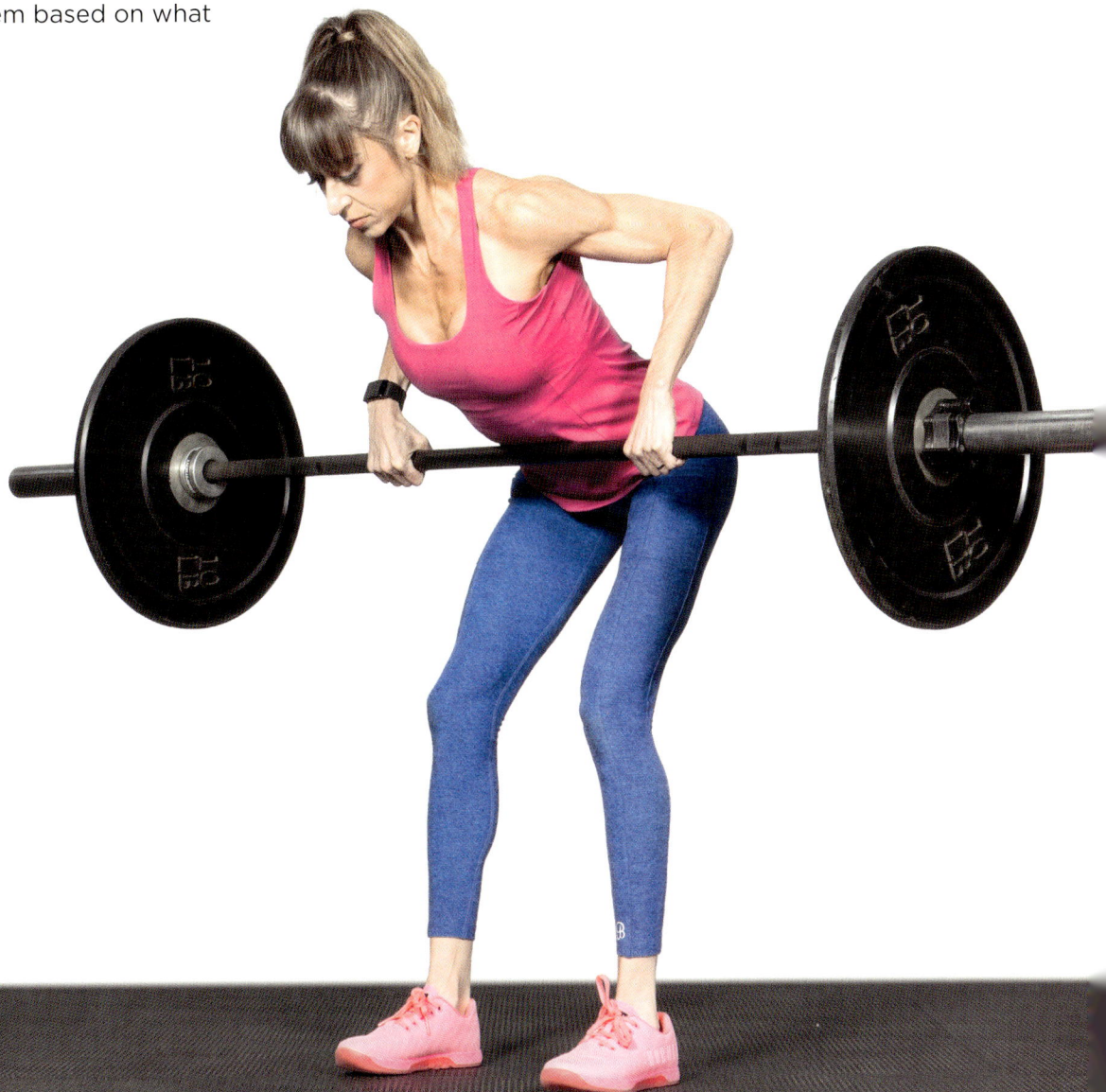

CREATING YOUR ROUTINE

Now the super fun part. It's time to pick a routine and put it on your calendar! To help you create your plan, recall a few key things from your STRONG system analysis:

? What is a realistic schedule for your training? Set this first in your mind to hold yourself to what is a doable change.

? What is your primary goal? Fat loss? Muscle gains? Hitting a performance PR?

? What is a secondary goal? Have this in the back of your mind.

? What does your current routine look like? You want to know where you're starting from to meet yourself where you are with moves but also to understand what you're doing and the results you're getting to decide what bigger shifts may be worthwhile, even if they're uncomfortable.

? What has changed in your lifestyle? If some of these protocols are very different from what used to work but now isn't working, *recognize* that to help you embrace a bigger shift rather than running from making the change. This will also help you determine which bonus cardio or adjusted schedule may work if you've been training five days a week and now are looking at a schedule that recommends four.

? What are you willing to sacrifice? This is where you have to consider the other activities you're doing and how they fit in and what you want to keep as nonnegotiable based on cost and reward and what you're going to choose to let go of.

After you've written these thoughts out, you can jump to Part 3 and select not only the design but the weekly schedule that works. You can also select any additional cardio sessions and recovery work. (I get into recovery work more in Chapter 13.) As you're selecting your workouts, keep in mind that you will want to stick with the same progression for at least three to six weeks.

There will be some final adjustments you will need to make to those routines as you review them, including selecting the moves. You may see an exercise in a routine you aren't comfortable with or don't have equipment for. The exercise library in Part 3 includes swaps so that you can fine-tune your routines.

Now, with your overall progression and schedule planned, you want to outline your diet to complement it! You're probably tempted to jump into training. I know; these designs are exciting! But still don't do it!

Many people are comfortable being uncomfortable in the gym but want to avoid nutritional changes at all costs. Buuuuuut the best results will happen when all your systems work together. You can't out-exercise your diet! Onward to those macros methods!

12 THE MACROS METHODS

I have a confession: I resisted adjusting my diet for as long as possible. When Ryan and I were first dating and he talked about his "clean eating" in relation to his boxing, I told him that I could never restrict myself. Of course, at that point, I was a college athlete who chowed down on burritos, pastries, and just about everything bad for me without really gaining weight, even though I was far from lean.

My tune changed when I gained a whole heck of a lot of weight with my first job out of college. I could no longer get away with massive Chinese food take-out meals and ice cream while lazing on the couch watching TV every weekend. It was time for a change. Of course, embracing change didn't happen overnight, and I'm quite familiar with the dieting roller coaster.

I learned a lot, and I want to save you a lot of time, wasted effort, frustration, and ... well ... wasted hope because you think that maybe you'll find a way around the challenging stuff. You won't.

The sooner you face the fundamentals of nutrition and own them, the sooner you'll find true food freedom. That's why I'm going to share the sucky, hard truth, and tell you the key to everything is macros—tracking macronutrients, the portions of your food that come from protein, carbs, and fats.

Tracking macros can stink. Doing it can feel overwhelming. Many people want to run from tracking like it's the plague. I did. I even wrote some blog posts about how I would *never* track.

Eventually, I realized you can't run from learning the fundamentals if you want to build a solid foundation and make a lasting change. Now, this doesn't mean everyone uses macros in the same way or that tracking in one particular way is right for you. But you do need to recognize the opportunity in learning the boring stuff if you want to see the sexy results. It's time you stopped going *on* a diet and instead learned to *adjust* your diet.

Get your STRONG system analysis ready, especially your nonnegotiables and your list of big-rock habits. It's time to jump headfirst into the nutritional changes most people want to resist.

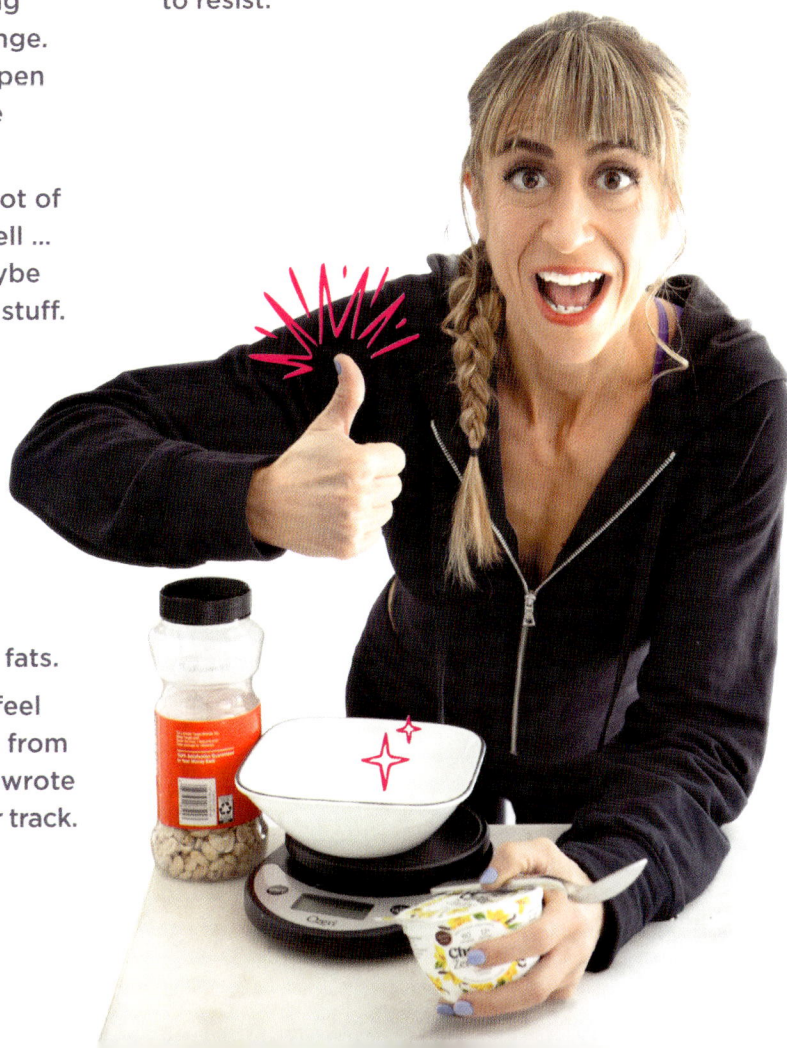

WHAT GETS MEASURED GETS MANAGED

I want to step back for a second. The more I tell you that you *should* do something you don't want to do, and the more you try to bully yourself into something that you hear you *should* do, the less likely you are to do it. Newton's third law, remember? Sometimes, things you feel you should do and even "want" to do are still big-rock habits.

However, sometimes a slight step back can propel you forward and help you take a sledgehammer to those habits to make them more manageable. In this case, I want to step back and talk about looking in a mirror. What is the mirror showing you? Merely your reflection, right? But what you "see" in your mind might be something more than that. Your thoughts tell you something else is there.

When you look in the mirror, an inner voice talks to you. *Judges* you. You tell yourself you're fat. You're ugly. You're weak. You're stupid.

And if that's what your mind is telling you when you look in the mirror, chances are good that you're going to *hate* your reflection. You'll avoid it at all costs. But the mirror isn't what's telling you these things. *You* are.

If you start looking in the mirror every day and say to yourself, "I'm fabulous. I'm strong. I'm beautiful. I'm intelligent. I can conquer anything," your feelings about the mirror will change. You're going to feel better about looking at it, not to mention you'll feel better about *yourself.*

You're going to make the mirror and this habit of looking in it positive forces for change in your life rather than negative ones. It all comes back to the fact that if you change the way you look at things, the things you look at change.

I mention this because people often develop negative feelings and associations with the tools, changes, and habits they need the most. They create these negative associations because of how they've used the tools in the past. Tracking is a perfect example.

Just the mention of tracking your food or macros may make you shudder. You may be tempted to skip this chapter and say, "Forget it." But that won't change anything. To empower yourself, you must face the situation and assess the why and the mindsets behind the habit changes. That's why the work you've already done with the STRONG system reflection is so valuable.

Now's the time to push back and reclaim these tools for your use.

When was the last time you tracked? Was it when you hated the weight you saw on the scale? Did you feel mad, miserable, and a bit disappointed in yourself? Did you feel unworthy? Were you frustrated that you just didn't have the willpower to make changes? Were you telling yourself all the negative things you see in yourself?

A negative mindset like this gets projected onto the tools and habit changes you make, especially if you use the tools from a negative angle. You track to restrict the things you love. You make yourself feel miserable and hungry. You overwhelm yourself with changes.

However, none of those issues are actually the fault of the tracker any more than the mirror was at fault. The mirror is just a reflection of what is there, and your tracker is just a reflection of the foods you ate.

All the judgment comes from you.

So that means you can change how you look at these tools and habits and embrace them to see the results you want and deserve. You can realize that tracking can help you eat *more*. It can help you fuel your amazing body to feel your most fabulous. It can give you the power not to wonder what is and isn't working. You can see it as the best way to create sustainable habit changes and work in foods you love rather than as judgment for being "bad" and a way to tell you to cut things out.

You can shift your mindset and the language you use to think and talk about tracking, which will ultimately help you see opportunity in the options. As I say in this section's title, what gets measured gets managed.

Tracking gives you an accurate picture of your lifestyle, which means you can more easily see where you are so you know how to make changes. You can figure out how to approach nutritional changes by addition. Sometimes, focusing on what you can *add* to make changes can help reduce a sense of negativity. It creates a key shift in your mindset and makes the process feel more empowering because the changes are stemming from adding instead of only subtracting!

Your thoughts, mindsets, and beliefs shape your actions by affecting how you feel about your habits and routines. Just like you can shift the language you use when looking in the mirror, you can shift your language and mindset related to dietary changes. You can stop seeing adjustments to your diet as impossible. You can stop feeling like making changes means restriction and hanger.

So, if you find yourself mentally resisting tracking, pause and breathe. Pay attention to the language you're using about tracking and get ready to shift it. Realize that one size doesn't fit all, and habits can be done in many ways. That's why I share three different macros methods later in this chapter.

No matter which method you choose, I want to help you shift your mindset around tracking. The first step in shifting your perspective starts with tracking without making changes.

DON'T CHANGE A THING!

When you've tracked in the past, you probably haven't been in a positive headspace or felt very good about why you're tracking. You've probably started tracking while trying to force other changes at the same time. On top of that, you were probably harshly judging how well you were doing with those changes.

Changes aren't easy, and they don't feel natural. If they were intuitive, you'd already be doing them! When I make changes, I struggle to step back and give myself grace with the learning process, and I think that's a common problem for others too.

The number one step to taking back power from your tracker is to log without any desire to make a change. Just simply record what you're currently doing, and don't have a view of it being "good" or "bad." You're just trying to see what you're doing.

This first step helps you realize that the tracker has no power. You're not removing or restricting anything. You're just gathering data, and your tracker can't judge you for it. It's just collecting data, and it's the data you've *chosen* to enter.

This data can be eye opening. It can make you realize why certain changes have been so hard to make in the past, and it can highlight where you can make immediate improvements to your nutritional habits. You can identify routines, habits, and foods that are important to you and may need to be included in your nonnegotiables.

The data you collect without making changes is part of your origin story. It shows what you're currently doing to create your current situation. With this clear picture established, you can use the power of the 1 percent to move forward.

The best part is that you've already overcome a huge hurdle in starting the habit of tracking macros—logging your food! By tracking without making changes, you've probably started to realize that tracking really isn't that bad. I know; you're never going to feel like it's "fun," but it's a process that's known to guarantee results, so you should embrace it. Good things happen when you use precision. You weigh and measure all the ingredients in a recipe for delicious, gooey chocolate chip cookies—at least that's what I do. I'm not winging it! I'm following the recipe exactly as it's laid out. The reward makes the effort of the process worth it.

From here, you can start to adjust your portions based on the meals and foods you enjoy eating. Stacking one habit on top of another can be helpful for making sustainable changes.

But tracking is really only part of the process, like having all the baking tools and ingredients you need to make the cookies only takes you part of the way to the finished product. You need the exact amounts of each ingredient to use. This is where macro ratios and portion guidelines come into play. They help you create the perfect recipe for ooey, gooey results. Once you have the basics down, you can adjust as your needs and goals change over time.

Before I dive into the different methods of tracking and why I don't recommend you just track calories or eliminate whole food groups, I want to talk about something I find can sabotage dietary changes in any circumstance: the pressure to eat clean.

Download it at
redefiningstrength.com/extras.

STOP THE CLEAN EATING PRESSURE

A couple quick questions for you: What's a "clean" food, and what's the definition of "eating clean"? The answer you get depends on who you talk to—for example, a vegan or an omnivore. Heck, if you have certain health conditions, you may label vegetables like broccoli as bad, although most of the world considers broccoli the epitome of a healthy food. I've even been told *water* isn't healthy.

My point is, there's no one definition of "clean eating." You'll stress yourself out and feel like you can't eat anything if you try to follow all definitions of clean eating.

This lack of definitiveness can not only be very annoying but also creates unnecessary pressure. Clean eating creates restriction. It creates deprivation. It demonizes foods. And often, it's what leads to people having a horrible relationship with food.

Most people have some food they've labeled "bad," "unclean," or "off-limits." You probably have a food you "know" you shouldn't eat but that haunts you until you ultimately cave and binge on it. When foods are "bad," you feel guilty for eating them. Ultimately, this holds you back from embracing balance.

This is one reason why tracking what you're currently doing (without making changes) can be so important. You take away any judgment or assignment of value. It's all just *food*. As you learn about its impact, you can make changes to what you do or do not consume. You can make a choice about how you fuel.

And you know what? There is a way to have balance! You *can* have cake and your results too! I mean, you can't have cake whenever you want in whatever quantity you want, but that's the case for everything in life. Yes, there are foods that are better for your health than others, but even this is nuanced and where that balance comes in.

Being healthy is a balance of many different factors, both mental and physical, including emotional enjoyment and stress. Constantly stressing yourself out, freaking out about whether foods are healthy, and draining your willpower isn't a recipe for a healthy, happy life.

You want to focus on whole natural foods, and I will discuss micronutrients in Chapter 13 where I cover the stuff people often ignore, but you also need to realize it's not only OK but good to strike a balance.

When I talk about "balance," I'm suggesting you sometimes have a food you enjoy without a side of guilt, rather than seeking perfection based on some arbitrary standard of clean eating that prevents you from repeating habits long enough for them to become sustainable or results to snowball. In some seasons of life, like the holidays, you may swing a bit more toward doing the minimum. At other times, you may choose to eliminate some foods that don't support improving your health. This balancing act over the year adds up.

Don't get caught up in just one meal, one day, or one week. Realize that balance happens over time as things ebb and flow. I suggest you try to apply the 80/20 rule.

Eighty percent of the time, focus on whole natural foods, and 20 percent of the time, don't give a flying fart in space about the healthfulness of foods; pick them because you mentally enjoy them. This may be a daily balance you strike, with about 20 percent of your calories coming from your favorite dessert or salty snack. Alternatively, your balance may play out over weeks or months as you work in cheat meals or days. The point is to embrace the idea that success isn't about perfection or "good" or "bad" foods but about consistency and mental balance.

This balance is why I so passionately push macros. Through tracking and adjusting your portions of protein, carbs, and fat, you can include the foods you love. You can tweak recipes you currently enjoy to still be delicious while helping you reach your goals. You don't have to feel like you have to cook one meal for yourself and one for your family; instead, you first plan for the meal you eat together and work your other meals around it.

Take some time to review your nonnegotiables. What have you usually cut out in the past that has made you miserable? Identify those things and be prepared to embrace having them as you add other things around them.

WHY MACROS MATTER MOST

Calories in versus calories out is all you need for *weight loss*, but most people aren't after only weight loss. Most people are after *body recomposition*.

The calories in versus calories out oversimplification keeps people stuck in the yo-yo dieting cycle. They cut calories to lose weight only to regain it when they increase calories for maintenance (because you can't stay in a deficit forever). It's also why people sometimes eat 800 calories *without* losing weight. (I'll cover more on undereating when I discuss each macros method.) Metabolism is an ever-adapting process, and a calorie is *not* just a calorie. The type of calorie matters!

Yes, one calorie is one calorie from an energy perspective, and one pound is one pound from a weight perspective. However, the effect can vary dramatically, which is why it's important not to oversimplify. One person can look very different from another at 120 pounds based on each person's body composition, and if you lose 1 pound of fat but gain 1 pound of muscle to stay at the same weight, that pound looks a whole heck of a lot different.

Where calories are concerned, it's not just that food quality matters, although it does. Quality fuel impacts the efficiency and balance of your body, leading to better and faster results. But the macronutrient breakdown of the foods you eat—how much protein, carbs, or fat it contains—affects how your body responds and utilizes it. Each macronutrient has a different role to play in your body, which is why you balance them based on your goals, activity level, age, and needs to see results as fast as possible. It is also why I'm going to harp on the importance of one specific macro throughout all three macros methods: PROTEIN!

PROTEIN

Losing muscle mass with age is a huge concern for your health and longevity and can hinder your aesthetic goals. (Not to be vain, but I plan to be a lean, mean fighting machine 'til I'm done on this earth!) Not only do you lose muscle more easily as you get older, but you also don't use protein as efficiently. To achieve the same muscle-building response you did as when you were younger, you need to increase your protein intake.

Protein literally makes up all of your tissues, so from a health perspective, it can't be overlooked. And from a recomp perspective, it's also significant because of protein's impact on muscle.

Protein is the macro that requires the most energy to digest. About 20 to 30 percent of the total calories in protein go toward its digestion, whereas 5 to 10 percent of carbs' calories are used for digestion, and fats use only 0 to 3 percent. In other words, if you want to burn more calories without training more, eat more protein because you'll burn more calories just to process it.

Now, I'm not telling you to fill your fridge with only protein. More is better—to a degree. But eventually you get to the point where restricting the other macros is to your detriment. Carbs are not evil, and neither are fats. You'll even benefit from cycling carbs and fats up and down. I will get into more about cycling when I cover the third macros method in the "Macro Cycling" section.

10 WAYS TO BUMP YOUR PROTEIN!

SERVING SIZE	ITEM	WHERE TO ADD IT
3 THUMBS	HEMP HEARTS/ CHIA SEEDS	Oats, yogurt, salads, peanut butter toast, avocado toast, rice bowls
2 1/2 THUMBS	SPIRULINA	Smoothies, dressings, oatmeal, fruit juice, water
3 THUMBS	POWDERED PEANUT BUTTER	Smoothies, yogurt, oatmeal
3 THUMBS	NUTRITIONAL YEAST	Popcorn, pasta, salad, eggs, roasted vegetables, soups
1/4 PALM	CHICKEN, TURKEY, LEAN BEEF, FISH	Add extra to any of your main protein portions. This boosts intake without overwhelming your meal.
2 THUMBS	CHEESE (cheddar, mozzarella)	Soups, salads, sandwiches, chili, eggs, veggies, tacos
1/4 PALM	COTTAGE CHEESE	Scrambled eggs, mashed potatoes, dips
1/2 SCOOP	PROTEIN POWDER OF CHOICE	Coffee, oatmeal, smoothies, pancake batter
1/2 FIST	LENTILS	Soups, stews, tacos, salads
1/2 FIST	LEGUMES	Soups, stews, tacos, salads

Small tweaks and changes add up. Instead of completely redoing your diet, make small additions and changes to what you're currently doing. Here are 10 ways to sneak in more protein to meals and dishes you may already be making and enjoying!

FAT

Dietary fat doesn't make you fat. It helps maintain hormonal balance and reduce inflammation, which is important as you get older and are more prone to aches and pains (especially for women during menopause). Often, increasing fat with protein results in decreasing carbs, and the lower carb ratios can be valuable for weight loss because they deplete your glycogen stores, which means you use your fat stores as energy.

Here's the *but* you probably knew was coming: Higher fat ratios can also work against you if you're super active and need immediate fuel for training. For building muscle, carbs are protein sparing and help create an anabolic environment, which basically means carbs create the right internal environment to optimize for muscle growth and allow you to use protein more efficiently, even as you get older.

CARBS

Many people rationalize cutting out carbs because there are no "essential" carbs like there are essential fats or essential amino acids (aka protein), but it's not necessary to eliminate or demonize carbs. The right amount of carbs for you might not be the right amount for another person, and insulin sensitivity and other health concerns may make you adjust carb type or timing (just like you may be conscious of different forms of fat) while someone else isn't concerned about those things.

Carbs play an integral role in keeping hormones (specifically T3 thyroid hormone, cortisol, and testosterone) at optimal levels. If T3 decreases, it can not only hinder your weight-loss results but also impact your energy levels, which can negatively impact your workouts. Thyroid hormone problems can also lead to anxiety issues and contribute to menstrual irregularities (aka missed periods).

When you consume enough carbs, especially if you're exercising regularly, you can keep your testosterone and other anabolic hormone levels higher and your cortisol levels lower. Basically, you create hormone levels that *promote* muscle growth.

I don't share this to make you freak out that a low carb ratio is bad for you. The important point is that no macro is evil, and you have to pay attention to what you have going on with your hormones, age, lifestyle, activity level, and goals and figure out what works best for you. Everyone has a different natural balance and responds differently to various ratios.

You may find that cycling macros can be key. (Read more about macro cycling on page 169.) It can help you bust through plateaus and tap into fat stores by depleting your glycogen. Then you can add carbs again to see the Whoosh Effect.

NOTE: *The Whoosh Effect is the name for something we see often but don't fully scientifically have an answer for. It's when carbs are increased after a lower carb or glycogen-depleted state, and we see fat cells release the water they have stored. If you feel like you look softer on a low-carb ratio and haven't lost, you may consider this switch in energy and see that definition pop!*

DETERMINING YOUR PERSONALIZED MACRO LEVELS

You may now be thinking, *Oh, gosh, so what do I do!? What macros are right for me?!* Don't worry. In each of the three macros methods, I'll break down how to calculate what you need. And remember that the thing you do right now isn't necessarily what you'll do forever. The STRONG system reflection you've done has shown you how habits need to evolve as you progress toward your goals or experience other changes.

Be ready to revisit these macros methods at different stages as you reassess, and don't see the need to change as a bad thing. Creating something sustainable and finding a forever lifestyle is about having the knowledge and tools to adjust—not about doing one thing forever!

With each method, I'll cover all of the following (not necessarily in this order):

» How it works

» Why you might use it

» Upsides and downsides of the method

» How to assess where you are now

» How to set your calories

» How to set your macros

» How to track it

» How to determine your first small changes

A key component of each method is first assessing where you are. You use your chosen method to measure what you're currently doing to understand your starting point. If you don't know that, you can't assess what "could" work or what may be "best" for your goals. So don't skip the assessment phase because it'll help you notice big-rock habits or small pebbles so you can make changes in a way that works for you!

It's time to plunge into the first of the macros methods, which is an amazing place to start if macros conjure up nightmares of calculus equations. If you're biting your nails thinking, *UGH! I don't know if this is for me*, don't stress!

HAND-SIZED HEALTH

The idea of logging everything in an app and weighing and measuring every morsel can feel overwhelming. I get how the idea of tracking may feel like a huge rock—or even a boulder—standing in your way.

The more you feel you should do something, the bigger the obstacle it can be. You may feel like there is no way it will work for you. This is where you have to see opportunity in the different ways of measuring as you start to learn about macros and portions.

In this first method, you use a simple tool—your hand!—as a visual reference to figure out portion sizes. For example, 1 tablespoon of peanut butter is the size of your thumb (which may seem pathetic, but at least it's relatively accurate). Portions of protein are the size of your palm.

PALM OF PROTEIN

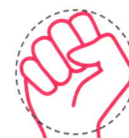

FIST OF CARBS

THUMBS OF FAT

Using your hand as a visual guide may not provide you the to-the-gram accuracy of full tracking, but it's a great way to get started and learn to see your portions more intuitively. It also isn't only for people who are hesitant to weigh and measure things or resistant to using a food tracker. It's also a great tool for when you travel or after you've really learned your portions and want a bit of a mental break while maintaining.

Balance isn't a set thing, so how you maintain balance should and will evolve over time. So don't skip this section just because you're planning to do macro cycling and are comfortable with macro tracking. This information may be extremely eye-opening and helpful if you "know macro tracking works BUT you fall off at some point."

How Hand-Sized Health Works

This macro method's title is very on the nose when it comes to describing what it is: You use your hand as a visual estimate for your portions. You still need to figure out what percentage of your calories will come from each macro (protein, carbs, and fats), but you do it by knowing how many palm-sized portions of protein you need, how many fists of carbs you need, and how many thumbs of fat you need.

To calculate the number of portions you need of each macro, you have to find your daily calories. Then you decide on a macro ratio and determine how many portions (palms of protein, fists of carbs, and thumbs of fat) you need. You'll also divide the carbs into two categories: carb dense and carb lite. These are not scientific terms, but they generally describe the "carbyness" of the foods. Carb-dense foods are things like starchy carbs, fruits, and the "fun" foods people like to eat that are sugar rich. Carb-lite foods are nonstarchy carbs.

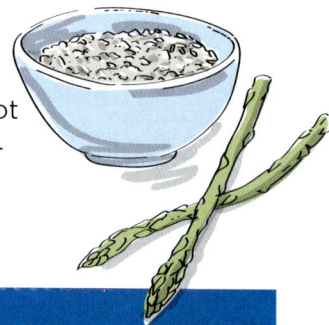

CARB-DENSE CARBS VERSUS CARB-LITE CARBS

These two categories separate carbs based on, well, "carbyness." The terms aren't scientific but focus more on how starchy or carb-dense the foods are for the calories. Breaking down your carbs into two types can help you better adjust your portions to match your needs and goals.

The "carb-dense" foods are things like starchy carbs, fruits, and those more "fun" foods we like to eat that are sugar rich. They're foods made up of long chains of glucose molecules. This gives these foods a more dense, calorie-rich carb structure that makes them amazing at delivering energy, and they can be key for performance. They're even in micronutrient-rich foods like fruits! As my RD Michelle says, they're the "heavyweights of the carb world!"

The "carb-lite" foods are those non-starchy carbs in general. They are shorter sugar chains (monosaccharides and disaccharides) that give you fiber and are rich in vitamins and minerals. They're generally lower in calories per serving than carb-dense carbs.

DENSE CARBS	LITE CARBS
BARLEY	ASPARAGUS
BEANS	ARTICHOKE
BREAD	BOK CHOY
CHIPS	BROCCOLI
CORN	BRUSSELS SPROUTS
GREEN PEAS	CABBAGE
LENTILS	CAULIFLOWER
OATMEAL	CELERY
PARSNIPS	CUCUMBER
PASTA	EGGPLANT
POPCORN	ENDIVE
POTATOES	LEAFY GREENS
PRETZELS	LEEKS
QUINOA	MUSHROOMS
RICE	ONION
RYE	PEPPERS
SQUASH (WINTER)	SAUERKRAUT
	SPROUTS
	TOMATO
	ZUCCHINI

You don't need to track your macros in grams, use a fitness app, or weigh your food. Instead, you can record everything in a notebook or on a sheet like the one I provide in the workbook at redefiningstrength.com/extras. If the idea of any macro math is still making your head spin and you're considering closing this book, don't! Another thing you can find at redefiningstrength.com/extras is a cheatsheet chart for different goals and calories so you can start without doing any math.

Now, take a breath and keep going to figure out how to calculate your hand-sized health portions.

Set Your Calories

Remember, you can use calorie calculations from any section in this chapter. I mention this because

A. I don't want you to avoid the other macros sections. I want you to embrace the knowledge there.

B. There is opportunity in having options.

If your activity level or goals dictate a different calorie intake than what's provided in this section, the calculations in the other sections will help you meet yourself where you are.

Your body doesn't like change any more than your mind does. So the more you can make small changes based on where you're starting, the more quickly the changes will feel natural. This is one reason I want to encourage you to take a week to record what you're already doing. The more you understand your origin story, the better equipped you are to create your roadmap toward your destination with as few wrong turns as possible! Recording without change can also help you lower your mental resistance against the protein increases or tweaks to carbs and fats you may need to make.

Ideally, you've tracked your current eating habits and you can use your current calorie intake as your starting point. If you haven't done that and you're curious where your calories may need to be based on your goals and activity level, multiply your goal weight by one of the caloric targeting factors in the following table. (This is the reason I encouraged you to set your workout programming first, so if you haven't worked through Chapter 11, stop and go back there now.) The result is your target number of daily calories.

If you're not sure what you use as your goal weight, consider these things:

» If you have quite a bit of weight to lose, pick a first goal weight that's midway between your current weight and your ultimate goal.

» If you're doing body recomp, your goal weight may be the same as your current weight or a higher weight.

» If you aren't sure what weight you should be, start with your current weight.

OPTION	A	B	C
GOAL/TARGET	I have 30 pounds to lose.* *If you have more than 30 pounds to lose, use the halfway mark for your goal body weight.*	I work out consistently and intensely three to five times a week	I am training hard five to seven times a week. I'm working on making my six-pack pop with only a few pounds to lose.
GOAL-BASED CALORIC TARGETING FACTOR	10	12	14

$$\text{Goal bodyweight (pounds)} \times \text{caloric targeting factor (A, B, or C)}$$

For example, if your goal weight is 150 and column B matches your activity level, your total daily calorie target is 1,800.

Remember, this calculation is a starting point. You'll adjust as you go based on your progress and increase your daily calories as you reach your goals to retrain your body to eat more. You may also find that you adjust your calories as your activity level changes.

Set Your Macros

This section is called "Set Your Macros" because with hand-size health you're using macros, but your brain doesn't have to go to crazy with math calculations! I want you to understand the principles behind the hand portions you're consuming. The more you see the workings behind what you're doing, the more you can value the changes.

I'm sharing four basic options for four different goals, but these certainly aren't the only options. You can use a different macro breakdown if you find it works better for you.

Identify which of the following macro splits matches your goal.

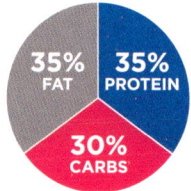

35% FAT · 35% PROTEIN · 30% CARBS	40% FAT · 35% PROTEIN · 25% CARBS	25% FAT · 35% PROTEIN · 40% CARBS	30% FAT · 40% PROTEIN · 30% CARBS
GOAL: Body recomp: burn fat and build muscle	**GOAL: Fat loss and hormonal balance**	**GOAL: Muscle and endurance training**	**GOAL: Faster fat loss**

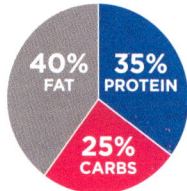

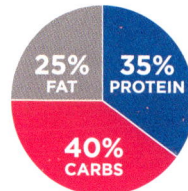

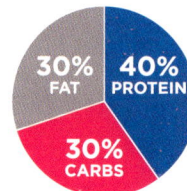

With that decision made, you can figure out how many portions of each macro you need for your daily calorie total.

Calculating Your Hand Portions

Macros and barbell math are the only two types of math I do, so I understand if you're freaking out about the math involved with tracking macros! You can skim this section quickly to see what the calculations are. At redefiningstrength.com/extras, I provide a chart with this math already done for each of the four ratios in the preceding section and an array of calorie ranges.

PROTEIN

To calculate the number of palms of protein to consume, multiply your total daily calories by the protein percentage in the macro breakdown you've chosen. Then divide that number by 4, which is the number of calories per gram of protein. The result of this calculation is the number of your daily calories that come from protein. (You can file this info away for later when you want to dip your toe into more macro tracking!)

Now, take the number of grams of protein and divide by 25 grams, which is the average palm portion size. *Boom!* You now know how many palm-sized portions of protein you need to eat.

Here's the formula:

NOTE: *While you can get as precise about portion estimates as you'd like, I recommend rounding up to the nearest half.*

$$\left(\text{Total calories} \times \text{\% protein} \right) / 4 = \text{total grams of protein} \qquad \text{total grams of protein} / 25g = \text{NUMBER OF PALMS OF PROTEIN}$$

Here's an example:

1,500 calories **X** **35%** protein **=** **525** calories from protein   **525** calories from protein **/** **4** calories per gram **=** **131.25** total grams of protein   **131.25** total grams of protein **/** **25** grams per portion **=** **5.25** *or* **5.5** palm-sized protein portions

If you're curious what this amount looks like, check out page 155, where I've included a protein portion guide.

PALM-SIZED PROTEINS

What does a "palm sized" serving of protein look like? Here are some visual reminders to help you adjust your protein portions on your plate and fuel your results. Mix and match different protein sources to increase your protein—don't feel like you just have to chow down on more chicken!

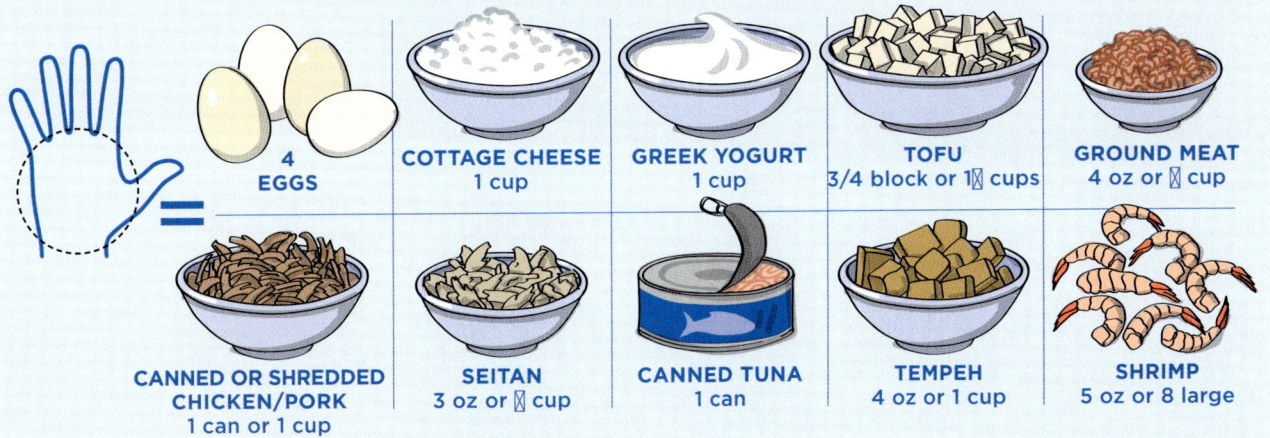

4 EGGS

COTTAGE CHEESE
1 cup

GREEK YOGURT
1 cup

TOFU
3/4 block or 1 cups

GROUND MEAT
4 oz or cup

CANNED OR SHREDDED
CHICKEN/PORK
1 can or 1 cup

SEITAN
3 oz or cup

CANNED TUNA
1 can

TEMPEH
4 oz or 1 cup

SHRIMP
5 oz or 8 large

CARB-DENSE CARBS

For your carbs, you will do two different calculations to differentiate between starchy (carb-dense) and nonstarchy (carb-lite) carbs. Starchy carbs—like potatoes, rice, bread, and pasta—contain a higher amount of starch and, well, have a higher carb count than nonstarchy carbs. Starchy carbs are the foods that more often get demonized but can be important in your diet, especially if you're active. Carb-dense carbs have a calculation of their own.

Nonstarchy carbohydrates often have less of an impact on blood sugar and are lower in carbohydrates. They're foods like broccoli, cauliflower, carrots, and a lot of other nutrient-dense veggies. They're also often lower in calories, which is part of the reason for the differentiation between the two. Carb-lite carbs are calculated separately after your fat amount is determined.

For a list of foods that fall into each category, check the "Carb-Dense vs. Carb-Lite" sidebar on page 152.

To calculate the portion for the starchy carbs, go back to your calorie calculation and the macro ratio you selected. Multiply your total calories by your carb ratio. Then divide the result by 4 (carbs' calories per gram) to get your total grams of carbs.

Next, divide your total grams by 40 (the grams per average fist-sized serving) to get the number of fists of starchy carbs you should consume. Round down to the nearest half rather than rounding up as you do for protein. This helps keep your calorie intake in line.

Here's the formula for starchy carbs:

NOTE: *If it seems weird that the carb-lite number is related to the fat number, here's the reason: Fat is often added to these carbs—in some cases, it should be added to them purposefully to help with nutrient absorption. Also, you want a huge portion of your plate to be occupied by these fiber-filled, nutrient-rich foods that help you feel fueled and full.*

$$\left(\text{Total calories} \times \text{\% carbs} \right) / 4 = \text{total grams of carbs}$$

$$\text{total grams of carbs} / 40g = \text{NUMBER OF FISTS OF CARBS}$$

Example:

1,500	x	30%	=	450		450	/	4	=	112.5		112.5	/	40	=	2.8 *or* 2.5
calories		carbs		calories from carbs		calories from carbs		calories per gram		total grams of carbs		total grams of carbs		grams per portion		fists of carbs

FAT

Multiply your total calories and the fat macro percentage you've selected. Divide the result by 9 (the calories per gram of fat). The result is your daily total for grams of fat.

Then divide the total grams of fat by 12, which is the number of grams per thumb-size serving. Again, I recommend rounding down to the nearest half. However, if you're using fractions of servings, you might inadvertently cut out too much by rounding down each time.

NOTE: *Remember, fats do not make you fat, although all fats are not created equal. For some amazing healthy fat-rich foods, check out page 156.*

Here's the formula for fat:

$$\left(\text{Total calories} \times \text{\% fat} \right) / 9 = \text{total grams of fat}$$

$$\text{total grams of fat} / 12g = \text{NUMBER OF THUMBS OF FAT}$$

Example:

1,500	x	35%	=	525		525	/	9	=	58.33		58.33	/	12	=	4.86 *or* 4.5
calories		fat		calories from fat		calories from fat		calories per gram		total grams of fat		total grams of fat		grams per portion		thumbs of fat

THUMBS UP FOR HEALTHY FATS

Fats do not make you fat! They are an essential macronutrient that helps you maintain hormonal balance and supports many bodily functions while keeping you feeling full and satisfied!

The key is focusing on quality fat sources to reduce inflammation and promote optimal health. Below are some visual portions of fats to help you dial in your hand-sized health tracking!

1 THUMB OF FAT = **ABOUT 1 TABLESPOON** (with some other measurements, see below)

SUNFLOWER SEEDS (1 tablespoon)

CHIA SEEDS (1 tablespoon)

FLAX SEEDS (1 tablespoon)

GUACAMOLE (1 tablespoon)

NUT/SEED BUTTER (1 tablespoon)

OLIVE OIL (1 tablespoon)

OLIVE TAPENADE (1 tablespoon)

PESTO (1 tablespoon)

1 THUMB OF FAT =

2 thin slices AVOCADO

1 square DARK CHOCOLATE

6 ALMONDS

7 CASHEWS

CARB-LITE CARBS

The last step is to calculate your portion of "carb-lite" carbs, which should take up a big portion of your plate. This number is based on the fat percentage for the ratio you're working with. Divide your fat percentage by 10 to get the number of fist-sized servings of nonstarchy carbs you need.

Here's the formula:

$$\frac{\%}{fat} \; / 10 \; = \; \text{number of fists of nonstarchy carbs}$$

Here's an example:

$$40\% \; / 10 \; = \; 4$$

40% fat / 10 = 4 fists of nonstarchy vegetables

At redefiningstrength.com/extras, you'll find a Hand-Sized Health Portions chart, which includes a chart where you can write out the portions you need per day and a tracking page to mark what you eat as you go.

How to Track

Once you've determined the portions for each macro, I recommend you record what you consume each day. You can do something simple like the template at redefiningstrength.com/extras. Just color in or cross off your portions as you go. Alternatively, you can write out meals and portions in a workbook. Even photos of your meals can hold you accountable.

Marking off what you've done (or having the picture proof) enables you to look back at the end of the day and know you ate the correct portions, and the accountability of tracking helps you follow through with the necessary habits. Seeing how well you're meeting your macro percentages helps you assess what changes you need to make.

Before you jump into using this macro method, I urge you to consider the pros and cons of this option and review the other sections to find out how the other methods work.

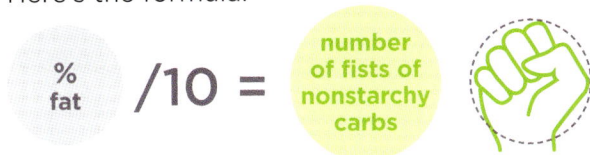

Download it at redefiningstrength.com/extras.

The Good and the Bad of Hand-Sized Health

This method is a great way to get started and learn what your portions should look like without having to weigh and measure everything, so don't fear that you can't lose weight or gain muscle with this method. However, you do need to embrace the fact that it's about creating a lifestyle balance more than achieving aggressive results.

The upside for hand-based portions is that it may be the step you need to break down a big-rock habit, shift your mindset, and gain momentum so you can eventually shift to tracking, but this method simply isn't as precise as full macro tracking and cycling. If you want to reach a new level of leanness and see that six-pack popping, I urge you to embrace full macro cycling (page 169) and then switch to hand-sized health macros when you reach your goals and are ready to maintain. Precision is the name of the game to reach elite level.

Your Origin Macros

I mentioned earlier that tracking what you're currently doing helps you adjust your calories based on your current intake. Tracking also helps you to see your portions of each macro. You may be surprised by how close to or far away from the target portions you are.

By taking seven to ten days to record your current diet without judging what you're doing or making any changes, you mentally separate tracking from any feelings of restriction or overwhelm. You get an accurate picture of where you're starting.

Your Small-Stone and Pebble Habits

Even three days of tracking will show you at least one area in which you need *lots* of improvement. What's one small way you could build toward it? *Note:* I didn't say do it all at once and double what you're doing. I just want you to look for one small change that would be so easy you could start it tomorrow.

Here's an example: Say you need six palm-sized portions of protein, and you're currently getting three. Is there a place you could add another half-palm portion? More chicken on your lunch salad? Tofu in your stir fry at dinner? Make a small portion adjustment and stick with that for a few days.

You build a wall not with one big block but brick by brick. Look at what small things you can add based on what you already enjoy.

Write three small pebbles and one slightly bigger small-stone adjustment you can make to work toward the guidelines for the macros you calculated. Also list a reason you like this method and a downside so that you can compare this process to the other options!

Remember, if you were already hitting these portions, you'd be seeing results. Later in the book, I explain why I avoid meal plans as much as possible, but I know they can be a way to carry pebbles while making other harder changes. To help you ease in to adjusting your macro distribution, don't sleep on the meal plans and meal plan builders at redefiningstrength.com/extras.

9 WAYS TO GET 20g OF PROTEIN

CHICKEN BREAST (4 oz)
CALORIES: 136	CARBS: 0g
PROTEIN: 26g	FAT: 3g

FLANK STEAK (4 oz)
CALORIES: 155	CARBS: 0g
PROTEIN: 24g	FAT: 6g

SALMON (4 oz)
CALORIES: 144	CARBS: 0g
PROTEIN: 23g	FAT: 5g

TEMPEH (4 oz)
CALORIES: 219	CARBS: 11g
PROTEIN: 21g	FAT: 12g

SIZE OF PALM

GREEK YOGURT (1 cup)
CALORIES: 142	CARBS: 9g
PROTEIN: 25g	FAT: 1g

EGG WHITES (1 cup)
CALORIES: 126	CARBS: 2g
PROTEIN: 27g	FAT: 1g

SIZE OF BASEBALL

TOFU (10 oz)
CALORIES: 176	CARBS: 7g
PROTEIN: 20g	FAT: 8g

SIZE OF GRAPEFRUIT

SIZE OF CARD DECK

GROUND TURKEY (93%) (3 oz)
CALORIES: 158	CARBS: 0g
PROTEIN: 20g	FAT: 9g

EDAMAME, unshelled (7 oz)
CALORIES: 216	CARBS: 17g
PROTEIN: 20g	FAT: 9g

SIZE OF ORANGE

Use this guide as a visual reference, weigh your food for best results.

MINIMALIST MACROS

If you've tried counting macros in the past, you may feel it's like doing a jigsaw puzzle with missing pieces. How do you lower your carbs and increase your protein? And can you boost your protein without making your fat go up?! GAH! You may feel like there are just too many things to worry about, so you might be inclined not to do any of it at all.

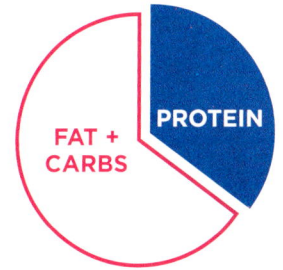

This is where minimalist macros can come to the rescue. If you've ever thought, *If I could just focus on one macro at a time, I'd be fine,* that's exactly what you will do with this minimalist approach. You're going to focus only on protein while hitting your calories. This is a great method to use to get started or when you're struggling to track because the effort doesn't feel worth it.

For example, during the holidays or when work has gotten stressful, you might need to focus less without completely abandoning everything. Or if you get overwhelmed every time you start a new program, this time, take a different approach by focusing on one macro.

This dialed-back version of tracking is a happy middle ground between visual portion guides and full tracking.

How Minimalist Macros Works

Your focus with this approach is on your protein and your calorie cap. Your carbs and fats can vary day to day and fall wherever as long as you hit your protein grams and are not going over your calorie intake. To make sure you're hitting your calories and your protein with this minimalist approach, you need to weigh and measure your food.

As you progress toward your goals, you use the mini targets and checkpoints you identified during your STRONG reflection to help you assess the protein and calorie amounts you're using. You may want to increase or lower protein at times or increase or lower calories for diet breaks or to gain muscle or expedite fat loss.

NOTE: *It's important to be conscientious that you don't undereat too much. It might seem like a bigger deficit is better, but it really isn't. (I touch on undereating a bit more in the next section.)*

Minimalist macros gives you the freedom to include a diversity of foods because you don't have specific fat or carb goals. This method provides an opportunity to see what you crave and what you feel best on. You may notice you always trend toward more fat or more carbs, which can be useful information as you consider more full ratios and further cycling in the future!

Set Your Calories

Do you know how many calories you're eating right now? Chances are, your guess is way off. I thought I was good at knowing my portions, and I found I wasn't. AT ALL.

Portion distortion happens for many reasons, including these:

» You view a food as healthy so assume it has fewer calories than it does.

» A portion seems small, so you assume it can't be that calorically dense. (Two mega-stuffed Oreos, which are like two bites of food that you don't feel full after eating, are 180 calories.)

» You don't feel full after eating, so you assume you didn't consume many calories.

» You don't realize the macro breakdown of the food, which affects the caloric density and even how your body processes it.

» Finally, you want to eat it, so the portion gets bigger!

While I *love* the idea of becoming a more intuitive eater, intuition for many people must be relearned because their intuitive mechanism has gotten busted because food tastes really good and can be comforting and enjoyable for a bazillion reasons outside of being fuel.

Tracking what you're currently doing is eye-opening, and it helps you to make accurate small changes rather than forcing some ideal. It can also help you see that tracking isn't restrictive or that it always means cutting foods out.

When you do your test run of tracking for seven to ten days, you find out how many calories you're currently consuming; then you adjust to create a deficit or surplus based on your goals. Later in this section, I share some calculations to give you an idea of numbers to shoot for. However, no calculation or "ideal" can fully account for your genetics, activity level, hormonal balance, or previous dieting practices.

I mention "previous dieting practices" for a reason. Your habits create what is "natural" for your body. In other words, you experience hunger cues at set times because you always eat at those times. You create cravings for specific foods because of what they're associated with in your life. You even train your body to function off of the calories you give it, which is why you may feel like your metabolism is broken. Your metabolism isn't broken; it's just adapted. If you've been underfueling, your body has learned to run off of too few calories, and you have to retrain it.

You have to determine whether you're eating the right amount, undereating, or overeating. Your calorie minimum should be ten times your goal body weight:

Goal bodyweight (pounds) X 10 = calorie minimum

For example, a goal weight of 120 multiplied by 10 is 1,200 calories.

If you've been eating fewer calories than that target, you first need to focus on a phase of metabolic healing, when you slowly increase your calories. The reason is that when you undereat, your body fights to conserve energy and put it toward the processes you need to survive. It will get the fuel it needs from the source that costs you the most energy—your muscle. Muscle costs more to maintain and is the best source of amino acids for your body to use to repair tissues. So, if you can conserve expending energy and get amino acids to rebuild tissues as needed, that means bye-bye muscle mass. All that hard work in the gym is only backfiring in muscle tissue breakdown with no repair.

To get out of this cycle of eating less to gain more, you have to embrace stepping back (and possibly seeing the number on the scale go up temporarily) to move forward by retraining yourself to eat more, especially if you've complained you can't build muscle.

To increase your calories, add 100 to your current daily intake. Do this for a week. Then increase by another 100 the next week. Do this week after week until you reach *at least* the minimum daily calories you calculated by multiplying your goal weight by 10. You may do this process more gradually to help yourself not feel too full and not freak out with the scale shifts, but you need to do this. I'm being a pushy coach here and not giving you an option. Otherwise, you'll end up stuck in the change loop forever and continue to see that middle-age spread ... well ... *spread*!

As hard as it can be to see the number on the scale go up, this process is essential if you want to restore hormonal balance and improve your metabolic health. If you're conscientious about your protein during this time, you'll be doing so much to avoid gaining fat.

The scale will change due to glycogen and water weight being stored and muscle mass being gained, but you'll help make these gains a positive by focusing on protein. You'll know you're on the right track because you may see other changes in your metabolism too:

- » Increased fidgeting
- » Better sleep
- » More energy
- » Stronger workouts
- » Hair and nail growth happening faster
- » Not feeling cold or sluggish

While your starting place is what you're currently eating, you'll have to adjust at some point, so having some idea of what to shoot for is key. So in the next sections, I explain how to figure out how much to add or subtract and give you some basic guidelines for adjusting over time.

Body Recomp: Fat Loss

For body recomp with a focus on fat loss, a great rule of thumb is to decrease calories by between 100 to 300 calories (and no more) from your current daily intake. Then maintain that change for at least one or two weeks before adjusting again. The more extreme the deficit, the more you risk losing muscle and experiencing performance decline and metabolic adaptations (especially the leaner you get).

Here are some general guidelines:

- » If you're more active, use a 100- to 200-calorie decrease from your current daily intake.
- » If you aren't currently training more than two times per week, go with a decrease of 200 to 300 off your daily intake.
- » If you have more than 50 pounds to lose, you can push the decrease to the 300- to 500-calorie range for a few weeks, especially if you need the motivation of fast progress to keep you going.

Table 12.1 shows three basic ranges. Multiply your goal weight (which can be your current weight if you're unsure) by the caloric targeting factor for your chosen progress category. If you have 30 or more pounds to lose, I suggest using a first goal weight that's about halfway to your ultimate goal. Each day, stay within 100 calories (plus or minus) of your goal calories while hitting your protein goal for the day.

Here's an example for a person who has more than 30 pounds to lose:

STARTING WEIGHT:	GOAL WEIGHT:	FIRST GOAL WEIGHT:		
200 pounds	**150** pounds	**175** pounds	**175 x 11 = 1,925** calories for fat loss	*This would give you a range of 1,825 to 2,025 calories.*

TABLE 12.1: BASIC RANGES FOR FAT LOSS

PROGRESS CATEGORY	Aggressive	Sustainable	Performance
WHEN TO USE	• Creating a bigger deficit to kickstart progress • Having more than 30 pounds to lose • Having an inactive exercise habit (less than three consistent workouts per week) and/or a very sedentary job	• Creating a sustainable deficit • Working on losing the last 15 pounds • Training consistently three to five times per week and/or a desk job with outside activity	• Working on losing the last few pounds • Focusing on fueling your training • Training hard five to seven times a week consistently and active daily
GOAL-BASED CALORIC TARGETING FACTOR	10 or 11	12 to 13	14 to 15

You may even find you move between these categories so you can create a bigger deficit to start and then back off as you progress or as your activity level changes. If you're between ranges, you can straddle the caloric targeting factor—for example, using 13 to 14 if you're between the sustainable and performance categories.

RELYING ON YOUR STRONG GOALS

Regardless of whether your goal is to lose fat, gain muscle, or both, use your STRONG systems assessment to consider what you've struggled with in the past and determine your caloric targeting factor number. Not seeing results fast enough? Then work within the aggressive range. Did you fall off because you felt too hungry and deprived? If so, you'll want more calories, so you should *not* be in the most aggressive category. Remember, you can adjust as you go, starting slower to ease in or doing more to capitalize on that motivation, but weigh the cost and reward of each!

Also remember that what got you to one goal, like losing fat, might hold you back from achieving a new goal, like gaining muscle, and you may find it difficult to embrace habits that you've never done before. Make sure to set complementary targets, especially with gaining muscle, so you can track progress in multiple ways; you won't be able to use only the scale. In fact, if your goal is to gain muscle, you may want to put the scale away for a while.

Body Recomp: Gaining Muscle

Have you ever struggled to add muscle no matter how hard you work in the gym? You're probably not fueling your gainzzz. (I had to add the Z's again!) The key is eating enough.

The metabolic processes to repair and rebuild are calorically costly. And while not a ton of calories are directly burned by each pound of muscle per day (it's around 6 calories), that still means extra calories are being burned at rest to maintain the muscle you're adding.

If your focus is on gaining muscle and improving performance, you need to make sure you're eating enough—at least enough calories for maintenance and maybe even a small surplus. Gaining muscle is *not*, however, an excuse to eat everything you can because you're "bulking," unless you want to add a ton of fat and see your performance decline.

Tracking what you're currently eating to get your baseline is ideal, especially if you've been maintaining your weight for a while. However, if you've been in a deficit to lose weight, your calories will be lower than what you need for maintenance. You first need to rebuild slowly out of this deficit by adding 100 calories to your daily intake and maintaining that new calorie level for a couple of weeks. Don't cycle macros while you do this. The goal is to increase at least 500 calories over a period of weeks to have a new maintenance level and build muscle.

If you're currently maintaining your weight with what you're eating, you'll want to create a small surplus of 100 to 300 calories to build muscle. If you add more than this, you won't really see gains faster, but you might see more fat creeping on. The only time you'll want to add 400 to 500 calories is if you're including a ton of cardio that's going to fight your muscle-building process.

Table 12.2 shows three basic ranges. Multiply your current weight by the caloric targeting factor for your chosen category. Although you may gain weight as you add muscle, and you may need to increase calories as you gain further, you can use your current weight to get a baseline. Each day, stay within 100 calories (plus or minus) of your goal calories while hitting your protein goal for the day.

Here's an example for a person who wants to gain muscle:

STARTING WEIGHT:
165
pounds

165 x 15 = 2,475
calories for lean performance and gaining muscle

This would give you a range of 2,375 to 2,575 calories.

TABLE 12.2: BASIC RANGES FOR GAINING MUSCLE

PROGRESS CATEGORY	Stay lean	Lean performance	Pure gainzzz
WHEN TO USE	• Coming out of a fat-loss phase to build back • Feeling nervous about gaining fat • Lifting only three times per week and having a sedentary job	• Looking to build and stay lean after maintaining • Focusing on strength and performance • Training consistently three to five times per week and having a desk job with outside activity	• Struggling to build and willing to accept a little fluff • Starting out as very lean and older than fifty • Training hard consistently five to seven times per week, active daily, and including more cardio
GOAL-BASED CALORIC TARGETING FACTOR	13 or 14	15 to 16	17 to 18

As you retrain your body to eat more or build more muscle, don't be afraid to increase calories more or move between calorie options. You can straddle the ranges for the caloric targeting factor to find the midpoint between the high number in one category (14, for example) and the low number in the next (15).

Set Your Macros

Now, you have your calories, so you need to determine your protein. How much protein do you currently consume? You may think that you focus on protein at each meal, but you might be surprised to discover how little you're truly consuming.

This is was eye-opening for me. I was eating far less protein than I thought I was. The struggle to increase it was real. Having a clear picture of your current intake is so important. You use your current protein intake from the two weeks of tracking you did to set your first goal.

You want to get a minimum of 30 percent of your calories from protein for body recomp, regardless of whether your primary focus is fat loss or gaining muscle. If you're starting at 10 or 15 percent, your body may rebel when you try to double the protein quantity! Make small changes so your body and digestion have time to adapt.

If the number you logged for protein during your two-week trial period is less than 20 percent, your first goal is to build to at least 20 percent of your calories coming from protein over the next two weeks.

From there, you will want to bump it to 30 percent for the next two to six weeks. Build up to this slowly. In this first week, simply increase your current intake by 5 percent.

After making these small changes, you will build up to the protein range for your selected goals. For fat loss, because of the calorie deficit, you will want your protein to be higher than it will if you're in a calorie surplus and working to gain muscle.

Protein Goals for Fat Loss

Your goal is to work toward a 30 percent protein minimum; however, achieving a protein intake of 40 to 45 percent while in a caloric deficit can give you an extra amazing kickstart and generate faster fat loss.

If you follow a plant-based diet, you may find that you stay in the 20 to 25 percent protein range during the first four weeks. Then you increase to 30 to 35 percent at points for a few weeks at a time as you feel more comfortable.

If you eat animal products, you will want to shoot for 30 to 35 percent consistently, with strategic bumps toward 40 percent as you feel comfortable or want to speed up your results. If you're really serious about getting a six-pack, you'll not only want to get above 40 percent, but it may be a time to dial in all three macros together. Table 12.3 gives you an at-a-glance overview of the protein targets for different goals.

TABLE 12.3: SNAPSHOT OF PROTEIN TARGETS

WHEN TO USE FOR FAT LOSS	PROTEIN TARGET
Plant-based minimum	20–25%
Optimized minimum	30%
Kickstart minimum	30–35%
Plant-based accelerate	30–35%
Lean accelerate	40%
Full shred mode	40–45%

Protein Goals for Gaining Muscle

Your goal is still a 30 percent protein minimum. If you're actually eating closer to eighteen to twenty times your body weight goal, though, you may find your protein can dip to 25 percent of your calories during your focused build.

If you follow a plant-based diet, you may find that you stay in the 20 percent protein range during the first four weeks. You then increase to 25 to 30 percent at some points for a few weeks at a time as you feel more comfortable.

If you eat animal products, you will want to shoot for 30 percent consistently, with strategic bumps toward 40 percent to help you avoid gaining unwanted fat while in a surplus. However, be conscientious of not overdoing the protein

TABLE 12.4: PROTEIN TARGETS FOR GAINING MUSCLE

WHEN TO USE FOR GAINING MUSCLE	PROTEIN %
Plant-based gains baseline	20%
Optimized gains baseline	25–30%
Lean gains baseline	30%
Plant-based lean gains accelerate	25–30%
Lean accelerate	40%

percentage because, in a surplus, even 30 percent can feel like a lot and more than when you were in a deficit! Table 12.4 shows some basic target percentages for different goals.

You'll often be getting more carbs and won't be deficient in anything, so you don't have to worry as much about not having an anabolic environment for muscle growth. Being conscientious about getting enough carbs will help because they're protein sparing! (See page 177 for an explanation of protein sparing.)

PROTEIN CHART

PROTEIN	20g	30g	40g
CHICKEN BREAST (cooked)	2.3 oz	3.5 oz	4.7 oz
LIQUID EGG WHITES	3/4 cup	11/4 cups	11/2 cups
93% lean GROUND TURKEY/BEEF (cooked)	2.6 oz	3.9 oz	5.3 oz
CANNED TUNA	3.7 oz	5.5 oz	7.3 oz
WILD SALMON (cooked)	2.8 oz	4.3 oz	5.6 oz
COD (cooked)	3.2 oz	4.8 oz	6.3 oz
WHEY PROTEIN	25g	38g	50g
TOFU (firm)	4.5 oz	6.8 oz	9 oz
SEITAN	3.3 oz	4.6 oz	6.3 oz
EDAMAME	11/4 cups	2 cups	21/2 cups
COTTAGE CHEESE (1% milk fat)	3/4 cup	1 cup	11/2 cups
GREEK YOGURT (nonfat)	1 cup	11/4 cups	12/3 cups
PEA PROTEIN	23g	34g	45g

What About the Other Macros?

With the minimalist approach, your focus is on hitting your protein minimum while staying in your calorie range, but you still weigh, measure, and log everything you eat. Don't worry about whether you're higher in carbs or fat for the day as long as you hit your protein and calories.

Look for patterns and trends with your carb or fat intake so you can begin to adjust based on how things are progressing. You can use this information to decide what full macro ratios to start with if you want to transition to macro cycling (page 169) to see results happen faster.

Remember, protein is the key with fat loss, and there's more leeway with carbs and fat. When you're focused on gaining muscle, emphasize carbs over fats whenever possible. But during menopause, when you may be more insulin resistant, an emphasis on fats may feel better. While you focus on specific protein and calorie numbers, vary your carbs and fat to see how you feel.

NOTE: *Make sure not to miss logging days! You want daily consistency in hitting your protein and for your weekly averages to balance, as shown in the graph. If you're constantly up and down in your intake, you can't tell what is or isn't working. You also can't strategically increase or decrease protein based on your progress. You want to focus on improving your daily consistency before making any changes.*

In your food tracking app, try screenshotting your weekly averages. This can show you the impact a single day can have as you're getting started! Shoot for always being within 2 percent of your protein goal, erring on the side of going over your goal rather than under, while keeping your calories within 100 plus or minus of your goal.

DAILY MACRO BREAKDOWN WITH NATURAL CALORIE VARIATION

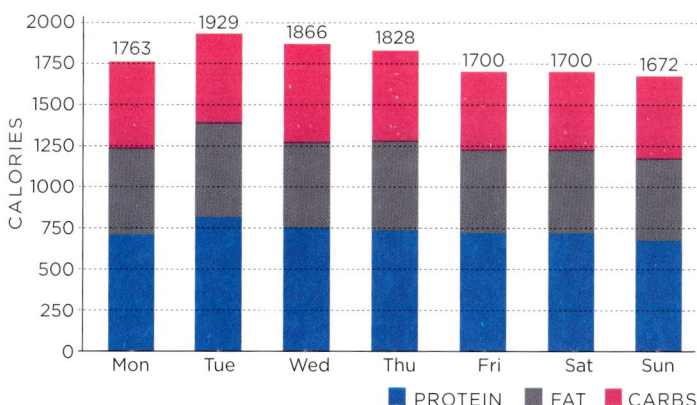

Bar chart showing calories (y-axis 0 to 2000) for days Mon–Sun with stacked PROTEIN, FAT, CARBS. Daily totals: Mon 1763, Tue 1929, Wed 1866, Thu 1828, Fri 1700, Sat 1700, Sun 1672.

PROTEIN · FAT · CARBS

How to Track

At the start, tracking takes some time because you have to find ingredients, save recipes and meals, and make changes to the portions you're currently eating. Let's face it, if you were hitting the macros you needed already, you'd be seeing the results you want. People often aren't intuitively near the macros they need.

Also, when people see how far off the numbers they are, the natural inclination is to defend their current habits. They might say things like

» "But it's healthy fats!"
» "But my carbs are high from fruits and veggies!"
» "But I can't eat more protein!"

These things might be true, but it doesn't mean they're in line with your goals. When you feel yourself push back on change, pause your brain and tell yourself to embrace it. Do something simple like figuring out a small swap that seems doable.

For example, add one more ounce of protein to one meal. Or swap one fattier cut of meat for a less fatty one, like a chicken thigh for a chicken breast. Logging everything without making changes helps create the habit of tracking and helps you prep your tracker with foods you enjoy, which then makes it easier to make changes in what you're eating.

Another "trick" is to plan! I know planning is annoying. Tedious. Boring. All the things. But in this case, you're creating your own meal plans with things you actually want to eat. You're not just going on another diet and using a meal plan someone else created. You get to adjust your diet to be sustainable. Don't demonize a specific food. Work it in. See where you can create balance.

I always used to plan my dessert first because dessert was a nonnegotiable for me. Don't forget to look back at your nonnegotiables to make sure you're finding a balance with them.

NOTE: *If you haven't already done so, download a food tracking app like MyFitnessPal or Cronometer. You might want to test out a few to see what you like before you commit to one.*

In your tracking app, enter your calories under goals and your protein percentage under goals and ratios (you can put carbs and fat there as well); then enter what you'd like to eat tomorrow. From there, you can tweak! Use the cheatsheets at redefiningstrength.com/extras to figure out how to adjust based on the areas you're over or under your targets.

NOTE: *If you want to log and need help building meals but are hesitant to use an app, check out the minimalist meal plan builder at redefiningstrength.com/extras. These can help you simplify doing the math by hand as you create some dishes you love to quickly add to your app later! You still have to weigh and measure every ingredient, just like when you make a recipe, but you can focus on your daily totals for calories and protein.*

Since the meal plan builders are based on grams of each macro, and you're just focusing on protein, you will multiply your protein percentage by your calories to figure out the calories that come from protein. Then you'll divide by 4 (calories per gram of protein) to get your total grams. Refer to the "Calculating Your Hand Portions" section on page 154 for more information on determining your protein target.

Give yourself grace as you learn. Focus on small changes! Realize you are creating the "recipe" for your results as you weigh and measure your foods!

MACRO ASSISTANCE CHART

So many food options! Where do I start?!
Select food items from the chart below to help you hit your macros!

NEED CARBS?

Bread	Juice
Cereal	Maple Syrup
Corn tortillas	Popcorn
Crackers	Potatoes
Dried fruit	Rice
Fruit	Root veggies
Honey	

NEED PROTEIN?

Buckwheat	Ground beef
Canned tuna	Ground turkey
Chicken breast	Shrimp
Cottage cheese (nonfat)	Tempeh
Edamame	Tilapia
Egg whites	Tofu
	Whey protein

NEED FAT?

Almonds	Hemp hearts
Avocado	Mayonnaise
Butter	Olive oil
Coconut milk	Olives
Fish oil	Sesame oil
Flaxseeds	Walnuts

NEED CARBS + FAT?

- Avocado + Toast
- Bagel + Cream cheese
- Berries + Coconut milk
- Bread + Butter
- Chips + Salsa
- Chocolate + Fruit
- Chocolate + Nuts
- Fruit + Nut butter
- Peanut butter + Banana
- Popcorn + Butter
- Toast + Peanut butter
- Veggies + Dip

NEED CARBS + PROTEIN?

- Beans/Lentils/Peas
- Cereal + Skim milk
- Chocolate milk
- Crackers + Deli meat
- Egg whites + Potatoes
- Flavored yogurt (nonfat)
- Fruit + Nonfat yogurt
- Poke + Rice
- Quinoa
- Veggie burger
- Whey + Fruit smoothie

NEED PROTEIN + FAT?

- Bacon
- Beef jerky
- Cheese
- Chorizo
- Cottage cheese (full fat)
- Eggs
- Hummus
- Nut butter
- Salmon
- Steak
- Whole milk
- Whole milk yogurt

MORE FOOD BUT LESS MACROS

Air-popped popcorn	Chicken broth	Lemon/Lime juice	Radishes
Almond milk	Coffee	Mushrooms	Rice cakes
Apple cider vinegar	Cucumbers	Mustard	Salsa
Blueberries	Hot sauce	Nutritional yeast	Seaweed snacks
Cabbage	Hot tea	PB2	Strawberries
Celery	Lemon	Pickles	Tamari

The Good and Bad of Minimalist Macros

One good aspect of this method is that you start dialing in precision for your portions, which will help you see better results faster than with the hand-sized health method. It also gives you a bit more food freedom because it'll be easier to factor in more foods you love, and that's good for sustainability.

Focusing on protein and calories is the key to seeing progress with your recomp while fueling your performance. This method simplifies tracking macros, which is especially helpful if tracking macros has been a big-rock habit in the past.

Another positive of the minimalist macros method is that it works especially well for fat loss/weight loss and maintaining your results, so it may be the version of tracking you shift to after you've reached your goals. Fat-loss studies have shown that with a focus on protein, people can see results with either low-carb or low-fat eating.*

Of course, there are downsides, too. One big downside is that tracking is required because you need precision for hitting your protein and calories. Weighing and measuring everything is important. Planning ahead and doing some meal prep can make things easier, but your willingness to do these things may factor into whether you choose this approach.

If your focus is on recomp to gain muscle, this approach is a bit less effective than full tracking, especially if you're really nervous about coming out of a weight-loss phase and don't want to gain fat. If your focus is on building muscle while staying lean, you want to consider your carb intake, especially for more intensive training and as you become a more advanced or experienced exerciser. In that case, working with full macro ratios may be better as you slowly increase calories.

If you struggle with severe symptoms of perimenopause or menopause, tracking full ratios could be valuable to see how higher fat or higher carbs impact you. Often, adjustments in those macros can have a huge impact on symptoms like inflammation.

Your Origin Macros

Use the data from your week of tracking without changes to determine what foods would be easy to eliminate and spot places where you can add other things. Remember, you're not looking for the final turn you have to make to get to your destination; you're looking for the first turn out of your driveway and onto the main street! Find those meals you love to eat and find one small swap so you can plan ahead.

Your Small-Stone and Pebble Habits

With this method, you should be able to see pretty quickly where you can make improvement. After tracking for just a few days or mapping out a day's worth of food you'd usually eat, can you see one area in which you need lots of improvement? Are you at 10 percent protein and want to shoot for 30 percent? What's one meal you could add just 5 or 10 grams of protein to? Maybe you could add Greek yogurt to your smoothie or another ounce of chicken to your salad. See page 149 for some ideas.

The more you feel successful with the changes, the more you will want to keep making changes. So, if you feel resistance against a change, ask yourself why you're reluctant. Is it because you've never done it? Or are you trying to adjust something you really care about? More assessment leads to more ways to make changes that work for you so you can build momentum.

Write three small pebbles and one slightly bigger small-stone adjustment you can make to work toward your calorie and protein goal. Stick with one of those habits for a week before adding new habits.

Pause and write some thoughts on those habits. List a reason you like this method and a downside so you can compare the minimalist macros method to the other options.

---

*Stijn Soenen et al., "Relatively High-Protein or 'Low-Carb' Energy-Restricted Diets for Body Weight Loss and Body Weight Maintenance?" *Physiology & Behavior* 107, no. 3 (2012): 374–80, https://pubmed.ncbi.nlm.nih.gov/22935440/.

MACRO CYCLING

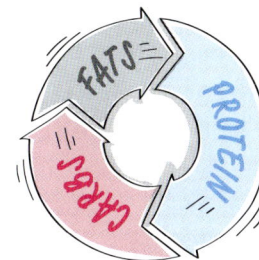

Macro cycling changed my life. It's helped me to fuel so I feel my best and get more definition than I ever thought possible while helping me strike a lifestyle balance to include foods I love. I've realized that it's my choice whether I include something, and my balance can shift as my lifestyle, body, and goals evolve. I can have my cake and my abs too.

I'm not saying I get to eat exactly what I want whenever I want in any portion I want, and not every day is easy. But the balance macro cycling has given me is tremendous, and I'll never ever stop. There's always sacrifice in life to get amazing rewards, but you can have control over your choices and an awareness of their impact, and you can determine your balance.

NOTE: *Even though I love macro cycling, I do use the other methods from time to time. I'm still focused on macros at the core, but occasionally trying the other methods adds to my belief that full macro tracking is the best way for me. I'm empowered and feeling fabulous. I've seen this same freedom and empowerment happen when my clients have pushed through the hard to learn to embrace macro cycling as well.*

If you've ever heard "knowledge is power," tracking macros is a perfect example of that statement. It gives you the power to adjust based on what you need when you need it!

Now, if you're wondering if this is the same as carb cycling, it's not. Let's dive into what macro cycling is.

How Macro Cycling Works

If you've ever tried tracking macros and thought it didn't work or were frustrated by it, what ratio did you try hitting? Why did you pick that ratio? How long did you do it? What other ratios did you try with it? What were your calories with that ratio?

Counting or tracking macros is a technique that can be used with sooooooo many different ratios, and the ratios that work for you aren't necessarily what works for someone else. In fact, ratios that work for you at one time may not work for you at another, either because your goals have shifted or your body and lifestyle have evolved!

Your needs can change over time. Each macro has a different benefit and purpose, and by cycling over the weeks, you can use these different purposes to your advantage. Sometimes, switching from a cycle lower or higher in one macro to the exact opposite can be what helps you see results snowball faster.

Your body adapts over time to what you give it, so these changes in energy sources not only create balance but help you avoid plateaus. The more you can avoid slashing your calories, the better you can maintain your metabolic health, which makes long-term maintenance easier.

Get ready to cycle ratios every few weeks, even when one ratio is working, especially at the start. While you may stay on ratios you enjoy as you learn what works for you and your lifestyle, cycling is key at the start. But note that you need to be consistent with your daily macros over the weeks you do them before you "earn" a switch.

With macro cycling, you set a macro ratio to hit daily within 2 or 3 percent and a calorie target you'll hit within 100 calories. You'll stick with that ratio for one to six weeks. Over the weeks, you may increase or decrease any of the three macros, cycling based on what your body responds to and what kind of results you want.

In terms of what foods you "have" to eat, *there are none.*

NOTE: *Macro cycling is* not *carb cycling, where you vary your macros day to day. That's just too much extra work for too little payoff. While a fitness or bodybuilding competitor may find that necessary for their sport, I like to be as lazy as possible while seeing the biggest benefit, and I find that keeping a consistent ratio over the week makes things more sustainable for most people.*

You get to find the balance that's right for you. Include foods you love. Focus on foods for your health. Realize that there will be times your food quality improves and times you need foods you know aren't that good for you. But through it all, you hit your ratios, and that leads to something sustainable.

You weigh and measure *everything* with this method. So, it will take time to fit all the pieces together. Planning ahead is the name of the game!

Before you set your ratios, you need to set your calories. You may find you need to adjust your calories as you shift your macros because different proportions of the macros can impact how full or fueled you feel. You may think 1,500 calories feels like a lot or like nothing based on the type of foods you fuel with.

Set Your Calories

If your ratios affect calorie intake, why do you need to establish calories first? The reason is that you may find adjusting your macros while consuming your current calories—that's right, making *no* changes to your calorie intake—can build some results for you.

The less you can change at once, the better! You want to try to change one thing at a time so you understand the impact of that factor, and then you continue to tweak. It allows your body and your mind to adjust to the changes slowly, and you often feel better in the process.

This brings me to something you've probably read multiple times now: Track your current intake! Don't make adjustments. Don't cut out. Don't change anything, and track without judgment. If you're new to tracking, this period helps you acquire the habit.

This period of tracking what you're already doing without trying to hit specific ratios is especially helpful if you're coming back to tracking after trying it before and not loving it or feeling like it was restrictive. It also helps you let go of "what used to work" and assess where you are right now. For example, maybe you didn't have a family when you tracked in the past. Maybe you didn't have your current sixty-hour-per-week job. Maybe you weren't traveling as much. Maybe you didn't have specific health concerns. Heck, maybe you were just younger and had different hormonal fluctuations.

Regardless of what's different, it's important to reassess based on where you are now. It helps you make the changes that matter in the present so you can accurately build and understand what your destination looks like.

After you've tracked for a week or ten days, try setting a macro ratio from the next section while sticking with your current calorie target for another week or two.

Earlier in this chapter, I went over what to do if your problem is undereating rather than overeating. If the problem is that you've roller-coaster dieted for long enough that your body is functioning off of a low calorie intake, you may find the weight is creeping on. Check the "Set Your Calories" section under "Minimalist Macros" for guidelines to help you know if this is you.

Instead of going straight to bumping up calories, I highly recommend switching macros first. The minimalist macros approach is a slow build in protein, so you can use your comfort or willingness to go all-in with tracking to help you quickly set a higher protein ratio. This can help expedite the muscle-gaining progress and prevent unwanted fat gain as you retrain your body to eat more.

Protein is very filling, and often in the retraining process, you may feel like you're eating when you aren't hungry. Switching macros allows you to give your body time to adapt to the protein before increasing the amount more. So if you're retraining your body to eat more, switch macros using the ratios in the next section.

Then, slowly, over the weeks, increase your current daily calorie intake by up to 100. Maintain each increase for a week. You might see an initial jump in the number on the scale as you store water and glycogen, but it should level out, and that's when you want to increase again. However, if you keep gaining over the week, switch ratios the next week and stay there for a week or two before you introduce another increase.

YOU MUST NOT AVOID THIS PROCESS! Yup, pushy coach is here again, giving you no option. Otherwise, you're going to end up stuck in the change loop, eating less and less as you feel like you gain more and more.

As hard as it can be to see the scale going up, if you want to restore hormonal balance and improve your metabolic health, you have to do it. You want to increase your calories to at least 10 (if not 11) times your goal bodyweight before you consider focusing on cycling macros.

In this section, I give you some basic guidelines to help you determine your calories. Small changes add up, and your genetics and previous dieting practices may mean what you need is different than an "ideal." Ideals are good to help you test out what may be best, but you still have to listen to your body so you can adjust and tweak as you go.

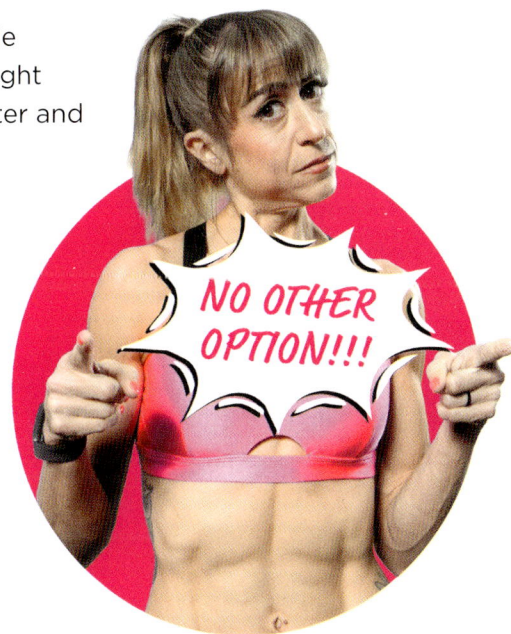

NOTE: *I highly recommend you check out Chapter 14, where I make a push to have you step off the scale while you're going through this process. Other forms of measurement and setting other complementary targets are where it's at!*

Body Recomp: Fat Loss

For body recomp with a focus on fat loss, a great rule of thumb is to decrease calories by no more than 100 to 300 from your current daily intake and then maintain that change for at least one or two weeks before making any other adjustments. I recommend doing this after adjusting macros with your current calorie intake. Macros can have a huge impact, and just a 100-calorie deficit can make a big difference.

The more you push that 300- to 500-calorie extreme deficit, the more you risk losing muscle, seeing performance decline, and experiencing metabolic adaptations, especially as you get leaner. When you have 50 or more pounds to lose, you may find you are able to "get away with" a more aggressive reduction, and doing so helps to build momentum, but be cautious of a long-term big deficit.

Based on your activity level, here are some ranges to consider for your calorie deficit:

» If you train four to seven days a week:

  100- to 200-calorie decrease

» If you train two to three days a week:

  200- to 300-calorie decrease

» If you have more than 50 pounds to lose:
  300- to 500-calorie decrease

NOTE: *The more weight you have to lose, the less risk there is for muscle loss, but you will also adapt to that lower intake faster. You can push that 300- to 500-calorie range for a few weeks, before a diet break or small calorie increase, especially if you need motivation of fast progress to keep you going.*

The only other time you may use an "extreme" deficit is with a mini cut, which is a very short, intensive fat-loss phase—something you might do before a vacation or to kickstart things after the holidays. Times to use it are when you've been maintaining or after a diet break, which I go over in the next chapter. But you don't want to cut an additional 300 to 500 calories off your deficit. You're taking 300 to 500 calories off your maintenance calories.

Table 12.5 shows basic ranges that are consistent with what you may have set if you started with minimalist macros. You will multiply your goal weight (or a first goal weight that's 10 to 15 pounds less than your current weight) by the caloric targeting factor for your chosen progress goal.

NOTE: *An "extreme" mini cut protocol lasts only one or two weeks and uses macro ratios that are, well, not fun. This is a straight-up fat-loss cut. It isn't meant to be sustainable; you use it for the last little intensive push to be extra lean or as a kickstart. It isn't something to do long term, even if it might be tempting to do so.*

TABLE 12.5: BASIC CALORIE GUIDELINES FOR FAT LOSS

PROGRESS CATEGORY	Aggressive	Sustainable	Performance
WHEN TO USE	• Create a bigger deficit to kickstart • More than 30 pounds to lose • Not active with less than three consistent workouts per week and a very sedentary job	• Create a sustainable deficit • Last 15 pounds to lose • Training consistently three to five times a week and a sedentary job with outside activity	• Last few pounds to lose • Focus on fueling your training • Training hard consistently five to seven times a week and active daily
GOAL-BASED CALORIC TARGETING FACTOR	10 or 11	12 to 13	14 to 15

As you start tracking, stay within 100 calories of your daily calorie goal while hitting your macros goal. The closer you stay to the calculated daily number, the faster your results will happen. More precision with these basics is key to efficiency in results.

Remember, these are *guidelines.* You may move between these ranges—for example, starting with a smaller deficit and then increasing the deficit before decreasing it again. If you feel you need to straddle ranges, don't hesitate to select a number from two categories and find the midpoint.

Don't get focused on an "ideal." Forcing yourself into a mold or onto a specific plan is why you've always gone *on* a diet, and it's never worked. This is about *adjusting* your diet and lifestyle.

> **Don't get focused on what you feel may be "ideal."**

Revisit your STRONG system assessment and consider what you've struggled with in the past. Did you not see results fast enough, which means you should try pushing the deficit to start and backing off as progress builds? Or did you fall off because you felt too hungry and deprived? That means you did too much too fast, and the restriction made you hate tracking. Start by doing less and add as you go. Weigh the cost and reward of how you approach change to fill your bag with the habit rocks that fit.

Body Recomp: Gaining Muscle

If you read the "Minimalist Macros" section, I'm not telling you anything new when I say this: You have to eat more to build. In the past, you may have struggled to see the muscle gainzzz you want because you weren't eating enough to support your recovery and growth. While this doesn't mean going crazy with surplus calories, it does mean you have to embrace eating more, even if you sometimes aren't hungry.

You need to be strategic with your calorie surplus to focus on recomp rather than putting on a ton of fat with the muscle. Even if you're willing to gain some fat, it's not an excuse to just pig out. Overeating will lead to lackluster performance and can negatively impact your recovery and energy. And generally, when people want to overeat, they don't overeat quality foods, which ultimately sabotages muscle gains and can leave you feeling like it's impossible to see the muscle and definition you want.

If you're coming out of a fat-loss phase, the increases to maintenance-level calories will be a "surplus" to start. If you're already tracking to lose, you will maintain the macro ratio you're on but increase calories; then you'll go back to cycling macros, much like you would rebuild if you'd been undereating. You want to try to increase by 500 and settle into that new maintenance before adding more calories.

NOTE: *Remember that each 100-calorie increase from your deficit gives your body more calories than it had previously been using—basically a "surplus" you need to adjust to! As your body adjusts to that, builds muscle, and increases your metabolic rate, you need to continue to add more calories.*

If you aren't currently coming out of a weight-loss phase but have been maintaining your weight, track your current calorie intake as you dial in your macros. Then create a small surplus of 100 to 300 calories. Adding more won't really result in faster gains, but you may see more fat creeping on. The only time you'll want to increase by 400 to 500 calories is if you're including a ton of cardio that will fight your muscle-building process.

Table 12.6 shows three basic ranges to guide you, which align with what you might have started with minimalist macros. They're "ideals," but they can help guide you if you've never rebuilt from a deficit or created a surplus strategically.

Multiply your current weight by the caloric targeting factor for your chosen progress goal. While you may gain weight as you add muscle and have to increase calories as you gain further, you can use your current weight to get a baseline.

NOTE: *Throwing away (or avoiding) your scale might be a good idea for this process. Read more in Chapter 14.*

You want to stay within 100 calories of your calculated calorie number while hitting your macros. The more precise you are, the faster results snowball!

TABLE 12.6: GUIDELINES FOR GAINING MUSCLE

PROGRESS CATEGORY	Stay lean	Lean performance	Pure gainzzz
WHEN TO USE	• Coming out of a fat-loss phase to build back • Hesitant to gain fat • Lifting only three times a week and having a desk job	• Looking to build and stay lean after maintaining • Focused on strength and performance • Training consistently three to five times a week and having a desk job with outside activity	• Struggling to build and willing to have a little fluff • Very lean to start and older than 50 • Training hard consistently five to seven times a week, active daily, and including more cardio
GOAL-BASED CALORIC TARGETING FACTOR	13 or 14	15 to 16	17 to 18

If you straddle ranges, you can find a midpoint by using the high point of one range and the low point of another—for example, 14 to 15.

The final note I want to make about creating a calorie surplus is that you have to embrace eating more, even if you see the number on the scale go up.

You have to remember that the habits that got you to one goal can hold you back from reaching the next goal. You have to shift how you've set targets and measured progress in the past. Reflecting on your mindsets about food and fueling will be key, especially if you've just been in a weight-loss phase and are fearful of losing everything you've worked hard for. Step back to reexamine your origin story and what you hope your destination will be.

Remember, you're not just jumping from goal to goal. There's always a slow build. You can pause to maintain (and often should maintain) rather than going straight from fat loss to muscle building. As I've mentioned before, you'll be surprised by the gains you see as you come out of a deficit while still continuing to lose fat. So, as you hit maintenance, know that it can be a "pit stop" on your journey. Maintenance can even be a first mini target.

I also want to remind you that the more you feel yourself pushing back on a habit, the more you can—and should—slow down to speed up. You can say, "Suck it up, buttercup!" all you want, but you have to take smaller steps and break down those big-rock habits to make progress.

Set Your Macros

To determine what your macro targets will be, you have to consider how much protein, carbs, and fat you're consuming currently. This is especially important if you've been overwhelmed by tracking in the past or you aren't motivated to go from zero to sixty. You want to take a small step onto a low box rather than attempting a full box jump onto a six-foot box. You're better off using the ratio closest to what you're currently doing than going for any ideal or specific guideline.

You don't want to fall into the trap of doing keto when your diet is straight up carb central. That would be dooming yourself to fail by getting caught in the change loop cycle. By understanding your current diet, you can "steer into the skid," as I like to say. (I actually said this so often for a period, I'm pretty sure Ryan never wanted to hear the expression again.)

Instead, you want to build off of what your "natural" inclination is because lowering your mental resistance to change is so important. As you assess your current macro breakdown, review your STRONG system nonnegotiables, the habits that felt super hard in the past, your past struggles, and what you value. From there, you can choose a six- to nine-week cycle to start with. As you track progress, you can adjust. The ratios are guides, not handcuffs. They're meant to be implemented in different ways.

At any point, if you feel that the effort isn't worth the outcome, ease back. Use a ratio that feels more manageable. Go back to minimalist macros for a bit. What feels good at one time of year may not fit another, so switch it up as needed. Even if you know one ratio will yield faster results, sometimes you have to own your priorities and lifestyle and adjust accordingly.

Body Recomp: Fat Loss

If your focus is fat loss, protein is key. Every ratio you use will focus on protein at 30 percent or more. If you're struggling currently to hit even 20 or 25 percent, I highly recommend you start with the minimalist macros approach I discuss earlier in this chapter. Once you're able to increase protein, add the other macros.

That 30 percent mark is where the magic really happens. The way carbs and fats are broken down is based on two main factors—activity level and age—and research has shown that high protein is really the key for fat loss.* The more active you are, the more you want to be conscious of eating more carbs, although if you're a woman in perimenopause or menopause, you may need to watch carbs because you can become more insulin-resistant. If you're in this category, you may need to test out a lower-carb option from the "less active" side of the chart (even if you're active), using a lower carb ratio for a one- to three-week stretch between higher-carb breakdowns.

Table 12.7 breaks down ratios into three levels of activity for the six- to nine-week cycles. You must hit these ratios *consistently* for that period to assess if they're working. If you're inconsistent—one day you're way over in fat, the next in carbs—you don't really know if that ratio breakdown works. So, really set your focus to be consistent for at least six of seven days.

NOTE: *Carb type and timing are also factors. In Chapter 13, I discuss carb type and meal timing, and I touch on intermittent fasting.*

*Alan A. Aragon et al., "International Society of Sports Nutrition Position Stand: Diets and Body Composition," *Journal of the International Society of Sports Nutrition* 14 (2017): 16, https://pubmed.ncbi.nlm.nih.gov/28630601/.

Also, note the impact that one day has on your overall averages. If you choose to include a day of off-macro eating, be conscious of how much those calories and macros can have an impact! The more "off-plan" you eat, the more you impact your weekly average.

The cruise control level is about lifestyle balance. These ratios are often easier to start with, and you might shift to them to maintain your results. This level can yield efficient results, but it won't result in the accelerated results that the next two ratio cycles—hit the accelerator and gunnin' it—provide.

Use your STRONG system reflection to assess which level is best for your starting point. You can always change to another set of cycles at another time. Remember that as tempting as it is to do what is fastest, you need to own your priorities and reality to create a plan truly built for you rather than an ideal.

You will want to change ratios when you've been consistent for two to three weeks, especially for your first round through them. So even if the ratio you've been using is working, switch to the next cycle. This helps you avoid plateaus and helps you build by changing energy sources slightly while maintaining balance.

After your first six- to nine-week cycle, you will determine which ratios you enjoyed more and which ratios yielded faster results. You may return to specific ratios based on what you need for longer cycles later. You may use ratios you enjoyed more during seasons you need something "easier." Alternatively, you may use ratios that led to faster results, even if you didn't like them as much, when you want an extra kickstart. You can decide whether to change ratios with workout progressions as needed if your activity level or type of training shifts.

One other thing to note: Always eating over in protein and under in calories does *not* mean you're hitting your macros. Hit *all* your numbers within 2 percent and your calories within 100. You aren't being "better" by not actually hitting your goals!

> **Remember that as tempting as it is to do what is fastest, you need to own your priorities and reality to create a plan truly built for you rather than an ideal.**

TABLE 12.7: GUIDELINES FOR FAT LOSS

CRUISE CONTROL

LESS ACTIVE

PROTEIN	CARBS	FAT
30%	35%	35%
30%	30%	40%
35%	30%	35%

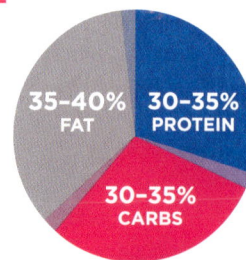

MORE ACTIVE

PROTEIN	CARBS	FAT
30%	35%	35%
30%	40%	30%
35%	35%	30%

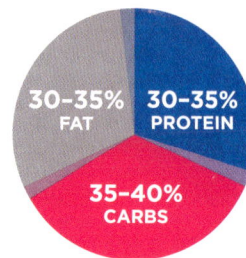

HIT THE ACCELERATOR

LESS ACTIVE

PROTEIN	CARBS	FAT
35%	30%	35%
35%	25%	40%
40%	30%	30%

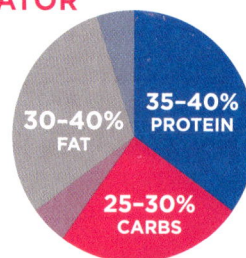

MORE ACTIVE

PROTEIN	CARBS	FAT
35%	35%	30%
35%	40%	25%
40%	30%	30%

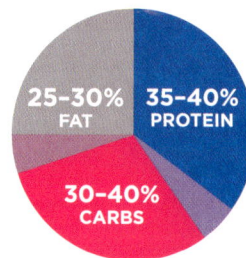

GUNNIN' IT

LESS ACTIVE

PROTEIN	CARBS	FAT
40%	30%	30%
40%	25%	35%
40%	20%	40%

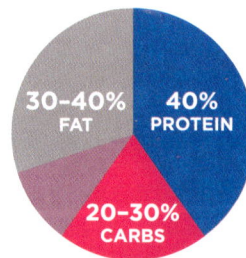

MORE ACTIVE

PROTEIN	CARBS	FAT
40%	30%	30%
40%	35%	25%
40%	40%	20%

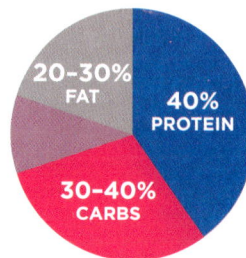

Plan ahead as you work your way through the cycles. Each time you change ratios, you have to step back and reassess your portions. A ratio that seems easier may be hard simply because it's different than what you've been doing. Also, give your body time to adjust. If the ratio includes lower or higher carbs, you may find it takes your body a few days to adjust to the new energy source.

Track how you feel using the questions at the bottom of this page. You don't want to stick with something that isn't prompting you to feel or move your best, but you don't want to just write it off. See the opportunity in some experimentation in the first round by testing out different options. You may be surprised by how a ratio that didn't work in the past now matches your activity level or hormonal balance.

MACROS JOURNAL REFLECTION

	CALORIES	PROTEIN	CARBS	FAT
RATIO USED				
WEEKLY AVERAGE				

Week:.................................

Date:.................................

Results (did you lose weight, inches, etc.?):..
....
....

Non-scale victories (did you sleep better, lift more, fit into clothes better, etc.?):..............
....
....

Reflection (how did you feel, did you like these ratios, etc.?):...................................
....
....

Don't forget to take measurements and progress photos!

Body Recomp: Gaining Muscle

With the strategic focus on macros, you'll find you build muscle with the fat-loss ratios, especially if you're staying consistent with a smaller deficit. However, what you prioritize as your primary goal will happen faster and more efficiently because all systems will drive toward it. So, if gaining muscle is your goal, you want to consider the lean build or pure gainzzz cycles.

As with the fat-loss macros, you may use the slightly less active ratios if you're in perimenopause or menopause, especially if you find fat wants to accumulate around your middle quickly. Just don't get carbophobia! Carbs are important because they're protein sparing and create the anabolic environment needed for muscle growth!

NOTE: *Remember that "protein sparing" means that when you consume enough carbs, they will be used as energy, which allows protein to be prioritized for other needs.*

If you're an endurance athlete, even if you want to lose a few pounds, consider these muscle-gaining ratios instead of the fat-loss options, especially if you're logging more miles or training for an endurance race. Carbs are key for you while keeping your protein high to retain your lean muscle and fuel your performance.

You may stay on these ratios for three to four weeks rather than changing every two weeks. You may change cycles only with a new workout progression. Because pushing progression in the gym is key, having a very consistent energy source and full glycogen stores is essential. Longer stays on specific ratios can help you make sure you're fueling properly to allow your muscles to repair and rebuild. However, cycling still helps you avoid seeing fat creep on as you gain some hard-earned muscle.

Make sure to be consistent with your ratios before you switch to a different breakdown. If you're struggling to hit your numbers, especially if you feel full from the carbs and calories, try adjusting your meal timing or focus on the size of your meals. Using smoothies and focusing on calorically dense foods rather than on food volume can make a difference.

Hit your ratios within 2 to 3 percent and stay within 100 calories of your target. Be very careful of any cheat days and going over on calories—even a little—because it can create a much bigger surplus than you're already in. If you want a cheat day or a day where you go a bit above, work it into your overall week by setting a smaller daily surplus (maybe just 100 calories over maintenance) with one day of a bigger surplus (more like 300 over).

Table 12.8 shows the ratio options for different progress goals.

If you're coming out of a fat-loss phase or deficit, these ratios will result in a weight jump on the scale. Seeing the number go up can make you want to panic after you've worked so hard to lose, but the increase is necessary and good for gaining muscle. The higher carb ratios mean fuller glycogen stores and water retention, which contribute to the bigger number on the scale.

Go into these cycles aware and prepared. Slowly increase calories while using your fat-loss ratios; then select the ratio closest to what you were doing, even if it isn't in the cycle you think may be the best fit for your activity level or goal. From there, you can adjust. Embrace the jump on the scale and then watch it level out.

Focus on the complementary targets you set and make sure you've set some performance goals because you will see great gains with these macros!

TABLE 12.8: GUIDELINES FOR GAINING MUSCLE

LEAN BUILD

LESS ACTIVE

PROTEIN	CARBS	FAT
45%	35%	20%
35%	40%	25%
40%	30%	30%

20–30% FAT | 35–45% PROTEIN | 30–40% CARBS

MORE ACTIVE

PROTEIN	CARBS	FAT
30%	40%	30%
35%	45%	20%
35%	40%	25%

20–30% FAT | 30–35% PROTEIN | 40–45% CARBS

PURE GAINZZZ

LESS ACTIVE

PROTEIN	CARBS	FAT
45%	35%	20%
35%	45%	20%
40%	40%	20%

20% FAT | 35–45% PROTEIN | 35–45% CARBS

MORE ACTIVE

PROTEIN	CARBS	FAT
30%	50%	20%
30%	40%	30%
35%	45%	20%

20–30% FAT | 30–35% PROTEIN | 40–50% CARBS

How to Track

A tracking app is the easiest way to handle macro cycling. You can make your own spreadsheet and do the math yourself, but even a macros nerd like me finds it helpful to have the database for finding ingredients and saving meals.

Enter your macro ratios and calories into your tracking app, which will calculate grams of each macro you need. The formula the app uses is this:

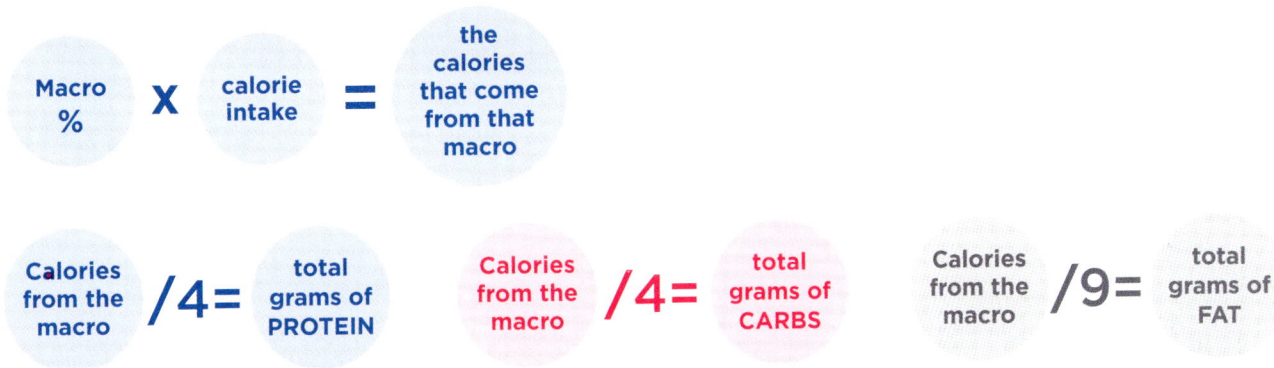

Macro % X **calorie intake** = **the calories that come from that macro**

Calories from the macro /4= **total grams of PROTEIN**   **Calories from the macro** /4= **total grams of CARBS**   **Calories from the macro** /9= **total grams of FAT**

Here's an example: You set your calorie intake at 1,500 and want to do a lean build but you're less active, so you choose the 40% protein/30% carbs/30% fat ratio:

1,500 X **40%** = **600**
calories · protein · calories from PROTEIN

1,500 X **30%** = **450**
calories · carbs · calories from CARBS

1,500 X **30%** = **450**
calories · fat · calories from FAT

600 / **4** = **150**
calories from PROTEIN · calories per gram · grams of PROTEIN

450 / **4** = **112.5**
calories from CARBS · calories per gram · grams of CARBS

450 / **9** = **50**
calories from FAT · calories per gram · grams of FAT

DAILY TOTALS: 1,500 calories from 150 grams of protein, 112.5 grams of carbs, and 50 grams of fat

These ratios are the daily totals you want to hit, not requirements for each meal. While you can make sure every meal hits the ratio, doing so may be more work, and just having a daily total you can hit allows for more food freedom and balance and can make things easier.

Also, planning ahead will help you be more successful. That way you have an idea of how your numbers are going to work out, and you can tweak things so you don't end up shoveling in chicken at the end of the day to hit your protein number. The more you plan ahead, the more you can work in things you love to make meals enjoyable.

You can work in the dessert you love or the crackers or chips you like to eat daily. You'll just plan more protein at another meal. The key is hitting your grams at the end of the day. (I say grams because hitting your gram totals means you hit your ratio and your calories.)

Over the course of your day, your ratio percentages will shift as those charts show the portion of calories consumed that come from each macro. At one point, you may be at 50 percent carbs because you have a banana at breakfast. But you aren't over your total carbs. You've just had more of your calories from carbs *so far* that day.

OATMEAL AND WHEY
BREAKFAST:

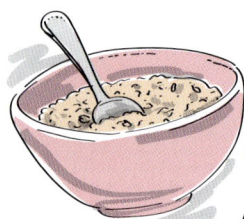

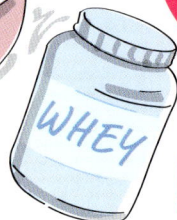

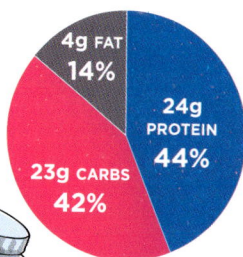

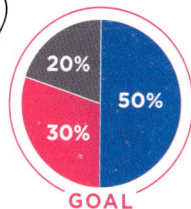

4g FAT
14%

24g
PROTEIN
44%

23g CARBS
42%

20%

50%

30%

GOAL

LUNCH OF GROUND BEEF,
SWEET POTATOES, AND
ASPARAGUS:

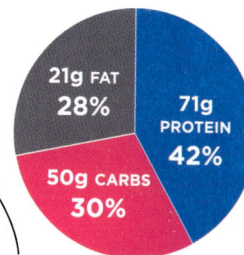

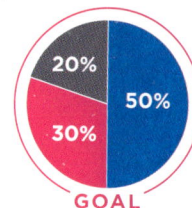

21g FAT
28%

71g
PROTEIN
42%

50g CARBS
30%

20%

50%

30%

GOAL

Balancing your macros will be a learning experience. You may have to step back and relearn how to manage your portions for a bit. It's the same as regressing to progress in your workouts. Sometimes, you have to be a beginner, have a learner's mindset, step back, and slow down to move forward. If you try to keep repeating the same meals, same snacks, and same way of eating without changing, it's like continuing to jam a square peg into a round hole. It's not going to work, and you're just going to waste time and effort.

Remember that story I brought up early in the book and have referred to many times? Be the woodcutter. Pause and sharpen your axe!

Look at the breakdown of your foods, try different ingredients, try the macro cycling meal plan builders at redefiningstrength.com/extras, test out different "puzzle pieces," and have fun learning! Realize it will take time. You're a baby learning to walk with macros. Celebrate your wins along the way but give yourself grace to have some missteps!

STRIKING A BALANCE

Faking habits and actions won't move you forward in any lasting way. That fake-it-'til-you-make-it attitude is what keeps people constantly doing twenty-one-day challenges and six-week programs. They get stuck in a loop of seeing results only to fall back into old patterns—repeating that change loop over and over and over again. Being stuck in that rut is what makes you feel like diet and workout changes need to be a full-time job to see results rather than being a component that fits into your lifestyle and priorities.

> " Sometimes, you have to be a beginner, have a learner's mindset, step back, and slow down to move forward. "

The Good and the Bad of Macro Cycling

Weighing the cost and reward of everything is key. Your budget for habit changes matters, and it can change over time. So, weigh the upsides and downsides over the course of your journey.

Sometimes, you may find you're spending more time and energy to track macros than you can really afford to and need to use the other macros methods. But don't be afraid to invest in yourself to see better results faster when you're ready for the change and sacrifice! Sometimes it's good to power through and show yourself your strength to overcome the challenge!

DO ALL CARBS COUNT?

I want to cover net carbs because it's a topic that comes up often. What are net carbs? They're the amount of carbohydrates in foods that are likely to be absorbed and affect blood sugar.

But with the rise in popularity of low-carb and keto diets for weight loss, *net carbs* has become a marketing term. Processed foods are always touting their net carb numbers. Fruits and vegetables, which are filled with fiber, aren't crowing about net carbs. The term has no "legal" definition to regulate it, so companies can use it to market as they'd like!

Many of these products have sugar alcohols that can impact your blood sugar, which can make them "sugar free," lower in carbs, and lower in calories. So they get the "net carb" label, and sometimes that means the calorie count can be lower because legally the product only has to list calories based on net, not total, carbs. Win-win for the manufacturer. But if net carbs are technically the amount of carbs that affect your blood sugar, and sugar alcohols *can* impact your blood sugar, this label is misleading.

Tracking net carbs and fiber can be significant for specific health issues, like diabetes, but for most, it shouldn't really matter. And when you set your calorie deficit or surplus, you're setting it with the assumption you're eating fiber.

As much as we say a calorie is just a calorie—which comes from the fact that one calorie is always one calorie from an energy standpoint—a calorie is *not* just a calorie. Protein has 4 calories per gram, but the thermic effect makes it less. Processed foods have a lower thermic effect than whole foods, but we don't try to subtract those extra calories burned to digest those foods from our logs.

It would be impossible to subtract the extra calories accurately. But generally speaking, it can create an extra deficit and is what you're considering when setting your calories. It's why I say macros can have a big impact on your calorie intake!

If you track only net carbs, you're basically doing the same thing as trying to subtract the thermic effect of protein or whole foods. The reason people do one thing and not the other is that calculating net carbs is easier to do and aids the trendy low-carb diets. It also allows food manufacturers to sell more processed foods. (It gives people an excuse to eat more carbs rather than sticking to the ratio they've set!)

While the argument to count only net carbs is that fiber doesn't impact blood sugar or contribute energy (so it shouldn't affect your calorie count or carb count), ratios and calories are set based on those overall totals. You're expected to consume fiber!

However, if you don't count all calories, you're allowing yourself to eat MORE than you'd planned.

So, here's my definitive statement on net carbs: *All carbs count.* There are no "free" foods. If a food has calories, you log it, and it counts. Plain and simple. Basically, count everything you eat. That way you can adjust based on totals. When presented with situations like this, I always think, "Why don't I want to count the carbs?" The answer is, "So I can eat more."

Macro cycling is the best way to get the results you want as fast as possible. It helps you to know exactly what is and isn't working. It also makes it possible to work in foods you love without feeling you have to eliminate anything.

While it can be challenging to learn at the start (yes, a downside), it also allows you to plan for the things you enjoy—even alcohol—and doesn't make foods you love off-limits. This doesn't mean you can and should include these foods all the time or can eat whatever you want whenever you want in any quantity, but no foods need to be demonized.

You can create a balance and have the power of choice rather than the feeling of restriction. You can work in family and restaurant meals without always feeling like a person on a diet!

Macro cycling is also a great way to address food intolerances and adjust your diet based on health concerns, hormonal changes, or changes in your activity level and goals.

Of course, macro cycling isn't without its downsides, the biggest of which is that you have to track. It can be annoying and tedious and time-consuming. It's not fun, but neither is balancing your checkbook (if you still even do that) or brushing your teeth. They're things you have to do to get the result that you want, but the habit isn't sexy or particularly enjoyable.

Learning how to hit your macros will take time. To start, it can be overwhelming and complicated, which might make you feel like giving up. If you've done your STRONG reflection, you should already know if this is likely to happen. If it is, start with one of the other methods instead. (Ahem, this is why the STRONG system works! Self-awareness and reflection are power!)

Meal planning and planning ahead are also crucial to easing the transition to tracking, so if you find this a challenge, start with a different method.

You do have to know your triggers, and if you have a history with disordered eating patterns, macro cycling may not be right for you. The hand-sized health method may be a better place to start to help you focus on your hunger cues and overall balance to your nutrition.

Otherwise, macro cycling can help you learn to fuel better and eat more. Tracking isn't just about weight loss. It can help you make sure you aren't underfueling, it can even help you know if you're hitting your micronutrients to improve your health!

Your Origin Macros

The thought of tracking macros, doing math, weighing, and measuring may make you want to back away from this method. You need to own your reluctance. You either realize you can budget for this and start with the ratio closest to what you're currently doing, or you realize you can't afford the cost right now and own that it's smarter to use the other macros methods.

No one way is more right or wrong than the others, and you can reassess at checkpoints as you go. Also, consider your destination and how quickly you want to get there. How lofty are your goals? Are they worth some effort? Sometimes, you have to push into the hard instead of shying away from it. You have to carry some heavy-rock habits to start, knowing that by going all-in, you will get more comfortable being uncomfortable.

Here are some other things to consider:

? Take a look at your nonnegotiables. Will full tracking allow you to work them in for better balance?

? Take a look at your targets. Will tracking allow you to hit them more quickly and see your success snowball? Will it create a ripple effect so that the more you do, the more you want to do?

? Take a look at what you've struggled with in the past. Will tracking allow you to optimize around those struggles by not feeling like foods are off-limits and by knowing that you can truly tell what is and isn't working? Or is the negative too great to start?

Pause, assess, and own where you are. Consider the significance of your goals. Realize you can start and adjust later. Set your first checkpoint to know you have a time frame for testing and trust in the process up to that point!

Your Small-Stone and Pebble Habits

After tracking for just three days, or after mapping out a day of food you'd usually eat, what's one area where you need lots of improvement? Which macro breakdown are you closest to and what would you need to do to hit those ratios?

Don't feel like you need to overhaul your diet. That's going *on* a diet rather than adjusting to create a meal plan based on your lifestyle. It's why things haven't worked in the past. You've gone on plan after plan after plan and have never adjusted for things you love so you can find balance.

Taking action is more important than being perfect. Action leads to greater improvements faster. If you use any of the ratios I suggested, you'll honestly start making progress if you do them consistently!

Small changes make a difference. One more ounce of protein in a meal, swapping a fruit for a veggie or a lower-carb fruit, or trading something as simple as brown rice for wild rice can have an amazing impact.

See the opportunity in trying new foods using the information on page 167 that breaks down ways to get your macros from many common grocery items. Make changes that make you feel excited. You won't like everything you do, but you can often find components that are fun. If you feel resistance against a change, ask yourself why you feel that way. You want to understand why you feel that way to address the root of the concern rather than trying to "sell" yourself on the change.

Make a list of three small pebbles and one small-stone adjustment. Focus on one of those things starting immediately (today) and outline how you can slowly implement the others, stacking them over the next few days or weeks. Let those habits become part of your routine. Then, continue to add; rock by rock, you'll build.

Pause and write some thoughts on the habit changes you'll need to make. List a reason you like this method and a downside in comparison to the other options.

If you skipped the other macros methods and came straight here because you thought this would be best, go back and read through the others. It will help you consider all the options to really know you're meeting yourself where you are so you can move forward most effectively.

As you read through the remaining chapters about the stuff people often ignore in their lifestyle, start taking action. Go ahead and start making small diet and workout changes.

13 THE STUFF WE IGNORE

There are many lifestyle factors that impact your results. People tend to focus on their diet and workouts because they're not only key but also easier to control. You can choose to pop those Reese's Pieces into your mouth as you walk to the couch, or you can tie your gym shoes, grab your protein shake, and hit the gym.

However, if I say, "Sleep better and you'll see better fat loss," you'd probably roll your eyes at me. But the reality is that you can't ignore these other lifestyle factors. They *do* affect your results. They can make your diet and workout changes easier or harder. They can make them pay off more or less.

I get that some lifestyle habits aren't that easy to change, but you still should try. I called this chapter "The Stuff We Ignore" because I talk about those factors that you know you "should" change but don't and the stuff you don't want to focus on, feel you don't fully have control over, or don't know how to change. On the other hand, these factors can also be the stuff you obsess over before it's time or the things you really push back against. Maybe I should have called this chapter "Unsexy, Hard Details That Are Key."

In this chapter, I cover the importance of sleep, recovery and rest days, micronutrients, fiber, hydration, and even diet breaks. I touch on meal timing because this is usually a detail that doesn't really matter, but people often get hung up on it. (Yup. I said it *doesn't* matter. Surprised?)

These are the lifestyle components that are more health and long-term focused or that come secondary to the macros and workouts. They are the lifestyle components that aren't in fads or quick fixes but are often what can bust plateaus or sticking points to help you feel your best!

When you're aware of the importance of these components, you might realize your other diet and workout changes positively affect them. These unsexy details can make for great complementary targets as well as ways to measure progress and know that your other habit changes are paying off. The point is, you definitely don't want to ignore them, and you also want to recognize how avoiding them may hold you back!

SLEEP: THE KEY TO IT ALL

Want to see better body recomp and improve your health and stress levels? Work to improve your sleep. That means focusing on getting not only more sleep but also higher-quality sleep. Of course, this is easier said than done. That's why I want to go over both why sleep quality is so important and what you can do to reduce your stress and create habits and routines that lead to better sleeping patterns.

THE SLEEP-STRESS LINK

"I know, I know. I need to get more sleep!" I'm pretty sure I've never heard someone say the opposite or complain about having too much time for getting too much quality sleep. Society oddly celebrates lack of sleep, and people often brag about how much caffeine they need to function.

Want to fit in that morning workout? Get up earlier. Want to meal prep for the next day? Stay up later. It seems even healthy habits are trying to sabotage your sleep. This is where the stuff you worked through in Part 1 plays a role. Your origin story needs to outline your current lifestyle from every angle—even how you're sleeping.

Honestly, a thirty-minute workout might be better for you right now than a one-hour session if it means you get thirty more minutes of sleep. Having a quick restaurant meal that you feel isn't as healthy may be better than having to go to bed an hour later so you have time to meal prep. Improving your health is about constantly balancing different lifestyle factors while acknowledging the stress involved in handling them all.

One way you might notice this stress accumulation is in your sleep. Not only do people tend to struggle to fall asleep and get less sleep, but sleep quality is also affected.

A lack of sleep can negatively impact hormone levels, leading to more stress and worse recovery. It can make you not want to do the healthy habits that would improve your stress and sleep, and it can even lead to changes in appetite, causing you to overeat. A lack of quality sleep makes sticking with healthy habit changes harder, not to mention that it also makes them pay off less. Then, because you don't stick with them, your sleep suffers further. Yikes! Talk about a catch-22!

Good news: You aren't doomed. Sleep is a hard thing to control directly, but there are small adjustments you can make to bedtime routines that can help. Being aware of the quality of your sleep and the impact it can have on your habits and goals, as well as when you're sacrificing sleep for other things that you perhaps shouldn't be, will help you start to find your balance.

Focus on your bedtime routine and how you're managing your stress. Be conscious of when you're drawing time for other habit changes from your sleep "time reserve." Is there really no other way you can squeeze in an early-morning workout? Is there no other time-suck in your day you could eliminate for extra time to meal prep? Consider where you want to end up, and ask yourself these questions:

? What would my sleep look like, ideally? **?** How would I wind down at the end of the day?

? When would I go to bed? **?** What other schedule changes may need to happen?

? How would that work? **?** What would my sleep environment look like?

Also reflect on the following lifestyle factors:

» Are you consuming caffeine later in the day (within six hours of going to bed)? Is it hidden in something you don't realize? You might feel you "need" caffeine to make it through the day, but that could be making you more dependent on it to survive. While breaking the cycle is hard, try cutting back just a little bit.

» Are you consuming a nightly glass of alcohol? You may think it helps you fall asleep, but really, it doesn't. You may feel more relaxed and like you fall asleep faster, but alcohol negatively impacts the quality of your sleep. So, what can seem like it's helping may actually be the culprit for why you feel so tired the next day, even though you've technically gotten enough sleep. Note: I'm not telling you not to drink at all; each person must find their balance, and I am a cocktail girl on a Friday night. (I especially like a super good margarita!) But try eliminating it for two or three weeks and see if you notice changes in your sleep. One night without won't do it. You have to run an experiment and let your body adjust. If you're drinking daily (even just one or two drinks per day), you may notice a bigger impact on your sleep than if you're only indulging in the occasional weekend drink.

» Are you eating close to bedtime? Sometimes, you have to because your schedule dictates eating late. If you hit your macros and calories, you'll be fine! But big late-night meals can sometimes negatively impact sleep, so if you can avoid late-night eating, do so.

» Are you training later in the evening? This might be the only time you feel you have, but pay attention to whether your late-night workouts are leaving you feeling revved up and struggling to relax for bed. If so, is there a way to try shorter routines earlier in the day? Maybe you can save only recovery workouts for later in the evening. Can you do a longer cool down to help?

The more you start to examine when shifts in your sleep have happened or which nights you've slept better (or worse), the more you can notice trends and make adjustments. Think small things. They add up!

Watch the impact that changing your macros and using the workouts in this program has on your sleep. This can be something you monitor as a complementary target even if you don't have a measurable goal of sleeping X more hours. Monitor how many days you wake up feeling refreshed. Or how many days you sleep through the night. Or how many days you get to bed earlier and fall asleep more easily. Not every target will have a fully objective data measurement as the goal.

With your answers to those questions, you can use the tips in the next section to improve your bedtime routine and address some common sleep struggles.

YOUR BEDTIME ROUTINE

Do you struggle to fall asleep? Feel like you just toss and turn and can't get comfortable? Like your mind starts going the second you lie down, and you could suddenly solve all of the world's problems (or at least see them!)?

Or maybe you're one of those people whose head hits the pillow, and you're *out*. Then, when the clock strikes 1 a.m., you're wide awake again. You try to go to the bathroom, thinking you'll get up and go back to bed relaxed, but nope. You're *up*. You doze a bit or finally drift off again an hour before your alarm goes off. But sleeping solidly through the night—ha! You wish!

The hard part is that you can't just command yourself to sleep. In fact, the more you stress and worry about your sleep, the worse it often gets. Instead, you want to focus on the routines before bed that make you feel good. You also want to assess the daily lifestyle factors that have an impact on your nightly sleep. The great part is that you're tracking and reflecting so much right now that you should be able to identify triggers. What gets measured, gets managed. (Sound familiar? I hope so!)

Now, let's talk bedtime routines. I want to focus on some basic sleep habits that are easy to start with, don't require you to buy anything, and have a positive payoff for the other lifestyle changes you're working to make with this program:

» **Brain dump**

» **One-minute mobility routine**

» **Distraction breathing** (I'll explain why I—as a bumblebee–brained person—call it this)

All three things can take you just five minutes in total. They're not fancy. They're simple, and they won't cut into your time reserves (aka your sleep).

The Brain Dump

I have a bumblebee brain to the extreme. The second I need it to quiet down and stop buzzing is the moment it seems to ramp up to double time. Right before bed is a prime time for this phenomenon to occur. I struggle to relax as I play through different scenarios, work through problems, and make my to-do list over and over again. There is no way I'll solve half of these things at that time of night, but I worry I won't remember something, which makes me repeat things and get stuck in a mental loop.

This is why doing a brain dump before bed is so helpful. You can have a note on your phone, make a to-do list on your computer, or have a notebook where you write everything down. Regardless of the tool you use, set a timer for a couple of minutes and write down anything you need to be organized for the next day. Write any earth-shattering thoughts you've had.

This mental clearing can help you relax and realize nothing is so important that it can't be done later. This dump can help you feel more organized for the next day.

It's also a way to mentally check out and set a finite end to your day. You're done. Everything is prepped for tomorrow. You can now relax.

After you get those thoughts out and slow the buzzing, your next thought should be to focus on the rest of your pre-bed routine, which continues with one minute of mobility work.

One-Minute Mobility Routine

After you've cleared your brain, you want to continue winding down by relaxing your body. When you physically relax, you help yourself mentally relax. It all relates to calming your nervous system.

Focusing on mobility also helps give your brain direction as you fully relax and prep yourself to wake up feeling refreshed the next day. This practice can help if you ever feel stiff or achy in the morning. This makes it a no-lose situation: Sleep better tonight and move better tomorrow!

This routine isn't time consuming. All you need is one minute. So, if you've ever thought, *I wish I had time to do more mobility work,* doing this daily helps you do 365 minutes per year.

Set a timer for one minute and pick one area to roll out. It can be your upper back, which is tense from a long day hunched over your computer. It can be your hips, which may be tight from a long commute. It can be something you're feeling from your workout.

Roll for thirty seconds (per side) and breathe as you focus on relaxing and releasing tension as you pause on any tight spots.

Often, one minute turns into five minutes, which not only helps you feel better for future workouts but can also make you feel very relaxed going to bed. If you're feeling tired or short on time, knowing you only need one minute puts no pressure on you.

Be very conscious of focusing on the muscle, relaxing it and releasing tension as you hold. Focus on the deep breaths. This helps you keep your mind from going back into buzz mode and even helps you feel relaxed as you move to the final step of distraction breathing.

Distraction Breathing

I'm easily distracted, especially when I'm trying my best *not* to be. I start trying to do something to relax, and all of a sudden, out of nowhere, my brain goes, "Squirrel!" like a dog distracted by the first thing it sees moving outside the window.

Breathing techniques that involve breathing with a simple count don't work for me. The more complicated the count, the better. I also set the number of breaths I "have" to take higher because it reduces the pressure to relax or fall asleep fast. It distracts my brain from any other thoughts and makes me fully engrossed in the process. I also feel no pressure to relax because I "expect" to have to do fifty breaths. I usually make it to ten at most.

Deep breathing fully relaxes you physically and mentally and is a great technique to use anytime you feel anxiety rising in everyday life. By slowing down and focusing on controlled, deep, and slow breaths, you'll find that you relax not only your body but also your mind.

I like to use a 4-7-8 breathing count. The variation in the numbers makes me focus on only the breathing. You'll take a four-count inhale, hold for seven counts, and do an eight-count exhale. Find a count that feels comfortable to you and keeps you focused on the breathing. Then set a number of breaths you "have" to complete before falling asleep. I like to give myself fifty breaths, knowing there is no way I'll get there; I don't feel pressure to get to the goal.

As you incorporate these bedtime routine changes, you may need a while to get in a flow and find the variations that resonate most with you. For example, you may find that doing mobility work before the brain dump helps you work through some thoughts as you physically relax; then you can write down the most important ones.

If you have enough time, maybe you can extend the mobility work and add in some stretching as well. The idea is to set a routine that you repeat consistently to promote relaxation and to have a finite end to your day. You're taking some time for you.

What would a good bedtime routine be for you to wake up feeling refreshed and ready to conquer the day? What changes would you have to make from where you are now? Don't write down the obvious stuff, like "Get more sleep," or "Go to bed earlier." Focus on how you can *relax* before bed to help yourself catch more quality Z's.

NUTRIENTS TO IMPROVE YOUR SLEEP

Later in this chapter, I will go over micronutrients (vitamins and minerals) more, but I want to mention them with regard to sleep because they can have a huge impact while being an easy change to implement. Micronutrients can provide great benefits, especially to perimenopausal and menopausal women.

Two foods and one nutrient that help to improve the quality of your sleep are kiwis, tart cherries, and magnesium.

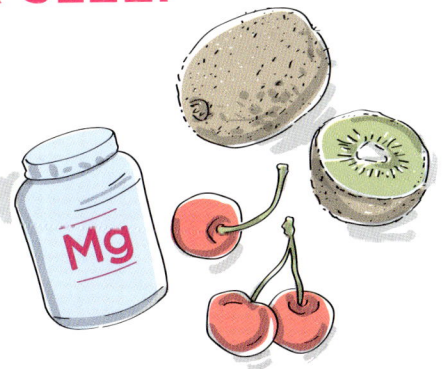

Kiwis

Kiwis are high in vitamins C and E and contain potassium and folate. These vitamins and minerals help promote melatonin production, improve neurotransmitter regulation and function, and can even help with night sweats (which can often impact the quality of your sleep during menopause).

Kiwis are also high in serotonin, which, together with dopamine, plays an important role in how well and long you sleep. Your brain needs serotonin to make melatonin, a hormone that regulates your sleep/wake cycle. A study of people who ate two kiwis one hour before bed found they fell asleep faster, slept more, and had higher-quality sleep![*]

Tart Cherries

Ever heard that turkey makes you sleepy because of tryptophan? Well, getting more tryptophan (an amino acid) is important if you want to improve the quality of your sleep. Tart cherries are rich in both this amino acid and melatonin. A study showed that consuming two servings of tart cherry juice could improve total sleep time

---

*Hsiao-Han Lin, Pei-Shan Tsai, Su-Chen Fang, and Jen-Fang Liu, "Effect of Kiwifruit Consumption on Sleep Quality in Adults with Sleep Problems," *Asia Pacific Journal of Clinical Nutrition* 20, no. 2 (2011): 169–74, https://pubmed.ncbi.nlm.nih.gov/21669584/.

and even lead to higher sleep efficiency.* This is most likely due to the fact that tart cherries increase the amount of melatonin available in the body.

An easy way to consume tart cherries is in juice form, although you can buy an extract or get a pill supplement. Drink up to 16 ounces of tart cherry juice or take 480 milligrams of tart cherry extract capsules once per day for up to two weeks before cycling off for a bit. For a real sleep "cocktail," mix a bit of magnesium powder (200 milligrams) into your tart cherry juice!

Magnesium

Magnesium is a mineral that plays a role in the production of serotonin and promotes relaxation and better circulation. It's essential for many processes throughout your body, including communication between cells in your nervous system. Because your nervous system largely controls sleep, magnesium can have a huge impact on your sleep health. While this micronutrient is easy to supplement, you can increase your natural consumption through foods like dark chocolate (yes, an excuse to include chocolate in your macros!), spinach, pumpkin seeds, bananas, and avocados.

Consider including a few of these foods in the latter half of your day but be conscious not to eat or drink too close to bed. You don't want to struggle to fall asleep because your body is processing a late meal, and you don't want to have to wake up extra to go to the bathroom! These foods make for a great dessert snack plate if you want a sweet treat to end your night.

REST TO REBUILD

Resting is the thing most people struggle to do when they're pushing hard with a workout routine. They can feel guilty for resting despite knowing they should *take time off.*

You probably know you should take recovery days, but the struggle to pause and rest is real. An object in motion tends to stay in motion, and you may have a fear that you'll backslide because of one day of doing nothing.

I have two things to say about that: 1) A rest day doesn't mean doing nothing. 2) This *exact* mindset often dooms people to repeat the change loop; people burn out from never slowing down.

People worry about burning calories. Building muscle. Working hard. They feel like if they do more, results will happen faster. This attitude is what makes people try to out-exercise their diets. This is short-term thinking because it ends with overestimating what can be accomplished in the short term while underestimating what can be accomplished long term with consistency.

That's why planning the rest and recovery is so key. When you strategically plan "deload" weeks, recovery days, or lower-intensity days, it doesn't feel like you're

---

*Wilfred R. Pigeon, Michelle Carr, Colin Gorman, and Michael L. Perlis, "Effects of a Tart Cherry Juice Beverage on the Sleep of Older Adults with Insomnia: A Pilot Study," *Journal of Medicinal Food* 13, no. 3 (2010): 579–83, https://pmc.ncbi.nlm.nih.gov/articles/PMC3133468/.

letting off the gas or slowing down for no reason. It doesn't feel like you're going easy on yourself. There isn't a shift in momentum to do less. In this section, I explain why recovery is so important and what it means to have a recovery, or deload, week.

WHY RECOVERY IS IMPORTANT

You need rest stops and refuel breaks on road trips. They're times to recharge and make sure you're going in the right direction. The same thing goes for planned periods of recovery and rest. This rest isn't only for your body; it's for your mind as well. You can't push at 100 percent intensity all of the time.

Often, when people hit burnout and feel like the effort isn't worth the outcome, it's because they've been pushing intensely for a while. Mental fatigue from the constant focus on new habits, the willpower they're exerting, and the discomfort in learning and making changes has added up. Lifestyle priorities may have shifted during that time as well.

If you're in this situation, you need to realize that easing off the gas for a bit and taking that rest stop may ultimately help you get back on track more quickly. For now, you may need to embrace doing the minimum. You can strategically plan recovery weeks into your routine if you know you usually hit the wall around six, twelve, or sixteen weeks into a new program or plan. You can also plan your recovery if you know you're going into a busy time of year.

"Slow down to speed up," and "Less is more," may be clichés, but they're spot on! That's why you'll find recovery days in each week of the workout progressions in Part 3. You'll also see full days of (gasp!) *nothing*! This doesn't mean I'm telling you not to be active or do some mobility work, but you must have rest days that make you crave the intensity and push of your training days.

Recovery days aren't only about resting a muscle group. You can rest a muscle by focusing on different areas each workout or even by working the same muscle in different ways. The point of recovery is not to create more stress on your body and mind for a day. Exercise is a good stressor, but it's still a stressor. Pushing hard in your training should wear you down mentally to some extent. You should be uncomfortable as you push the progression to see results.

If you haven't felt the need for a recovery day, assess whether you're really maximizing your current training sessions. Could you give it more? If a feeling of guilt stops you from taking a day off, I'd challenge you with this question: Why do you feel guilty about allowing your body a day to rest and repair?

Any guilt you feel probably comes back to how you pressure yourself to do more and a desire to see results faster. But remember: You can't out-exercise or out-diet time!

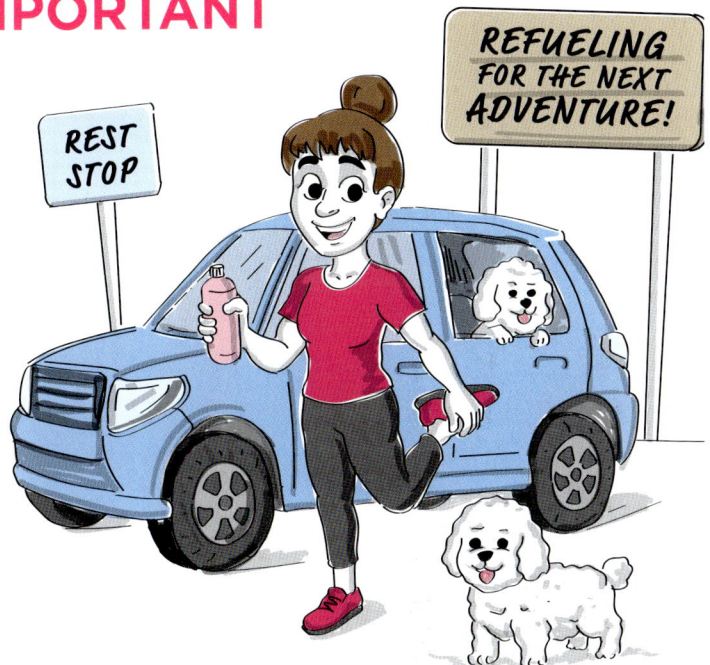

Take the rest days. Do your mobility work to move better during other training sessions. Go for walks. Stay active. And if you've ever used the excuse, "I don't have enough time to meal prep or plan out my macros ahead of time," take the rest day and use that hour you would have worked out to do those things.

HOW TO INCORPORATE RECOVERY WEEKS

The workouts I offer include a recovery, or "deload," week. Switching progressions every three to six weeks allows you to change intensity that first week on the new progression and can keep you charging ahead. If you feel good and aren't seeing diminishing returns from your training or aches and pains popping up, there may be no need for an official recovery week just yet. You don't need to include deload weeks at set intervals, but be on the lookout for both physical and mental burnout so you can take advantage of recovery when you need it.

Unless you're training for a specific race date, you usually aren't trying to peak for something specific. Consequently, you have the flexibility to press the gas when you're motivated and feeling good but ease back or take a rest stop when you need it so you don't crash your car into the guardrail.

The deload week is a week involving restorative prehab work. It isn't a week of doing nothing but lounging on the couch as you lose the habit and routine of training. Honestly, a recovery week doesn't even have to mean easy workouts. You could do something as simple as go very light with the next progression you're going to start so you move and train those movement patterns without stress. You can do all bodyweight workouts if you usually use weight. You can do only prehab work, isometrics, and walking.

You can vary what you do based on what you need. Whatever you do, it should feel good mentally, and you should feel your body getting a break from the consistent intensity and pushing of your usual workouts. You can time these weeks with vacations when you'll be active but would have trouble getting to the gym. Some added mobility work will only help with travel aches and pains. Another approach is to strategically plan your recovery weeks for when you know you'll have an extra busy week at work or a stressful family week.

Around the holidays, when you know your workouts will be inconsistent, you can adjust to a three-day-a-week training schedule. It keeps you doing something—a training minimum—that ultimately moves you forward and can even make you crave doing more.

Much of how you shift habits is based on the mindset momentum they create, and too often, people forget the importance of this.

Do this assessment to start considering the perfect times for recovery weeks:

» Consider the reflection you did for O in your STRONG system reflection and recognize and assess the struggles that popped up in the past.

» Assess what wall you usually hit that leads to you quitting.

» Assess what training habits haven't felt repeatable at certain times of year and *why* they've felt that way.

» Assess your nonnegotiables and the impact they have on your training.

Plan ahead so you don't feel guilty or like you're "letting yourself off the hook" with a recovery day or week.

In case you're concerned, no, you won't eat less on days off from training. Your body often needs that fuel to repair, and it's best to have full energy stores for your next workout. When you track macros (using any method), you want your daily intake to remain consistent. Do not cut calories just because you didn't exercise!

Even though you don't cut calories for a recovery day, you may consider a shift in macros with a full recovery week. For example, you might use the minimalist macros method (page 159) or reduce carbs for that week because you've wanted to try going lower carb but usually gas out when you're more active. Find a balance and focus on feeling fully recharged. Don't starve yourself because you're worried you aren't burning enough calories. This week is meant to help you prepare to hit the gas mentally and physically the next week!

MICRONUTRIENTS: QUALITY MATTERS

Demonizing foods isn't part of the STRONG system, but you still need to remember that everything in your body is built from the foods you consume and that vitamins and minerals matter. The quality of your fuel can have an impact on your health and your fat loss and muscle-building results.

I know very little about cars, but I know this: Give a nice car low-grade fuel, and it's eventually going to break down. Give it the high-quality fuel it needs, and its engine will run well. Your body is the same way. When you avoid nutritional gaps and deficiencies, your body will function better, leading to faster results.

As you get older, your nutritional needs evolve due to shifting hormone levels, bone density changes, and metabolic adaptations. You simply don't absorb or utilize micronutrients as efficiently, so you need more to stay healthy.

Many vitamins and minerals become more crucial to consume at higher levels later in life, especially for women during menopause and into the postmenopausal years, to support healthy aging, muscle function, mood regulation, body composition, and health in general. A study by the CDC has shown that 75 percent of women don't get enough calcium and that 90 percent of women need more folate and vitamin E.* The CDC standards are based on minimums for preventing disease rather than on optimal levels, so you want to do even better than those recommendations. You don't just want to avoid being ill and frail; you want to be *strong* and *thrive*!

To help you feel your most fabulous until your final day on this planet, I want to touch on eleven micronutrients (plus one fat, so I'm cheating a little bit here) you should pay

---

*Christine M. Pfeiffer et al., "The CDC's Second National Report on Biochemical Indicators of Diet and Nutrition in the U.S. Population Is a Valuable Tool for Researchers and Policy Makers," *The Journal of Nutrition* 143, no. 6 (2013): 938S–47S, https://pubmed.ncbi.nlm.nih.gov/23596164/.

attention to as you get older to build your leanest, strongest, fittest, healthiest body at any age. Your primary goal is to get the following nutrients by consuming whole, natural foods, but you can consider a supplement if you're struggling to hit your daily intake. (This is another great thing you can easily monitor by tracking macros!)

Alpha-Lipoic Acid (ALA)

ALA is a powerful antioxidant that improves metabolic health and insulin sensitivity, lowers inflammation and oxidative stress, and combats fatigue and cognitive decline. It keeps the brain and body healthy and helps you see better fat-loss results, especially during menopause.

It supports mitochondrial health, which declines as you get older. Consequently, you can see improvement in your energy levels, which can help during menopause if you're feeling fatigued and unmotivated to train. If you're going through an especially stressful time, increasing your intake of this powerful antioxidant can improve your fat-loss results while helping you manage sugar cravings! Focus on spinach, broccoli, tomatoes, and potatoes. Organ meats are also great if you enjoy them.

B Vitamins

Especially in a fat-loss phase, you may find your recovery is a bit impaired. Making sure you're not low in B vitamins, specifically B6, B9, and B12, is key because low levels can lead to poor muscle recovery, low energy, and negatively impact protein synthesis. If you're struggling to maintain your calorie deficit for fat loss, check your vitamin B levels!

To consume more B6, include more chicken, turkey, potatoes, bananas, and spinach. Leafy greens will also increase B9 (folate), as will beans, peas, lentils, and asparagus. You can get vitamin B12 from poultry, fish, and dairy products. If you're plant based, you might find it harder to get B12, so consider fortified foods, supplementation, or including nutritional yeast on a regular basis. (Bonus: Nutritional yeast is a great way to boost protein!)

Calcium

Most people are aware of the important role calcium, along with vitamin D, plays in bone health, but low calcium levels can also reduce muscle contraction strength, which takes away from the muscle gains you may want. There are even some studies linking low calcium levels to negative impacts on metabolic health and fat metabolism.

Don't fear dairy! Include things like milk and yogurt in your diet if you're not lactose intolerant. The probiotics in yogurt have added gut health benefits to improve overall health and fat loss. And if you can't consume dairy, eat fortified tofu, leafy greens, broccoli, and almonds.

Iodine

This mineral is often not discussed but is crucial for the thyroid, which regulates metabolism, to function properly. An underactive thyroid can lead to low energy, which can contribute to not only difficulty losing weight but also unwanted fat creeping on. Cod, fortified salt, and seaweed are great sources. If you're a sushi lover, this is a win-win! (I know—salt often gets a bad rap, but you do need some of it in your diet; there is nuance to everything!)

Iron

Iron is a key mineral to pay attention to if you're plant based, an endurance athlete, or a premenopausal woman who still has a regular cycle. Low iron levels negatively impact endurance and recovery. You may find you're constantly tired and fatigued. Also, low iron levels can lead to a slower metabolism, making it harder for you to burn fat and build muscle. There are two forms of iron: heme iron, which is more easily absorbed, and non-heme iron. Heme iron can be consumed through red meat, poultry, fish, and shellfish, while non-heme iron can be consumed in lentils, beans, tofu, spinach, quinoa, and pumpkin seeds.

Magnesium

I mentioned magnesium a bit when it comes to improving sleep, but it's also responsible for helping regulate insulin levels, stress levels, adrenal function, and anxiety. Low levels of magnesium not only negatively impact sleep but also increase cortisol levels, which can lead to a struggle to lose fat or gain muscle. You may even suffer from chronic headaches and mood swings. If you experience an increase in any of these symptoms with menopause, it may be time to check your magnesium levels and increase your intake of nuts and seeds.

Selenium

You've probably heard about the importance of antioxidants, and selenium is a powerful one! It supports thyroid and heart health and helps reduce inflammation. This makes it an extra important micronutrient for anyone in menopause or postmenopause. It helps keep your metabolism healthy, improves energy levels, and even helps reduce brain fog. It can lower your risk for heart disease, which increases after menopause. Selenium promotes joint health and supports a healthy immune system to help you recover faster and train harder. It even improves skin and hair health, which can be helpful as skin becomes drier, and hair often becomes thinner, during menopause.

The best part? You can consume two Brazil nuts per day and hit your quota! If you don't like Brazil nuts, eat more seafood, eggs, or even whole grains.

WARNING: More is not better with Brazil nuts. Eat no more than two per day!

Vitamin D3

While vitamin D is the sunshine vitamin, most people unfortunately don't get enough through sunlight alone. Beyond that, as you get older, your skin's ability to absorb and produce vitamin D from the sun declines.

Vitamin D is essential to help absorb calcium, which supports bone health. It regulates blood sugar to improve insulin sensitivity, which is helpful, especially during menopause. It also supports thyroid function, boosts immune function, and improves mood and mental health. It's a key vitamin to pay attention to if you've struggled to lose weight, especially due to an increase in inflammation during menopause or an autoimmune condition. Sunlight is a great way to increase your vitamin D levels, but fatty fish, egg yolks, and fortified foods can also help; you may need a supplement during the winter months.

Vitamin E

As you get older, oxidative stress increases. Vitamin E is a powerful antioxidant that can help protect your cells, improve your immune function, and even keep your brain healthier! It can also improve your metabolic health by improving your insulin sensitivity and reducing inflammation. To get more vitamin E, focus on foods like almonds, avocados, kiwis, salmon, sunflower seeds, and trout.

Vitamin K

This is the under-discussed third wheel for bone health along with calcium and vitamin D. It's also often the missing link! Menopausal women will want to pay attention to this micronutrient.

Vitamin K strengthens bones by activating proteins that bind calcium to them, reducing fracture risk. It can help lower the risk for heart disease and even reduce inflammation, supporting brain health while also helping reduce joint pain so you can train harder. Less inflammation and better joint health mean more quality training sessions and better recovery. To get your vitamin K, focus on leafy greens, fermented foods, and things like egg yolks and liver (ugh, not my favorite!).

Zinc

If you are in a calorie deficit for fat loss, you want to be especially conscious of your immune system health, which is why zinc is important as you get older. It plays a role in your testosterone and estrogen balance, which affects muscle growth and fat storage distribution. Zinc also supports adrenal and thyroid function, which both impact your energy levels and metabolic health. Low zinc levels can slow fat loss and negatively impact recovery and strength gains. It's essential for skin health. To increase your zinc intake, consider things like oysters (or seaboogers, as I lovingly call them) and beef, although nuts and seeds are also great sources.

Omega-3 Fatty Acids

Here's the thing: Omega-3 fatty acids are not technically a micronutrient. They're a type of fat, so I'm cheating by putting them here. But I've included them because I think their nutritional value is so significant.

This healthy fat improves heart health, brain function, skin health, and hormonal balance. It also helps keep joints healthy, and some interesting research has been done on its ability to improve recovery.* Focusing on healthy fats is important if you want to feel and look your best, especially as you get older and inflammation levels rise. For women, omega-3s can help reduce symptoms of menopause, such as hot flashes, mood swings, and sleep disturbances. Focus on omega-3s by consuming fatty fish, such as salmon and sardines, or take a fish oil or algae supplement (especially the latter if you're plant based).

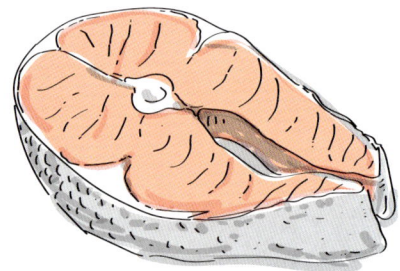

*Trisha A. VanDusseldorp et al., "Impact of Varying Dosages of Fish Oil on Recovery and Soreness Following Eccentric Exercise," *Nutrients* 12, no. 8 (2020): 2246, https://pubmed.ncbi.nlm.nih.gov/32727162/.

EAT THE RAINBOW

Now, if your head is spinning and you feel like you have to start adjusting everything in your diet and managing every detail—stop. Pause and breathe.

Note the foods you like for each color in the chart. There's a lot of overlap, so you can focus on those foods first and maybe add one that you're not consuming much of right now. From there, you can add others if you'd like.

RED	ORANGE	YELLOW	GREEN	BLUE/PURPLE
APPLE	CARROT	BANANA	APPLE	BLACKBERRIES
CHERRY	GRAPEFRUIT	CORN	ASPARAGUS	BLUEBERRIES
CRANBERRIES	MANGO	LEMON	AVOCADO	EGGPLANT
PEPPER	NECTARINE	PEPPER	BROCCOLI	FIG
POMEGRANATE	ORANGE	PINEAPPLE	CABBAGE	GRAPES
RASPBERRY	PEACH	POTATO	CELERY	PLUM
STRAWBERRY	PEPPER	SQUASH	CUCUMBER	PRUNES
TOMATO	PUMPKIN	STARFRUIT	GREEN BEAN	RAISINS
WATERMELON	SWEET POTATO	YELLOW ONION	KIWI	RED CABBAGE
	TANGERINE		LETTUCE	RED ONION
	YAM		PEAS	TURNIPS
			SPINACH	

EAT AS MANY COLORS OF THE RAINBOW AS YOU CAN EACH DAY!

FIBER: THE FAT LOSS MAGIC PILL

When you think fat loss, you probably don't think fiber. I don't know about you, but when I think of fiber, the first word that pops into my head is *poop*! Second, I think *gut health*.

Fiber helps you maintain balance in your gut microbiome, and if your gut microbiome isn't healthy, the rest of your body won't function optimally. A healthy gut helps reduce inflammation, keeps your metabolic rate higher to burn more fat, and helps reduce cravings. An increase in "bad" bacteria has been shown to trigger an overproduction of insulin, leading to insulin resistance, which causes your body to stop burning fat and start storing it. The more insulin-sensitive you are, the more likely you are to have a leaner body due to insulin's anabolic properties—replenishing fuel stores while reducing the rate of protein degradation or breakdown.

Increasing your fiber intake and taking care of your gut can also help you feel fuller and balance your appetite, which is super helpful when you're in a calorie deficit. When the bacteria in your gut ferment fiber, leptin is released, which can help suppress appetite and make you feel more satisfied. Soluble fiber—from oats, legumes, lentils, and apples, for example—ferments in the gut and feeds the good gut bacteria.

This good bacteria then produces short-chain fatty acids, like butyrate, propionate, and acetates, that stimulate the release of glucagon-like peptide-1 (GLP-1) in the intestines. This increases satiety, slows gastric emptying, and regulates blood sugar by stimulating insulin release.

As amazing as fiber is, most people don't get anywhere close to meeting the daily requirements. The general recommendation is 25 grams per day for women and 38 grams per day for men, and most people are well below that. (Another great part about tracking macros is that you can easily monitor your fiber intake in your food tracker!)

Most of the time, people don't notice (or care) that they're not getting enough fiber. Stomach or digestion issues are usually the only reasons people think about fiber, and the solution is often to turn to a supplement. Instead, you should focus on getting quality fuel and examine how you're hitting your macros.

The hand-sized health macros method has an emphasis on nonstarchy carbs. This can help you start to adjust your fiber intake and include more nutrient-dense foods. You can maintain this same focus on carb sources with the other two macros methods.

This focus on whole foods that are fiber- and nutrient-rich makes the weight-loss process easier for two other big reasons besides your gut health:

» They have a higher thermic effect, meaning you burn more calories at rest to digest them than processed foods.

» They're often less calorically dense and more nutrient dense, meaning you can eat a larger volume of them to feel fuller and more satisfied even while in a deficit.

Don't look at your current fiber intake, freak out if you're only getting 10 grams a day, and try to jump straight to 25 grams. Your stomach will *not* appreciate that. Instead, find ways to increase your daily intake by just 5 grams, and maintain that single 5-gram increase for a week before increasing further. Bodies don't like change, and while fiber is amazing for the body, it can cause bloat or discomfort if you make dramatic shifts in your intake quickly.

Small tweaks add up. Balance is what helps you get better results from your macro changes, so focus on whole, natural foods to improve your results. Fiber is a key component of this. Aim to consume foods rich in probiotics and prebiotics, such as yogurt, fermented foods, garlic, potatoes, bananas, and legumes, to aid in optimal gut health for body recomp. Pay attention to eating that rainbow.

NOTE: *Eating a variety of fruits and vegetables is also important. Research shows that consuming at least thirty different types of plants per week can lead to a stronger and more diverse gut microbiome.* This can be a great complementary target to set for yourself as you get consistent with your macros and want to optimize your results.*

INCREASING YOUR FIBER INTAKE

The fiber intake you want to shoot for is 25 grams per day for women (or 21 grams if you're older than 50) or 38 grams per day for men (or 30 grams if you're older than 50).

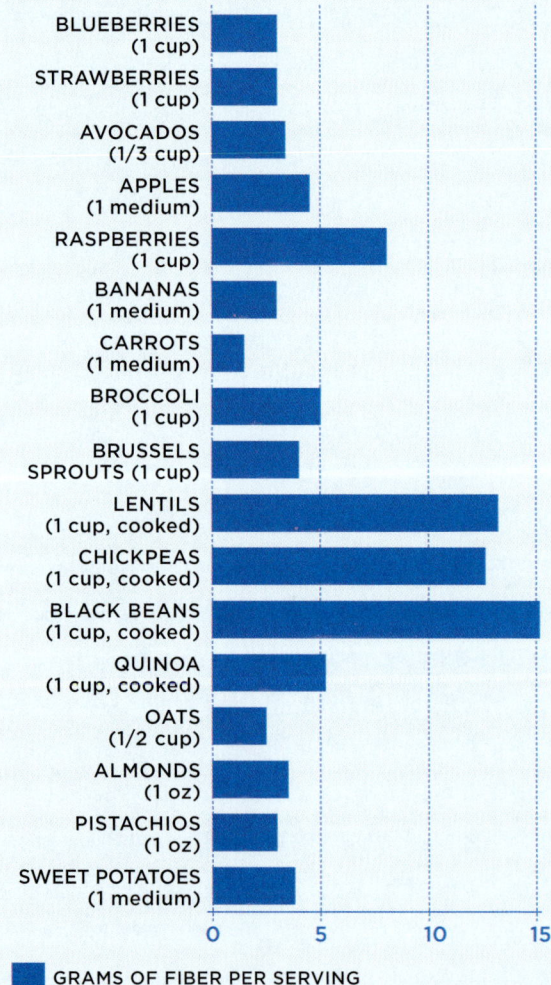

BLUEBERRIES (1 cup)	
STRAWBERRIES (1 cup)	
AVOCADOS (1/3 cup)	
APPLES (1 medium)	
RASPBERRIES (1 cup)	
BANANAS (1 medium)	
CARROTS (1 medium)	
BROCCOLI (1 cup)	
BRUSSELS SPROUTS (1 cup)	
LENTILS (1 cup, cooked)	
CHICKPEAS (1 cup, cooked)	
BLACK BEANS (1 cup, cooked)	
QUINOA (1 cup, cooked)	
OATS (1/2 cup)	
ALMONDS (1 oz)	
PISTACHIOS (1 oz)	
SWEET POTATOES (1 medium)	

■ GRAMS OF FIBER PER SERVING

*Daniel McDonald et al., "American Gut: An Open Platform for Citizen Science Microbiome Research," *mSystems* 3, no. 3 (2018): e00031-18, https://pmc.ncbi.nlm.nih.gov/articles/PMC5954204/.

THE BODY RECOMP ELIXIR

You can't talk about health or body recomp without talking about the importance of the body recomp elixir everyone needs to drink: water.

Most of us have thought, *I need to drink more water!* because we know we don't drink enough. I speak from experience because I've struggled with the hydration habit. It's funny how something so simple but so valuable can still be so hard to do!

Drinking more water is a habit that's hard to implement, and it's easy to abandon it the second something changes in your routine. Travel, a busy day at work, being on the go from activity to activity—that's all it takes to throw your hydration off.

Being dehydrated may be the reason you aren't seeing the muscle gains or fat-loss results you want. Proper hydration can help improve your overall metabolic health. Water is required for many metabolic and hydrolysis reactions, meaning that water helps your body burn fat.

Lipolysis is how the body breaks down and burns fat, and it begins with hydrolysis. Water molecules interact with triglycerides and break them down into two main components: glycerol and fatty acids. Then, through the process of lipolysis, these fatty acids are used as energy. For your body to burn fat as fuel, you need to be hydrated.

Water is also key for gaining muscle because it's required for transporting nutrients needed to produce protein and glycogen structures, which are the building blocks of muscle. Basically, you're killing your gains if you're dehydrated!

Your hydration needs only increase as you get older, especially as you increase your protein intake. Dehydration may negatively impact your energy, sleep, and skin health, and while we often want to blame negative side effects—like bloat or constipation—on protein, they're actually due to a lack of proper hydration. (Decreasing your fiber intake as you shift macros could also be to blame; fiber and water go hand in hand!) Proper hydration, which balances drinking enough water with getting enough electrolytes, is what keeps your body functioning optimally.

So, how much water do you need?

A great place to start is to drink about 50 percent of your body weight (in pounds) in ounces of water per day. So, if you weigh 150 pounds, you'd try to drink 75 ounces of water (150 x 50%) per day. However, this isn't necessarily "optimal." What's optimal can vary based on your activity level and age, and even your macros have an impact.

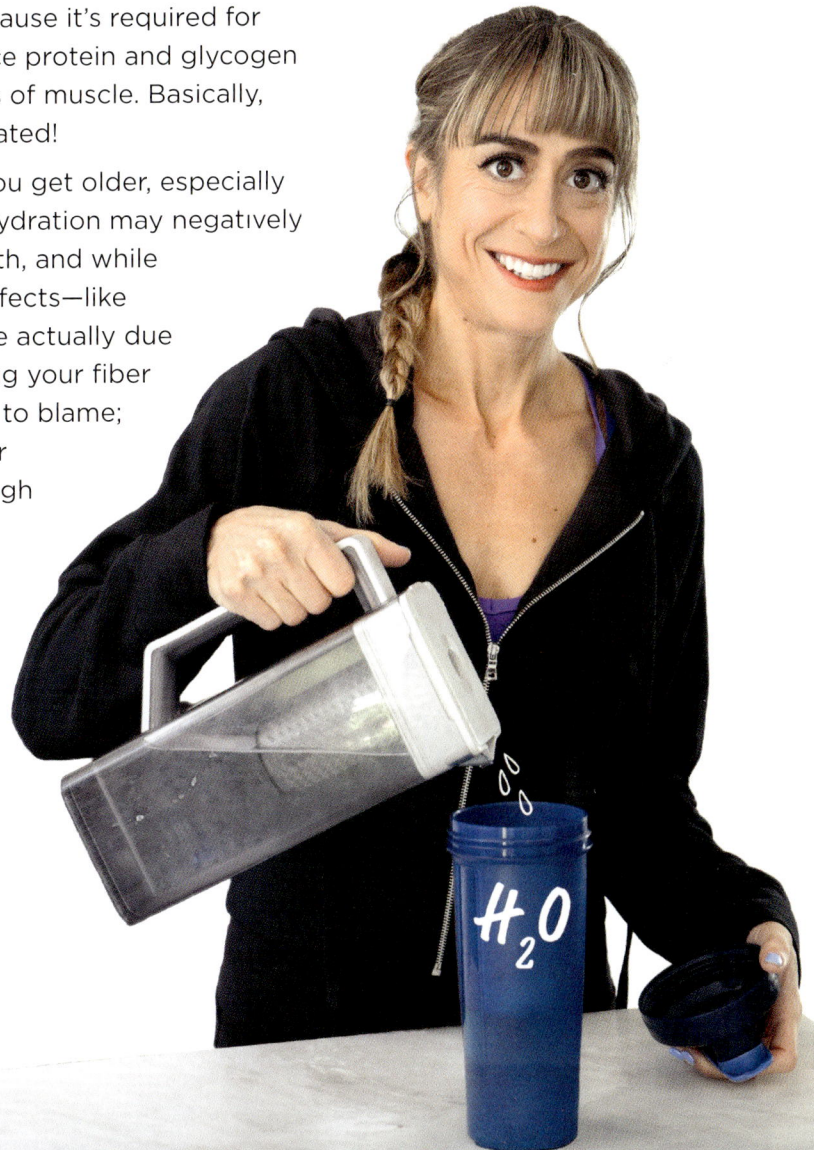

As you get older, and especially with higher protein intakes of 35 percent or greater, you may want to consider increasing your water intake to 70 percent of your body weight. In this scenario, someone weighing 150 pounds would try to drink 105 ounces of water (150 x 70%) per day.

A great way to determine your hydration status is from the color of your urine. The goal isn't to have clear urine; that's a sign that your electrolyte balance is off. The goal is for it to be a light lemonade color.

This focus on hydration really pays off during perimenopause and menopause because women often see an increase in dryness. Try not to drink too much water close to bed. You don't want one healthy habit (drinking enough water) to negatively impact another (getting good sleep).

The real challenge: How do you drink more water if this is a habit you've struggled with? Here are a few ideas. Consider which of these may be easier to work in if the habit of drinking water is a bigger stone than it should be and you need to break it down into pebbles, and check out the fun water recipes in the nearby sidebar:

» Buy a fun water bottle you want to use.

» Fill that fun water bottle and put it by your coffee maker to drink first thing in the morning.

» Set an alarm to remind you to drink water throughout the day.

» Make your water more interesting by adding things like a zero-calorie electrolyte mix or fruits or herbs. (Cucumbers or oranges infused into your water can help boost your electrolyte intake and improve your hydration as well!)

» Connect drinking water with other habits, putting it before the thing you enjoy.

» Know how many refills of your water bottle you need to hit your intake and use refilling the bottle as an excuse to also get more steps. (Connecting one habit with others to have multiple payoffs can help!)

List some other easy ways to slowly increase your water. If you're barely drinking 10 ounces and need to get to 70 ounces, focus not on the goal number but on how you can add just 5 or 10 ounces more to start.

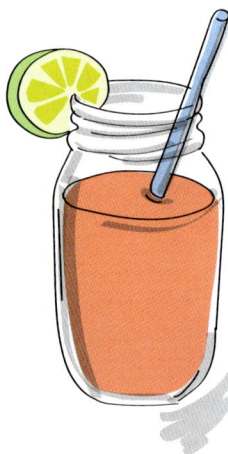

HYDRATION RECIPES

Electrolyte Drink
Makes 6 cups

34 fl oz club soda (1 kg)
1/2 cup slices cucumber (52 g)
1 lime (67 g)
3 tbsp spearmint (17 g)
1/4 tsp salt (1.5 g)

Cut cucumber and limes in slices, leave peel. Mix rest of ingredients with the sparkling water, leave in fridge overnight to macerate. Add optional no-calorie sweeteners. Drink throughout the next day.

Per 1 cup (1 serving): 6 CALORIES
1.7g CARBS (0.5g FIBER) | 0g FAT | 0.2g PROTEIN

Fresh Strawberry Limeade
Makes 8 cups

1 cup whole strawberries (144 g)
3 limes (201 g)
2 1/2 oz raw agave nectar (71 g)
2 cups water (473 g)
34 fl oz club soda (1 kg)

1. Add fresh strawberries, limes, agave, and water to a blender. Blend until smooth.

2. Using a strainer to catch all the chunks, pour strawberry lime mixture into a pitcher.

3. Add club soda to strawberry limeade and finish off with ice. Serve!

Per 1 cup (1 serving): 39 CALORIES
10.8g CARBS (1.1g FIBER) | 0.1g FAT | 0.3g PROTEIN

TAKE A DIET BREAK

A diet break is basically a recovery week for your weight-loss or fat-loss diet. If you're focused on building muscle right now, you won't make use of this, although you could back off the surplus for a bit if you're feeling a bit burned out by trying to pack in extra calories daily. This break is more about coming out of a deficit.

I do not usually recommend this diet break in combination with a recovery week, partly because you're going to be eating more and feeling really good, which makes it easier to train and push hard.

A diet break is often a nutritional slow down so you can speed up. It's the rest stop you need on your road trip to results not only to make better progress but also create sustainable and lasting results.

You're reading this program because you want to lean down, and nothing has worked to help you maintain your results in the past. So, instead of trying to keep white-knuckling your way through habit changes—only to end up stuck in the change loop when you hit habit overload and emotional sabotage and eventually quit—try doubling down to break free by doing less for a bit.

REASONS TO TAKE A DIET BREAK

Your body adapts to what you're doing, which is the reason you can hit plateaus during your weight- or fat-loss plan, even when you're doing everything "right." Cycling macros (page 169) can help you stick with things, mentally and physically, for a while, but you might eventually need a more significant break, especially if you need a longer dieting period to lose more or you're pushing your body's set point to get leaner than you ever have been.

A diet break can help you bust through plateaus, stay consistent for longer, avoid burnout, and create some balance when you may need to "steer into the skid." It can give you a little mental break from full cycling if you're feeling burned out on tracking. Or it can be a time to switch to a ratio you find easier to do. Whatever your reason for a break, it's a break for your body from the deficit and also for your mind from the more focused dieting.

Habits may become routine, but that doesn't mean you always want to do what you should. Pushing yourself to stay consistent through long, hard, stressful days wears on you. A break is sometimes necessary so you don't end up saying, "Forget everything!" and not only slashing the other three tires but also lighting the car on fire. (If you don't recall my analogy about slashing your car's tires, check out Chapter 1.)

Now, you may be thinking, *But if my results have slowed, shouldn't I decrease my calories or do more exercise?* The answer is often no. Typically, when you've been dieting for a while and cycled macros while in a deficit, you can only push those systems so far before they break. While you can be strategic with moving toward an extreme deficit of 500 calories, the harder you're pushing your training, the more creating a bigger deficit will backfire. It's not always wise to keep lowering calories because your energy, hormones, and even mental clarity can suffer.

Here are some scenarios when you should consider a diet break:

» You've been in a calorie deficit for three or more months and have lost 10 or more pounds.

» You've hit a *true* plateau. This means you haven't seen any results despite being consistent and having adjusted macros for three or four weeks (four weeks if you're a female with a regular period).

» You've hit mental burnout or are starting to feel habit overload. If you have been dieting and tracking for a while and are having doubts about whether this is truly sustainable, use a diet break to mentally recharge and be able to feel motivated to start pushing again.

HOW TO TAKE A DIET BREAK

Diet breaks are seven to fourteen straight days of eating at about your maintenance calorie intake. This isn't just your "cheat day" or macro cheat day or carb refeed, which are "mini breaks" done weekly or every few weeks for an entire day or meal. A diet break is an extended period with specific macro goals and a 400- to 500-calorie increase, which may even be 200 or 300 calories higher than your original "maintenance" calories.

This is not an excuse to eat anything you want and not care for a few weeks. You still want to focus on quality fuel and hitting specific macros. One strategy is to use a diet break on vacations or holidays when you know you will want more food flexibility or when it may be more sustainable to increase calories and back off your intensive weight-loss goals and macros.

You will want to keep a 30 percent protein minimum with the calorie increase. You may find that when you first bump up your calories, you keep your current macro ratio for the first one to three days to adjust; then you may also adjust your macros. A more even thirds split of macros works well for overall balance and fueling. You can also choose to go higher in a macro you were previously lower with to make sure you aren't deficient in anything. To use this period to optimize muscle gains, going slightly higher in carbs than fat can be ideal.

Consider putting your macros in the following ranges. Once you select a ratio, use it for the entire diet break. If you're just using a protein minimum, let carbs and fats fall as you'd like, but keep protein consistent daily:

» **PROTEIN: 30 to 35 percent**   » **CARBS: 30 to 40 percent**   » **FATS: 30 to 40 percent**

If this is your first diet break and you're nervous about gaining weight, you can go as high as 40 percent protein, but focus on those other two macros to use the increase in protein strategically as you move back to your deficit.

You'll see an initial jump on the scale or even some bloat come on when you increase your calories from your deficit numbers, but this isn't fat being gained overnight. You want your glycogen stores to become full, which means you're gaining water weight. This is what helps you push your training for muscle gains, optimize hormonal balance, and improve metabolic health.

When returning to your deficit level, consider a few things:

? How much did you initially gain during the diet break?

? Did you continue to gain over the diet break?

? Did only the scale weight change, or did inches change in areas where you didn't want to gain fat? (For example, compare your waist to areas like your biceps, where you may not mind gaining a bit of muscle.)

These questions will help you determine if you can go back to your previous calorie intake or need to adjust. Use the following guidelines:

» If you initially saw an increase on the scale but didn't gain the remainder of the break, consider not dropping more than 200 calories off of your diet-break intake. Your maintenance has increased.

» If you lost during the diet break, do not drop calories. Begin to cycle macros. Consider a further increase in calories after a few weeks. You've gained muscle, and your metabolism is telling you that you need more fuel!

» If you gained on the scale but inches didn't change or even went down, don't drop calories. This is also a sign you've gained muscle, and you should begin to cycle macros at this calorie intake.

» If you continued to gain weight over the course of the diet break, go back to your previous deficit and begin to cycle macros again. If you find the big change in fuel leaves you super hungry after three or four days, consider a slight bump to a midpoint before fully dropping back down.

WHAT ABOUT CHEAT DAYS AND REFEEDS?

I want to touch briefly on "cheat days" and refeeds. If you hate the name "cheat day," you can call it an "off-macro day" or whatever works for you mentally. You aren't cheating on anything; you're creating balance. A "cheat" can be a single meal per week or per month or even a full day.

The important thing to note is that the more "off" your macros and calories are, and the more frequently you include cheat days or refeeds, the slower your progress will be because they can have an impact on your overall weekly macro and calorie averages. But they may be what you need to stay consistent long term. You can experiment with them and exclude them to start if you want faster results. Later, you can work them in more when you need that sustainable balance.

Cheat Days

Cheat days often get a bad rap because of the "mindset" associated with them and their name. But you aren't actually cheating on anything.

A cheat day can be a day where you eat things you choose not to include on other days because they aren't as easy to work in or because you want them in quantities that don't generally fit your macros. These days can also give you a mental reset because you aren't having to hit any specific numbers.

If you want to see faster results at the start and ensure you aren't throwing yourself out of your weekly calorie deficit, you may want to track and record these break days. You may still want to stay within a calorie cap for the day. (This is also where you may decide to start with a single cheat meal rather than a full day of eating.)

Another alternative is to implement what I call the "macro cheat day." This day has specific macro boundaries, such as a protein minimum and a calorie cap. These bumpers keep you in line without limiting you.

Don't feel guilty on these days as you enjoy foods that maybe aren't as nutrient dense as you normally shoot for. Enjoy meals out. Have a cocktail, wine, or beer. These days give you mental balance so you don't always feel like you're a person on a diet, but you're still focused on fueling for your goals.

Whether you include these days once a week or plan ahead to have them once or twice a month for specific events is up to you. Again, the more cheat days you include, and the more the calories and macros deviate from your current goals, the more progress slows down. Whether, and even how, you include them will be based on the "budget" you assessed when you did your STRONG system reflection.

NOTE: *If you're nervous about including a cheat day but feel balance has been missing in the past (leading to habit overload and falling back into the change loop), consider the macro cheat day variation or just start with a single meal.*

Refeed Days

If you've hit a plateau or results have slowed down but you haven't been dieting for long enough to feel the need for a diet break, a refeed day is a great option! Unlike a cheat day, a refeed day is a day when you still strategically track macros and calories while you increase your calories—like a mini diet break. It can be good to coordinate a refeed day with your hardest workout day once a week or a couple of times a month, especially if that muscle group is one you'd like to see muscle gains in as you lean down.

Refeed days can help kick-start your metabolism and increase your energy levels so you can train hard and bust through a plateau. When you adjust your macros and calories, you will want to increase your calories by 200 to 300 and bump carbs accordingly. If you aren't doing refeed days weekly, you can use them once a month for up to five days, but only extend a refeed to five days if you've hit a true three- or four-week plateau or have been in a deficit for six weeks or longer.

Refeeds become increasingly useful when you hit a dead zone, or a period where it feels like nothing is budging as you try to lose those last few percentages of body fat. The carb increase can lead to the "whoosh effect," or the release of water from fat cells. Also, carbohydrates increase leptin levels to help you feel fuller, so you don't get to the point where your brain is telling you you're hungrier than you are causing you to eat more than you meant to.

The following are some signs you may need a refeed:

» You've hit a true plateau.

» You've been in a deficit for longer than six weeks and have the last few percentages of body fat to lose.

» You constantly crave carbs and sweets.

» You suddenly want to snack frequently.

» Your energy levels have dipped.

WHY MEAL TIMING ISN'T IMPORTANT

When I say that meal timing doesn't matter, what I mean is that lots of meal timings can work. The more you focus on what makes you feel best and allows you to manage your schedule with less stress, the better the results.

Lots of conflicting information about meal timing is circulating out there. People tout all types of fasting as the secret to fat loss and longevity, or they say that your muscle will decline and your metabolism will break if you don't eat six small meals a day and time macros perfectly after your workouts. Both camps are right, and both are wrong.

What truly matters is that you hit your total macros and calories consistently. Every. Single. Day. If you hit your macros and calories, you'll see fabulous results. *Period.* But your muscles won't melt off if you miss a meal. You won't gain fat just because you ate outside of a specific window. Meal timing should make you feel better and make life easier. It shouldn't be something you stress over.

In the next sections, I touch on a few popular meal timings, as well as some meal-timing myths.

INTERMITTENT FASTING VERSUS SIX SMALL MEALS A DAY

Should you skip breakfast? Should you eat more frequently? Should you eat fewer meals? What's the best number of meals and the best window to eat in? The honest answer is that *one size doesn't fit all.*

Ask yourself these questions to determine the best meal timing for you:

? How do I feel about my current meals? Am I full? Or am I hungry?

? Do I like the amount of meal prep I have to do?

? Do I like to be able to snack?

? Do I feel more satisfied with big meals?

? Do I like to skip breakfast? Or do I like to eat first thing?

? Do I feel I get too hungry if I fast and eat later?

? Will skipping a meal work with the timing of my training? Or will it have a negative impact? Will I feel depleted and have low energy?

How you time your meals should depend on what makes you feel best and what you're doing currently. The fewer changes you can make at once, the better!

If you naturally like to skip breakfast, don't force breakfast on yourself to start. You may decide later that you want to include it, but it isn't necessary. If you like to snack, don't force fewer meals. Steer into this and prep snacks to hit your macros. If you like to have big meals and would rather prep only one or two meals, try fasting and larger, less frequent meals. If you train early in the morning, don't force yourself to fast until the afternoon. You can break your fast before you train or right after. On the other hand, if you like to train at night and only eat right before as your first meal, great!

The point is to make sure you feel full and fueled and to create sustainable eating habits. You never want to force something that makes you focus even more on food or that causes you to feel so hungry that you overeat.

For instance, don't skip meals as a way to cut calories. This approach often leads to overeating. Also, don't force yourself to eat if you know you'll never be able to keep prepping all of those meals.

The best approach—especially when it comes to weight loss—is the habit you'll do consistently that allows you to hit your total macros and calories for the day. Studies have shown that the benefits of intermittent fasting can be achieved through calorie restriction alone.* (Read more about the benefits and downsides of intermittent fasting on pages 207 to 209.)

I CAN'T EAT AFTER *X* P.M.

Ever heard that if you eat carbs after a certain time—say, 5 p.m.—they'll be stored as fat? Well, that is 100 percent *not* correct. You can eat at any time and see results. If you train at night, eating later may not only be more convenient but also essential. If you need the calories and macros to hit your goals for the day, it doesn't matter if you have to eat them later. *You just need to eat them*!

If you overeat at *any* time of day, that will backfire. But this myth about not eating after a certain time came about due to the rise of popular diets that told people to eat that way. Those diets used that limitation to help create the calorie deficit people needed to see results.

Why did it create that deficit for many people? The cutoff time eliminated much of the mindless snacking people do at night while watching TV! If thinking you can't eat after a certain time helps you to break a snacking habit, go ahead and tell yourself that. But from a scientific standpoint, there is simply no cutoff time where you will magically gain fat if you eat after it. Focus on hitting your ratios and calories, and you'll see results.

NOTE: *If you eat later than usual or have a bigger meal later than usual (especially something more carb-heavy), you will see a gain on the scale the next day, but that's not fat gain. The food had less time to be fully digested and … well … pooped out. The scale shows that you still have food in your system from eating closer to the time you weighed. So, know that eating later will probably mean a temporary weight fluctuation, but don't stress about it. Make sure you're fueling based on your schedule!*

WHAT ABOUT PRE- AND POST-WORKOUT NUTRITION?

Your muscles will not melt off if you don't eat right after your workout, and fasted training isn't bad, although it may work for fat loss better than for muscle building. There can be value in tweaking your pre- and post-workout nutrition, especially if you're trying to get ab definition or get rid of those last few percentages of body fat, but again, what matters most is hitting your calories and macros for the day.

*Joseph J. Cynamon, "Is Intermittent Fasting a Better Option Than Continuous Calorie Restriction?" *The Science Journal of the Lander College of Arts and Sciences 16*, no. 2 (2023), https://touroscholar.touro.edu/sjlcas/vol16/iss2/12/?utm_source=touroscholar.touro.edu%2Fsjlcas%2Fvol16%2Fiss2%2F12&utm_medium=PDF&utm_campaign=PDFCoverPages.

I say this because that anabolic window everyone worries about is much bigger than most people realize. Consuming a meal three hours after training can provide the same value! However, you may want to consider "optimizing" your meal timing around your workouts as you get older. As people age, they become less able to utilize protein efficiently, so increasing the amount of protein per meal and timing it to when your body is more primed to use it can only help.

If you're fasting prior to your training during a fat-loss phase, make sure to break your fast right after your workout to help ensure you're getting your muscles the fuel they need, especially because you're already in a calorie deficit.

Fueling around your workouts as you get closer to your goal can also be helpful because you're in that deficit where you're not really getting "enough" of anything. Making sure your muscles have fuel when they're primed to use it can be helpful for retaining and building muscle while in a deficit. But don't worry; your muscles will not melt away if you don't chug a protein shake right after your workout.

If you eat prior to your workout session, focus on simple carbs and protein, keeping fat and fiber lower to avoid delaying digestion; you definitely don't need to stress about eating post workout because you'll go into your training already fueled. However, if you train fasted, a post-workout meal may be more important. When you eat after a workout, focus on getting 30 to 40 grams of protein to really maximize muscle gains, especially as you get older.

INTERMITTENT FASTING: YEA OR NAY?

While many people call intermittent fasting (IF) a "diet," it's actually a type of meal timing. That meal timing can be used with a variety of dietary preferences and macro breakdowns. You can eat keto and do IF or eat high carb and do IF. I want to discuss the upsides, downsides, and options with this meal timing so you can determine if the hype you've heard is worth it for you.

What Is Intermittent Fasting?

There are a few different types of IF:

» **Time-restricted eating:** A set daily eating window

» **The 5:2 method**: Two days of a 500-calorie cap

» **24-hour fasts:** A full twenty-four-hour fast once or twice a week

While you can include different fasting lengths, a very common form of IF is the 16:8 time-restricted fast. You will fast for sixteen hours and then have an eight-hour eating window. You can think of this as skipping breakfast, although technically you can skip any meal. The idea is to have all of your meals in a shortened window each day.

If you do one of the other setups, you may have a calorie allotment or full day of not eating rather than skipping one meal.

What Are the Benefits of IF?

IF has gained mainstream attention over the years as a great thing to do not only for your health but also for fat loss. A big reason why it became so popular is because people claimed you didn't have to change what you were eating to see results. You only had to eat within this set window and—*poof*—the weight would melt off magically.

Having a set eating window does often help people get started with losing weight. It creates a calorie deficit without tracking, just like cutting out a food group can often do with other diets. It can help cut out mindless snacking, and when you're restricted to only a set amount of time, it's easier to fill up as you eat your daily calorie intake in a condensed period. When you're in a calorie deficit, it can feel more satisfying to have bigger meals rather than snack frequently. You can get that "eat until you're full" feeling.

Also, there's simply not as much meal planning to do, which can make it easier to stick with the healthy habits. Many people find the simple lifestyle change sustainable while leading to the habits they need to lose weight.

From a more "scientific" perspective, it's argued that IF is helpful for weight loss because it can promote stronger insulin sensitivity and increased growth hormone secretion, both of which can also help with gaining muscle. That, in turn, leads to better fat-loss results. The more you're able to focus on muscle mass retention, the less metabolic adaptations you suffer from as you lose weight. Muscle mass is metabolically costly, meaning it needs a lot of energy to be maintained.

In a deficit, you can often end up using muscle mass for fuel, especially if the deficit is too great. By promoting an anabolic environment, you can prevent metabolic adaptations and burn more calories at rest by promoting better muscle mass retention and growth.

IF can also lead to better fat-burning results, especially at the end of a longer fast, which is part of why twelve to eighteen hours is recommended for IF. Some people even argue that it's especially helpful when you have that last little bit you want to lose off of stubborn areas.

The argument for IF is that spending more time in the low-insulin state reached during a fast equates to spending more time where fat can be mobilized from stubborn areas. This state is different from the one seen with a low-carb diet because when you're eating low carb, triglycerides inhibit hormone-sensitive lipase (HSL) in a similar manner to insulin. HSL is basically activated to shuttle the fat out of the cell to be burned off.

Because of this fatty acid mobilization and the fact that some studies have shown fasting to increase abdominal subcutaneous blood flow, the case has been made that IF can promote better loss of stubborn belly fat.* This may be a reason for women, especially during menopause, to consider trying IF while dialing in their macros because decreasing estrogen levels during menopause can lead to more stubborn belly fat accumulating.

---

*Marjolein P. Schoonakker et al., "A Fasting-Mimicking Diet Programme Reduces Abdominal Adipose Tissue While Preserving Abdominal Muscle Mass in Persons with Type 2 Diabetes," *Nutrition, Metabolism and Cardiovascular Diseases* (2025): 104111, https://www.nmcd-journal.com/article/S0939-4753%2825%2900265-0/fulltext.

While many turn to fasting for the weight-loss benefits, other benefits people tout with fasting include

» Reducing cancer risk

» Decreasing triglycerides and LDL as well as cholesterol and inflammation markers

» Reducing blood pressure

» Improving cardiovascular function

» Improving brain function and preventing conditions such as Parkinson's, dementia, and Alzheimer's

But, as you know, nothing is a magic pill. Some of the benefits associated with fasting may be achieved by creating a calorie deficit and then maintaining a healthy weight overall regardless of your meal timing. The benefits some people see from any lifestyle or dietary changes always rely on multiple factors and don't apply to everyone. It's why you want to build a plan around *your* lifestyle, body, needs, and goals—not force yourself into a mold.

What Are the Downsides of IF?

In terms of serious negative consequences from fasting, there aren't any, especially when it comes to weight loss. That still does *not* mean it is a magic pill or right for you.

You can't just eat whatever you want in whatever quantity you want simply because you are eating in a set window. Macros and calories still matter. If you dial those in, any meal timing that fits your lifestyle will work. Forcing a meal timing that doesn't fit your schedule or lifestyle will backfire no matter how magical it's supposed to be. That's often the main reason why IF doesn't work for people. They force a meal timing that isn't realistic or sustainable for them, and then they don't know how to truly dial in their nutrition to match their needs and goals when they remove the restriction of an eating window.

If you train first thing in the morning, trying to fast until the afternoon probably won't work well. While you can make your eating window earlier, you might not find that lifestyle sustainable because it means you're eating dinner earlier than you'd like. Fasting can even result in overeating. People become so hungry that they end up overeating during the eating window, and their cravings increase.

Fasting may also not be right for you if you're chronically stressed or if you've seen your cortisol levels rise during menopause. High stress levels and skipping breakfast may prolong cortisol elevation. This can lead to chronic fatigue, blood sugar dysregulation, and even feeling more stressed.

So, if you aren't finding that fasting makes your life *easier*, there is no point in doing it. Adding in something that increases your stress will backfire. You can achieve the same benefits through a calorie deficit and by dialing in your macros.

Also, if fat loss isn't your goal, fasting may not be the ideal meal schedule, especially if you aren't training late enough in the day to break your fast before your workout. Instead, it may backfire when trying to gain muscle.

Having full glycogen stores to create an anabolic environment and help your body repair and rebuild can be key, especially if you're a hard gainer or advanced lifter who won't see those newbie gains. Gaining muscle is a slow process, and for many of us, it requires creating the right environment and having fuel readily available. Not to mention, fasting may mean your energy levels are lower than ideal, so you can't push your training in the gym as hard as you'd like to create that progressive overload.

Should You Do IF?

There are two main reasons I use IF with my clients:

» To help them better understand their hunger cues and break the habit of always eating at set times rather than really understanding what their bodies are telling them

» To make it easier to work around their schedule so they can hit their macros and feel full and satisfied

If IF meal timing feels right for you, great. Use it. Everything you include in your lifestyle should be focused on your needs and goals. For many people, fasting allows them to eat when they're hungry and maintain the macros and calories they need to feel fueled while seeing results. Whatever your fitness goal, no meal schedule is going to get you results if your calories and macros aren't in line with your needs and goals.

If your goal is gaining muscle and you've found you're really struggling, sticking with IF, no matter how much you loved it for fat loss, may work against you. Change requires change, and you may need to adjust your meal timing to help make sure you're creating an anabolic environment. While this could just mean a pre-workout meal to break your fast instead of eating first thing after, you may find you need to swap to a longer eating window and include more meals. The key is finding what works for your current needs and goals.

IF FOR WOMEN

Women respond differently to IF than men do. Studies have shown potentially fewer benefits from IF for women and more adverse effects in terms of adrenal stress and muscle mass loss, especially in premenopausal women.[*] If you aren't naturally a meal skipper, start with a shorter fast and only build up to a longer length if it feels right.

Because of the hormonal changes women go through in menopause, IF may become a more useful tool for females during this time. It may complement changes in macro ratios to help prevent that dreaded menopausal weight gain, especially for people who aren't as active.[**]

Studies have shown that IF may also have some heart health benefits and reduce inflammation—both of which can be especially beneficial for women in menopause. It has also been shown to improve mood, mental clarity, and focus, as well as reduce stress levels. So, if you're struggling with changes in your mood or increased brain fog during menopause and want to test out a different eating window, IF may work well for you.

All that said, if you're a very active woman going through perimenopause or menopause, you may still find that IF is not for you.[***] It can raise cortisol levels and hurt performance, and it can make it a challenge to fuel properly. IF can lead to dysregulation of your appetite and even negatively impact your hormone levels and thyroid health.

One size doesn't fit all!

Always consider your personal needs and goals. If something is "popular" or works for someone else, go ahead and test it, but don't be afraid to ditch it if it doesn't work for you.

[*]Patricia L. Brubaker and Alexandre Martchenko, "Metabolic Homeostasis: It's All in the Timing," Endocrinology 163, no. 1 (2022): bqab199, https://academic.oup.com/endo/article/163/1/bqab199/6371839; Faiza Kalam et al., "Effect of Time-Restricted Eating on Sex Hormone Levels in Premenopausal and Postmenopausal Females," *Obesity* 31, no. S1 (2023): 57–62, https://onlinelibrary.wiley.com/doi/10.1002/oby.23562; Franck Mauvais-Jarvis, "Sex Differences in Energy Metabolism: Natural Selection, Mechanisms and Consequences," *Nature Reviews Nephrology* 20 (2024): 56–69, https://www.nature.com/articles/s41581-023-00781-2.

[**]Jip Gudden, Alejandro Arias Vasquez, and Mirjam Bloemendaal, "The Effects of Intermittent Fasting on Brain and Cognitive Function," *Nutrients* 13, no. 9 (2021): 3166, https://pmc.ncbi.nlm.nih.gov/articles/PMC8470960/; Stephan Schleim, "Cognitive or Emotional Improvement Through Intermittent Fasting? Reflections on Hype and Reality," *Journal of Trial and Error* (2024), https://journal.trialanderror.org/pub/cognitive-fasting/release/2.

[***]James Frampton et al., "The Acute Effect of Fasted Exercise on Energy Intake, Energy Expenditure, Subjective Hunger and Gastrointestinal Hormone Release Compared to Fed Exercise in Healthy Individuals: A Systematic Review and Network Meta-Analysis," *International Journal of Obesity* 46 (2022): 255–68, https://www.nature.com/articles/s41366-021-00993-1; Alexa Govette and Jenna B. Gillen, "At-Home Bodyweight Interval Exercise in the Fed Versus Fasted State Lowers Postprandial Glycemia and Appetite Perceptions in Females," *Applied Physiology, Nutrition, and Metabolism* 49, no. 9 (2024): 1217–27, https://cdnsciencepub.com/doi/10.1139/apnm-2023-0485.

14 HELP! HOW DO I KNOW IF IT'S WORKING?

Wanna know the hardest part about achieving results? Trusting the process! You know you can't just jump from thing to thing. But you also don't want to be "stupid" and keep doing something that isn't working.

How do you find balance between sticking with something long enough for results to snowball and abandoning something that isn't moving you forward? This is where complementary targets come into play in a big way. Because you know when you're doing things that lead to improvements (as long as you're honest about your consistency with the habits), you just have to pause to notice the other ways success is snowballing. You can't get so caught up in measuring progress in one specific way that you miss out on all of the signs that something is working!

Notice what you think when you read this statement: "It isn't even working. I don't get why I'm trying so hard to cram in all of these fruits and vegetables. The scale hasn't changed." Do you think of all of the health benefits of fruits and veggies? I know I do, and I consider how important this shift is for quality fueling. I also know that this change will ultimately lead to achieving weight-loss goals.

But maybe you still want to give up because the scale isn't changing yet. Logically, you may "know" how important dietary changes can be for your long-term health, but that doesn't always make you motivated now.

You need to break down the other benefits you're seeing. Consider these things:

- Is your digestion better? Are you pooping more regularly? (You'd be amazed at how often you'll find yourself thinking about your poop with dietary changes!)
- Are you sleeping better?
- Is your skin looking clearer?
- Are your energy levels better?
- Has your mood changed? Has brain fog or mental clarity improved?
- Are you feeling fuller?
- Have your workouts improved?
- Have your clothes started fitting better?
- Can you celebrate a habit win, like being consistent with eating X number of servings of veggies daily? And for how long?

The answers to these questions can show you that the habits are paying off. When you see these positive changes, you know you're on the right track. You just need to keep going.

Results leave clues, but you can't ignore them and get too focused on only one goal. Remember, your expectations can determine your success. They can blind you to improvements, especially if you have tunnel vision about losing weight and the number on that dang horrible scale.

STEP AWAY FROM THE SCALE

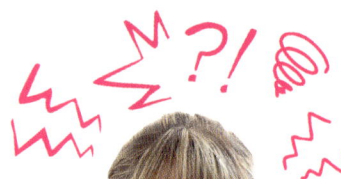

Have you ever seen that comic where the kids are looking at the scale, and one says, "Don't step on it. It makes you cry"? While there are a bazillion funny scale comics and memes, that one always makes me chuckle, shake my head, and groan at the same time.

I think that comic speaks to me because so many people are way too emotionally attached to a number that technically means less than nothing. That's how I was for the longest time. Not only does the scale dictate how people feel about themselves far too often, but (as the comic shows) this scale obsession is inadvertently being passed on to the next generation as well.

Now, if you're about to defend how important your goal weight is to you—don't. Because it isn't the number that's important. It isn't the weight you really care about. It's how you *felt* at that weight in the past that makes that number matter so much.

It's how your clothes fit. How much you could lift. How you looked in a particular vacation photo. How you felt at your wedding. How your spouse or friends looked at you. You're searching for that feeling again.

The weight signifies a feeling. The scale can be helpful for that reason. It can show you the number of a desired aesthetic you want to maintain and then help you create systems to maintain those results. But it can't be the end-all, be-all goal.

While that "ideal" weight can help guide you back to the identity and lifestyle you want, it's easy to get so stuck on seeing the scale change in that direction that you sabotage your own efforts. You may ignore the progress you're making and the healthy habits you're implementing if the scale isn't changing. Ultimately, you may give up when you could look and feel fabulous without ever seeing that number you have in your head reflected on the scale.

So, what does all of this mean? That you can't have a goal weight? That you shouldn't weigh? I know I said, "Step away from the scale," but that doesn't mean you have to stop using it. You just have to know the limitations of this form of measurement.

Heck, sometimes when I recommend "stepping away" from the scale, I actually suggest you weigh yourself more so you can see how easily that gosh darn thing fluctuates and how important it is to watch trends. Weighing daily can help desensitize you to the constant fluctuations and help you pay more attention to the overall trend. It can be helpful to see that the one day a week you would have normally weighed in might be the one day that week you somehow gained!

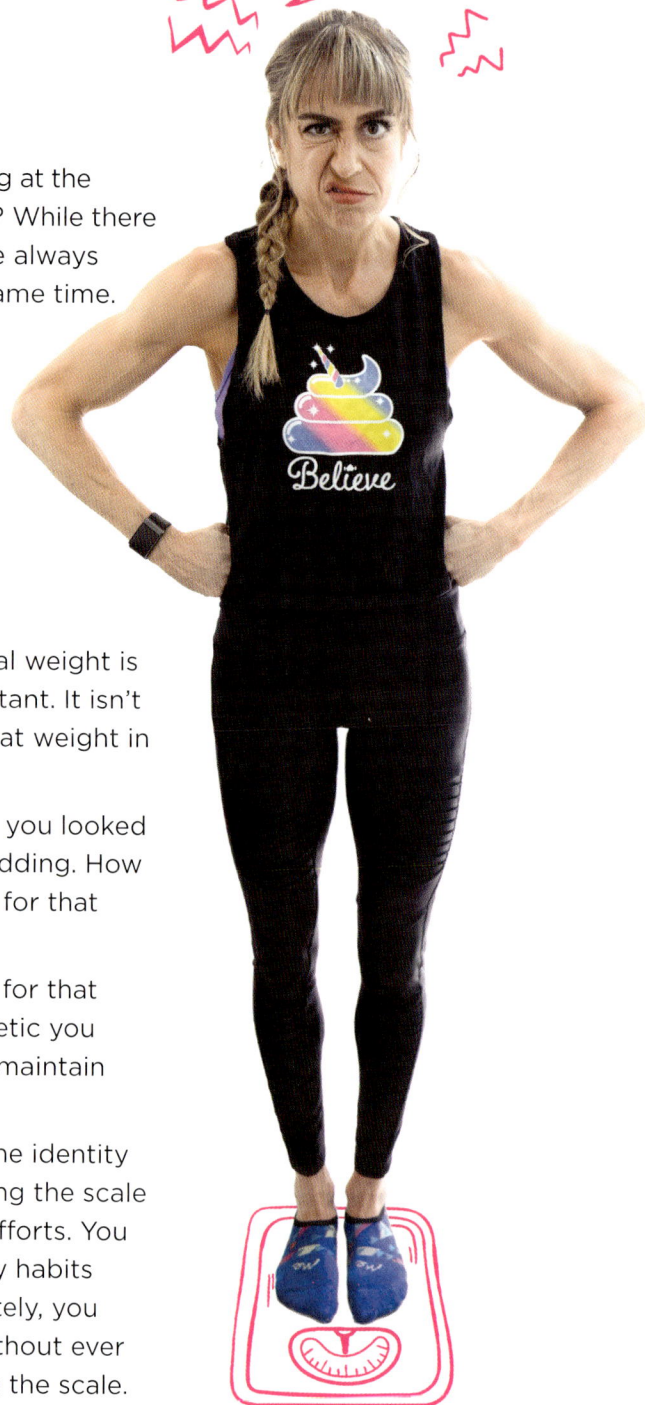

For example, you could have

- » Eaten later at night
- » Had more water
- » Eaten more salt
- » Not pooped yet
- » Slept poorly
- » Soreness from your workouts
- » Sneezed wrong

Any one of these things can make you see an increase on the scale the next morning. If that one morning was your only weigh-in, you would have thought you'd gone backward. You could have been down every day up to that point but ended up believing you'd gained! That's why weighing more frequently can help you see those daily fluctuations so you avoid getting sabotaged by one deviation.

The flip side is that you may find you need to step away completely and not weigh at all because you can't get off the emotional roller coaster the scale creates. You feel great if it goes down and like slashing every tire on any car you find if it goes up! This mindset can lead to self-sabotaging even if you see it go down because you feel like you "deserve" to celebrate.

To know what "stepping away from the scale" means for you, you need to assess your triggers. Consider your origin story. How does the scale impact you currently? Is it keeping you stuck in the change loop because you hit emotional sabotage? Do your particular struggles mean you should or shouldn't use it?

Also, think about your destination. Is the scale really the best measurement of your success? Is your weight really going to matter at your goal? Or will feeling fabulous in a little black dress that shows off your arms or kayaking and hiking through picturesque scenery with your family matter more?

If the answer to that last question is yes, consider what "measurement" will actually show you that progress is happening and keep you accountable.

THE WAYS YOU MEASURE PROGRESS

The more ways you measure progress, the more ways you can see things are working!

Think about your complementary targets—those are all ways to see that your habits are building in the right direction. Are you getting stronger? Are you consistently hitting your nutritional goals? If your main goal is body recomp of some sort, how can you measure that?

Taking progress pictures and body measurements can be alternatives to the scale. Or you can get one of those fancy scales that measures body fat, but those are typically still going to be impacted by hydration. Honestly, no form of measurement is perfect or without blips. I'll say it again: You have to watch trends.

If you take progress photos, always do it in the same light, in the same outfit, and at set intervals. I recommend weekly or at least every four weeks so you can do a side-by-side comparison. Take a front, side, and back view. You can do it in selfie mode with the timer on your phone, in a mirror, or have someone else take them.

NOTE: *The reason you use the same lighting and the same clothing is that those things affect how you view definition. If you use different lighting, you could get really good lighting one week and really bad lighting the next.*

If you're going to do measurements, check the guide in the workbook at redefiningstrength.com/extras. I recommend you measure at least your chest, glutes/hips, waist (whether you do the narrowest part, belly button, or both), thigh, and biceps. It's best to take the measurements with those areas relaxed. Do it once a week or at least every four weeks. Doing it more frequently makes it easier to see trends than when you have a single measurement day that ends up being the one day things went "backward."

Checkpoint dates give you set times to reflect and tweak the process while allowing enough time for results and trends to develop. They help you to know how long you have to "trust the process" before making a change if something isn't working. You don't worry you'll be going the wrong way forever, which can often help you stay more focused on the habits until the check-in.

Checkpoints can also be a good time to journal. When you reach a checkpoint, you have a chance to step back and see opportunities to improve, especially if you feel things aren't happening fast enough. You can also see all of the ways habits are paying off. Although most people don't set a complementary goal of overall health or more energy, those things *do* show the habits are working.

You can't control how long results take or how fast your body responds to changes and reaches a weight-loss goal, performance goal, or improvement in health markers. Therefore, you need to assess (in a truthful way) your consistency with doing healthy habits because habits and actions are something you can truly control. The more you monitor all of the things that healthy habits can impact, the more you can help yourself see what is and isn't working.

Honestly, the number one reason people don't see results? *They quit!*

Here's a list of things to assess at checkpoints. You can even ask yourself these questions weekly for more accountability:

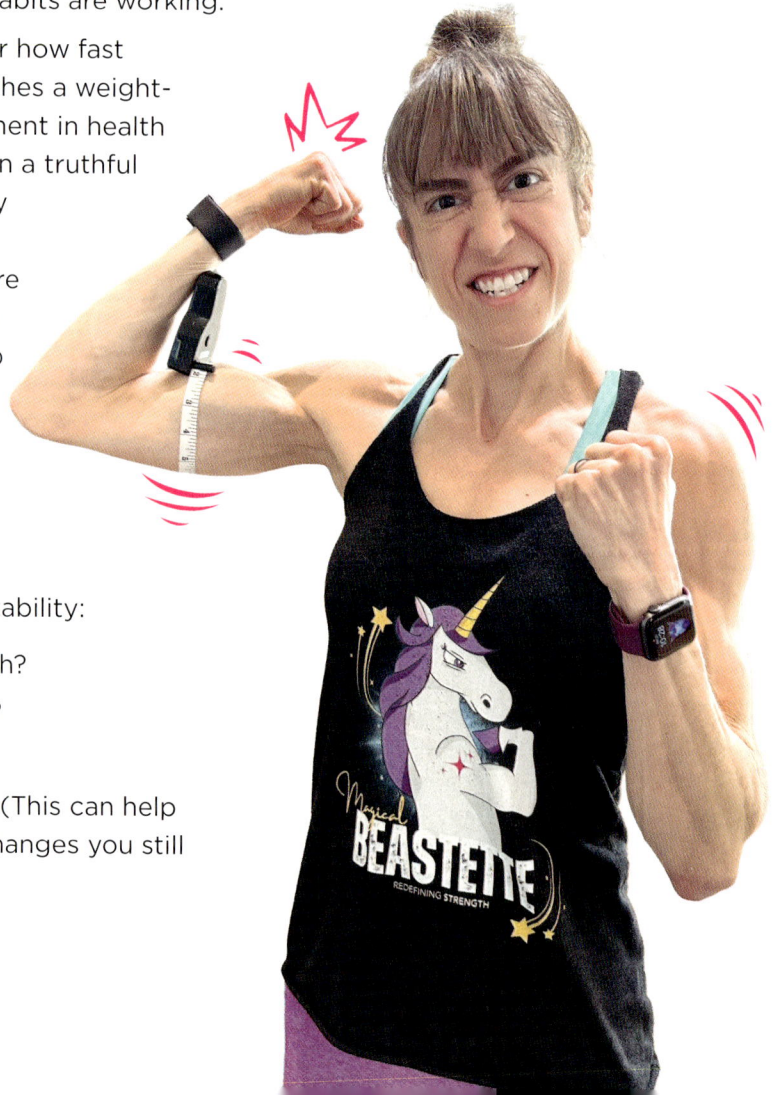

? What have I been super consistent with?

? What could I be more consistent with?

? What do I feel good doing?

? What do I not feel good doing? Why? (This can help you see where you may be resisting changes you still need to make.)

? How has my sleep been?

? How has my energy been?

? How has my mood been?

? How have my workouts felt?

? What changes to my skin, hair, nails, and such have I seen?

? How has my digestion been? Any bloating? Constipation? Gas?

? How has my confidence been?

? How have my mental clarity and focus been?

? How sustainable do the habits feel and why? (This can help you assess if any big rocks have been broken down or if there are any pebbles that have grown into medium stones.)

> **Honestly, the number one reason people don't see results? *They quit!***

You can reflect on countless other things based on "symptoms" or struggles you'd like to address or health and digestive issues that have popped up other times you've tried to make a change. But you want to reflect on how the habits are paying off even if they aren't directly related to your goal, and you need to consider your consistency with the habits. Often, realizing the wins that come with being consistent and pushing through the hard is enough to help you keep going and finally bust that change loop. This reflection can help you double down where needed to see progress snowball!

Take some time to use the NSVs Reflection Journal in the workbook at redefiningstrength.com/extras. It can help you take time to pause and celebrate those nonscale victories and trust the process when you feel like nothing is working. Don't miss the signs!

WHAT IF IT'S NOT WORKING?

There is no perfect plan. Your body, lifestyle, and needs evolve. Things aren't always going to work, even if they worked in the past. Nothing works forever. It sucks, but it's true.

With the STRONG system, you aren't just throwing spaghetti at a wall, hoping something sticks. You're working through the chapters and creating a plan. You have a clear roadmap to results. You'll make wrong turns and have to reassess the course, but when you have a plan in place, you have something to make adjustments to. You have focus and purpose in everything you do.

You can even see when you're not doing something you should be—because the plan doesn't work if you don't work the plan. Having a clear roadmap only helps if you follow the course. If you somehow take a wrong turn, you can reflect on it and adjust course.

You won't get anywhere if you just get in the car and never turn it on. You won't get to your destination if you choose to drive really fast in reverse. It can feel hard just loading up the car for your trip. It can feel fast driving backward. But you have to realize where your energy is going. You have to assess whether you're putting your efforts and actions in the right direction.

You might think I'm not answering the question, "What if it's not working?" but I am. You have to assess whether you're not moving forward *despite* following the plan or if you're not moving forward because you *aren't* following the plan. Only reflection and assessment can help you determine that.

What you uncover with your reflection influences the course corrections you make. If you could improve your implementation, you simply need to refocus. Assess why you haven't been able to stick with the plan. Are there too many big-rock habits? Too many small pebbles that aren't adding up? Are you ignoring the fact that priorities and nonnegotiables have shifted?

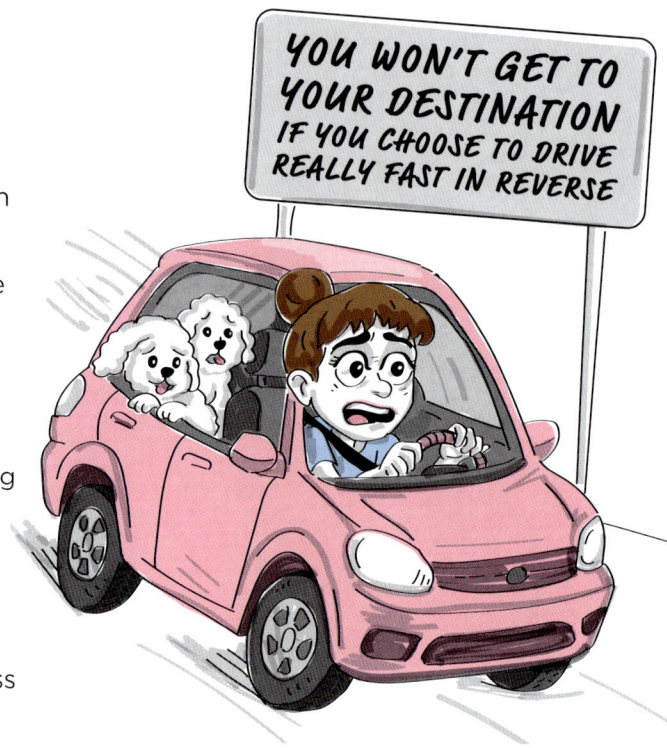

YOU WON'T GET TO YOUR DESTINATION IF YOU CHOOSE TO DRIVE REALLY FAST IN REVERSE

Or are you making progress and just ignoring the results that are building? Have you stopped focusing on your complementary targets or measuring success in multiple ways?

If you do this assessment and can honestly say you're consistently hitting things close to 90 percent, you may need to adjust. I say 90 percent rather than 80 percent because even though 80 percent does mean you're consistent, there's still lots of opportunity for growth.

At 90 percent consistency, you should make one change and map out the impact and future steps. It's like your GPS gives you the first turn back on track, but then it also maps out future turns that may potentially be different. You don't take all of those turns at once. Just one at a time.

This is where having exercise progressions you repeat and commit to switching at specific times helps. You'll stay on one for three to six weeks and then change, no matter what. The same goes for macro cycling, whichever method you implement.

The more you have set points when you will shift, especially in this initial season of your journey, the more you can test out what works best for you. Think of it like an experiment to find what makes you feel best and discover how your body responds to shifts in your energy source.

For example, embrace a lower carb ratio after a higher carb one. If it doesn't work? You have that checkpoint when you can make a change. This will help you learn what ratios work and what don't. Often, you don't know until you've tried.

The more you feel yourself resisting a change, the more that change is probably the one you need. And if it isn't working, you shift. Plain and simple. You will make lots of shifts as results slow and you find that what used to work no longer does because something else changed.

That's why there are only two key things to remember:

» Track what's going on.

» Pause to reflect on the "data" you've collected.

NOTE: *Something that doesn't seem like it's working on the surface can be what allows the next thing to launch you forward. Life doesn't start over. Every new thing is just building off the previous thing. So, keep going!*

TRUST THE PROCESS

When I say, "Trust the process," I don't mean I want you to follow what I say blindly. If that was my plan, I wouldn't have included so much why behind the what and how. But too often, doubt dooms the best intentions. When you don't believe something will work or doubt that it's right, you don't embrace the habit changes in the way that you need. You can't just dip your toe in; you've got to cannonball in with commitment.

The more you immerse yourself in the new identity and lifestyle, the more you shift mindsets and give change a chance. Is it scary as all get-out? *Yup.* The changes you need the most will be the scariest. But remember, you don't need to change everything at once to grow into your new identity. You just need to embrace the habit changes (even those small pebbles) by taking action and believing in those actions.

You can't hedge your bets. If you do, you go in looking to be proven right, and the "I told you so" attitude you have after a failed attempt is why that attempt never had a chance from the start. You weren't looking to really understand and embrace the change. You weren't looking to evolve who you are.

If you want your results to last, you must build a new identity with these lifestyle changes, and it takes time.

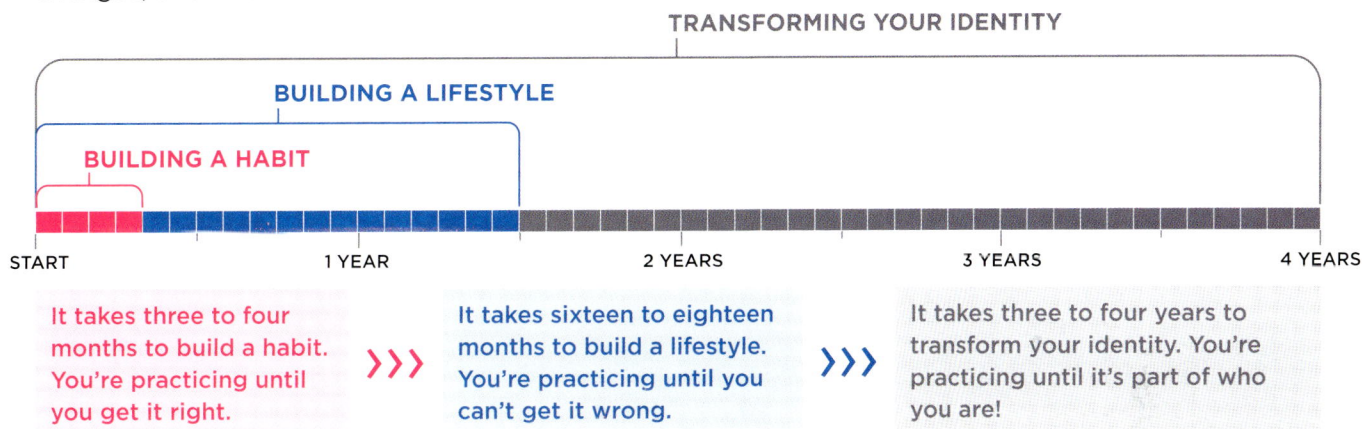

TRANSFORMING YOUR IDENTITY

BUILDING A LIFESTYLE

BUILDING A HABIT

START — 1 YEAR — 2 YEARS — 3 YEARS — 4 YEARS

It takes three to four months to build a habit. You're practicing until you get it right.

>>>

It takes sixteen to eighteen months to build a lifestyle. You're practicing until you can't get it wrong.

>>>

It takes three to four years to transform your identity. You're practicing until it's part of who you are!

How many people last the three months, let alone years?

IS THIS SUSTAINABLE?

People have to be "parented" into many sustainable habits, like toothbrushing. As an adult, you do those habits because you always have, and you understand their value even if you don't really find them fun or like them. Those habits are sustainable.

That's what making a change is: Parenting yourself into doing new habits you don't really want to do at the start. It's about teaching yourself the value of the habit so you find a way to prioritize it. (I talked more about this in Chapter 6 when I talked about the R [repeatable] in STRONG.)

If you're questioning whether your habit changes are sustainable, consider the following:

» Assess why you feel the changes may not be sustainable to learn more about their value.

» When you're pinched for time, put those habits you aren't currently prioritizing first so you don't skip them at the end of the day when you're tired.

» Find ways to connect the more difficult habit changes, or changes you don't enjoy, with habits you do enjoy.

» Most importantly? Set a time frame and make the goal to be consistent with your habits. Too often, people stop when they're still practicing to get them right. So, of course, they haven't started feeling natural.

Sustainability = Consistent Habit Repetition + Time

Set firm checkpoints and embrace the habits and routines until the designated date *without* shifting or changing them. Then reassess and make a small, 1 percent change. Break things down further if you've struggled with your consistency or continue to add on if things feel good. Focus on stacking those habits and building!

Sustainability happens when you *make* something a habit. And what makes that habit sustainable will evolve over your life. You can't just set it and forget it.

You may have this idea that a habit, routine, or lifestyle has to be *forever*, which is what sabotages you when it doesn't feel repeatable for that long. But nothing is done in one form forever. What you do to reach a goal is not what you do to maintain it. And maintaining your results doesn't mean standing still—you're a living organism, which means things are changing, growing, and dying every single day!

Y-E-T

"I can't do it … *yet*." This three-letter word takes a door you've slammed closed on yourself and pushes it open just slightly. The simple fact is, you don't know what is possible until you prove it's possible.

Change takes time, and too often, you might be limiting yourself when the limitation doesn't really have to hold you back. You have to pause to reassess and reflect. You need to give yourself permission to test limits, adjust what you're doing, and even reconsider what you want out of life.

I once again want you to keep your destination in mind and reflect on the lifestyle you want to lead and the goals you want to achieve. Are they *big enough*? Have you tied "yet" to things you haven't thought possible?

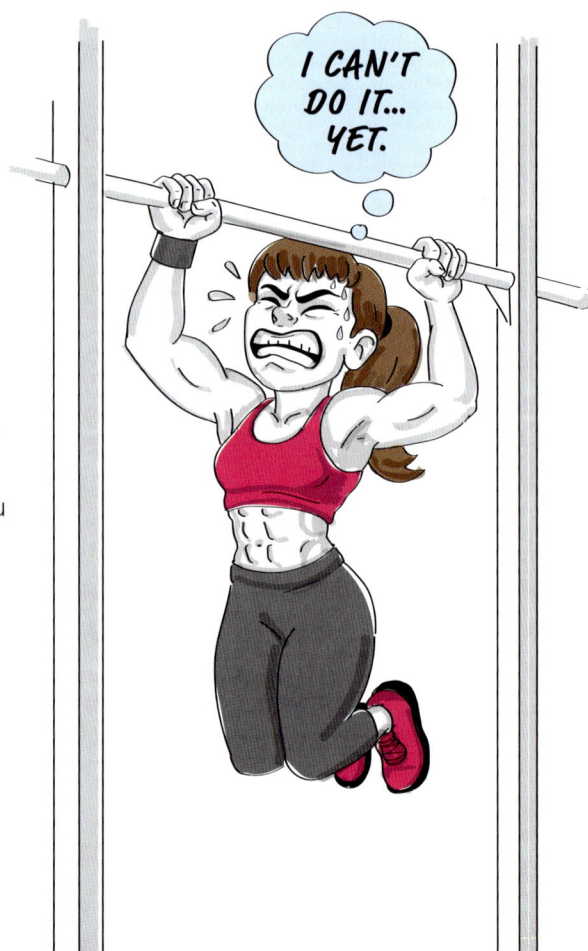

If you can see yourself at your destination, you're going to push harder, believe more, embrace the process, and keep going through the ups and downs. You will ultimately get further than you could have if you aimed for less. When you see yourself at your destination, you believe you deserve to have the life and reach the goals you want.

And I'm telling you that you do. You *deserve* to achieve success.

It won't be easy. You'll struggle. You'll have doubts. But every time you say, "I can't," or "It's not possible," mentally pause and add "yet!" Often, the only reason people haven't reached a goal is that they've only stuck with it up to the point of wanting to quit. Remember the miner in Chapter 5 who digs and digs only to give up because they feel like they haven't made progress? When they actually had made progress and just needed to stick with it? Keep going!

The STRONG system isn't something you do once. It's something you do along your journey, and you sometimes have to pause and reflect. That's where the STRONG Refocus comes in. It's a shorter reflection that allows you to assess the small changes in what you want and what you need that are appropriate based on what's changed in your life. I recommend doing it every three to six weeks, especially as you consider changing macros or workouts. You can find a place to record your reflections in the workbook at redefiningstrength.com/extras.

Reflection is the secret sauce to help you trust the process, so here are some key questions you can reflect on every few weeks (or even weekly):

? What positive changes have I seen this week?

? Where could I still improve and do better?

? What doesn't feel like it "fits"?

? What am I fighting against doing, and why am I fighting it?

? What am I holding on to that isn't serving me?

? What do I really enjoy that I want to do more of?

In addition to asking yourself those questions, list all of your wins since your last reflection and write down one or two things to adjust and change.

Recognize that having a plan is a way to help yourself trust the process; it keeps you from continuing down the wrong path when you should turn around. The checkpoints you've built for reflection and assessment help you avoid getting too far off course and give results time to build.

Don't become blind to all of the signals around you that you're on the right path, and don't ignore when your lifestyle, needs, or goals have become misaligned. The more you don't fall into the trap of letting feelings cause a knee-jerk reaction, and the more you use the power of pausing to reflect, the faster you're going achieve even more than you thought possible.

To help you pause and reflect, check out the STRONG Refocus and journal pages in the workbook at redefiningstrength.com/extras. Get a journal, create some of your own questions or "prompts," and write down your answers so you can reflect on what you need or what you feel has sabotaged you in the past. Just keeping a daily list of habit wins and NSVs can be that pause you need to keep going!

15 DON'T SET IT AND FORGET IT

You're feeling good. Your pants are looser. You're seeing definition in your arms when you flex. You have your habits dialed in. You're tracking and following your workout routine to a T. You're thinking to yourself, *Cori is my hero. She changed my life with her STRONG system! I have everything dialed in. This is a lifestyle!*

Then you mentally find yourself going on cruise control. You think, *Oh my gosh! Dirty Dough has my favorite Kooky Monster cookie right now! I'll have one!* Why does it feel like you all of a sudden get to this point, and— *bam*—the habits start to slide?

You try to excuse the "deviation." Progress, not perfection, right? Consistency and balance are key. Sure, your macros won't be perfect today, but they're close enough. And you should get to celebrate your results, right?

The next day, you notice Cold Stone Creamery has a new Nutter Butter flavor, and Reed avocados, which go so well with a margarita, are now in season. That one little deviation because you're feeling good becomes two, then three, then ten. You start out celebrating your success, but you ultimately fall back into old patterns.

Why does success bring self-sabotage to the party?!

This is such a common occurrence. You get *sooo* close to your goal. Results are snowballing, and you're getting in a groove with a new routine that's starting to feel sustainable. You've been conscious of stepping back to reflect and adjust. Then you start to let old habits creep in, and you begin a slow slide back into old patterns and routines.

All of a sudden, you feel like you're starting over. You may feel like you're constantly holding yourself back from finally seeing the results you want. You work really hard just to get to the same sticking point, and you can't seem to keep pushing forward.

Is it that you lack willpower? Did you run out of motivation? I'd argue it isn't a lack of willpower or motivation. It's simply an unconscious pattern that you need to be aware of before it's too late to control and change.

You might have doubled down and seen results snowball, but you can still find yourself curving back around the bend in the change loop cycle at any time. To prevent this, you need to embrace the new identity you've created. You need to double down again to recognize the new you that you've become. Your identity *has* changed in the process of achieving your goals. You've created new habits and routines and developed new mindsets, and you need to keep yourself in touch with those so you avoid the slide back into old patterns.

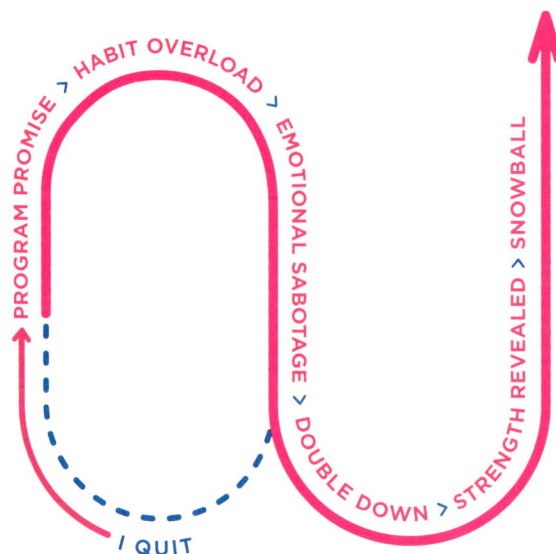

PROGRAM PROMISE > HABIT OVERLOAD > EMOTIONAL SABOTAGE > DOUBLE DOWN > STRENGTH REVEALED > SNOWBALL

I QUIT

So, if you feel those results snowballing, step back. Appreciate your success and then recognize the habits and mindsets that got you there. Realize the identity shift you've undergone and remind yourself of its importance.

Plan how you can keep pushing forward, shifting your habits and routines slightly so you don't start to backslide. Also, realize that taking a step back helps you evaluate what you need to do to keep moving forward. You have the power to change this pattern and embrace your new identity!

THE DANGERS OF HABIT AUTOPILOT

When you put your car on cruise control, you can't then just fall asleep at the wheel. You still have to look around and be conscious of where you're going. The same thing can be said as you create new habits. As they start to feel natural, you have to stay alert and adjust rather than allowing habit autopilot to take over.

The complacency often sets in right before the seasons change. You get comfortable and in a groove with the habits that fit your current lifestyle and priorities. But as things start to feel easy, you loosen the reins a bit and feel overly confident in your abilities. You may not notice the backslide or the shifts going on around you.

A 1 percent deviation from what you need can be your undoing. One percent seems like very little, but over time, a series of 1 percent shifts that you ignore will take you more and more off course. A plane that is 1 degree off course as it heads from New York to Japan will end up landing smack dab in the middle of the ocean!

This is the reason you can't reach your goals and then go on autopilot with the thought that something will work forever. That's a self-sabotaging pattern you might not often catch yourself in until it's too late. Instead, pay attention to your checkpoints and end dates. Your goals may shift to maintaining your results, but you still need goals and habits to focus on.

Performance might become your primary focus. Perhaps you'll concentrate on new ways to create a better balance, work to include more foods you love, or find ways to do the minimum while maintaining. Whatever your focus, you still need targets and checkpoints because the idea of forever isn't motivating. Life is about driving toward something, and if you feel like you aren't going somewhere, it's easy to let yourself off the hook. In every area of your life, you're planning or working toward the next thing, and your health and fitness goals are no different.

Of course, other life priorities will sometimes become more important, and that will affect your motivation and willingness to make sacrifices. Owning this fact is important because it can factor into how you choose to set your goals and adjust your habits.

For example, perhaps you recognize that during the holidays, you struggle to care as much about your weight-loss goals, aren't motivated to work out, or will be devouring those holiday cookies that call your name. That's not only OK—it's *good*. Recognizing that you won't always feel the same motivation and drive isn't quitting. You're not being soft or weak or lacking willpower. You're giving yourself the power to plan.

When you recognize a change in your priorities or focus, you can adjust your habits to match. This goes back to Chapter 6 and what's *repeatable*. Sometimes, small stones become larger because lifestyle factors have shifted. Sometimes, big-rock habits become easier because your habit budget has increased and the sacrifices feel worth it. You need to own that life is evolving so you can plan for it. You need that constant assessment and reflection.

You can't just go on habit autopilot! You're not driving at one speed on an endless highway. There are stop signs, stop lights, speed limit changes, and even traffic jams popping up. Motivation shifts. Burnout happens. Priorities evolve. And your goals do change. Embrace the fun in being able to tweak and adjust with the tools you've developed through building out your STRONG system, and plan ahead to have checkpoints with each new season, when you know your habits and lifestyle often evolve.

Maintaining your results doesn't mean you're done. It just means shifting gears. Life is constant evolution, and the second you become complacent—often when you least expect it—habit relapse can occur!

> " **Maintaining your results doesn't mean you're done. It just means shifting gears.** "

HABIT RELAPSE

Old habits are like weeds with roots that are deceptively hard to get rid of. When you go on a new program or plan, you're basically breaking off the weed without also pulling out the roots. That's why you tend to fall right back into old habits and see your results slide the second the twenty-one-day fix or six-week plan is done. But the STRONG system reflection is what makes this time different.

To ensure its success, you have to take time to dive into the uncomfortable reflection. You can't just breeze past it and go straight to the workouts and macros, thinking that's all you need. Even with this reflection, the roots of old habits typically run deep. Often, you might think you've pulled everything out when you've just broken the weed off at the stem, and only a few measly roots are coming with it.

It takes time to kill some of those deep roots, and that's why you have to be conscious of old habits rearing their ugly heads long after you think you've conquered them. You have to be mindful of the connections between old habits and the new ones you're creating. You have to be aware of old mindsets popping up because of priorities shifting or stress intensifying. You have to notice when your environment is shifting and the new patterns you've created are starting to slide.

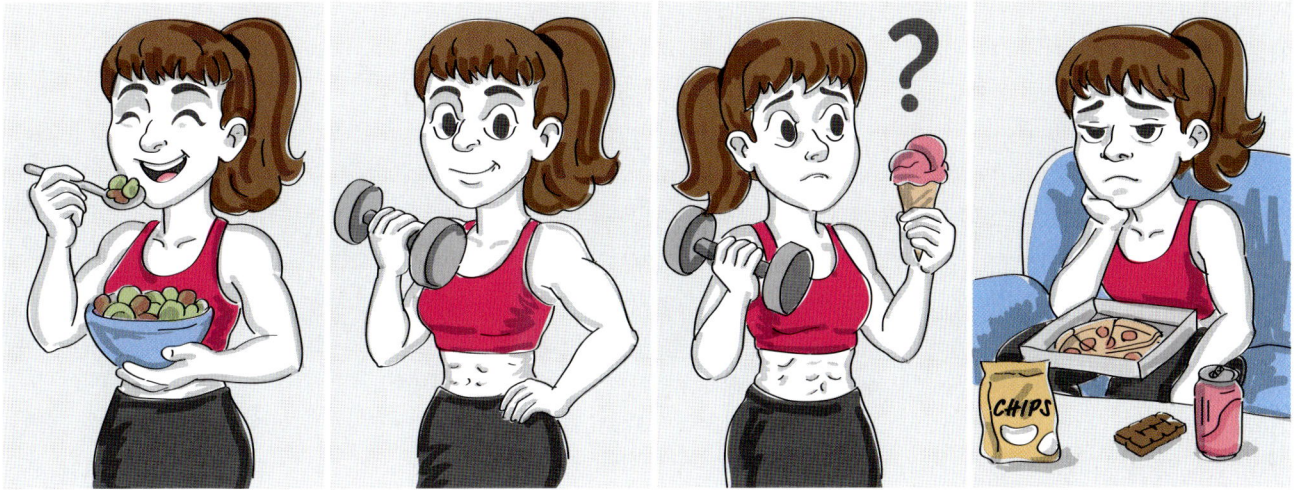

Always be vigilant of habit creep and relapse. Even if you've repeated the new habits enough for them to feel comfortable, you've still done them for only, what—a few months? A year? How long have you repeated some of your other old habits and patterns? Years? Decades? They're not gone; you've just buried them in a shallow grave.

Habits are like injuries: You can never stop doing what healed you or made you better, or you'll default to old movement and recruitment patterns. Have you ever noticed that the second you stop mobility work or rehab, you start to feel old aches and pains crop up? The same thing can be said for old habits and mindsets.

The old you will always call you back. The more you recognize this, and the more awareness you have, the more you give yourself the power to prevent it.

When you feel the slide happening and see yourself relapsing, ask yourself this one important question: Why?

> **When you feel the slide happening and see yourself relapsing, ask yourself this one important question: Why?**

Why is such a powerful word of reflection. It can help you assess what in your lifestyle, priorities, environment, or goals has led to old habits and mindsets creeping back in. Your answer can enable you to adjust and meet yourself where you are right now.

MAINTAINING YOUR RESULTS

Have you ever thought, *Yay! I reached my goal! Now what?!* That feeling of "now what?" is a pretty common reaction, even if you haven't thought it in precisely that way.

When you've reached your goal, you're not just done. There's always something more you want to achieve or accomplish. You may not have considered "finding more of a lifestyle balance" a goal, but it is. To get where you are, you've made some sacrifices you were OK with for the short term. Now, you have to find a long-term way to live without making those same sacrifices.

You can't just go back to what you were doing. Your lifestyle has changed. At the beginning, you envisioned your destination; now, you should see much of it in your daily actions, mindsets, and lifestyle. If you don't, assess where you still have room to grow into the new you.

The more you embrace your new lifestyle balance, the easier it will be to maintain your results. Find areas for growth and set your sights on where you still want to go now that you've shown yourself this is possible.

Learn to love the fact that there is always more you can improve upon and achieve. Having new challenges to overcome and basics that can be perfected can be an exciting part of life. It's why Olympic athletes always look for ways to improve; they want a new PR even when they win the race.

You are *never* done because this is a forever process. But systems shift. Goals change. What you want out of life evolves. And you have the opportunity at each checkpoint and with each goal you achieve to reassess and reset your GPS with a new destination in mind.

> **You are *never* done because this is a forever process.**

So, what do you want now?

The STRONG Refocus in the workbook at redefiningstrength.com/extras can play a role here. It can help you see what habits helped you reach your current goal but won't serve you for the next. Yup. That's right. Often, the exact thing that made you successful is the thing you need to tweak to reach your next goal.

For example, if you want to lose fat and successfully used sprint interval training (SIT) and high-intensity interval training (HIIT) but now want to build extra muscle, you might need to drop the SIT and HIIT sessions for a while. If you increased your calories to build muscle but now want to lose a little extra fluff before vacation, a deficit may be needed.

The STRONG system has given you the foundation on which to build. You have the power to assess what you need. Don't get married to a tool or tactic. No matter how much you loved the 6-12-25 method, it may now be time for timed strength work techniques.

As you shift to maintaining your results, embrace the transition. Maintenance is a learned process. You don't just flip a switch. But the great part is, the exact mechanisms that made it hard to lose the weight or gain the muscle are also what will help you maintain your results more easily the longer you've repeated the new habits. Your body wants to maintain the new balance and set point you've created!

Give yourself time to transition, and don't fear the changes. Set new targets and checkpoints to help you keep assessing and trusting the process while tweaking as you go. Rebuild out of the calorie deficit you've been in. Include more foods you love. Cycle your workout techniques. Embrace the evolution and fun in the next challenge!

PUTTING YOUR PLAN IN ACTION

Say it with me: Nothing changes if nothing changes! The essential final step in the STRONG system is you taking *action*. It's time to get going!

Doing so means that you have to use everything you've learned about yourself to make this time different. You aren't fitting yourself into a plan; you're building the plan around you.

MEETING YOURSELF WHERE YOU ARE

You've done the reflection. You know where you're starting from. Now, it's time to create the plan that addresses what you need so you can head in the right direction with your first step.

I want you to pause for just a second to appreciate the work you've already done to help create your plan:

1. **BREAKING THE CHANGE LOOP:** You're done with the same old pattern. You're ready to step back to move forward. You've considered where and why habit overload and emotional sabotage have occurred in the past to prepare yourself to double down through those struggles.

2. **ORIGIN STORY:** You've assessed your current lifestyle and the changes you need and want. You've created your "budget." You've weighed the pain of staying stuck to help you overcome the pain of change.

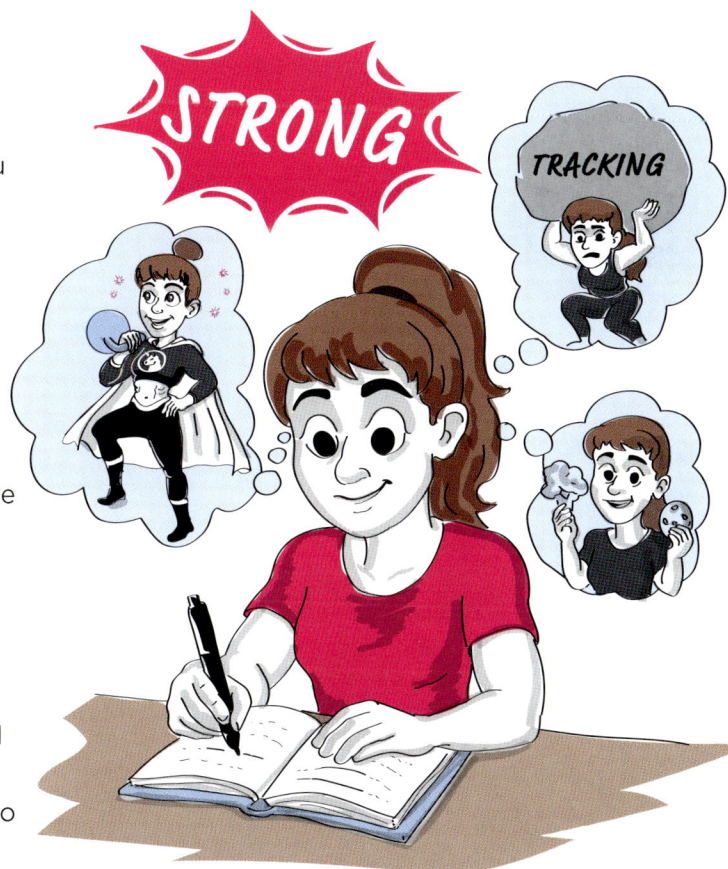

3. **SIGNIFICANT:** You know why your goal matters. You've owned all of the far-reaching benefits and the huge impact it can have in many areas of your life.

4. **TARGETED:** You've set checkpoints and targets toward your main goal and complementary goals. You've recognized that the more ways you measure success, the more successful you will be, so you can trust the process and see changes working and building even before you've reached your goal.

5. **REPEATABLE:** You've assessed the habits you need and what is truly doable, meeting yourself where you are right now. You've recognized the mindsets and feelings associated with certain habits to account for how you implement them. You're ready to break things down and stack those habit changes based on your lifestyle, priorities, and the excuses you've seen popping up in the past. You have a big-rock habit you'll work to break down, a couple of stones, and even a few pebbles you know you can implement immediately.

6. **OPTIMIZED:** You've accepted ownership for everything you're planning to do and that's happened in past attempts. You've mentally prepared for struggles and setbacks. You're not looking for a perfect plan; you're tailoring the plan to what you need.

7. **NONNEGOTIABLE:** You've assessed what you value in order to own the choices you will have to make as you build your habit changes. You've gone back to reassess what habits may be bigger rocks than you thought. You've recognized what is truly important to you to strike a balance and determine what sacrifices are worth it, especially to start. This will help you determine the best workout schedule and macros method because now it's time to …

8. **GO!** Nothing worth having ever comes easy. You can do hard things, and you know you deserve the results and success you're working toward. Now's the time to own what you need, select your workouts, and tailor your macros to match. Then you can dive into the details and make tweaks to the stuff people often ignore. Focus on those big fundamentals first and add as you progress. You eat an elephant one bite at a time (as gross as that analogy is!).

Right now, take out a calendar to write down your workouts. (You can also find a page for writing them in the workbook at redefiningstrength.com/extras. Write dates to reassess your macro changes. Plan your weekly or monthly check-ins and set your target checkpoints.

Writing everything down, marking on a calendar, and tying it to reminders and alerts provides accountability. It helps you know how long you're "trusting the process" before making changes, which enables you to focus on consistency without repeating something that isn't working for too long.

Don't wait to write out your action steps. Build your plan based on what you need so you have a solid roadmap you can be reminded of daily. Doing so makes it easier to track how you feel so you can make changes and hold yourself accountable. Knowing some dates when you'll check in can be motivation to get started now. You won't be nearly as motivated without a deadline.

REMEMBER: *Just because something is working doesn't mean you can set the habit and forget it. Your lifestyle, needs, goals, schedule, and body will change, and you have to be prepared to reassess. Reflection and the STRONG Refocus (see page 219) are powerful tools to keep you achieving more than you thought possible!*

NOTHING WORKS FOREVER

Sorry to be a Debbie Downer, but nothing works forever. (I know. I say that a lot.) But that's not a bad thing! It's just the reality, because life is constantly evolving, which gives you opportunities to do something new. Embrace the idea that making changes can be fun!

Try different macros. Try different workouts. Mix up moves. Test out different meal timings. Use those diet breaks or cheat days. Embrace balance.

Be excited that you can shift and adjust as your priorities and lifestyle evolve. You can work in cocktails and relax on vacation, but you can also dial things in further and push extra hard to PR in a race or build a little extra muscle.

You have the tools and reflection assessments you need to meet yourself where you are and keep moving forward!

Take action, reflect, and tweak. Then do it again and again and again! Love that you can constantly strike a new balance to enjoy life while seeing results!

NOTE: *As you move into selecting your workout progression and start tracking your macros and changing your workout habits, embrace the learning process. If you feel stress or overwhelm rising at any time,* tweak before you freak! *Pause and find a way to break down a habit that may be a bigger rock than you first realized. There can be a steep learning curve no matter how much you try to tailor a program for your needs. Don't let that throw you back into the change loop.* Own it! *You've got this!*

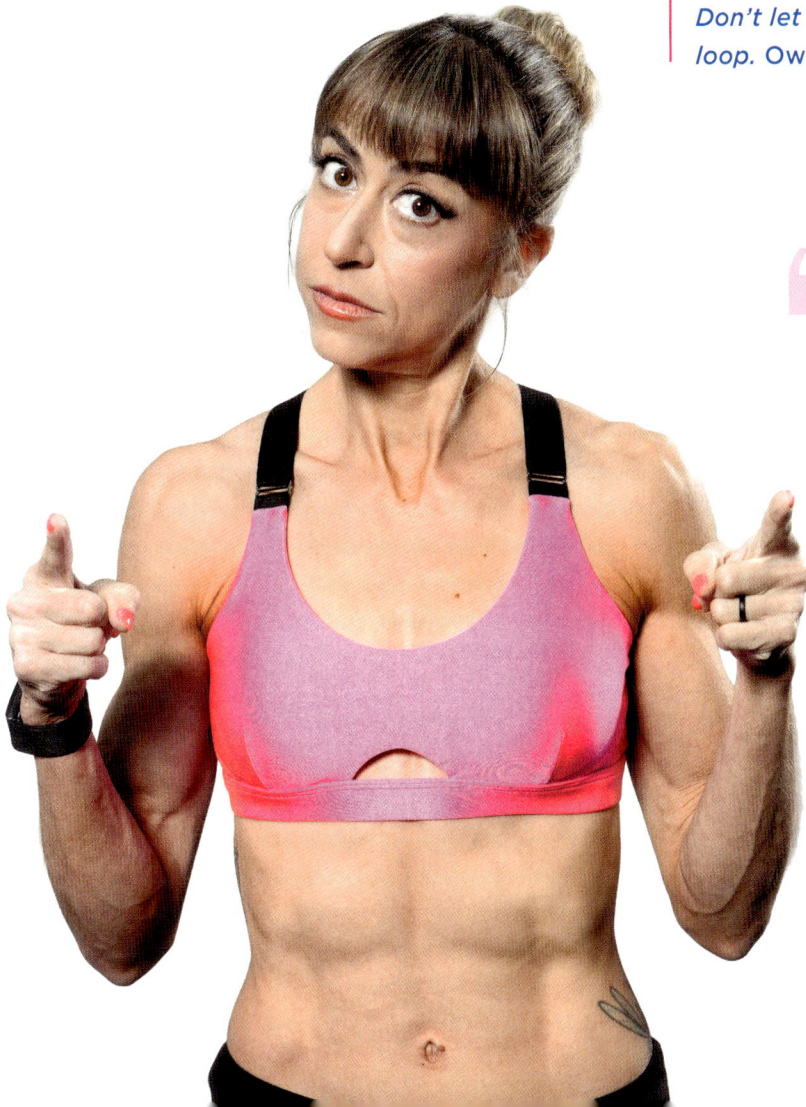

> **Take action, reflect, and tweak. Then do it again and again and again!**

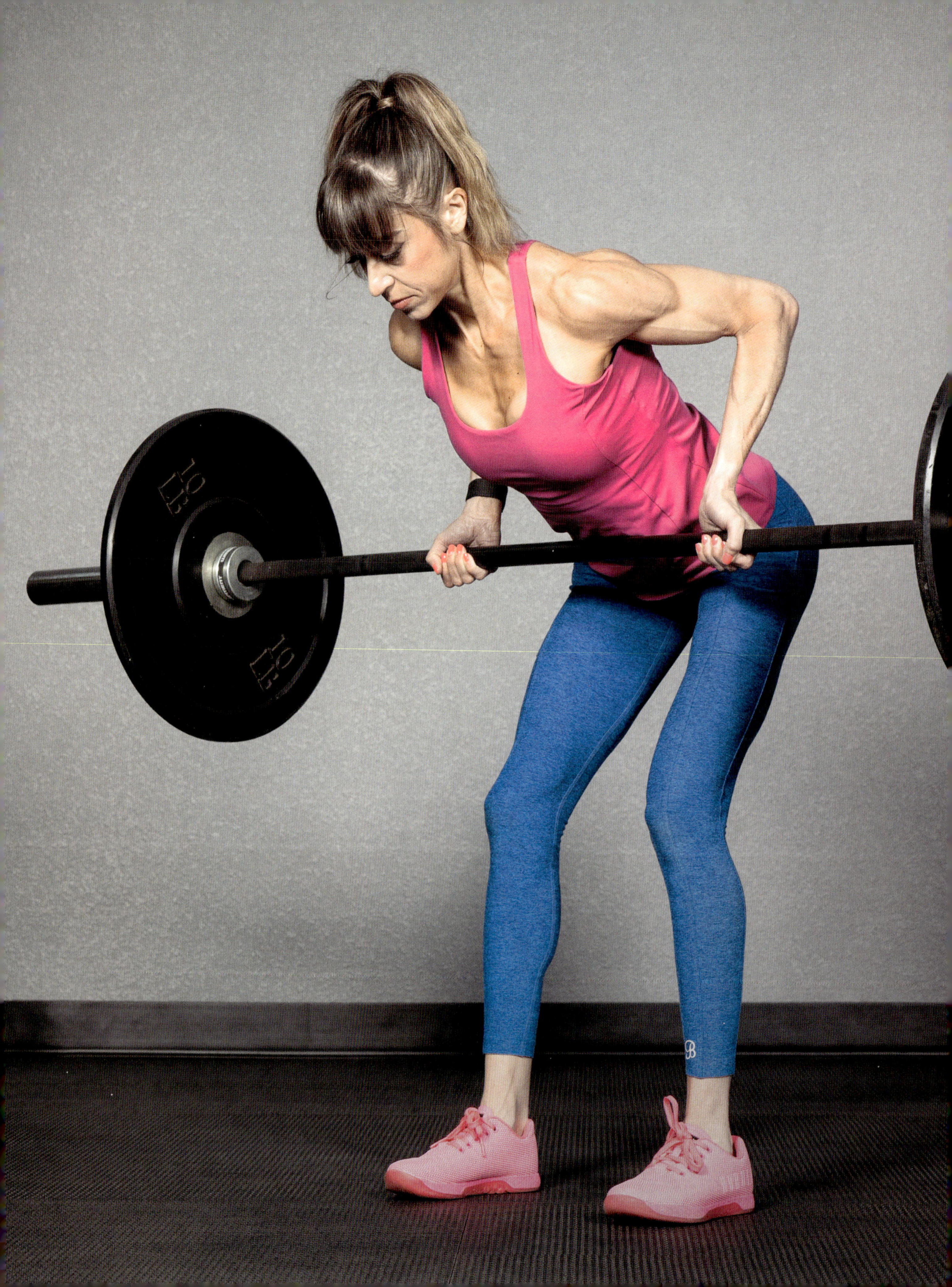
10 LB
10 LB

EXERCISE
PROTOCOLS
AND LIBRARY

17 WORKOUT TIME: PUTTING TOGETHER YOUR PLAN

My mean and nerdy trainer heart loves this part. It's the time I get to finally say, "Good … suffer!" And it's your chance to finally take the action you've wanted to. But before you jump in and feel overwhelmed by the options, I want to go over the best way to approach these plans because they're built like puzzle pieces.

One size doesn't fit all.

Each muscle-building protocol (the 6-12-25 method, compound burner sets, timed strength work techniques) has a few different split options:

- **Full-body schedules**
- **Anterior/posterior schedules**
- **Hemisphere schedules**

Based on your STRONG system reflection and the information about the protocols in Chapter 11, you should have an idea of which one you want to jump to. Now, you'll find how to lay out your week and see that each workout you'll need to do is outlined.

You will repeat this schedule for three to six weeks. If after at least three weeks, you feel you're not able to keep progressing or mentally need a change-up, you can move on to a different protocol or simply switch up movement variations in those routines.

The Exercise Library that starts on page 301 includes options to help you adjust the workouts based on the tools you have and your fitness level or injuries. Don't write off a workout just because it has a move you can't do. Swap it with something else in the library.

Use a workout log like the one in the workbook at redefiningstrength.com/extras to keep track of your progress.

I've offered tips about the different protocols, which will help you tweak the weekly schedule and workouts to fit your main goal or fitness level. I've even suggested "accelerated" options for advanced lifters.

Once you've selected your overall progression, you then need to add the warm-ups and any cardio or recovery workouts you want to include to create your perfect workout puzzle. I've listed each component separately so you can adjust and add or subtract as you need! Have fun seeing the opportunity in these options and knowing you can tweak based on how things are progressing!

NOTE: *If you want more variations of these protocols or are interested in using a video exercise library to swap in more fun moves, check out the seven-day free trial to Dynamic Strength by visiting redefiningstrength.com/extras.*

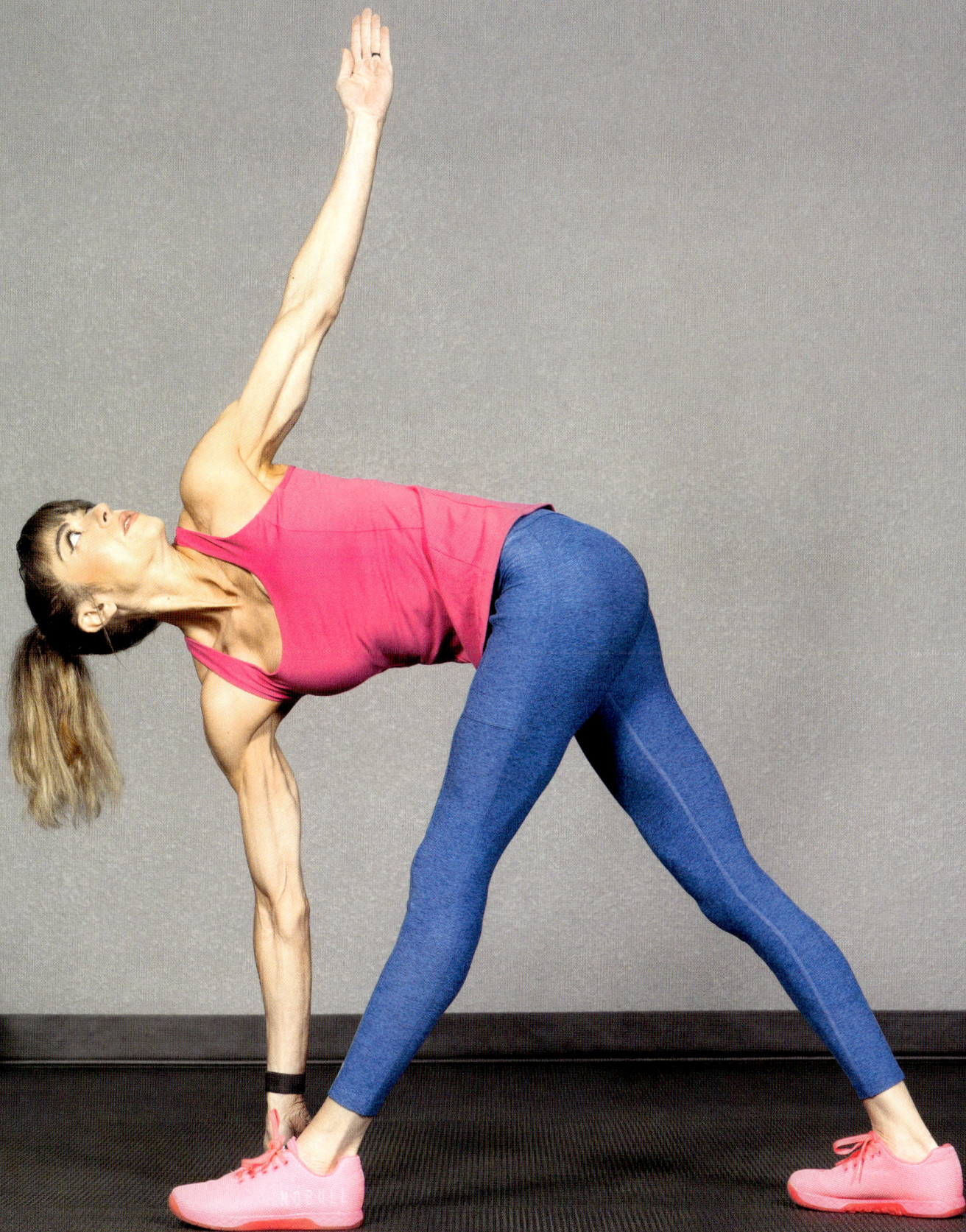

18 THE 6-12-25

ANTERIOR/POSTERIOR PROGRESSION

This progression is best if you have four or five days to train. If you have only three days to train, you'll pick either an anterior or posterior workout for the third day based on your "stubborn" areas or where you want to focus on building muscle. You can switch to a different progression after three to six weeks. While you don't want to ignore the recovery work, sneaking in even a 5-minute session on off days can create balance if you have only three days to train.

If you're doing six days a week, I do *not* recommend another lifting day, because the four days hit everything with enough volume. The sixth day is best used for a run—if you enjoy it and your goal isn't pure muscle gains—or a recovery session. You may do a very short ab finisher or 5-minute "trouble zone" bonus with a recovery session and SIT or power protocol. If you push hard with the four lifts, you shouldn't want to do more.

With this progression, you will want to use the full-body or anterior/ posterior prehab warm-ups as well as the suggested cooldowns.

3 DAYS A WEEK	4 DAYS A WEEK	5 DAYS A WEEK	6 DAYS A WEEK
DAY 1	**DAY 1**	**DAY 1**	**DAY 1**
Posterior 6-12-25 #1	Posterior 6-12-25 #1	Posterior 6-12-25 #1	Posterior 6-12-25 #1
DAY 2	**DAY 2**	**DAY 2**	**DAY 2**
Off	Anterior 6-12-25 #1	Anterior 6-12-25 #1	Anterior 6-12-25 #1
DAY 3	**DAY 3**	**DAY 3**	**DAY 3**
Anterior 6-12-25 #1	Off	Off	Recovery workout *or* Cardio
DAY 4	**DAY 4**	**DAY 4**	**DAY 4**
Off	Posterior 6-12-25 #2	Posterior 6-12-25 #2	Posterior 6-12-25 #2
DAY 5	**DAY 5**	**DAY 5**	**DAY 5**
Posterior 6-12-25 #2 *or* Anterior 6-12-25 #2	Anterior 6-12-25 #2	Anterior 6-12-25 #2	Anterior 6-12-25 #2
DAY 6	**DAY 6**	**DAY 6**	**DAY 6**
Off	Off	Recovery workout	Recovery workout
DAY 7	**DAY 7**	**DAY 7**	**DAY 7**
Off	Off	Off	Off

In the schedules for five and six days a week, do not skip the recovery workouts! If you find you aren't recovering from the volume of these sessions, move to the hemisphere progression in the next chapter. You can change the order of these workouts, but do not put two posterior or anterior days back to back.

6-12-25 WORKOUT BUILDER

You can build out your own 6-12-25 workouts from this template. Each series focuses on one area/hemisphere of the body (lower or upper). I recommend alternating which you put first or prioritizing the area you most want to build so you will be freshest for that series.

MUSCLE FOCUSED: Focus on longer rest periods and going heavier, even if that means having to pause during the reps assigned to finish them as you go up in weight over the weeks. Exclude any SIT except on the recovery workout day, but you may include one or two power sessions. For a six-day schedule, walking can be great extra cardio to go with the recovery sessions. Check out the Bonus Accelerate Strength Builder on page 235 to take your strength up an extra notch.

FAT LOSS: Rest may be shorter, like 90 seconds to 2 minutes. Include SIT two or three days a week or one or two SIT sessions and one power session. Include SIT on recovery workout days. Keep long runs or rides to one or two days between lifts and make sure to still have a day off.

BEGINNERS: Start with lower volume to let your connective tissues adjust and maintain proper form and recruitment patterns. Use the three-day schedule with one or two recovery sessions. Don't be afraid to start with just 2 rounds through each series.

WARM-UP
Make sure to choose the warm-up that addresses the areas you plan to work.

Optional POWER SESSION

SERIES #1: Upper or lower body
Complete 2 to 4 rounds through the series, resting 90 seconds to 3 minutes between rounds and up to 3 minutes between series. Over the moves, you are going to home in on one muscle worked in the main 6-rep lift.

- 6 reps **heavy big compound lift***
- 12 reps **accessory lift (homing in)**
- 25 reps **isolation move for main stubborn muscle**

SERIES #2: Upper or lower body
Complete 2 to 4 rounds through the series, resting 90 seconds to 3 minutes between rounds.

- 6 reps **heavy big compound lift***
- 12 reps **accessory lift (homing in)**
- 25 reps **isolation move for main stubborn muscle**

Optional SIT**

COOLDOWN

---

*With any lift where you're getting under heavy loads, you want to do 2 or 3 warm-up sets first, building up with 50 percent (8 to 10 reps), 75 percent (6 to 8 reps), and 85 percent (4 to 6 reps) of your working weight. You may then increase after that first round. The heavier you go, the more you want to do those warm-up rounds before the series.

**If possible, it's recommended to do these on the recovery days. You may consider only adding this to your progression after you've done three to four weeks of adapting first.

POSTERIOR
6-12-25 #1

WARM-UP

Optional **POWER SESSION**

SERIES #1

Complete 2 to 4 rounds through the series, resting 90 seconds to 3 minutes between rounds and up to 3 minutes between series.

- 6 reps **hip thrusts***
- 12 reps (per side) **single-leg deadlifts**
- 25 reps (per side) **cable seated hamstring curls**

SERIES #2

Complete 2 to 4 rounds through the series, resting 90 seconds to 3 minutes between rounds.

- 6 reps **overhand rows***
- 12 reps **back flys**
- 25 reps **back shrugs**

Optional **SIT****

COOLDOWN

POSTERIOR
6-12-25 #2

WARM-UP

Optional **POWER SESSION**

SERIES #1

Complete 2 to 4 rounds through the series, resting 90 seconds to 3 minutes between rounds and up to 3 minutes between series.

- 6 reps **lat pulldowns***
- 12 reps **underhand rows**
- 25 reps **lat pushdowns**

SERIES #2

Complete 2 to 4 rounds through the series, resting 90 seconds to 3 minutes between rounds.

- 6 reps (per side) **reverse lunges***
- 12 reps **pull-throughs**
- 25 reps **hyperextensions**

Optional **SIT****

COOLDOWN

ANTERIOR
6-12-25 #1

WARM-UP

Optional **POWER SESSION**

SERIES #1

Complete 2 to 4 rounds through the series, resting 90 seconds to 3 minutes between rounds and up to 3 minutes between series.

- 6 reps **bench presses***
- 12 reps **chest press to skull crushers**
- 25 reps **triceps pushdowns**

SERIES #2

Complete 2 to 4 rounds through the series, resting 90 seconds to 3 minutes between rounds.

- 6 reps (per side) **front lunges***
- 12 reps **front squats**
- 25 reps (per side) **cable seated quad extensions**

Optional **SIT****

COOLDOWN

ANTERIOR
6-12-25 #2

WARM-UP

Optional **POWER SESSION**

SERIES #1

Complete 2 to 4 rounds through the series, resting 90 seconds to 3 minutes between rounds and up to 3 minutes between series.

- 6 reps **back squats***
- 12 reps (per side) **step-ups**
- 25 reps **kneeling lean backs**

SERIES #2

Complete 2 to 4 rounds through the series, resting 90 seconds to 3 minutes between rounds.

- 6 reps **overhead presses***
- 12 reps **dips**
- 25 reps **lateral raises**

Optional **SIT****

COOLDOWN

Perform the warm-up sets prior to starting your rounds of the 6-12-25.

**If possible, it's recommended to do these on the recovery days. You may consider only adding this to your progression after you've done three to four weeks of adapting first.*

ACCELERATE STRENGTH BUILDER

Use this template to build out your own 6-12-25 workouts with an extra strength focus. This is an extra intensive and long workout design. I recommend using this most often when you're lifting only four times a week and for no longer than a three- to four-week progression. Use it to push for recomp when you're focused on strength and muscle or if you're an experienced trainee who's really struggling to move to the next level. Extra cardio is not recommended, especially on lifting days.

WARM-UP: Make sure to choose the warm-up that addresses the areas you plan to work.

LIFT*

Complete 3 to 5 rounds, usually of 3 to 10 reps in that space that crosses between maximal strength and hypertrophy work. If this is an upper body move, include your lower body series next, or vice versa. If you use this design more than one day in your week, I recommend doing a heavy lift in one workout for your upper body and one for your lower body. If you only do one day, pick a heavy lift to target your most stubborn area or the area you want to build.

- 3 to 10 reps **heavy big compound lift** (e.g., squats, deadlifts, bench presses, back rows)**
- 2 to 5 minutes **rest**

SERIES #1: Upper or lower body

Complete 2 to 4 rounds through the series, resting 90 seconds to 3 minutes between rounds and up to 3 minutes between series. Over the moves, you're going to home in on one muscle worked in the main 6-rep lift.

- 6 reps **heavy big compound lift**
- 12 reps **accessory lift (homing in)**
- 25 reps **isolation move for main stubborn muscle**

SERIES #2: Upper or lower body

Complete 2 to 4 rounds through the series, resting 90 seconds to 3 minutes between rounds.

- 6 reps **heavy big compound lift**
- 12 reps **accessory lift (homing in)**
- 25 reps **isolation move for main stubborn muscle**

COOLDOWN

*You can do fun things like cluster sets, drop sets, 10-7-3-1, and such for this first lift based on your goals. See the bonus workouts on page 236 for these three techniques.

**Perform the warm-up sets prior to your working rounds of the first lift. You may want to do 2 or 3 warm-up sets, building up with 50 percent (8 to 10 reps), 75 percent (6 to 8 reps), and 85 percent (4 to 6 reps) of your working weight. The heavier you go, the more you want to do those warm-up rounds before the series.

18 THE 6-12-25 235
ANTERIOR/POSTERIOR PROGRESSION

POSTERIOR ACCELERATE 6-12-25

BONUS

WARM-UP

LOWER LIFT: CLUSTER SETS

Complete 3 to 5 working rounds. For each round, you will complete 6 to 10 reps. But those reps will be broken down into mini sets of just 2 or 3 reps with 15 to 30 seconds of rest between sets. This should allow you to use a heavier weight for the full 6 to 10 reps than you could without the mini breaks. This can also help you maintain better form while using heavier loads for more reps.

- **6 to 10 reps deadlifts***
- **2 to 5 minutes rest**
  OR

UPPER LIFT: DROP SETS

Do 3 or 4 rounds of max pull-ups at the hardest variation you can possibly do with a 4-rep minimum. If you can't hit 4 reps, pause only 15 seconds to finish with that same variation or modify immediately if you'd need to rest longer. On your final round, modify the move to complete 10 reps without resting after your first 4 to 8 reps. This may mean modifying a couple of times. If you can do 10 pull-ups in a row, you should be doing weighted pull-ups to try to force yourself to max out around 4 or 5 reps on each round. You'll then lower the weight for the drop sets to complete 10 total reps.

- **4 to 8 reps pull-ups*** + 1 drop set on the final set for 10 reps
- **90 seconds to 2 minutes rest**

SERIES #1**

Complete 2 to 4 rounds through the series, resting 90 seconds to 3 minutes between rounds and up to 3 minutes between series.

- **6 reps (per side) single-arm rows***
- **12 reps chest-supported rows**
- **25 reps biceps curls**

SERIES #2**

Complete 2 to 4 rounds through the series, resting 90 seconds to 3 minutes between rounds.

- **6 reps (per side) curtsy lunges***
- **12 reps weighted glute bridges**
- **25 reps (per side) cable abductions**

COOLDOWN

ANTERIOR ACCELERATE 6-12-25

BONUS

WARM-UP

LOWER LIFT: 10-7-3-1

Complete 2 to 4 rounds through the 10-7-3-1 squats, resting 90 seconds to 2 minutes between rounds. Do not shorten the rest period between rounds; at the end of the rest, you should crave more of the lift. To do the 10-7-3-1, you will pick a weight that you max out on at about 10 to 12 reps. You will do 10 reps and rest 10 seconds, putting the weights down or in the rack. Then do 7 reps and rest 7 seconds. Do 3 reps and rest 3 seconds. Then do 1 rep and completely rest before repeating the 21-rep series. Basically, you're performing 21 reps with a weight you can barely do for 10 reps! For the warm-up rounds, build up to a weight you can do 12 reps with to start your first working round.

- **10-7-3-1 back squats**
- **90 seconds to 2 minutes rest**
  OR

UPPER LIFT

Complete 3 to 5 rounds, resting 2 to 4 minutes between rounds. It's better to rest longer and keep the weight heavier or even go up as you work toward that 5-rep max.

- **5 to 8 reps bench presses**
- **2 to 4 minutes rest**

SERIES #1*

Complete 2 to 4 rounds through the series, resting 90 seconds to 3 minutes between rounds and up to 3 minutes between series.

- **6 reps (per side) deficit split squats****
- **12 reps goblet squats**
- **25 reps squat pulses**

SERIES #2*

Complete 2 to 4 rounds through the series, resting 90 seconds to 3 minutes between rounds.

- **6 reps incline bench presses****
- **12 reps chest flys**
- **25 reps push-ups**

COOLDOWN

NOTE: *SIT and power work is not recommended on this day.*

Perform the warm-up sets prior to your working rounds of the first lift. You may do weighted pull-ups or use assistance, using the warm-up rounds to find an appropriate weight.

**You will determine which series is first based on the lift.*

***Do warm-up rounds if needed before starting the series.*

19 THE 6-12-25
HEMISPHERE PROGRESSION

This progression is best if you have five or six days to train because you want to hit both the upper and lower body twice as well as include at least one active recovery day. I've included bonus upper- and lower-focused workouts that you can include to start the week if you're going super heavy on the lift for maximal strength work. If you want to lift five days a week because you're focused on building muscle in a stubborn area, pick the bonus session that targets the hemisphere you want to focus on.

With this progression, you will want to use the upper and lower prehab warm-ups as well as the suggested cooldowns.

Here, I give you schedules for five and six days a week. Do not skip the recovery workouts! If you find you can only do three or four days a week, check the 6-12-25 Anterior/Posterior Progression in Chapter 18. You can change the order of these workouts, but do not put two lower or two upper workouts back to back without at least one rest day between. The more rest you get between hitting the same hemisphere (twenty-four hours minimum), the better; just don't be too inconsistent.

5 DAYS A WEEK	6 DAYS A WEEK (upper body focused)	6 DAYS A WEEK (lower body focused)
DAY 1	**DAY 1**	**DAY 1**
Lower body 6-12-25 #1	Upper body 6-12-25 bonus*	Lower body 6-12-25 bonus*
DAY 2	**DAY 2**	**DAY 2**
Upper body 6-12-25 #1	Lower body 6-12-25 #1	Upper body 6-12-25 #1
DAY 3	**DAY 3**	**DAY 3**
Off	Upper body 6-12-25 #1	Lower body 6-12-25 #1
DAY 4	**DAY 4**	**DAY 4**
Lower body 6-12-25 #2	Lower body 6-12-25 #2	Upper body 6-12-25 #2
DAY 5	**DAY 5**	**DAY 5**
Upper body 6-12-25 #2	Upper body 6-12-25 #2	Lower body 6-12-25 #2
DAY 6	**DAY 6**	**DAY 6**
Recovery workout	Recovery workout**	Recovery workout**
DAY 7	**DAY 7**	**DAY 7**
Off	Off	Off

*This first workout in both the upper body and lower body schedules will be the bonus session included in this chapter.

**The recovery day could be the third day instead of the sixth day.

6-12-25 WORKOUT BUILDER

You can build out your own 6-12-25 workouts based on this template.

MUSCLE FOCUSED: Focus on longer rest periods and going heavier, even if that means having to pause during the reps assigned to finish them as you go up in weight over the weeks. Exclude any SIT except on the recovery workout day, but you may include one or two power sessions. Consider following a six-day schedule rather than the five-day schedule. Check out the Bonus Accelerate Strength Builder on page 241.

FAT LOSS: Focus on maximizing the two series and include SIT at the end of your workout two or three days a week. You can also do two SIT sessions and include one power session. If you're doing an endurance sport, include your longer distances on off days or on days when you don't work that hemisphere. Consider doing just four days of lifting and including a bonus SIT session on a sixth day if you want to train six days a week!

BEGINNERS: Start with lower volume to let your connective tissues adjust and maintain proper form and recruitment patterns. You may start with just one 6-12-25 series that's more like the bonus day on page 240 or do only 2 rounds through each series.

BONUS

BONUS SESSIONS: On the bonus day, which may be done first in your weekly schedule if maximal strength is part of your focus, you will see a lift included prior to a single 6-12-25 series. This maximal strength work helps with hypertrophy and, ultimately, recomp.

WARM-UP
Make sure to choose the warm-up that addresses the areas you plan to work.

Optional POWER SESSION

SERIES #1
Complete 2 to 4 rounds through the series, resting 90 seconds to 3 minutes between rounds and up to 3 minutes between series. Over the moves, you are going to home in on one muscle worked in the main 6-rep lift.

- **6 reps heavy big compound lift***
- **12 reps accessory lift (homing in)**
- **25 reps isolation move for main stubborn muscle**

SERIES #2
Complete 2 to 4 rounds through the series, resting 90 seconds to 3 minutes between rounds.

- **6 reps heavy big compound lift***
- **12 reps accessory lift (homing in)**
- **25 reps isolation move for main stubborn muscle**

Optional SIT

COOLDOWN

With any lift where you're getting under heavy loads, especially in the first 6-rep series, you may want to do 2 or 3 warm-up sets first, building up with 50 percent (8 to 10 reps), 75 percent (6 to 8 reps), and 85 percent (4 to 6 reps) of your working weight. You may then increase after that first round. The heavier you go, the more you want to do those warm-up rounds before the series.

LOWER BODY
6-12-25 #1

WARM-UP

Optional **POWER SESSION**

SERIES #1

Complete 2 to 4 rounds through the series, resting 90 seconds to 3 minutes between rounds and up to 3 minutes between series.

- 6 reps hip **thrusts***
- 12 reps (per side) **single-leg deadlifts**
- 25 reps (per side) **cable seated hamstring curls**

SERIES #2

Complete 2 to 4 rounds through the series, resting 90 seconds to 3 minutes between rounds.

- 6 reps (per side) **front lunges***
- 12 reps **front squats**
- 25 reps (per side) **cable seated quad extensions**

Optional **SIT**

COOLDOWN

UPPER BODY
6-12-25 #1

WARM-UP

Optional **POWER SESSION**

SERIES #1

Complete 2 to 4 rounds through the series, resting 90 seconds to 3 minutes between rounds and up to 3 minutes between series.

- 6 reps **bench presses***
- 12 reps **chest press to skull crushers**
- 25 reps **triceps pushdowns**

SERIES #2

Complete 2 to 4 rounds through the series, resting 90 seconds to 3 minutes between rounds.

- 6 reps **overhand rows***
- 12 reps **back flys**
- 25 reps **back shrugs**

Optional **SIT**

COOLDOWN

LOWER BODY
6-12-25 #2

WARM-UP

Optional **POWER SESSION**

SERIES #1

Complete 2 to 4 rounds through the series, resting 90 seconds to 3 minutes between rounds and up to 3 minutes between series.

- 6 reps **back squats***
- 12 reps (per side) **step-ups**
- 25 reps **kneeling lean backs**

SERIES #2

Complete 2 to 4 rounds through the series, resting 90 seconds to 3 minutes between rounds.

- 6 reps (per side) **reverse lunges***
- 12 reps **pull-throughs**
- 25 reps **hyperextensions**

Optional **SIT**

COOLDOWN

UPPER BODY
6-12-25 #2

WARM-UP

Optional **POWER SESSION**

SERIES #1

Complete 2 to 4 rounds through the series, resting 90 seconds to 3 minutes between rounds and up to 3 minutes between series.

- 6 reps **lat pulldowns***
- 12 reps **underhand rows**
- 25 reps **lat pushdowns**

SERIES #2

Complete 2 to 4 rounds through the series, resting 90 seconds to 3 minutes between rounds.

- 6 reps **overhead presses***
- 12 reps **dips**
- 25 reps **lateral raises**

Optional **SIT**

COOLDOWN

Perform the warm-up sets prior to starting your rounds of the 6-12-25.

LOWER BODY
6-12-25

BONUS

WARM-UP

LIFT: Cluster sets

Complete 3 to 5 working rounds. For each round, you will complete 6 to 10 reps. But those reps will be broken down into mini sets of just 2 or 3 reps with 15 to 30 seconds of rest between sets. This should allow you to use a heavier weight for the full 6 to 10 reps than you could without the mini breaks. This can also help you maintain better form while using heavier loads for more reps.

- 6 to 10 reps **deadlifts***
- 2 to 5 minutes **rest**

SERIES #1

Complete 2 to 4 rounds through the series, resting 90 seconds to 3 minutes between rounds.

- 6 reps (per side) **curtsy lunges****
- 12 reps weighted **glute bridges**
- 25 reps (per side) **cable abductions**

Optional WALK***

COOLDOWN

UPPER BODY
6-12-25

BONUS

WARM-UP

LIFT: Drop sets

Do 3 or 4 rounds of max pull-ups at the hardest variation you can possibly do with a 4-rep minimum. If you can't hit 4 reps, pause only 15 seconds to finish with that same variation or modify immediately if you'd need to rest longer. On your final round, modify the move to complete 10 reps without resting after your first 4 to 8 reps. This may mean modifying a couple of times. If you can do 10 pull-ups in a row, you should be doing weighted pull-ups to try to force yourself to max out around 4 or 5 reps on each round. You'll then lower the weight for the drop sets to complete 10 total reps.

- 4 to 8 reps **pull-ups*** + 1 drop set on the final set for 10 reps
- 90 seconds to 2 minutes **rest**

SERIES #1

Complete 2 to 4 rounds through the series, resting 90 seconds to 3 minutes between rounds.

- 6 reps (per side) **single-arm rows****
- 12 reps **chest-supported rows**
- 25 reps **biceps curls**

Optional WALK***

COOLDOWN

---

*Perform the warm-up sets prior to your working rounds of the first lift.

**Do warm-up rounds if needed before starting the series.

***SIT and power work is not recommended on this day; however, walking is if fat loss is the goal because it can help utilize mobilized fatty acids to help with definition!

ACCELERATE STRENGTH BUILDER

Use this template to build out your own 6-12-25 workouts with an extra strength focus for either hemisphere. This is an extra intensive and long workout design. I recommend using this most often when you're lifting only four times a week and for no longer than a three- to four-week progression. Use it to push for recomp when you're focused on strength and muscle or if you're an experienced trainee who's really struggling to move to the next level. Extra cardio is not recommended on lifting days, but you may include walks or SIT on one or two days around your lifts with some recovery work.

WARM-UP
Make sure to choose the warm-up that addresses the areas you plan to work.

LIFT*
Complete 3 to 5 rounds, usually of 3 to 10 reps in that space that crosses between maximal strength and hypertrophy work.

- **3 to 10 reps heavy big compound lift** (e.g., squats, deadlifts, bench presses, back rows)**
- **2 to 5 minutes rest**

SERIES #1
Complete 2 to 4 rounds through the series, resting 90 seconds to 3 minutes between rounds and up to 3 minutes between series. Over the moves, you're going to home in on one muscle worked in the main 6-rep lift.

- **6 reps heavy big compound lift**
- **12 reps accessory lift (homing in)**
- **25 reps isolation move for main stubborn muscle**

SERIES #2
Complete 2 to 4 rounds through the series, resting 90 seconds to 3 minutes between rounds.

- **6 reps heavy big compound lift**
- **12 reps accessory lift (homing in)**
- **25 reps isolation move for main stubborn muscle**

COOLDOWN

You can do fun things like the cluster sets, drop sets, and such for this first lift based on your goals. See the bonus workouts on page 240 for these two techniques.

**Perform the warm-up sets prior to your working rounds of the first lift. You may want to do 2 or 3 warm-up sets, building up with 50 percent (8 to 10 reps), 75 percent (6 to 8 reps), and 85 percent (4 to 6 reps) of your working weight. The heavier you go, the more you want to do those warm-up rounds before the series.*

20 THE COMPOUND BURNER SETS

ANTERIOR/POSTERIOR PROGRESSION

This progression is best if you have four to six days to train. If you only have three days, check the Compound Burner Sets Full-Body Progression on page 253. While you don't want to ignore the recovery work, sneaking in even a 5-minute session on the off days can create balance if you're limited to three or four days to train.

If you're doing six days a week, I do *not* recommend another lifting day; the four days hit everything with enough volume. This sixth day is best used for a run—if you enjoy it and your goal isn't pure muscle gains—or a recovery session. You may do a very short ab finisher or 5-minute "trouble zone" bonus with a recovery session and SIT or power protocol. But if you push hard with the four lifts, you shouldn't want to do more.

With this progression, you will want to use the full-body or anterior/posterior prehab warm-ups as well as the suggested cooldowns.

Here, I give schedules for four to six days a week. Do *not* skip the recovery workouts! You can change the order of the workouts, but don't put two posterior or anterior days back to back. Repeat this progression using the same moves each week for three to six weeks before switching up the exercises or trying another workout design or split!

4 DAYS A WEEK	5 DAYS A WEEK	6 DAYS A WEEK
DAY 1	**DAY 1**	**DAY 1**
Posterior compound burner sets #1	Posterior compound burner sets #1	Posterior compound burner sets #1
DAY 2	**DAY 2**	**DAY 2**
Anterior compound burner sets #1	Anterior compound burner sets #1	Anterior compound burner sets #1
DAY 3	**DAY 3**	**DAY 3**
Off	Off	Recovery workout *or* Cardio
DAY 4	**DAY 4**	**DAY 4**
Posterior compound burner sets #2	Posterior compound burner sets #2	Posterior compound burner sets #2
DAY 5	**DAY 5**	**DAY 5**
Anterior compound burner sets #2	Anterior compound burner sets #2	Anterior compound burner sets #2
DAY 6	**DAY 6**	**DAY 6**
Off	Recovery workout	Recovery workout
DAY 7	**DAY 7**	**DAY 7**
Off	Off	Off

COMPOUND BURNER SETS
WORKOUT BUILDER

You can build out your own compound burner sets workouts from this template. The muscles targeted in the single heavy lift that starts the workout should only be worked again in 1 compound burner set. So, if you lift heavy for the upper body, only do upper body in 1 compound burner set while including 2 compound burner sets for your lower body.

MUSCLE FOCUSED: Focus on longer rest periods and going heavier, even if that means having to pause during the reps assigned to finish them as you go up in weight over the weeks. Exclude any SIT except on the recovery workout day. Walking is recommended.

FAT LOSS: Rest may be shorter, closer to just 90 seconds. Include SIT two or three days a week. Power work is not recommended for this progression. Keep long runs or rides to days between lifts while still making sure to have a day off each week. For a pure fat-loss focus, check out the Bonus Accelerate Fat Loss Builder options on page 246 with 4 compound burner sets and no lift.

BEGINNERS: Start with lower volume to let your connective tissues adjust and maintain proper form and recruitment patterns. Don't be afraid to start with just 2 rounds through each set and no primary lift. For more of a muscle-building focus, include the lift but just 2 compound burner sets.

I've included other training techniques in the bonus workouts on page 247 to give you options for this first lift, including 10-7-3-1, cluster sets, and drop sets.

**With any lift where you're getting under heavy loads, you want to do 2 or 3 warm-up sets first, building up with 50 percent (8 to 10 reps), 75 percent (6 to 8 reps), and 85 percent (4 to 6 reps) of your working weight. You may then increase after that first round. The heavier you go, the more you want to do those warm-up rounds before the sets.*

WARM-UP
Make sure to choose the warm-up that addresses the areas you plan to work.

LIFT: Upper or lower body
Complete 3 to 5 rounds, usually of 3 to 10 reps in that space that crosses between maximal strength and hypertrophy work. If this is an upper body move, include your lower body set next, or vice versa. Do both an upper and a lower for each split.*

- 3 to 10 reps **heavy big compound lift** (e.g., squats, deadlifts, bench presses, back rows)**
- 2 to 5 minutes **rest**

COMPOUND SET #1: Upper or lower body
Complete 2 to 4 rounds through the set, resting 90 seconds to 2 minutes between rounds and up to 2 minutes between sets.

- 6 to 12 reps **heavy compound lift**
- 15 to 25 reps **isolation exercise for muscle worked in compound lift**

COMPOUND SET #2: Upper or lower body
Complete 2 to 4 rounds through the set, resting 90 seconds to 2 minutes between rounds and up to 2 minutes between sets.

- 6 to 12 reps **heavy compound lift**
- 15 to 25 reps **isolation exercise for muscle worked in compound lift**

COMPOUND SET #3: Upper or lower body
Complete 2 to 4 rounds through the set, resting 90 seconds to 2 minutes between rounds.

- 6 to 12 reps **heavy compound lift**
- 15 to 25 reps **isolation exercise for muscle worked in compound lift**

Optional SIT

COOLDOWN

POSTERIOR COMPOUND BURNER SETS #1

WARM-UP

LIFT: CLUSTER SETS

Complete 3 to 5 working rounds. For each round, you will complete 6 to 10 reps of pull-ups. But those reps will be broken down into mini sets of just 2 or 3 reps with 15 to 30 seconds of rest between sets. This should allow you to use a harder, more advanced variation of the pull-up for the full 6 to 10 reps than you could without the mini breaks. This can also help you maintain better form while building up your pull-ups, whether you want to achieve your first full pull-up, do double digits, or even add weight! Rest 2 to 3 minutes after all 6 to 10 reps in that round are complete.

- 6 to 10 reps pull-ups*
- 2 to 3 minutes rest

COMPOUND SET #1

Complete 2 to 4 rounds through the set, resting 90 seconds to 2 minutes between rounds and up to 2 minutes between sets.

- 6 to 12 reps deadlifts**
- 15 to 25 reps glute bridge and curls

COMPOUND SET #2

Complete 2 to 4 rounds through the set, resting 90 seconds to 2 minutes between rounds and up to 2 minutes between sets.

- 6 to 12 reps underhand rows**
- 15 to 25 reps biceps curls

COMPOUND SET #3

Complete 2 to 4 rounds through the set, resting 90 seconds to 2 minutes between rounds.

- 6 to 12 reps (per side) side lunges**
- 15 to 25 reps (per side) cable abductions

Optional SIT

COOLDOWN

ANTERIOR COMPOUND BURNER SETS #1

WARM-UP

LIFT

Complete 3 to 5 rounds, resting 2 to 4 minutes between rounds. It's better to rest longer and keep the weight heavier or even go up as you work toward a 5-rep max. If you work with heavier weights and prefer a 5x5 design (5 rounds of 5 reps), consider resting the full 4 minutes.

- 5 to 10 reps back squats***
- 2 to 4 minutes rest

COMPOUND SET #1

Complete 2 to 4 rounds through the set, resting 90 seconds to 2 minutes between rounds and up to 2 minutes between sets.

- 6 to 12 reps overhead presses**
- 15 to 25 reps lateral raises

COMPOUND SET #2

Complete 2 to 4 rounds through the set, resting 90 seconds to 2 minutes between rounds and up to 2 minutes between sets.

6 to 12 reps (per side) deficit split squats**

15 to 25 reps (per side) cable seated quad extensions

COMPOUND SET #3

Complete 2 to 4 rounds through the set, resting 90 seconds to 2 minutes between rounds.

- 6 to 12 reps incline bench presses**
- 15 to 25 reps overhead triceps extensions

Optional SIT

COOLDOWN

*Perform the warm-up sets prior to your working rounds of the first lift. You may do weighted pull-ups or use assistance, using the warm-up rounds to find an appropriate weight.

**You may perform warm-up sets for each primary lift in the compound burner sets depending on the weights you're using.

***Perform the warm-up sets prior to your working rounds of the first lift.

POSTERIOR
COMPOUND BURNER SETS #2

WARM-UP

LIFT: 10-7-3-1
Complete 2 to 4 rounds through the 10-7-3-1 hip thrusts, resting 90 seconds to 2 minutes between rounds. Do not shorten the rest period between rounds; at the end of the rest, you should crave more of the lift. To do the 10-7-3-1, you will pick a weight that you max out on at about 10 to 12 reps. You will do 10 reps and rest 10 seconds, putting the weights down. Then do 7 reps and rest 7 seconds. Do 3 reps and rest 3 seconds. Then do 1 rep and completely rest before repeating the 21-rep series. Basically, you're performing 21 reps with a weight you can barely do for 10 reps! For the warm-up rounds, build up to a weight you can do 12 reps with to start your first working round.

- 10-7-3-1 hip **thrusts***
- 90 seconds to 2 minutes **rest**

COMPOUND SET #1
Complete 2 to 4 rounds through the set, resting 90 seconds to 2 minutes between rounds and up to 2 minutes between sets.

- 6 to 12 reps **pullovers****
- 15 to 25 reps **lat pushdowns**

COMPOUND SET #2
Complete 2 to 4 rounds through the set, resting 90 seconds to 2 minutes between rounds and up to 2 minutes between sets.

- 6 to 12 reps **Romanian deadlifts****
- 15 to 25 reps **hyperextensions**

COMPOUND SET #3
Complete 2 to 4 rounds through the set, resting 90 seconds to 2 minutes between rounds.

- 6 to 12 reps **overhand rows****
- 15 to 25 reps **back flys**

Optional SIT

COOLDOWN

ANTERIOR
COMPOUND BURNER SETS #2

WARM-UP

LIFT: DROP SETS
Do 3 to 5 rounds of bench presses. If you do 8 to 10 reps, complete 3 rounds plus the drop set, resting 90 seconds to 2 minutes between rounds. If you do 5 to 8 reps, consider 4 or 5 rounds plus the drop set, resting at least 2 minutes between rounds. On your final round, modify the move to complete 10 reps without resting after your first 5 to 10 reps. This may mean modifying a couple of times to hit 10 reps.

- 5 to 10 reps **bench presses*** + 1 drop set on the final set for 10 reps
- 90 seconds to 4 minutes **rest**

COMPOUND SET #1
Complete 2 to 4 rounds through the set, resting 90 seconds to 2 minutes between rounds and up to 2 minutes between sets.

- 6 to 12 reps (per side) **step-ups****
- 15 to 25 reps (per side) **cable lying quad extensions**

COMPOUND SET #2
Complete 2 to 4 rounds through the set, resting 90 seconds to 2 minutes between rounds and up to 2 minutes between sets.

- 6 to 12 reps **dips****
- 15 to 25 reps **chest flys**

COMPOUND SET #3
Complete 2 to 4 rounds through the set, resting 90 seconds to 2 minutes between rounds.

- 6 to 12 reps **front squats****
- 15 to 25 reps (per side) **cable adductions**

Optional SIT

COOLDOWN

Perform the warm-up sets prior to your working rounds of the first lift.

**You may perform warm-up sets for each primary lift in the compound burner sets depending on the weights you're using.*

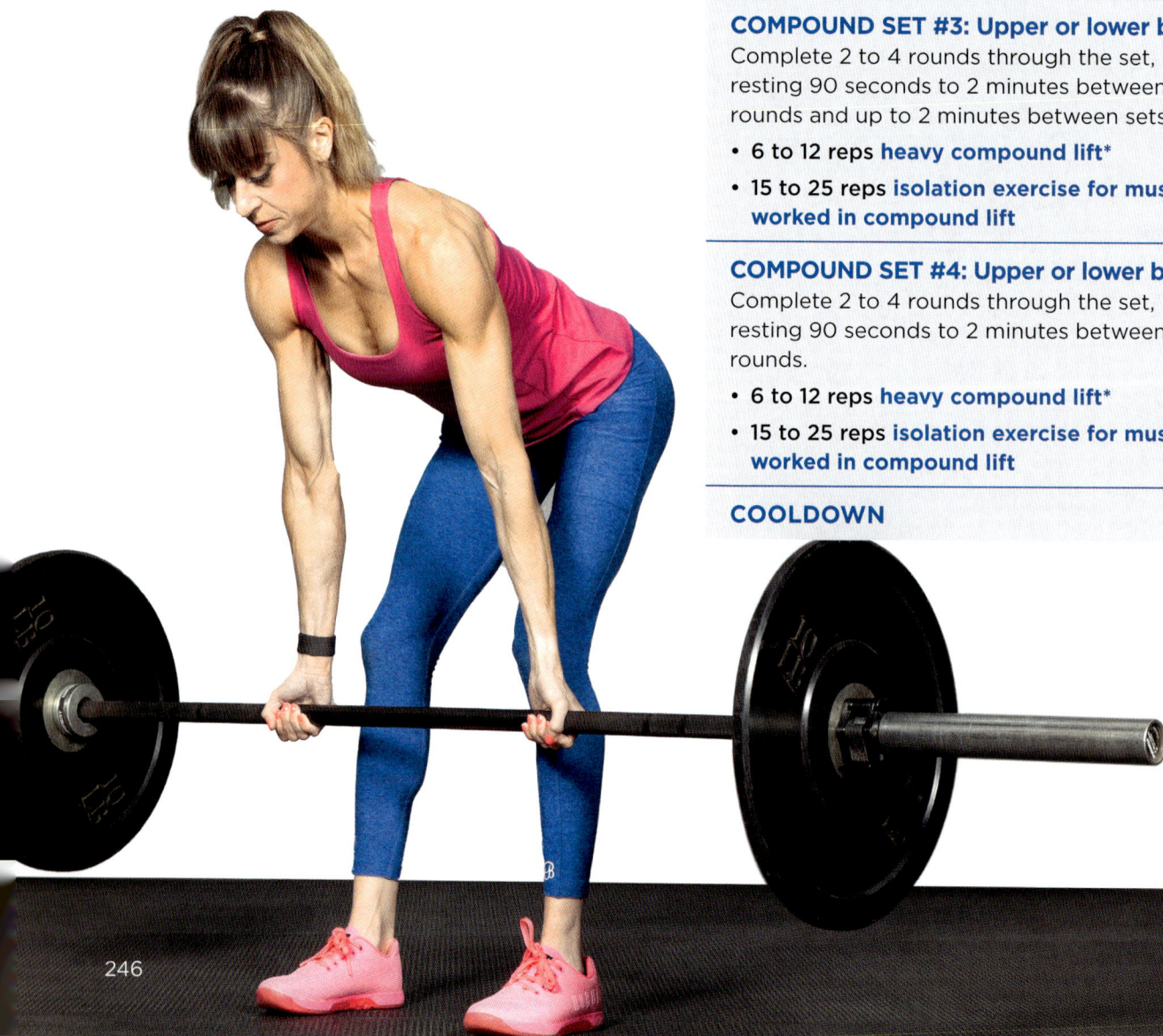

Use this template to build out your own compound burner sets workouts with an extra fat-loss focus. This is an extra intensive and long workout design. I recommend using this most often when you're lifting only four times a week and for no longer than a three- to four-week progression. Use it to push for recomp, focus on fat loss while still maintaining muscle in stubborn areas, or if you're an experienced trainee who's really struggling to move to the next level. Extra cardio is not recommended, especially on lifting days. Alternate the hemisphere worked for each compound set.

WARM-UP

Make sure to choose the warm-up that addresses the areas you plan to work.

COMPOUND SET #1: Upper or lower body

Complete 2 to 4 rounds through the set, resting 90 seconds to 2 minutes between rounds and up to 2 minutes between sets.

- **6 to 12 reps heavy compound lift***
- **15 to 25 reps isolation exercise for muscle worked in compound lift**

COMPOUND SET #2: Upper or lower body

Complete 2 to 4 rounds through the set, resting 90 seconds to 2 minutes between rounds and up to 2 minutes between sets.

- **6 to 12 reps heavy compound lift***
- **15 to 25 reps isolation exercise for muscle worked in compound lift**

COMPOUND SET #3: Upper or lower body

Complete 2 to 4 rounds through the set, resting 90 seconds to 2 minutes between rounds and up to 2 minutes between sets.

- **6 to 12 reps heavy compound lift***
- **15 to 25 reps isolation exercise for muscle worked in compound lift**

COMPOUND SET #4: Upper or lower body

Complete 2 to 4 rounds through the set, resting 90 seconds to 2 minutes between rounds.

- **6 to 12 reps heavy compound lift***
- **15 to 25 reps isolation exercise for muscle worked in compound lift**

COOLDOWN

POSTERIOR ACCELERATE COMPOUND BURNER SETS

BONUS

WARM-UP

COMPOUND SET #1
Complete 2 to 4 rounds through the set, resting 90 seconds to 2 minutes between rounds and up to 2 minutes between sets.

- **6 to 12 reps hip thrusts***
- **15 to 25 reps pull-throughs**

COMPOUND SET #2
Complete 2 to 4 rounds through the set, resting 90 seconds to 2 minutes between rounds and up to 2 minutes between sets.

- **6 to 12 reps lat pulldowns***
- **15 to 25 reps lat pushdowns**

COMPOUND SET #3
Complete 2 to 4 rounds through the set, resting 90 seconds to 2 minutes between rounds and up to 2 minutes between sets.

- **6 to 12 reps (per side) single-leg deadlifts***
- **15 to 25 reps (per side) cable seated hamstring curls**

COMPOUND SET #4
Complete 2 to 4 rounds through the set, resting 90 seconds to 2 minutes between rounds.

- **6 to 12 reps overhand rows***
- **15 to 25 reps back flys**

COOLDOWN

ANTERIOR ACCELERATE COMPOUND BURNER SETS

BONUS

WARM-UP

COMPOUND SET #1
Complete 2 to 4 rounds through the set, resting 90 seconds to 2 minutes between rounds and up to 2 minutes between sets.

- **6 to 12 reps bench presses***
- **15 to 25 reps push-ups**

COMPOUND SET #2
Complete 2 to 4 rounds through the set, resting 90 seconds to 2 minutes between rounds and up to 2 minutes between sets.

- **6 to 12 reps front squats***
- **15 to 25 reps pulse squats**

COMPOUND SET #3
Complete 2 to 4 rounds through the set, resting 90 seconds to 2 minutes between rounds and up to 2 minutes between sets.

- **6 to 12 reps overhead presses***
- **15 to 25 reps overhead triceps extensions**

COMPOUND SET #4
Complete 2 to 4 rounds through the set, resting 90 seconds to 2 minutes between rounds.

- **6 to 12 reps (per side) front lunges***
- **15 to 25 reps (per side) cable seated quad extensions**

COOLDOWN

*You may perform warm-up sets for each primary lift in the compound burner sets depending on the weights you're using.

21 THE COMPOUND BURNER SETS

HEMISPHERE PROGRESSION

This progression is best if you have five or six days to train. However, the workouts are shorter than the Compound Burner Sets Anterior/Posterior Progression in Chapter 20, making them good if you have less time each day. If you have only three days to train, check the Compound Burner Sets Full-Body Progression in Chapter 22. While you don't want to ignore the recovery work, sneaking in even a 5-minute session on those off days can create balance if you only have four days to train.

I've included bonus upper- and lower-focused workouts that you can include to start the week if you're going super heavy on the lift for maximal strength work. If you want to lift five days a week because you're focused on building muscle in a stubborn area, pick the bonus session that targets the hemisphere you want to focus on.

With this progression, you will want to use the upper and lower prehab warm-ups as well as the suggested cooldowns.

Here are schedules for five and six days a week. Do *not* skip the recovery workouts! You can change the order of these workouts, but do not put two lower or two upper workouts back to back without at least one rest day between. It's best to rest at least twenty-four hours between workouts for the same hemisphere. Repeat this progression using the same moves each week for three to six weeks before switching up the exercises or changing to another workout design or split!

5 DAYS A WEEK	6 DAYS A WEEK (upper body focused)	6 DAYS A WEEK (lower body focused)
DAY 1 Lower body compound burner sets #1	**DAY 1** Upper body compound burner sets bonus*	**DAY 1** Lower body compound burner sets bonus*
DAY 2 Upper body compound burner sets #1	**DAY 2** Lower body compound burner sets #1	**DAY 2** Upper body compound burner sets #1
DAY 3 Off	**DAY 3** Upper body compound burner sets #1	**DAY 3** Lower body compound burner sets #1
DAY 4 Lower body compound burner sets #2	**DAY 4** Lower body compound burner sets #2	**DAY 4** Upper body compound burner sets #2
DAY 5 Upper body compound burner sets #2	**DAY 5** Upper body compound burner sets #2	**DAY 5** Lower body compound burner sets #2
DAY 6 Recovery workout	**DAY 6** Recovery workout**	**DAY 6** Recovery workout**
DAY 7 Off	**DAY 7** Off	**DAY 7** Off

*This should be the bonus workout design, including the heavy lift to start the week.

**The recovery day could be the third day instead of the sixth day.

COMPOUND BURNER SETS
WORKOUT BUILDER

You can build out your own compound burner sets workouts from this template. Be sure to alternate the muscle groups worked over the compound burner sets; for example, you can do chest and triceps one set and then back and biceps the next, or you can do a lower body glute set followed by a lower body quad set.

MUSCLE FOCUSED: Focus on longer rest periods and going heavier, even if that means having to pause during the reps assigned to finish them as you go up in weight over the weeks. Exclude any SIT except on the recovery workout day, but you may include one or two power sessions. Walking is recommended.

FAT LOSS: Rest may be shorter, closer to just 90 seconds. Include SIT at the end of your workout two or three days a week, especially on days that hit your more stubborn areas. You can also do two SIT sessions and include one power session. If you're doing an endurance sport, include your longer distances on off days or on days when you don't work that hemisphere.

BEGINNERS: Start with lower volume to let your connective tissues adjust and maintain proper form and recruitment patterns. You may start with just 2 rounds through each set or even do just 2 compound burner sets.

SHORT ON TIME: If you're short on time and want to focus on strength, consider using the Bonus Short-on-Time Workout Builder on page 252 with 2 sets and a lift instead of the 3 compound burner sets!

WARM-UP
Make sure to choose the warm-up that addresses the areas you plan to work.

Optional POWER SESSION

COMPOUND SET #1
Complete 2 to 4 rounds through the set, resting 90 seconds to 2 minutes between rounds and up to 2 minutes between sets.
- 6 to 12 reps **heavy compound lift***
- 15 to 25 reps **isolation exercise for muscle worked in compound lift**

COMPOUND SET #2
Complete 2 to 4 rounds through the set, resting 90 seconds to 2 minutes between rounds and up to 2 minutes between sets.
- 6 to 12 reps **heavy compound lift***
- 15 to 25 reps **isolation exercise for muscle worked in compound lift**

COMPOUND SET #3
Complete 2 to 4 rounds through the set, resting 90 seconds to 2 minutes between rounds.
- 6 to 12 reps **heavy compound lift***
- 15 to 25 reps **isolation exercise for muscle worked in compound lift**

Optional SIT

COOLDOWN

*With any lift where you're getting under heavy loads, you want to do 2 or 3 warm-up sets first, building up with 50 percent (8 to 10 reps), 75 percent (6 to 8 reps), and 85 percent (4 to 6 reps) of your working weight. You may then increase after that first round. The heavier you go, the more you want to do those warm-up rounds before the sets.

LOWER BODY #1
COMPOUND BURNER SETS

WARM-UP

Optional **POWER SESSION**

COMPOUND SET #1
Complete 2 to 4 rounds through the set, resting 90 seconds to 2 minutes between rounds and up to 2 minutes between sets.

- 6 to 12 reps **back squats***
- 15 to 25 reps **kneeling lean backs**

COMPOUND SET #2
Complete 2 to 4 rounds through the set, resting 90 seconds to 2 minutes between rounds and up to 2 minutes between sets.

- 6 to 12 reps **Romanian deadlifts***
- 15 to 25 reps **glute bridge and curls**

COMPOUND SET #3
Complete 2 to 4 rounds through the set, resting 90 seconds to 2 minutes between rounds.

- 6 to 12 reps (per side) **curtsy lunges***
- 15 to 25 reps **weighted glute bridges**

Optional **SIT**

COOLDOWN

UPPER BODY #1
COMPOUND BURNER SETS

WARM-UP

Optional **POWER SESSION**

COMPOUND SET #1
Complete 2 to 4 rounds through the set, resting 90 seconds to 2 minutes between rounds and up to 2 minutes between sets.

- 6 to 12 reps **lat pulldowns***
- 15 to 25 reps **lat pushdowns**

COMPOUND SET #2
Complete 2 to 4 rounds through the set, resting 90 seconds to 2 minutes between rounds and up to 2 minutes between sets.

- 6 to 12 reps **bench presses***
- 15 to 25 reps **triceps pushdowns**

COMPOUND SET #3
Complete 2 to 4 rounds through the set, resting 90 seconds to 2 minutes between rounds.

- 6 to 12 reps **chest-supported rows***
- 15 to 25 reps **back flys**

Optional **SIT**

COOLDOWN

LOWER BODY #2
COMPOUND BURNER SETS

WARM-UP

Optional **POWER SESSION**

COMPOUND SET #1
Complete 2 to 4 rounds through the set, resting 90 seconds to 2 minutes between rounds and up to 2 minutes between sets.

- 6 to 12 reps **hip thrusts***
- 15 to 25 reps **pull-throughs**

COMPOUND SET #2
Complete 2 to 4 rounds through the set, resting 90 seconds to 2 minutes between rounds and up to 2 minutes between sets.

- 6 to 12 reps (per side) **step-ups***
- 15 to 25 reps (per side) **cable lying quad extensions**

COMPOUND SET #3
Complete 2 to 4 rounds through the set, resting 90 seconds to 2 minutes between rounds.

- 6 to 12 reps (per side) **single-leg deadlifts***
- 15 to 25 reps (per side) **cable seated hamstring curls**

Optional **SIT**

COOLDOWN

You may perform warm-up sets for each primary lift in the compound burner sets depending on the weights you're using.

UPPER BODY COMPOUND BURNER SETS #2

WARM-UP

Optional POWER SESSION

COMPOUND SET #1

Complete 2 to 4 rounds through the set, resting 90 seconds to 2 minutes between rounds and up to 2 minutes between sets.

- 6 to 12 reps **incline bench presses***
- 15 to 25 reps **chest press to skull crushers**

COMPOUND SET #2

Complete 2 to 4 rounds through the set, resting 90 seconds to 2 minutes between rounds and up to 2 minutes between sets.

- 6 to 12 reps **underhand rows***
- 15 to 25 reps **biceps curls**

COMPOUND SET #3

Complete 2 to 4 rounds through the set, resting 90 seconds to 2 minutes between rounds.

- 6 to 12 reps **pullovers***
- 15 to 25 reps **decline push-ups**

Optional SIT

COOLDOWN

LOWER BODY COMPOUND BURNER SETS **[BONUS]**

WARM-UP

Optional POWER SESSION

LIFT

Complete 3 to 5 rounds, resting 2 to 4 minutes between rounds. It is better to rest longer and keep the weight heavier or even go up as you work toward that 5-rep max. If you work with heavier weights and prefer a 5x5 design (5 rounds of 5 reps), consider resting the full 4 minutes.

- 5 to 10 reps **deadlifts****
- 2 to 4 minutes **rest**

COMPOUND SET #1

Complete 2 to 4 rounds through the set, resting 90 seconds to 2 minutes between rounds and up to 2 minutes between sets.

- 6 to 12 reps (per side) **front lunges*****
- 15 to 25 reps (per side) **cable seated quad extensions**

COMPOUND SET #2

Complete 2 to 4 rounds through the set, resting 90 seconds to 2 minutes between rounds.

- 6 to 12 reps (per side) **reverse lunges*****
- 15 to 25 reps (per side) **cable abductions**

Optional SIT

COOLDOWN

UPPER BODY COMPOUND BURNER SETS **[BONUS]**

WARM-UP

Optional POWER SESSION

LIFT: Drop sets

Do 3 to 5 rounds of overhead presses. If you do 8 to 10 reps, complete 3 rounds plus the drop set, resting 90 seconds to 2 minutes between rounds. If you do 5 to 8 reps, consider 4 or 5 rounds plus the drop set, resting at least 2 minutes between rounds. On your final round, modify the move to complete 10 reps without resting after your first 5 to 10 reps. This may mean modifying a couple of times to hit 10 reps.

- 5 to 10 reps **overhead presses**** + 1 drop set on the final set for 10 reps
- 90 seconds to 4 minutes **rest**

COMPOUND SET #1

Complete 2 to 4 rounds through the set, resting 90 seconds to 2 minutes between rounds and up to 2 minutes between sets.

- 6 to 12 reps **overhand rows*****
- 15 to 25 reps **back shrugs**

COMPOUND SET #2

Complete 2 to 4 rounds through the set, resting 90 seconds to 2 minutes between rounds.

- 6 to 12 reps **chest flys*****
- 15 to 25 reps **push-ups**

Optional SIT

COOLDOWN

---

*You may perform warm-up sets for each primary lift in the compound burner sets depending on the weights you're using.

**With any lift where you're getting under heavy loads, you want to do 2 or 3 warm-up sets first, building up with 50 percent (8 to 10 reps), 75 percent (6 to 8 reps), and 85 percent (4 to 6 reps) of your working weight. You may then increase after that first round. The heavier you go, the more you want to do those warm-up rounds before the sets.

***You may perform warm-up sets for each primary lift in the compound burner sets depending on the weights you're using.

Use this template to build out your own compound burner sets workouts that are great if you want to train six days a week but are more limited on time per day. Use this to push for recomp and especially to focus on gaining strength. If the lift is more posterior chain, I recommend targeting the posterior chain more in the second compound burner set while targeting the anterior chain in the first set.

WARM-UP

Make sure to choose the warm-up that addresses the areas you plan to work.

Optional POWER SESSION

LIFT

Complete 3 to 5 rounds, usually of 3 to 10 reps in that space that crosses between maximal strength and hypertrophy work. If this is an upper body move, include an upper body move for the opposing muscle group in the next set. For example, if you do bench presses, work your back in the first compound set.*

- 3 to 10 reps **heavy big compound lift (e.g., squats, deadlifts, bench presses, back rows)**

- 2 to 5 minutes **rest**

COMPOUND SET #1

Complete 2 to 4 rounds through the set, resting 90 seconds to 2 minutes between rounds and up to 2 minutes between sets.

- 6 to 12 reps **heavy compound lift*****
- 15 to 25 reps **isolation exercise for muscle worked in compound lift**

COMPOUND SET #2

Complete 2 to 4 rounds through the set, resting 90 seconds to 2 minutes between rounds.

- 6 to 12 reps **heavy compound lift*****
- 15 to 25 reps **isolation exercise for muscle worked in compound lift**

Optional SIT

COOLDOWN

---

*I've included other training techniques in the bonus workouts on pages 244 and 245 to give you options for this first lift, including 10-7-3-1, cluster sets, and drop sets.

**With any lift where you're getting under heavy loads, you want to do 2 or 3 warm-up sets first, building up with 50 percent (8 to 10 reps), 75 percent (6 to 8 reps), and 85 percent (4 to 6 reps) of your working weight. You may then increase after that first round. The heavier you go, the more you want to do those warm-up rounds before the sets.

***You may perform warm-up sets for each primary lift in the compound burner sets depending on the weights you're using.

22 THE COMPOUND BURNER SETS
FULL-BODY PROGRESSION

This progression is best if you have three or four days to train. While you don't want to ignore the recovery work, sneaking in even a 5-minute session on those off days can create balance if you are limited to three workout days.

This three-day schedule can be amazing if you're trying to maintain strength and muscle while logging more miles. It's also a great option if you're starting back to training and want to maintain the quality of your workouts with slightly lower volume that is spread out over the week.

With this progression, you'll want to use the full-body or anterior/posterior prehab warm-ups as well as the suggested cooldowns.

You can change the order of the workouts, but give yourself a day of rest between each session. Repeat this progression using the same moves each week for three to six weeks before switching up the exercises or changing to another workout design or split!

3

DAY 1
Full-body compound burner sets #1

DAY 2
Off

DAY 3
Full-body compound burner sets #2

DAY 4
Off

DAY 5
Full-body compound burner sets #3

DAY 6
Recovery workout

DAY 7
Off

COMPOUND BURNER SETS
WORKOUT BUILDER

You can build out your own compound burner sets workouts based on this template. Each compound set will focus on a different area of the body or muscle group. I recommend alternating which you put first or prioritizing the area you most want to build so you will be freshest for that set.

MUSCLE FOCUSED: Focus on longer rest periods and going heavier, even if that means having to pause during the reps assigned to finish them as you go up in weight over the weeks. Exclude any SIT except on the recovery workout day, but walking is recommended. You may include one or two power sessions. If you're a more advanced trainee looking to build muscle, the anterior/posterior and hemisphere progressions (see pages 242 and 248) are recommended if your schedule allows.

FAT LOSS: Rest may be shorter, closer to just 90 seconds. Include SIT two or three days a week or one or two SIT sessions and one power session. Keep long runs or rides to one or two days between lifts and make sure to still have a day off.

BEGINNERS: Start with lower volume to let your connective tissues adjust and maintain proper form and recruitment patterns. Don't be afraid to start with just 2 rounds through each set.

WARM-UP
Make sure to choose the warm-up that addresses the areas you plan to work.

Optional POWER SESSION

COMPOUND SET #1
Complete 2 to 4 rounds through the set, resting 90 seconds to 2 minutes between rounds and up to 2 minutes between sets.
- 6 to 12 reps **heavy compound lift***
- 15 to 25 reps **isolation exercise for muscle worked in compound lift**

COMPOUND SET #2
Complete 2 to 4 rounds through the set, resting 90 seconds to 2 minutes between rounds and up to 2 minutes between sets.
- 6 to 12 reps **heavy compound lift***
- 15 to 25 reps **isolation exercise for muscle worked in compound lift**

COMPOUND SET #3
Complete 2 to 4 rounds through the set, resting 90 seconds to 2 minutes between rounds.
- 6 to 12 reps **heavy compound lift***
- 15 to 25 reps **isolation exercise for muscle worked in compound lift**

Optional SIT

COOLDOWN

*With any lift where you're getting under heavy loads, you want to do 2 or 3 warm-up sets first, building up with 50 percent (8 to 10 reps), 75 percent (6 to 8 reps), and 85 percent (4 to 6 reps) of your working weight. You may increase after that first round. The heavier you go, the more you want to do those warm-up rounds before the sets.

FULL-BODY COMPOUND BURNER SETS #1

WARM-UP

Optional **POWER SESSION**

COMPOUND SET #1
Complete 2 to 4 rounds through the set, resting 90 seconds to 2 minutes between rounds and up to 2 minutes between sets.

- 6 to 12 reps **deadlifts***
- 15 to 25 reps (per side) **cable lying hamstring curls**

COMPOUND SET #2
Complete 2 to 4 rounds through the set, resting 90 seconds to 2 minutes between rounds and up to 2 minutes between sets.

- 6 to 12 reps **bench presses***
- 15 to 25 reps **chest flys**

COMPOUND SET #3
Complete 2 to 4 rounds through the set, resting 90 seconds to 2 minutes between rounds.

- 6 to 12 reps **overhand rows***
- 15 to 25 reps **back shrugs**

Optional **SIT**

COOLDOWN

FULL-BODY COMPOUND BURNER SETS #2

WARM-UP

Optional **POWER SESSION**

COMPOUND SET #1
Complete 2 to 4 rounds through the set, resting 90 seconds to 2 minutes between rounds and up to 2 minutes between sets.

- 6 to 12 reps **lat pulldowns***
- 15 to 25 reps **lat pushdowns**

COMPOUND SET #2
Complete 2 to 4 rounds through the set, resting 90 seconds to 2 minutes between rounds and up to 2 minutes between sets.

- 6 to 12 reps **back squats***
- 15 to 25 reps (per side) **cable seated quad extensions**

COMPOUND SET #3
Complete 2 to 4 rounds through the set, resting 90 seconds to 2 minutes between rounds.

- 6 to 12 reps **overhead presses***
- 15 to 25 reps **lateral raises**

Optional **SIT**

COOLDOWN

FULL-BODY COMPOUND BURNER SETS #3

WARM-UP

Optional **POWER SESSION**

COMPOUND SET #1
Complete 2 to 4 rounds through the set, resting 90 seconds to 2 minutes between rounds and up to 2 minutes between sets.

- 6 to 12 reps **incline bench presses***
- 15 to 25 reps **triceps pushdowns**

COMPOUND SET #2
Complete 2 to 4 rounds through the set, resting 90 seconds to 2 minutes between rounds and up to 2 minutes between sets.

- 6 to 12 reps **underhand rows***
- 15 to 25 reps **biceps curls**

COMPOUND SET #3
Complete 2 to 4 rounds through the set, resting 90 seconds to 2 minutes between rounds.

- 6 to 12 reps **hip thrusts***
- 15 to 25 reps **pull-throughs**

Optional **SIT**

COOLDOWN

You may perform warm-up sets for each primary lift in the compound burner sets depending on the weights you're using.

23 THE TIMED STRENGTH WORK

ANTERIOR/POSTERIOR PROGRESSION

This progression uses all three timed strength work techniques to help you achieve amazing results while training four to six times a week. If you're limited to three days, use the full-body progression (see page 253). If you have four days, it may be ideal to use the full-body progression with a recovery day! The six-day schedule is a great fat-loss accelerator schedule. If your goal is muscle gains, you may want to use a recovery workout on Day 3 instead or do a non-sweat variation of density sets. For this progression, I included both strength-focused density sets and a sweat variation that includes HIIT and is great for fat loss.

Workouts in this progression are bodyweight based and use sliders or towels, but you can check out the Exercise Library that begins on page 301 to swap for other tools you have at home.

4 DAYS A WEEK	5 DAYS A WEEK	6 DAYS A WEEK (muscle focused)	6 DAYS A WEEK (fat-loss accelerator)
DAY 1	**DAY 1**	**DAY 1**	**DAY 1**
Anterior strength intervals supersets	Anterior strength intervals supersets	Posterior strength intervals trisets	Anterior strength intervals supersets
DAY 2	**DAY 2**	**DAY 2**	**DAY 2**
Posterior strength intervals trisets	Posterior strength intervals trisets	Anterior strength intervals supersets	Posterior strength intervals trisets
DAY 3	**DAY 3**	**DAY 3**	**DAY 3**
Off	Off	Posterior density sets*	Anterior density intervals*
DAY 4	**DAY 4**	**DAY 4**	**DAY 4**
Anterior density intervals	Anterior density intervals	Anterior density intervals	Posterior density sets
DAY 5	**DAY 5**	**DAY 5**	**DAY 5**
Posterior density sets	Posterior density sets	Posterior density intervals	Density sets + sweat
DAY 6	**DAY 6**	**DAY 6**	**DAY 6**
Off	Recovery workout	Recovery workout	Recovery workout
DAY 7	**DAY 7**	**DAY 7**	**DAY 7**
Off	Off	Off	Off

* If your goal is muscle gains, you may want to use a recovery workout on Day 3 instead or do a non-sweat variation of density sets.

With this progression, you will want to use the full-body or anterior/posterior prehab warm-ups as well as the suggested cooldowns. You can even use the quick prehab options if you're really looking to keep your workouts short!

You can change the order of the workouts, but give yourself a day of rest between each session that works the same areas. Repeat this progression using the same moves each week for three to six weeks before switching up the exercises or trying another workout design or split.

STRENGTH INTERVALS SUPERSETS
WORKOUT BUILDER

You can build out your own strength intervals supersets workouts based on this template. Alternate the areas or hemispheres worked in each superset.

MUSCLE FOCUSED: Focus on pausing during intervals of work rather than being able to bust out reps quickly for the entire interval. Do not include SIT or steady-state cardio, especially if you're limited to bodyweight or very light resistance tools.

FAT LOSS: Don't let this strength work become cardio. Use variations and forms of progression like tempo or the tools you have to create pauses during intervals of work. Include SIT one or two days a week. Endurance training is best only with three or four days of training.

BEGINNERS: Start with lower volume to let your connective tissues adjust and maintain proper form and recruitment patterns. Don't be afraid to start with shorter intervals of work (even 20 seconds, if needed) or fewer rounds and supersets (2 or 3).

WARM-UP
Make sure to choose the warm-up that addresses the areas you plan to work.

SUPERSET #1: Upper or lower body
Complete 3 to 6 rounds through the superset, resting 30 seconds to 1 minute between rounds and up to 90 seconds between supersets.

- **30 seconds to 1 minute compound exercise**
- **30 seconds to 1 minute compound exercise for different muscle group**

SUPERSET #2: Upper or lower body
Complete 3 to 6 rounds through the superset, resting 30 seconds to 1 minute between rounds and up to 90 seconds between supersets.

- **30 seconds to 1 minute compound exercise**
- **30 seconds to 1 minute compound exercise for different muscle group**

SUPERSET #3: Upper or lower body
Complete 3 to 6 rounds through the superset, resting 30 seconds to 1 minute between rounds and up to 90 seconds between supersets.

- **30 seconds to 1 minute compound exercise**
- **30 seconds to 1 minute compound exercise for different muscle group**

SUPERSET #4: Upper or lower body
Complete 3 to 6 rounds through the superset, resting 30 seconds to 1 minute between rounds.

- **30 seconds to 1 minute compound exercise**
- **30 seconds to 1 minute compound exercise for different muscle group**

Optional SIT

COOLDOWN

STRENGTH INTERVALS TRISETS
WORKOUT BUILDER

You can build out your own strength intervals trisets workouts based on this template. Alternate the areas or hemispheres worked in each triset. These are great for getting in extra core work!

MUSCLE FOCUSED: Focus on pausing during intervals of work rather than being able to bust out reps quickly for the entire interval. Do not include SIT or steady-state cardio, especially if you are limited to bodyweight or very light resistance tools.

FAT LOSS: Don't let this strength work become cardio. Use variations and forms of progression like tempo or the tools you have to create pauses during intervals of work. Include SIT one or two days a week. Endurance training is best only with three or four days of training.

BEGINNERS: Start with lower volume to let your connective tissues adjust and maintain proper form and recruitment patterns. Don't be afraid to start with shorter intervals of work (even 20 seconds, if needed) or fewer rounds and trisets (2 or 3).

WARM-UP
Make sure to choose the warm-up that addresses the areas you plan to work.

TRISET #1: Upper or lower body
Complete 2 to 5 rounds through the triset, resting 30 seconds to 1 minute between rounds and up to 90 seconds between trisets. You may find you can cut the rest period between rounds by using a core exercise as active rest during the third move. However, if you work the same area as the first move, the full rest period is ideal.

- 30 seconds to 1 minute **compound exercise**
- 30 seconds to 1 minute **compound exercise for different muscle group**
- 30 seconds to 1 minute **compound exercise for different muscle group**

TRISET #2: UPPER OR LOWER BODY
Complete 2 to 5 rounds through the triset, resting 30 seconds to 1 minute between rounds and up to 90 seconds between trisets.

- 30 seconds to 1 minute **compound exercise**
- 30 seconds to 1 minute **compound exercise for different muscle group**
- 30 seconds to 1 minute **compound exercise for different muscle group**

TRISET #3: UPPER OR LOWER BODY
Complete 2 to 5 rounds through the triset, resting 30 seconds to 1 minute between rounds.

- 30 seconds to 1 minute **compound exercise**
- 30 seconds to 1 minute **compound exercise for different muscle group**
- 30 seconds to 1 minute **compound exercise for different muscle group**

Optional SIT

COOLDOWN

DENSITY INTERVALS WORKOUT BUILDER

You can build out your own density intervals workouts for an anterior/posterior focus based on this template. Each set will have two or three intervals of work focused on one area of the body. Alternate the areas or hemispheres worked in each set.

MUSCLE FOCUSED: Focus on pausing during intervals of work rather than being able to bust out reps quickly for the entire interval. Do not include SIT or steady-state cardio. It may be key to include isolation moves, or even holds, to target stubborn areas.

FAT LOSS: Don't let this strength work become cardio. Use variations and forms of progression like tempo or the tools you have to create pauses during intervals of work. Include SIT one or two days a week. Endurance training is best only with three or four days of training.

BEGINNERS: Start with lower volume to let your connective tissues adjust and maintain proper form and recruitment patterns. Don't be afraid to start with just 2 rounds through each set. You may also focus more on compound burner sets (see page 241) rather than trisets.

WARM-UP
Make sure to choose the warm-up that addresses the areas you plan to work.

SET #1: Upper or lower body
Complete 2 to 6 rounds through the set, resting up to 90 seconds between sets.
- 20 seconds to 1 minute **compound exercise**
- 20 seconds to 1 minute **compound or isolation exercise** to target same muscle group
- 20 seconds to 1 minute **compound or isolation exercise** to target same muscle group (optional)
- 20 seconds to 1 minute **rest**

SET #2: Upper or lower body
Complete 2 to 6 rounds through the set, resting up to 90 seconds between sets.
- 20 seconds to 1 minute **compound exercise**
- 20 seconds to 1 minute **compound or isolation exercise** to target same muscle group
- 20 seconds to 1 minute **compound or isolation exercise to target same muscle group** (optional)
- 20 seconds to 1 minute **rest**

SET #3: Upper or lower body
Complete 2 to 6 rounds through the set, resting up to 90 seconds between sets.
- 20 seconds to 1 minute **compound exercise**
- 20 seconds to 1 minute **compound or isolation exercise to target same muscle group**
- 20 seconds to 1 minute **compound or isolation exercise to target same muscle group** (optional)
- 20 seconds to 1 minute **rest**

SET #4: Upper or lower body
Complete 2 to 6 rounds through the set.
- 20 seconds to 1 minute **compound exercise**
- 20 seconds to 1 minute **compound or isolation exercise** to target same muscle group
- 20 seconds to 1 minute **compound or isolation exercise to target same muscle group** (optional)
- 20 seconds to 1 minute **rest**

Optional SIT

COOLDOWN

DENSITY SETS WORKOUT BUILDER

You can build out your own density sets workouts based on this template. This variation is best for home workouts. Alternate the areas or hemispheres worked in each density set to reduce rest time.

MUSCLE FOCUSED: Focus on doing fewer reps and maintaining more advanced variations of the moves over the course of the set, even if it means performing fewer than 5 reps. Do not include SIT or steady-state cardio, especially if you're limited to bodyweight or very light resistance tools.

FAT LOSS: Work down in reps, pushing the variations to create progressive overload. Include SIT one or two days a week. Keep long runs or rides to one or two days between lifts and make sure to still have a day off. If you aren't including any bonus SIT sessions or long runs or rides, you may consider including the accelerate fat loss option for a bonus HIIT session (see page 246).

BEGINNERS: Start with lower volume to let your connective tissues adjust and maintain proper form and recruitment patterns. Don't be afraid to start with just 1 density set if needed.

NOTE: *With all bodyweight moves, you may do up to 15 reps, as needed.*

WARM-UP
Make sure to choose the warm-up that addresses the areas you plan to work.

DENSITY SET #1: Upper or lower body
Complete as many rounds of the set as you can, challenging yourself and resting as little as possible between rounds. It's better to lower the number of reps per move or—if you really need to—modify a move rather than rest. Set your timer to work for 5 to 15 minutes.* Rest 1 to 2 minutes between sets.

- 5 to 10 reps **compound exercise**
- 5 to 10 reps **compound exercise for different muscle group**
- 5 to 10 reps **compound exercise for different muscle group** (optional)

DENSITY SET #2: Upper or lower body
Complete as many rounds of the set as you can, challenging yourself and resting as little as possible between rounds. Set your timer to work for 5 to 15 minutes. Rest 1 to 2 minutes between sets.

- 5 to 10 reps **compound exercise**
- 5 to 10 reps **compound exercise for different muscle group**
- 5 to 10 reps **compound exercise for different muscle group** (optional)

DENSITY SET #3: Upper or lower body
Complete as many rounds of the set as you can, challenging yourself and resting as little as possible between rounds. Set your timer to work for 5 to 15 minutes.

- 5 to 10 reps **compound exercise**
- 5 to 10 reps **compound exercise for different muscle group**
- 5 to 10 reps **compound exercise for different muscle group** (optional)

Optional SIT

COOLDOWN

If you do 10 to 15 minutes per set, you will want to do only 2 or 3 density sets. You may do less than 10 minutes and include up to 4 or 5 sets, but then SIT is not recommended, even for fat loss.

DENSITY SETS + SWEAT WORKOUT BUILDER

You can build out your own density sets workouts with HIIT based on this template. This variation is best for home workouts. Alternate the areas or hemispheres worked in each density set to reduce rest time.

MUSCLE FOCUSED: Unless this is absolutely your only cardio, this version isn't recommended when you're focused on muscle-building, especially if you aren't training with more tools at the gym.

FAT LOSS: Work down in reps, pushing the variations to create progressive overload, especially with the first 2 density sets. In the third set, your goal is conditioning, so you want to move quickly to get your blood pumping. Additional SIT is not recommended on this day, and this option is best when you're not really logging a ton of extra miles.

BEGINNERS: Start with lower volume to let your connective tissues adjust and maintain proper form and recruitment patterns. It may also be better to start with the basic density sets on page 260 rather than this layout. If you want to start back with HIIT, include exercises that match your fitness level and consider doing just 2 density sets for 8 to 10 minutes or a shorter HIIT set for 5 minutes.

WARM-UP
Make sure to choose the warm-up that addresses the areas you plan to work.

DENSITY SET #1: Upper or lower body
Complete as many rounds of the set as you can, challenging yourself and resting as little as possible between rounds. It's better to lower the number of reps per move or—if you really need to—modify a move rather than rest. Set your timer to work for 8 to 15 minutes. Rest 1 to 2 minutes between sets.

- 5 to 10 reps **compound exercise**
- 5 to 10 reps **compound exercise for different muscle group**
- 5 to 10 reps **compound exercise for different muscle group** (optional)

DENSITY SET #2: Upper or lower body
Complete as many rounds of the set as you can, challenging yourself and resting as little as possible between rounds. Set your timer to work for 8 to 15 minutes. Rest 1 to 2 minutes between sets.

- 5 to 10 reps **compound exercise**
- 5 to 10 reps **compound exercise for different muscle group**
- 5 to 10 reps **compound exercise for different muscle group** (optional)

DENSITY SET #3/AMRAP: Upper or lower body
Complete as many rounds of the set as you can, challenging yourself and resting as little as possible between rounds. Set your timer to work for 8 to 15 minutes.

- 5 to 15 reps **compound exercise**
- 5 to 15 reps **compound exercise for different muscle group**
- 5 to 15 reps **compound exercise for different muscle group**
- 5 to 15 reps **compound exercise for different muscle group** (optional)*

COOLDOWN

Three moves are recommended for the third set, although four can also work well. For the HIIT density set, you may perform higher reps of the cardio exercises.

ANTERIOR
STRENGTH INTERVALS SUPERSETS

WARM-UP

SUPERSET #1

Complete 3 to 5 rounds through the superset, resting 30 seconds to 1 minute between rounds and up to 1 minute between supersets.

- 1 minute **get-up lunges**
- 1 minute **push-ups***

SUPERSET #2

Complete 3 to 5 rounds through the superset, resting 30 seconds to 1 minute between rounds and up to 1 minute between supersets.

- 1 minute **alternating front-angled lunges**
- 1 minute **wide-grip push-ups**

SUPERSET #3

Complete 3 to 5 rounds through the superset, resting 30 seconds to 1 minute between rounds and up to 1 minute between supersets.

- 1 minute **alternating step-ups**
- 1 minute **plank with shoulder taps**

SUPERSET #4: AB BURNER

Complete 1 to 3 rounds through the superset, resting 30 seconds to 1 minute between rounds.

- 1 minute **slider plank jacks**
- 1 minute **lying knees**

Optional SIT

COOLDOWN

POSTERIOR
STRENGTH INTERVALS TRISETS

WARM-UP

TRISET #1

Complete 3 to 5 rounds through the triset, resting 30 seconds between rounds and up to 1 minute between trisets.

- 30 seconds (per side) **airborne lunges**
- 30 seconds **doorway rows**
- 30 seconds **glute bridges and curls**

TRISET #2

Complete 3 to 5 rounds through the triset, resting 30 seconds between rounds and up to 1 minute between trisets.

- 30 seconds **alternating curtsy lunges**
- 30 seconds (per side) **lying side slides**
- 30 seconds **posterior plank**

TRISET #3

Complete 3 to 5 rounds through the triset, resting 30 seconds between rounds.

- 30 seconds (per side) **single-leg hip thrusts**
- 30 seconds **lying scapular presses**
- 30 seconds **slider ab extensions**

Optional SIT

COOLDOWN

During the 1 minute of work, do a push-up variation you have to take breaks with. If you can't perform another rep with good form after pausing a few seconds, modify to do push-ups on an incline or your knees.

ANTERIOR
DENSITY INTERVALS

SET #1

Complete 2 to 4 rounds through the set, resting 40 seconds to 1 minute between sets. Do not cut out rest. To make this set harder, do all three moves on one side, then switch, resting no more than 20 seconds between rounds. One side will get some rest as the other works!

- 20 seconds (per side) front lunges
- 20 seconds (per side) split squats
- 20 seconds (per side) standing quad kickouts
- 40 seconds to 1 minute rest

SET #2

Complete 2 to 4 rounds through the set, resting 40 seconds to 1 minute between sets. Do not cut out rest.

- 20 seconds close-grip push-ups
- 20 seconds bench dips
- 20 seconds body saws
- 40 seconds to 1 minute rest

SET #3

Complete 2 to 4 rounds through the set, resting 40 seconds to 1 minute between sets. Do not cut out rest.

- 20 seconds sumo squats
- 20 seconds pulse sumo squats
- 20 seconds kneeling adductor slides
- 40 seconds to 1 minute rest

SET #4

Complete 2 to 4 rounds through the set. Do not cut out rest.

- 20 seconds pike push-ups
- 20 seconds plank with two-way taps
- 20 seconds T sit-ups
- 40 seconds to 1 minute rest

Optional SIT

COOLDOWN

POSTERIOR
DENSITY SETS

WARM-UP

DENSITY SET #1

Complete as many rounds of the set as you can, challenging yourself and resting as little as possible between rounds. It's better to lower the number of reps per move or—if you really need to—modify a move rather than rest. Set your timer to work for 10 minutes. Rest 1 to 2 minutes between sets.

- 5 to 10 reps (per side) balance lunges
- 5 to 10 reps (per side) single-arm doorway rows
- 5 to 10 reps glute bridges to sit-ups

DENSITY SET #2

Complete as many rounds of the set as you can, challenging yourself and resting as little as possible between rounds. Set your timer to work for 10 minutes. Rest 1 to 2 minutes between sets.

- 5 to 10 reps (per side) side-to-curtsy lunges
- 5 to 10 reps band/towel pulldowns*
- 5 to 10 reps (per side) alternating-arm plank rows

DENSITY SET #3

Complete as many rounds of the set as you can, challenging yourself and resting as little as possible between rounds. Set your timer to work for 10 minutes.

- 5 to 10 reps (per side) alternating slider reverse lunges
- 5 to 10 reps scapular wall reps*
- 5 to 10 reps (per side) side plank hip dips with rotational reach

Optional SIT

COOLDOWN

NOTE: *Beginners can start with just 2 sets.*

With moves like the pulldowns or scapular wall reps, if you don't have added weights or resistance and 10 in a row becomes easily doable, increase the reps to 15.

POSTERIOR
DENSITY INTERVALS

WARM-UP

SET #1

Complete 2 to 4 rounds through the set, resting 30 seconds between sets. Do not cut out rest. To make this set harder, do all three moves on one side, then switch, resting no more than 20 seconds between rounds. One side will get some rest as the other works!

- 30 seconds (per side) **single-leg deadlift holds**
- 30 seconds (per side) **single-leg deadlifts**
- 30 seconds (per side) **single-leg deadlift squats**
- 30 seconds **rest**

SET #2

Complete 2 to 4 rounds through the set, resting 30 seconds between sets. Do not cut out rest.

- 30 seconds **scapular wall holds**
- 30 seconds **doorway rows**
- 30 seconds **lying scapular presses**
- 30 seconds **rest**

SET #3

Complete 2 to 4 rounds through the set, resting 30 seconds between sets. Do not cut out rest. To make this set harder, do all three moves on one side, then switch, resting no more than 20 seconds between rounds. One side will get some rest as the other works!

- 30 seconds (per side) **side lunge holds**
- 30 seconds (per side) **side lunges**
- 30 seconds (per side) **fire hydrants**
- 30 seconds **rest**

SET #4

Complete 2 to 4 rounds through the set. Do not cut out rest.

- 30 seconds **extended plank holds**
- 30 seconds **slider ab extensions**
- 30 seconds **lying W pulldowns**
- 30 seconds **rest**

Optional SIT

COOLDOWN

NOTE: *Beginners can start with just 2 sets.*

DENSITY SETS
+ SWEAT

WARM-UP

DENSITY SET #1

Complete as many rounds of the set as you can, challenging yourself and resting as little as possible between rounds. It is better to lower the number of reps per move or—if you really need to—modify a move rather than rest. Set your timer to work for 10 minutes. Rest 1 to 2 minutes between sets.

- 5 to 10 reps (per side) **single-leg squats**
- 5 to 10 reps **decline push-ups**
- 5 to 10 reps (per side) **climber planks**

DENSITY SET #2

Complete as many rounds of the set as you can, challenging yourself and resting as little as possible between rounds. Set your timer to work for 10 minutes. Rest 1 to 2 minutes between sets.

- 5 to 10 reps (per side) **slider side lunges**
- 5 to 10 reps (per side) **triceps push-ups**
- 5 to 10 reps **plank knee tucks**

DENSITY SET #3/AMRAP

Complete as many rounds of the set as you can, challenging yourself and resting as little as possible between rounds. Really focus on getting your heart rate up by moving quickly through these exercises. Set your timer to work for 10 minutes.

- 5 to 10 reps **burpees**
- 5 to 10 reps (per side) **skater hops**
- 5 to 10 reps (per side) **sit-thrus**

COOLDOWN

24 THE TIMED STRENGTH WORK

SHORT-ON-TIME PROGRESSION

This progression uses all three timed strength work techniques to help you achieve amazing results while doing roughly 30-minute sessions at home three or four days a week. While you don't want to ignore the recovery work, sneaking in even a 5-minute session on off days can create balance if you're limited to three workout days.

This three-day schedule and timed work is great if you train at home with minimal equipment or are traveling and want to stay in a groove and maintain your body composition. It can also be a great way to start back to training and focus on movement and recruitment patterns.

Workouts in this progression are bodyweight based and use sliders or towels, but you can check out the Exercise Library that begins on page 301 to swap for other tools you have at home.

With this progression, you will want to use the full-body or anterior/posterior prehab warm-ups as well as the suggested cooldowns. You can even use the quick prehab options if you're really looking to keep your workouts short!

You can change the order of the workouts, but give yourself a day of rest between each session. Repeat this progression using the same moves each week for three to six weeks before switching up the exercises or trying another workout design or split.

3 DAYS A WEEK

DAY 1
Full-body density intervals

DAY 2
Off

DAY 3
Full-body density sets

DAY 4
Off

DAY 5
Full-body strength intervals circuit

DAY 6
Recommended recovery workout

DAY 7
Off

DENSITY INTERVALS WORKOUT BUILDER

You can build out your own density intervals workouts based on this template. Each set will have two or three intervals of work focused on one area of the body. Alternate the areas or hemispheres worked in each set.

MUSCLE FOCUSED: Focus on pausing during intervals of work rather than being able to bust out reps quickly for the entire interval. Do not include SIT or steady-state cardio, especially if you're limited to bodyweight or very light resistance tools. It may be key to include isolation moves, or even holds, to target stubborn areas.

FAT LOSS: Don't let this strength work become cardio. Use variations and forms of progression like tempo or the tools you have to create pauses during intervals of work. Include SIT one or two days a week. Keep long runs or rides to one or two days between lifts and make sure to still have a day off.

BEGINNERS: Start with lower volume to let your connective tissues adjust and maintain proper form and recruitment patterns. Don't be afraid to start with just 2 rounds through each set. You may also focus more on compound burner sets (see page 254) rather than trisets.

NOTE: *Based on whether you include SIT and the number of intervals of work you include, you can adjust the length of the workout to fit what you need. Because it's timed, you can know exactly how long it will take!*

WARM-UP
Make sure to choose the warm-up that addresses the areas you plan to work.

SET #1
Complete 2 to 8 rounds through the set, resting up to 90 seconds between sets.
- 20 seconds to 1 minute **compound exercise**
- 20 seconds to 1 minute **compound or isolation exercise to target same muscle group**
- 20 seconds to 1 minute **compound or isolation exercise to target same muscle group** (optional)
- 20 seconds to 1 minute **rest**

SET #2
Complete 2 to 8 rounds through the set, resting up to 90 seconds between sets.
- 20 seconds to 1 minute **compound exercise**
- 20 seconds to 1 minute **compound or isolation exercise to target same muscle group**
- 20 seconds to 1 minute **compound or isolation exercise to target same muscle group** (optional)
- 20 seconds to 1 minute **rest**

SET #3
Complete 2 to 8 rounds through the set.
- 20 seconds to 1 minute **compound exercise**
- 20 seconds to 1 minute **compound or isolation exercise to target same muscle group**
- 20 seconds to 1 minute **compound or isolation exercise to target same muscle group** (optional)
- 20 seconds to 1 minute **rest**

Optional SIT

COOLDOWN

DENSITY SETS WORKOUT BUILDER

You can build out your own density sets workouts based on this template. This variation is best for home workouts. Alternate the areas or hemispheres worked in each density set to reduce rest time.

MUSCLE FOCUSED: Focus on doing fewer reps and maintaining more advanced variations of the moves over the course of the set, even if it means performing fewer than 5 reps. Do not include SIT or steady-state cardio, especially if you're limited to bodyweight or very light resistance tools.

FAT LOSS: Work down in reps, pushing the variations to create progressive overload. Include SIT one or two days a week. Keep long runs or rides to one or two days between lifts and make sure to have a day off. If you aren't including any bonus SIT sessions or long runs or rides, you may consider including the accelerate fat loss option for a bonus HIIT session (see page 246).

BEGINNERS: Start with lower volume to let your connective tissues adjust and maintain proper form and recruitment patterns. Don't be afraid to start with just 1 density set if needed.

> **NOTE:** *With all bodyweight moves, you may do up to 15 reps, as needed.*

WARM-UP
Make sure to choose the warm-up that addresses the areas you plan to work.

DENSITY SET #1
Complete as many rounds of the set as you can, challenging yourself and resting as little as possible between rounds. It's better to lower the number of reps per move or—if you really need to—modify a move rather than rest. Set your timer to work for 5 to 15 minutes.* Rest 1 to 2 minutes between sets.

- **5 to 10 reps compound exercise**
- **5 to 10 reps compound exercise for different muscle group**
- **5 to 10 reps compound exercise for different muscle group** (optional)

DENSITY SET #2
Complete as many rounds of the set as you can, challenging yourself and resting as little as possible between rounds. Set your timer to work for 5 to 15 minutes.

- **5 to 10 reps compound exercise**
- **5 to 10 reps compound exercise for different muscle group**
- **5 to 10 reps compound exercise for different muscle group** (optional)

Optional SIT

COOLDOWN

If you do 10 to 15 minutes per set, you will want to do only 2 or 3 density sets. You may do less than 10 minutes and include up to 4 or 5 sets, but then SIT is not recommended, even for fat loss.

STRENGTH INTERVALS CIRCUIT
WORKOUT BUILDER

You can build out your own strength intervals circuit workouts from this template. Alternate the areas or hemispheres worked in each circuit to reduce rest time. For other options, like supersets and trisets, check the Timed Strength Work Anterior/Posterior Progression in Chapter 23.

MUSCLE FOCUSED: Focus on pausing during intervals of work rather than being able to bust out reps quickly for the entire interval. Do not include SIT or steady-state cardio, especially if you're limited to bodyweight or very light resistance tools. Focus on the hardest compound exercises you can.

FAT LOSS: Don't let this strength work become cardio. Use variations and forms of progression like tempo or the tools you have to create pauses during intervals of work. Include SIT one or two days a week. Keep long runs or rides to one or two days between lifts and make sure to have a day off.

BEGINNERS: Start with lower volume to let your connective tissues adjust and maintain proper form and recruitment patterns. Don't be afraid to start with just 2 or 3 rounds through a single circuit.

> **NOTE:** *Based on whether you include SIT and the number of circuits and rounds you include, you can adjust the length of the workout to fit what you need. Because it's timed, you can know exactly how long it will take!*

WARM-UP
Make sure to choose the warm-up that addresses the areas you plan to work.

CIRCUIT #1
Complete 3 to 6 rounds through the circuit, resting 20 to 90 seconds between rounds and up to 90 seconds between circuits. This is the only workout design where you may cut the full rest period between rounds if you're short on time, as long as you're strategic in cycling the areas you work over the circuit.

- **20 seconds to 1 minute compound exercise**
- **20 seconds to 1 minute compound exercise for different muscle group**
- **20 seconds to 1 minute compound exercise for different muscle group**
- **20 seconds to 1 minute compound exercise for different muscle group**
- **20 seconds to 1 minute compound exercise for different muscle group**
- **20 seconds to 1 minute compound exercise for different muscle group**

CIRCUIT #2*
Complete 3 to 6 rounds through the circuit, resting 20 to 90 seconds between rounds. This is the only workout design where you may cut the full rest period between rounds if you're short on time, as long as you're strategic in cycling the areas you work over the circuit.

- **20 seconds to 1 minute compound exercise**
- **20 seconds to 1 minute compound exercise for different muscle group**
- **20 seconds to 1 minute compound exercise for different muscle group**
- **20 seconds to 1 minute compound exercise for different muscle group**

Optional SIT

COOLDOWN

One circuit is usually best, especially for quick routines. However, if you perform only 2 or 3 rounds of 4 exercises, you may choose to do 2 circuits to really target muscles from multiple angles!

FULL-BODY DENSITY INTERVALS

WARM-UP

SET #1
Complete 2 to 5 rounds through the set, resting 40 seconds to 1 minute between sets. Do not cut out rest.

- 20 seconds **doorway rows**
- 20 seconds **lying scapular presses**
- 20 seconds **scapular wings**
- 40 seconds to 1 minute **rest**

SET #2
Complete 2 to 5 rounds through the set, resting 40 seconds to 1 minute between sets. Do not cut out rest.

- 20 seconds **get-up lunges**
- 20 seconds **squat pulses**
- 20 seconds **kneeling lean backs**
- 40 seconds to 1 minute **rest**

SET #3
Complete 2 to 5 rounds through the set. Do not cut out rest.

- 20 seconds **pike push-ups**
- 20 seconds **bench dips**
- 20 seconds **plank climbers**
- 40 seconds to 1 minute **rest**

Optional SIT

COOLDOWN

FULL-BODY DENSITY SETS

WARM-UP

DENSITY SET #1
Complete as many rounds of the set as you can, challenging yourself and resting as little as possible between rounds. It's better to lower the number of reps per move or—if you really need to—modify a move rather than rest. Set your timer to work for 12 minutes. Rest 1 to 2 minutes between sets.

- 5 to 10 reps (per side) **airborne lunges**
- 5 to 10 reps (per side) **single-arm doorway rows**
- 5 to 10 reps **fly push-ups**

DENSITY SET #2
Complete as many rounds of the set as you can, challenging yourself and resting as little as possible between rounds. Set your timer to work for 12 minutes.

- 5 to 10 reps (per side) **side-to-curtsy lunges**
- 5 to 10 reps **close-grip push-ups**
- 5 to 10 reps (per side) **lying side slides**

Optional SIT

COOLDOWN

FULL-BODY STRENGTH INTERVALS CIRCUIT

WARM-UP

CIRCUIT #1
Complete 3 to 5 rounds through the circuit, resting up to 1 minute between rounds. Because you're cycling the areas you work, you can cut rest to 30 seconds to do a fifth round if you're really short on time.

- 1 minute **alternating slider reverse lunges**
- 1 minute **scapular wall reps**
- 1 minute **triceps push-ups***
- 1 minute **glute bridges and curls**
- 1 minute **alternating arm plank rows**

Optional SIT

COOLDOWN

Complete 30 seconds per side, depending on the amount of time you plan to work and the number of rounds you plan to complete.

ANTERIOR/POSTERIOR PROGRESSION

This progression is best if you have four or five days to train. If you only have three days, use the full-body progression in Chapter 26. You don't want to ignore the recovery work, so if you have only three days to train, sneaking in even a 5-minute session on your off days can create balance.

If you're doing six days a week, I do *not* recommend another lifting day, because the four days hit everything with enough volume. The sixth day is best used for a run—if you enjoy it and your goal isn't pure muscle gains—or a recovery session. You may do a very short ab finisher or 5-minute "trouble zone" bonus with a recovery session and SIT or power protocol. But if you push hard with the four lifts, you shouldn't want to do more. If you do the fat loss–accelerator schedule, be conscious that this is a *super intensive push*. Do only three or four weeks on this schedule.

With this progression, you will want to use the full-body or anterior/posterior prehab warm-ups as well as the suggested cooldowns (see pages 287–288 and 291–292).

4 DAYS A WEEK	5 DAYS A WEEK	6 DAYS A WEEK (muscle focused)	6 DAYS A WEEK (fat-loss accelerator)
DAY 1	**DAY 1**	**DAY 1**	**DAY 1**
Posterior density sets #1	Posterior density sets #1	Posterior density sets #1	Posterior density sets #1 or #2
DAY 2	**DAY 2**	**DAY 2**	**DAY 2**
Anterior density sets #1	Anterior density sets #1	Anterior density sets #1	Anterior density sets + sweat
DAY 3	**DAY 3**	**DAY 3**	**DAY 3**
Off	Off	Recovery workout or Cardio	Recovery workout
DAY 4	**DAY 4**	**DAY 4**	**DAY 4**
Posterior density sets #2	Posterior density sets #2	Posterior density sets #2	Posterior density sets + sweat
DAY 5	**DAY 5**	**DAY 5**	**DAY 5**
Anterior density sets #2	Anterior density sets #2	Anterior density sets #2	Anterior density sets #1 or #2
DAY 6	**DAY 6**	**DAY 6**	**DAY 6**
Off	Recovery workout	Recovery workout	Recovery workout
DAY 7	**DAY 7**	**DAY 7**	**DAY 7**
Off	Off	Off	Off

Here, I give schedules for four to six days a week. Do *not* skip the recovery workouts! You can change the order of these workouts, but don't put two posterior or anterior days back to back. Repeat this progression using the same moves each week for three to six weeks before switching up the exercises or moving to another workout design or split.

DENSITY SETS WORKOUT BUILDER

You can build out your own density sets workouts by using this template. This variation is best for full-body or anterior/posterior workouts. Alternate the areas or hemispheres worked in each density set to reduce rest time.

MUSCLE FOCUSED: Focus on working down in reps and up in weight, even if it means doing fewer than 5 reps toward the end. If you include any SIT or power work, keep it to one session a week and perform it on your recovery day. Walking should be your main cardio.

FAT LOSS: Work down in reps, pushing the variations to create progressive overload. Include SIT one or two days a week. Keep long runs or rides to just one day between lifts and make sure to still have a day off. If you aren't including any bonus SIT sessions or long runs or rides, you may consider including the fat loss–accelerator option for a bonus HIIT session one or two days a week (see page 246).

BEGINNERS: Start with lower volume to let your connective tissues adjust and maintain proper form and recruitment patterns. Don't be afraid to start with just 1 density set if needed.

WARM-UP
Make sure to choose the warm-up that addresses the areas you plan to work.

DENSITY SET #1: Upper or lower body
Complete as many rounds of the set as you can, challenging yourself and resting as little as possible between rounds. It's better to lower the number of reps per move or—if you really need to—modify a move rather than rest. Set your timer to work for 10 to 15 minutes. Rest 1 to 2 minutes between sets.
- 5 to 10 reps **compound exercise***
- 5 to 10 reps **compound exercise for different muscle group**

DENSITY SET #2: Upper or lower body
Complete as many rounds of the set as you can, challenging yourself and resting as little as possible between rounds. Set your timer to work for 10 to 15 minutes. Rest 1 to 2 minutes between sets.
- 5 to 10 reps **compound exercise***
- 5 to 10 reps **compound exercise for different muscle group**

DENSITY SET #3: Upper or lower body
Complete as many rounds of the set as you can, challenging yourself and resting as little as possible between rounds. Set your timer to work for 10 to 15 minutes.
- 5 to 10 reps **compound exercise***
- 5 to 10 reps **compound or isolation exercise for different muscle group**
- 5 to 15 reps **compound or isolation exercise for different muscle group (optional)****

Optional SIT

COOLDOWN

*With any lift where you're getting under heavy loads, you want to do 2 or 3 warm-up sets first, building up with 50 percent (8 to 10 reps), 75 percent (6 to 8 reps), and 85 percent (4 to 6 reps) of your working weight. You may then increase after that first round. The heavier you go, the more you want to do those warm-up rounds before the sets. Start with a weight that is about your 10-rep max.

**For this final move, a more isolated exercise may be used, so reps may increase. You may do up to two isolation exercises in the third density set.

POSTERIOR DENSITY SETS #1

WARM-UP

DENSITY SET #1
Complete as many rounds of the set as you can, challenging yourself and resting as little as possible between rounds. It's better to lower the number of reps per move or—if you really need to—modify a move rather than rest. Set your timer to work for 10 minutes. Rest 1 to 2 minutes between sets.

- 5 to 10 reps deadlifts*
- 5 to 10 reps pull-ups

DENSITY SET #2
Complete as many rounds of the set as you can, challenging yourself and resting as little as possible between rounds. Set your timer to work for 10 minutes. Rest 1 to 2 minutes between sets.

- 5 to 10 reps (per side) reverse lunges
- 5 to 10 reps overhand rows

DENSITY SET #3
Complete as many rounds of the set as you can, challenging yourself and resting as little as possible between rounds. Set your timer to work for 10 minutes.

- 5 to 10 reps (per side) side lunges
- 5 to 10 reps back flys
- 5 to 15 reps biceps curls**

Optional SIT**

COOLDOWN

ANTERIOR DENSITY SETS #1

WARM-UP

DENSITY SET #1
Complete as many rounds of the set as you can, challenging yourself and resting as little as possible between rounds. Its better to lower the number of reps per move or—if you really need to—modify a move rather than rest. Set your timer to work for 10 minutes. Rest 1 to 2 minutes between sets.

- 5 to 10 reps back squats*
- 5 to 10 reps bench presses

DENSITY SET #2
Complete as many rounds of the set as you can, challenging yourself and resting as little as possible between rounds. Set your timer to work for 10 minutes. Rest 1 to 2 minutes between sets.

- 5 to 10 reps (per side) deficit split squats
- 5 to 10 reps overhead presses

DENSITY SET #3
Complete as many rounds of the set as you can, challenging yourself and resting as little as possible between rounds. Set your timer to work for 10 minutes.

- 5 to 10 reps goblet squats
- 5 to 10 reps decline push-ups
- 5 to 15 reps triceps pushdowns**

Optional SIT**

COOLDOWN

*With any lift where you're getting under heavy loads, you want to do 2 or 3 warm-up sets first, building up with 50 percent (8 to 10 reps), 75 percent (6 to 8 reps), and 85 percent (4 to 6 reps) of your working weight. You may then increase after that first round. The heavier you go, the more you want to do those warm-up rounds before the sets. Start with a weight that is about your 10-rep max.

**You may find you need slightly higher reps with this isolation move.

POSTERIOR
DENSITY SETS #2

DENSITY SET #1
Complete as many rounds of the set as you can, challenging yourself and resting as little as possible between rounds. It's better to lower the number of reps per move or—if you really need to—modify a move rather than rest. Set your timer to work for 10 minutes. Rest 1 to 2 minutes between sets.

- 5 to 10 reps **hip thrusts***
- 5 to 10 reps **underhand rows**

DENSITY SET #2
Complete as many rounds of the set as you can, challenging yourself and resting as little as possible between rounds. Set your timer to work for 10 minutes. Rest 1 to 2 minutes between sets.

- 5 to 10 reps **Romanian deadlifts**
- 5 to 10 reps **lat pulldowns**

DENSITY SET #3
Complete as many rounds of the set as you can, challenging yourself and resting as little as possible between rounds. Set your timer to work for 10 minutes.

- 5 to 10 reps (per side) **curtsy lunges**
- 5 to 10 reps **chest-supported rows**
- 5 to 15 reps **pull-throughs****

Optional SIT**

COOLDOWN

ANTERIOR
DENSITY SETS #2

WARM-UP

DENSITY SET #1
Complete as many rounds of the set as you can, challenging yourself and resting as little as possible between rounds. It's better to lower the number of reps per move or—if you really need to—modify a move rather than rest. Set your timer to work for 10 minutes. Rest 1 to 2 minutes between sets.

- 5 to 10 reps (per side) **front lunges***
- 5 to 10 reps **incline bench presses**

DENSITY SET #2
Complete as many rounds of the set as you can, challenging yourself and resting as little as possible between rounds. Set your timer to work for 10 minutes. Rest 1 to 2 minutes between sets.

- 5 to 10 reps **front squats**
- 5 to 10 reps **dips**

DENSITY SET #3
Complete as many rounds of the set as you can, challenging yourself and resting as little as possible between rounds. Set your timer to work for 10 minutes.

- 5 to 10 reps (per side) **step-ups**
- 5 to 15 reps **lateral raises****
- 5 to 15 reps **kneeling lean backs****

Optional SIT**

COOLDOWN

With any lift where you're getting under heavy loads, you want to do 2 or 3 warm-up sets first, building up with 50 percent (8 to 10 reps), 75 percent (6 to 8 reps), and 85 percent (4 to 6 reps) of your working weight. You may then increase after that first round. The heavier you go, the more you want to do those warm-up rounds before the sets. Start with a weight that is about your 10-rep max.

**You may find you need slightly higher reps with this glute-focused move.*

DENSITY SETS + SWEAT
WORKOUT BUILDER

You can build out your own density sets workouts with HIIT by using this template. Alternate the areas or hemispheres worked in each density set to reduce rest time.

MUSCLE FOCUSED: Unless this is absolutely your only cardio, this version isn't recommended when you're focused on muscle-building.

FAT LOSS: Work down in reps, pushing the variations to create progressive overload, especially with the first 2 density sets. In the third set, your goal is conditioning, so you want to move quickly to get your blood pumping. Additional SIT is not recommended on this day, and this option is best when you're not really logging a ton of extra miles otherwise.

BEGINNERS: Start with lower volume to let your connective tissues adjust and maintain proper form and recruitment patterns. It may also be better to start with the basic density sets on page 260 rather than this layout. If you want to start back with HIIT, include exercises that match your fitness level and consider doing just 2 density sets for 8 to 10 minutes or a shorter HIIT set for 5 minutes.

If you do 10 to 15 minutes per set, you will want to do only 2 or 3 density sets. You may do less than 10 minutes and include up to 4 or 5 sets, but then SIT is not recommended, even for fat loss.

**Three moves are recommended for the third set, although four can also work well. For the HIIT density set, you may perform higher reps of the cardio exercises.

WARM-UP
Make sure to choose the warm-up that addresses the areas you plan to work.

DENSITY SET #1: Upper or lower body
Complete as many rounds of the set as you can, challenging yourself and resting as little as possible between rounds. It's better to lower the number of reps per move or—if you really need to—modify a move rather than rest. Set your timer to work for 5 to 15 minutes.* Rest 1 to 2 minutes between sets.

- 5 to 10 reps **compound exercise**
- 5 to 10 reps **compound exercise for different muscle group**
- 5 to 10 reps **compound exercise for different muscle group** (optional)

DENSITY SET #2: Upper or lower body
Complete as many rounds of the set as you can, challenging yourself and resting as little as possible between rounds. Set your timer to work for 5 to 15 minutes. Rest 1 to 2 minutes between sets.

- 5 to 10 reps **compound exercise**
- 5 to 10 reps **compound exercise for different muscle group**
- 5 to 10 reps **compound exercise for different muscle group** (optional)

DENSITY SET #3/AMRAP: Upper or lower body
Complete as many rounds of the set as you can, challenging yourself and resting as little as possible between rounds. Set your timer to work for 5 to 15 minutes.

- 5 to 15 reps **compound exercise**
- 5 to 15 reps **compound exercise for different muscle group**
- 5 to 15 reps **compound exercise for different muscle group**
- 5 to 15 reps **compound exercise for different muscle group** (optional)**

COOLDOWN

POSTERIOR
DENSITY SETS
+ SWEAT

BONUS

WARM-UP

DENSITY SET #1
Complete as many rounds of the set as you can, challenging yourself and resting as little as possible between rounds. It's better to lower the number of reps per move or—if you really need to—modify a move rather than rest. Set your timer to work for 10 minutes. Rest 1 to 2 minutes between sets.

- 5 to 10 reps (per side) **single-leg deadlifts***
- 5 to 10 reps (per side) **single-arm rows**

DENSITY SET #2
Complete as many rounds of the set as you can, challenging yourself and resting as little as possible between rounds. Set your timer to work for 10 minutes. Rest 1 to 2 minutes between sets.

- 5 to 15 reps **weighted glute bridges****
- 5 to 10 reps **pullovers**

DENSITY SET #3/AMRAP
Complete as many rounds of the set as you can, challenging yourself and resting as little as possible between rounds. Really focus on getting your heart rate up by moving quickly through these exercises. Set your timer to work for 10 minutes.

- 10 to 15 reps **kettlebell swings**
- 10 to 15 reps **med ball slams**
- 10 to 15 reps **incline abs**

COOLDOWN

ANTERIOR
DENSITY SETS
+ SWEAT

BONUS

WARM-UP

DENSITY SET #1
Complete as many rounds of the set as you can, challenging yourself and resting as little as possible between rounds. It's better to lower the number of reps per move or—if you really need to—modify a move rather than rest. Set your timer to work for 10 minutes. Rest 1 to 2 minutes between sets.

- 5 to 10 reps (per side) **split squats***
- 5 to 10 reps **chest flys**

DENSITY SET #2
Complete as many rounds of the set as you can, challenging yourself and resting as little as possible between rounds. Set your timer to work for 10 minutes. Rest 1 to 2 minutes between sets.

- 5 to 10 reps **sumo squats**
- 5 to 15 reps **push-ups*****

DENSITY SET #3/AMRAP
Complete as many rounds of the set as you can, challenging yourself and resting as little as possible between rounds. Really focus on getting your heart rate up by moving quickly through these exercises. Set your timer to work for 10 minutes.

- 5 to 10 reps **burpees**
- 5 to 10 reps **squats to presses**
- 5 to 10 reps (per side) **sit-thrus**

COOLDOWN

---

*With any lift where you're getting under heavy loads, you want to do 2 or 3 warm-up sets first, building up with 50 percent (8 to 10 reps), 75 percent (6 to 8 reps), and 85 percent (4 to 6 reps) of your working weight. You may then increase after that first round. The heavier you go, the more you want to do those warm-up rounds before the sets. Start with a weight that is about your 10-rep max.

**I recommend higher reps for this move because while you can go heavy, it's a bit more isolated

***You can go higher in reps with these or progress the move by using bands.

26 THE DENSITY SETS
FULL-BODY PROGRESSION

This progression is best if you have three or four days to train. You don't want to ignore the recovery work, so if you have only three days to train, sneaking in even a 5-minute session on your off days can create balance.

This three-day schedule can be amazing if you're trying to maintain strength and muscle while logging more miles. The volume of these workouts can easily add up, so be conscious of starting lighter if you're just starting back to training.

With this progression, use the full-body or anterior/posterior prehab warm-ups as well as the suggested cooldowns (pages 287–288 and 291–292).

You can change the order of the workouts, but give yourself a day of rest between each session. Repeat this progression using the same moves each week for three to six weeks before switching up the exercises or moving to another workout design or split!

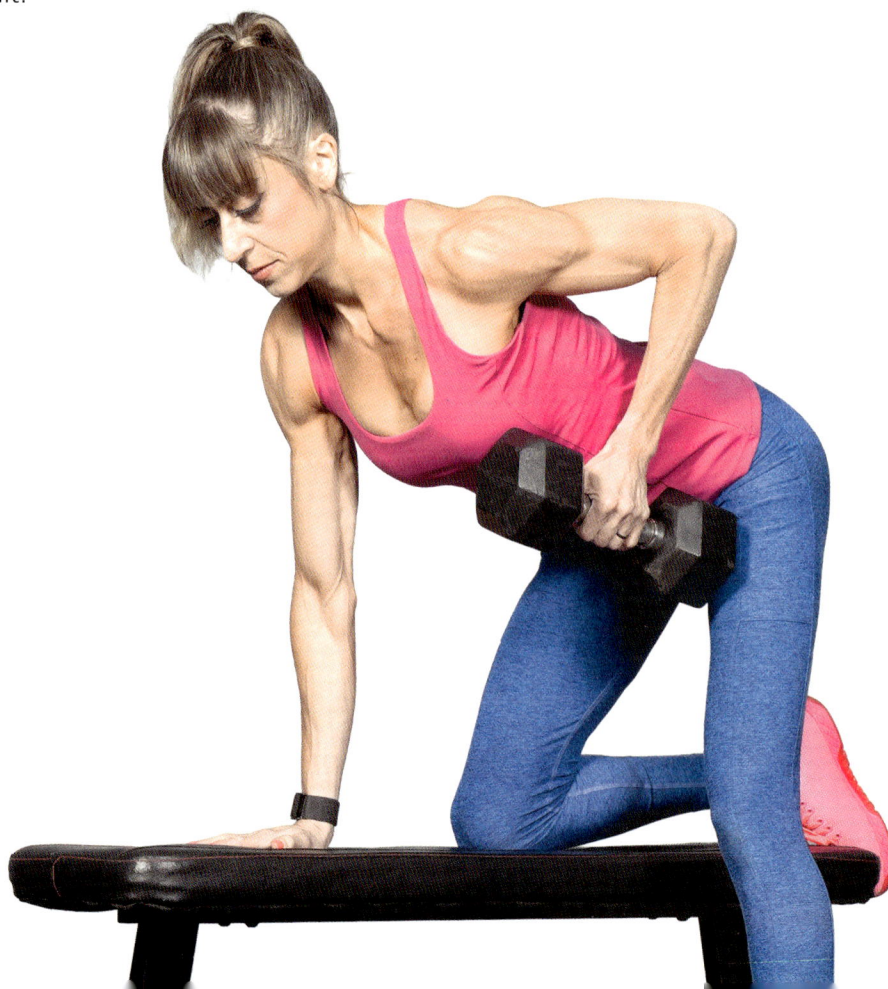

3 DAYS A WEEK

DAY 1
Full-body density sets #1

DAY 2
Off

DAY 3
Full-body density sets #2

DAY 4
Off

DAY 5
Full-body density sets #3

DAY 6
Recommended recovery workout

DAY 7
Off

DENSITY INTERVALS WORKOUT BUILDER

You can build out your own density sets workouts by using this template. This variation is best for full-body workouts. Alternate the areas or hemispheres worked in each density set to reduce rest time.

MUSCLE FOCUSED: Focus on working down in reps and up in weight, even if it means doing fewer than 5 reps toward the end. Do not include SIT or steady-state cardio. You may include power work one or two times a week.

FAT LOSS: Work down in reps, pushing the variations to create progressive overload. Include SIT one or two days a week. Keep long runs or rides to one or two days between lifts and make sure to have a day off. If you aren't including any bonus SIT sessions or long runs or rides, you may consider including the fat loss–accelerator option for a bonus HIIT session one day a week (see page 246).

BEGINNERS: Start with lower volume to let your connective tissues adjust and maintain proper form and recruitment patterns. Don't be afraid to start with just 1 density set if needed.

WARM-UP
Make sure to choose the warm-up that addresses the areas you plan to work.

Optional POWER SESSION

DENSITY SET #1
Complete as many rounds of the set as you can, challenging yourself and resting as little as possible between rounds. It's better to lower the number of reps per move or—if you really need to—modify a move rather than rest. Set your timer to work for 10 to 15 minutes. Rest 1 to 2 minutes between sets.

- 5 to 10 reps **compound exercise***
- 5 to 10 reps **compound exercise for different muscle group**

DENSITY SET #2
Complete as many rounds of the set as you can, challenging yourself and resting as little as possible between rounds. Set your timer to work for 10 to 15 minutes. Rest 1 to 2 minutes between sets.

- 5 to 10 reps **compound exercise***
- 5 to 10 reps **compound exercise for different muscle group**

DENSITY SET #3
Complete as many rounds of the set as you can, challenging yourself and resting as little as possible between rounds. Set your timer to work for 10 to 15 minutes.

- 5 to 10 reps **compound exercise***
- 5 to 10 reps **compound exercise for different muscle group**
- 5 to 15 reps **compound or isolation exercise for different muscle group** (optional)**

Optional SIT

COOLDOWN

With any lift where you're getting under heavy loads, you want to do 2 or 3 warm-up sets first, building up with 50 percent (8 to 10 reps), 75 percent (6 to 8 reps), and 85 percent (4 to 6 reps) of your working weight. You may then increase after that first round. The heavier you go, the more you want to do those warm-up rounds before the sets. Start with a weight that is about your 10-rep max.

**For this final move, a more isolated exercise may be used, so reps may increase.*

FULL-BODY DENSITY SETS #1

WARM-UP

Optional POWER SESSION

DENSITY SET #1
Complete as many rounds of the set as you can, challenging yourself and resting as little as possible between rounds. It's better to lower the number of reps per move or—if you really need to—modify a move rather than rest. Set your timer to work for 10 minutes. Rest 1 to 2 minutes between sets.

- 5 to 10 reps **deadlifts***
- 5 to 10 reps **bench presses**

DENSITY SET #2
Complete as many rounds of the set as you can, challenging yourself and resting as little as possible between rounds. Set your timer to work for 10 minutes. Rest 1 to 2 minutes between sets.

- 5 to 10 reps (per side) **front lunges**
- 5 to 10 reps **lat pulldowns**

DENSITY SET #3
Complete as many rounds of the set as you can, challenging yourself and resting as little as possible between rounds. Set your timer to work for 10 minutes.

- 5 to 10 reps (per side) **step-ups**
- 5 to 10 reps (per side) **single-arm rows**
- 5 to 10 reps **chest flys**

Optional SIT

COOLDOWN

FULL-BODY DENSITY SETS #2

WARM-UP

Optional POWER SESSION

DENSITY SET #1
Complete as many rounds of the set as you can, challenging yourself and resting as little as possible between rounds. It's better to lower the number of reps per move or—if you really need to—modify a move rather than rest. Set your timer to work for 10 minutes. Rest 1 to 2 minutes between sets.

- 5 to 10 reps **front squats***
- 5 to 10 reps **overhand rows**

DENSITY SET #2
Complete as many rounds of the set as you can, challenging yourself and resting as little as possible between rounds. Set your timer to work for 10 minutes. Rest 1 to 2 minutes between sets.

- 5 to 10 reps (per side) **curtsy lunges**
- 5 to 10 reps **overhead presses**

DENSITY SET #3
Complete as many rounds of the set as you can, challenging yourself and resting as little as possible between rounds. Set your timer to work for 10 minutes.

- 5 to 10 reps (per side) **single-leg deadlifts**
- 5 to 10 reps **back flys**
- 5 to 10 reps **chest presses to skull crushers**

Optional SIT

COOLDOWN

FULL-BODY DENSITY SETS #3

WARM-UP

Optional POWER SESSION

DENSITY SET #1
Complete as many rounds of the set as you can, challenging yourself and resting as little as possible between rounds. It's better to lower the number of reps per move or—if you really need to—modify a move rather than rest. Set your timer to work for 10 minutes. Rest 1 to 2 minutes between sets.

- 5 to 10 reps **hip thrusts***
- 5 to 10 reps **incline bench presses**

DENSITY SET #2
Complete as many rounds of the set as you can, challenging yourself and resting as little as possible between rounds. Set your timer to work for 10 minutes. Rest 1 to 2 minutes between sets.

- 5 to 10 reps (per side) **deficit split squats**
- 5 to 10 reps **underhand rows**

DENSITY SET #3
Complete as many rounds of the set as you can, challenging yourself and resting as little as possible between rounds. Set your timer to work for 10 minutes.

- 5 to 10 reps (per side) **side lunges**
- 5 to 12 reps **lateral raises****
- 5 to 12 reps **biceps curls****

Optional SIT

COOLDOWN

With any lift where you're getting under heavy loads, you want to do 2 or 3 warm-up sets first, building up with 50 percent (8 to 10 reps), 75 percent (6 to 8 reps), and 85 percent (4 to 6 reps) of your working weight. You may then increase after that first round. The heavier you go, the more you want to do those warm-up rounds before the sets. Start with a weight that is about your 10-rep max.

**You may find you need slightly higher reps with this isolation move.*

DENSITY SETS + SWEAT
WORKOUT BUILDER

You can build out your own density sets workouts with HIIT by using this template. Alternate the areas or hemispheres worked in each density set to reduce rest time.

MUSCLE FOCUSED: Unless this is absolutely your only cardio, this version isn't recommended when you are focused on muscle-building.

FAT LOSS: Work down in reps, pushing the variations to create progressive overload, especially with the first 2 density sets. In the third set, your goal is conditioning, so you want to move quickly to get your blood pumping. Additional SIT isn't recommended on this day, and this option is best when you're not really logging a ton of extra miles.

BEGINNERS: Start with lower volume to let your connective tissues adjust and maintain proper form and recruitment patterns. It may also be better to start with the basic density sets on page 260 rather than this layout. If you want to start back with HIIT, include exercises that match your fitness level and consider doing just 2 density sets for 8 to 10 minutes or a shorter HIIT set for 5 minutes.

If you do 10 to 15 minutes per set, you will want to do only 2 or 3 density sets. You may do less than 10 minutes and include up to 4 or 5 sets, but then SIT is not recommended, even for fat loss.

**Three moves are recommended for the third set, although four can also work well. For the HIIT density set, you may perform higher reps of the cardio exercises.*

WARM-UP
Make sure to choose the warm-up that addresses the areas you plan to work.

DENSITY SET #1
Complete as many rounds of the set as you can, challenging yourself and resting as little as possible between rounds. It's better to lower the number of reps per move or—if you really need to—modify a move rather than rest. Set your timer to work for 5 to 15 minutes.* Rest 1 to 2 minutes between sets.

- 5 to 10 reps **compound exercise**
- 5 to 10 reps **compound exercise for different muscle group**
- 5 to 10 reps **compound exercise for different muscle group** (optional)

DENSITY SET #2
Complete as many rounds of the set as you can, challenging yourself and resting as little as possible between rounds. Set your timer to work for 5 to 15 minutes. Rest 1 to 2 minutes between sets.

- 5 to 10 reps **compound exercise**
- 5 to 10 reps **compound exercise for different muscle group**
- 5 to 10 reps **compound exercise for different muscle group** (optional)

DENSITY SET #3/AMRAP
Complete as many rounds of the set as you can, challenging yourself and resting as little as possible between rounds. Set your timer to work for 5 to 15 minutes.

- 5 to 15 reps **compound exercise**
- 5 to 15 reps **compound exercise for different muscle group**
- 5 to 15 reps **compound exercise for different muscle group**
- 5 to 15 reps **compound exercise for different muscle group** (optional)**

COOLDOWN

FULL-BODY
DENSITY SETS
+ SWEAT

BONUS

DENSITY SET #1

Complete as many rounds of the set as you can, challenging yourself and resting as little as possible between rounds. It's better to lower the number of reps per move or—if you really need to—modify a move rather than rest. Set your timer to work for 10 minutes. Rest 1 to 2 minutes between sets.

- 5 to 10 reps **back squats***
- 5 to 10 reps **chest-supported rows**

DENSITY SET #2

Complete as many rounds of the set as you can, challenging yourself and resting as little as possible between rounds. Set your timer to work for 10 minutes. Rest 1 to 2 minutes between sets.

- 5 to 10 reps **Romanian deadlifts**
- 5 to 10 **reps dips**

DENSITY SET #3/AMRAP

Complete as many rounds of the set as you can, challenging yourself and resting as little as possible between rounds. Really focus on getting your heart rate up by moving quickly through these exercises. Set your timer to work for 10 minutes

- 5 to 10 reps **burpees**
- 10 to 15 reps **kettlebell swings**
- 10 to 15 reps **med ball slams**
- 5 to 10 reps (per side) **sit-thrus**

COOLDOWN

With any lift where you're getting under heavy loads, you want to do 2 or 3 warm-up sets first, building up with 50 percent (8 to 10 reps), 75 percent (6 to 8 reps), and 85 percent (4 to 6 reps) of your working weight. You may then increase after that first round. The heavier you go, the more you want to do those warm-up rounds before the sets. Start with a weight that is about your 10-rep max.

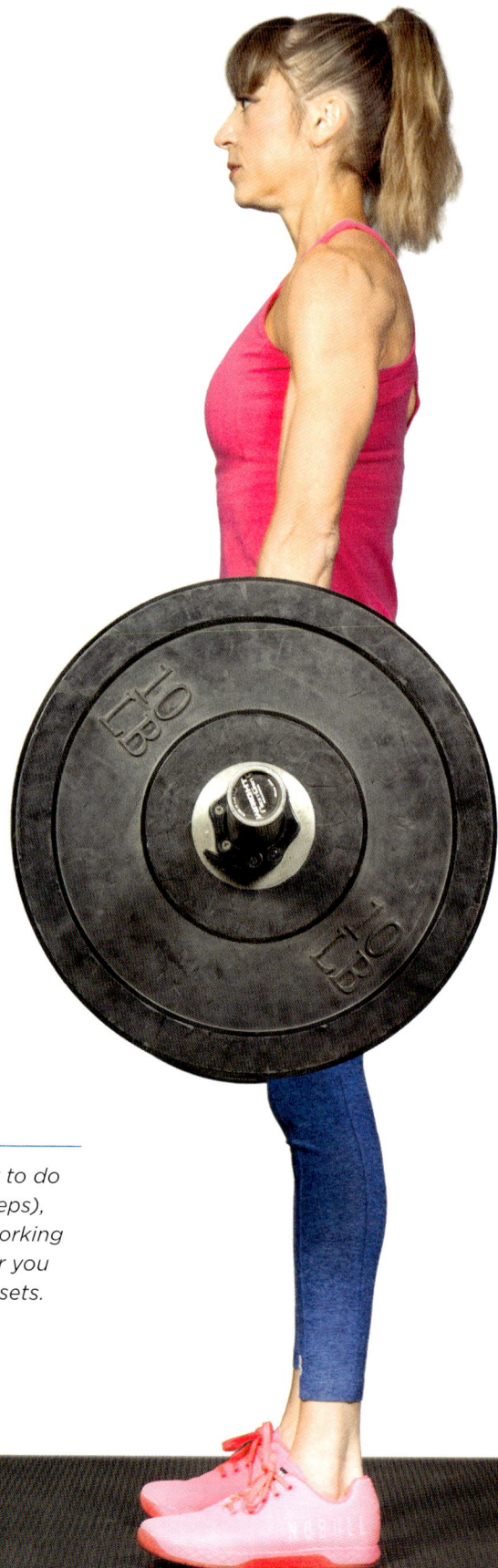

27 POWER AND SIT PROTOCOLS

Power work and sprint interval training (SIT) are short intervals of high-intensity, maximum-effort work. They're quick bursts that can be done along with your strength training and are key if you want to improve your body composition, performance, and health.

This type of training becomes even more valuable as you get older, but it's often the stuff people stop doing because they believe it's "too intense." It's not. Use it or lose it! These quick and dirty intervals are often what you need to age well and look your most fabulous. They're especially helpful for women who have to navigate the hormonal changes of menopause. These protocols help address changes in insulin sensitivity that often occur starting with perimenopause, and they may help you avoid gaining the dreaded stubborn belly fat associated with middle age. They're helpful for maintaining your metabolic health and lean muscle mass.

Using the power and SIT protocols in this chapter, you can customize your workout routines to match your specific needs and goals. Power work can be included after your warm-up before your main workout. SIT sessions may be included after your strength work is complete.

POWER SESSION BUILDER

This template allows you to customize your power sessions to what you need. These are best included after your warm-up before a strength session. They're meant to be explosive periods of work that help improve your reaction time, so you don't want to be fatigued for them.

Design your sessions to include 5 to 8 rounds, but you can occasionally do up to 10 rounds if needed. Include one to three sessions, preferably with different intervals, every week. These one to three sessions are combined with your SIT protocols, not added on top of them. You may choose to do two SIT and one power, two power and one SIT, or all three of one or the other based on your goals. For more pure muscle gains, consider only power work. If fat loss is your focus, consider more SIT.

POWER PROTOCOL
- 8 to 12 seconds **sprint exercise**
- 40 seconds to 1 minute **full rest**

RECOMMENDED EXERCISES
- **Air bike**
- **Rower**
- **Treadmill sprints**
- **Med ball drills**
- **Burpees**
- **Sled sprints**
- **Plyo push-ups**

For the work-to-rest intervals, you want to rest three to five times the length you worked. This recovery is crucial because you don't want to train slowness. You want explosiveness and 100 percent intensity each and every time you work. If you feel like you really start to decline in output, don't do 10 rounds just for the sake of doing 10 rounds. Stop when you're no longer giving 100 percent and make it your goal to do another round the next week or week after.

For the rest periods, full rest is always recommended. You want to be completely rested and itching to go again. If your tendency is to rest three times the length you work, consider increasing it to five times to maintain true explosiveness over more rounds. You can walk around rather than sitting down, but focus on fully bringing your heart rate down while relaxing the muscles you've worked.

Each week, your goal is to be able to do more during the work interval, recover faster so you see your heart rate come down quicker with rest, or complete another round in the range with the same intensity.

POWER SESSIONS

10/30 POWER SESSION
Complete 5 to 8 rounds through the protocol.

Power protocol
- 10 seconds **sprint exercise**
- 30 seconds **full rest**

12/60 POWER SESSION
Complete 8 to 10 rounds through the protocol.

Power protocol
- 12 seconds **sprint exercise**
- 1 minute **full rest**

8/32 POWER SESSION
Complete 6 to 8 rounds through the protocol.

Power protocol
- 8 seconds **sprint exercise**
- 32 seconds **full rest**

12/36 POWER SESSION
Complete 5 to 7 rounds through the protocol.

Power protocol
- 12 seconds **sprint exercise**
- 36 seconds **full rest**

10/50 POWER SESSION
Complete 8 to 10 rounds through the protocol.

Power protocol
- 10 seconds **sprint exercise**
- 50 seconds **full rest**

Pick one to three sessions to repeat on the same weekly schedule for the full length of your progression. Do *not* vary the exercises or intervals used. You want that consistency to see progress week after week. To track your progress, record how many reps you can do, if your intensity has increased, or if you're recovering faster.

SIT SESSION BUILDER

This template allows you to customize your SIT sessions to what you need. These are best included after a strength session before your cooldown. You can also include them after isometrics or activation on a recovery day if you're getting enough overall rest for the week. They can be a satisfying little burst!

Design your sessions to include 5 to 8 rounds, but you can occasionally do up to 10 rounds if needed. Include one to three sessions, preferably with different intervals, every week. These one to three sessions are

SIT PROTOCOL
- 8 to 30 seconds **sprint exercise**
- 12 to 90 seconds **rest (full or active)**

RECOMMENDED EXERCISES
- Air bike
- Rower
- Treadmill sprints
- Battle ropes
- Burpees
- Sled sprints
- Squat jumps
- Kettlebell swings

combined with your power protocols, not added on top of them! You may choose to do two SIT and one power, two power and one SIT, or all three of one or the other based on your goals. If you're more focused on building muscle, include just one SIT session per week (or even no sessions).

For the work-to-rest intervals, you want to rest half to three times the length you worked. I don't recommend having a work-to-rest interval of less than 8 seconds on, 12 seconds off. You want 100 percent intensity each and every time you work. If you feel like you really start to decline in output, don't do 10 rounds just for the sake of doing 10 rounds. Stop when you're no longer giving 100 percent and make it your goal to do another round the next week or week after, even if it means doing only 4 or 5 rounds this week.

For the rest periods, active or full rest can be appropriate. The longer the work interval, the more I recommend full rest so you recover for 100 percent intensity each round. With shorter work-to-rest intervals, you can include active rest to allow you to sprint hard when the timer goes off; for example, you can continue moving the pedals on the bike very slowly during the rest interval. With active rest, you want to recover. It's not the time to keep pushing.

Each week, your goal is to be able to do more during the work interval, recover faster so you see your heart rate come down quicker with rest, or complete another round in the range with the same intensity. Sometimes, you may even adjust from full rest to active rest if you've maxed out rounds and seen your recovery really improve, especially with shorter work intervals.

SIT SESSIONS

8/12 SIT SESSION
Complete 6 to 10 rounds through the protocol.

SIT protocol
- 8 seconds **sprint exercise**
- 12 seconds **rest** (active recommended)

30/30 SIT SESSION
Complete 5 to 8 rounds through the protocol.

SIT protocol
- 30 seconds **sprint exercise**
- 30 seconds **rest** (full recommended)

20/10 SIT SESSION
Complete 8 to 10 rounds through the protocol.

SIT protocol
- 20 seconds **sprint exercise**
- 10 seconds **rest** (active recommended)

20/40 SIT SESSION
Complete 5 to 8 rounds through the protocol.

SIT protocol
- 20 seconds **sprint exercise**
- 40 seconds **rest** (full recommended)

15/45 SIT SESSION
Complete 5 to 8 rounds through the protocol.

SIT protocol
- 15 seconds **sprint exercise**
- 45 seconds **rest** (active recommended)

Pick one to three sessions to repeat on the same weekly schedule for the full length of your progression. Do *not* vary the exercises or intervals used. You want that consistency to see progress week after week. To track your progress, record how many reps you can do, if your intensity has increased, or if you're recovering faster.

WARM-UP BUILDER

Use this template to customize your warm-ups to what you need. With some of the activation exercises, you may shorten them to 20 seconds if you find yourself getting fatigued. For the foam rolling, you may find yourself only rolling one side if the other isn't tight.

For both foam rolling and stretching, you'll do 1 round through the moves you select. Consider doing just one or two moves for foam rolling if you're not doing a full-body workout, especially if you're short on time. For the dynamic stretches, pick two to six, depending on how much of a full-body workout you're doing.

For activation, you can do 1 to 3 rounds through one to four moves, depending on how much of a full-body workout you're doing and how stubborn the muscle group is. It's especially good to do a couple of rounds for glute activation.

FOAM ROLLING

Complete 1 round through the moves.

- 30 seconds to 1 minute (per side) **foam rolling move #1**
- 30 seconds to 1 minute (per side) **foam rolling move #2**
- 30 seconds to 1 minute (per side) **foam rolling move #3**
- 30 seconds to 1 minute (per side) **foam rolling move #4**

STRETCHING

Complete 1 round through the stretches.

- 30 seconds or 8 to 15 reps (per side) **dynamic stretch #1**
- 30 seconds or 8 to 15 reps (per side) **dynamic stretch #2**
- 30 seconds or 8 to 15 reps (per side) **dynamic stretch #3**
- 30 seconds or 8 to 15 reps (per side) **dynamic stretch #4**

ACTIVATION

Complete 1 to 3 rounds through the exercises. Pay attention to what you feel working; include rest and quickly address anything that's tight by doing a little bonus rolling.

- 30 seconds or 15 to 30 reps **activation exercise #1**
- 30 seconds or 15 to 30 reps **activation exercise #2**
- 30 seconds or 15 to 30 reps **activation exercise #3**
- 30 seconds or 15 to 30 reps **activation exercise #4**

NOTE: *For a whole library of additional moves and options, visit redefiningstrength.com/extras.*

LOWER BODY #1 WARM-UP

This lower body warm-up is perfect for a session focused on the posterior chain or glutes and hamstrings.

FOAM ROLLING
Complete 1 round through the moves.

- 30 seconds to 1 minute (per side) **quad foam rolling**
- 30 seconds to 1 minute (per side) **QL foam rolling**

STRETCHING
Complete 1 round through the stretches.

- 10 to 15 reps **bear squats to foot stretches**
- 10 to 15 reps (per side) **crescents to hamstring stretches**
- 8 to 12 reps (per side) **alternating pigeon poses**

ACTIVATION
Complete 1 or 2 rounds through the series. Do not rest between moves on the same side. Perform them all back to back, resting up to 30 seconds between rounds.

- 15 to 25 reps (per side) **side-lying series**

LOWER BODY #2 WARM-UP

This lower body warm-up is perfect for a session focused on the anterior chain or quads and adductors.

FOAM ROLLING
Complete 1 round through the moves.

- 30 seconds to 1 minute (per side) **hamstring foam rolling**
- 30 seconds to 1 minute (per side) **piriformis foam rolling**
- 30 seconds to 1 minute (per side) **calf foam rolling**

STRETCHING
Complete 1 round through the stretches.

- 10 to 15 reps (per side) **ankle mobility and groin stretches**
- 10 to 15 reps (per side) **bench hip stretches**
- 10 to 15 reps **dynamic squat stretches**

ACTIVATION
Complete 1 or 2 rounds through the exercises, resting up to 30 seconds between rounds.

- 30 seconds **wall sit**
- 30 seconds (per side) **side plank clams**
- 30 seconds **glute bridges with squeeze**

UPPER BODY #1 WARM-UP

This upper body warm-up is perfect for a session focused on the anterior chain or chest, shoulders, and triceps.

FOAM ROLLING
Complete 1 round through the moves.

- 30 seconds to 1 minute (per side) **levator scapulae foam rolling**
- 30 seconds to 1 minute (per side) **lat foam rolling**
- 30 seconds to 1 minute **thoracic extensions/upper back peanut foam rolling**

STRETCHING
Complete 1 round through the stretches.

- 30 seconds **wrist flexion stretches**
- 30 seconds (per side) **quadruped thoracic rotations**
- 30 seconds suspension **trainer snow angels**

ACTIVATION
Complete 1 or 2 rounds through the exercises, resting up to 30 seconds between rounds.

- 15 to 20 reps roller **serratus anterior extensions**
- 5 to 10 reps (per side) **halos***
- 15 to 20 reps **prone snow angels**

The reps are lower here because this move is deceptively hard, and it's better to do fewer and focus on that full range of motion!

UPPER BODY WARM-UP #2

This upper body warm-up is perfect for a session focused on the posterior chain or back, lats, and biceps.

FOAM ROLLING

Complete 1 round through the moves.

- 30 seconds to 1 minute (per side) **chest foam rolling**
- 30 seconds to 1 minute (per side) **teres minor foam rolling**

STRETCHING

Complete 1 round through the stretches.

- 30 seconds **wrist extension stretches**
- 30 seconds (per side) **half-kneeling thoracic rotations**
- 30 seconds **kneeling thoracic extensions and lat stretch**

ACTIVATION

Complete 1 or 2 rounds through the exercises, resting up to 30 seconds between rounds.

- 30 seconds (per side) **single-arm scapular push-ups**
- 30 seconds **planks with toe touches**
- 30 seconds **lying W pulldowns**

FULL-BODY WARM-UP #1

This full-body warm-up touches on key joints and muscles from head to toe.

FOAM ROLLING

Complete 1 round through the moves.

- 30 seconds to 1 minute (per side) **levator scapulae foam rolling**
- 30 seconds to 1 minute (per side) **TFL foam rolling**
- 30 seconds to 1 minute (per side) **QL foam rolling**

STRETCHING

Complete 1 round through the stretches.

- 10 to 15 reps **wrist extension stretches**
- 10 to 15 reps **bear squats to foot stretches**
- 8 to 15 reps (per side) **world's greatest stretches**
- 10 to 15 reps **inchworms**

ACTIVATION

Complete 1 or 2 rounds through the exercises, resting up to 30 seconds between rounds.

- 15 to 20 reps **camel bridges**
- 15 to 20 reps (per side) **fire hydrants**
- 15 to 20 reps **scapular wings**

FULL-BODY WARM-UP #2

This full-body warm-up touches on key joints and muscles from head to toe.

FOAM ROLLING

Complete 1 round through the moves.

- 30 seconds to 1 minute **thoracic extensions/upper back peanut foam rolling**
- 30 seconds to 1 minute (per side) **posterior adductor foam rolling**
- 30 seconds to 1 minute (per side) **peroneal foam rolling**

STRETCHING

Complete 1 round through the stretches.

- 30 seconds **standing hamstring and calf stretches**
- 30 seconds **standing quad stretches with reach**
- 30 seconds **side lunges with rotational reach**
- 30 seconds **wings chest stretches**

ACTIVATION

Complete 1 or 2 rounds through the exercises, resting up to 30 seconds between rounds.

- 30 seconds **sit-thrus to thoracic bridges**
- 30 seconds (per side) **3-way hip circles**
- 30 seconds **cobra wings**

ANTERIOR WARM-UP #1

This anterior warm-up is perfect for a session focused on building strength in your chest, shoulders, triceps, quads, and adductors.

FOAM ROLLING
Complete 1 round through the moves.

- 30 seconds to 1 minute (per side) lat foam rolling
- 30 seconds to 1 minute (per side) hamstring foam rolling

STRETCHING
Complete 1 round through the stretches.

- 8 to 12 reps (per side) 3-way leg swings
- 10 to 15 reps (per side) wrist flexion stretches
- 10 to 15 reps (per side) half-kneeling hip to hamstring stretches
- 10 to 15 reps suspension trainer snow angels

ACTIVATION
Complete 1 or 2 rounds through the exercises, resting up to 30 seconds between rounds.

- 30 seconds bulldog shoulder taps
- 30 seconds tabletop bridges
- 30 seconds seated leg rainbows

ANTERIOR WARM-UP #2

This anterior warm-up is perfect for a session focused on building strength in your chest, shoulders, triceps, quads, and adductors.

FOAM ROLLING
Complete 1 round through the moves.

- 30 seconds to 1 minute (per side) levator scapulae foam rolling
- 30 seconds to 1 minute (per side) piriformis foam rolling
- 30 seconds to 1 minute (per side) calf foam rolling

STRETCHING
Complete 1 round through the stretches.

- 30 seconds wrist extension stretches
- 30 seconds (per side) ankle mobility and groin stretches
- 30 seconds downward dogs to upward dogs
- 30 seconds dynamic squat stretches

ACTIVATION
Complete 1 or 2 rounds through the exercises, resting up to 30 seconds between rounds.

- 15 to 20 reps (per side) rock lunges
- 15 to 20 reps downward dog scapular presses
- 15 to 20 reps glute bridges with squeeze

POSTERIOR WARM-UP #1

This posterior warm-up is perfect for a session focused on building strength in your back, biceps, lats, glutes, and hamstrings.

FOAM ROLLING
Complete 1 round through the moves.

- 30 seconds to 1 minute (per side) chest foam rolling
- 30 seconds to 1 minute (per side) quad foam rolling
- 30 seconds to 1 minute (per side) QL foam rolling

STRETCHING
Complete 1 round through the stretches.

- 10 to 15 reps bear squats to foot stretches
- 10 to 15 reps wrist extension stretches
- 5 to 10 reps (per side) half-kneeling thoracic rotations*
- 10 to 15 reps (per side) crescents to hamstring stretches

ACTIVATION
Complete 1 or 2 rounds through the exercises, resting up to 30 seconds between rounds.

- 30 seconds (per side) plank with reaches back and out
- 30 seconds scapular wings
- 30 seconds frog bridges

*Because 1 rep includes both sides, the reps are lower for this move.

#2 POSTERIOR WARM-UP

This posterior warm-up is perfect for a session focused on building strength in your back, biceps, lats, glutes, and hamstrings.

FOAM ROLLING
Complete 1 round through the moves.

- 30 seconds to 1 minute (per side) teres minor foam rolling
- 30 seconds to 1 minute thoracic extensions/upper back peanut foam rolling
- 30 seconds to 1 minute (per side) TFL foam rolling

STRETCHING
Complete 1 round through the stretches.

- 30 seconds (per side) active foam roller star stretches
- 30 seconds wrist flexion stretches
- 30 seconds downward dogs to runner's lunges
- 30 seconds standing hamstring and calf stretches

ACTIVATION
Complete 1 or 2 rounds through the exercises, resting up to 30 seconds between rounds.

- 15 to 20 reps scapular push-ups
- 15 to 20 reps (per side) side plank clams
- 20 to 30 reps (per side) single-leg reverse hyperextensions

QUICK PREHAB WARM-UP #1

This full-body warm-up touches on key joints and muscles from head to toe.

FOAM ROLLING
Complete 1 round through the moves.

- 30 seconds (per side) chest foam rolling
- 30 seconds (per side) TFL foam rolling

STRETCHING
Complete 1 round through the stretches.

- 30 seconds (per side) world's greatest stretches

ACTIVATION
Complete 1 round through the exercises.

- 30 seconds camel bridges
- 30 seconds (per side) side plank clams
- 30 seconds lying W pulldowns

QUICK PREHAB WARM-UP #2

This full-body warm-up touches on key joints and muscles from head to toe.

FOAM ROLLING
Complete 1 round through the moves.

- 30 seconds (per side) levator scapulae foam rolling
- 30 seconds (per side) hamstring foam rolling

STRETCHING
Complete 1 round through the stretches.

- 30 seconds dynamic squat stretches
- 30 seconds inchworms

ACTIVATION
Complete 1 round through the exercises.

- 30 seconds downward dog scapular presses
- 30 seconds sit-thrus to thoracic bridges
- 30 seconds glute bridges with squeeze

Use this template to customize your cooldowns to what you need. The point of a cooldown is to help everything relax after your workout. First, you stretch, then you foam roll. Focus on deep inhales and long exhales as you hold the stretch or relax on the trigger point tool. Do not tense through the stretch or while rolling.

For both stretching and foam rolling, you'll do 1 round through the moves you select. For the stretches, pick two to six, depending on how full-body your workout was. Focus more on static stretching variations. Consider doing just one or two moves for foam rolling if you didn't do a full-body workout, especially if you're short on time. Address not only the muscles that feel tight from being worked in the session but also areas you know may impact your next workout.

STRETCHING
Complete 1 round through the stretches.
- 30 seconds to 1 minute (per side) **static stretch #1**
- 30 seconds to 1 minute (per side) **static stretch #2**
- 30 seconds to 1 minute (per side) **static stretch #3**
- 30 seconds to 1 minute (per side) **static stretch #4**

FOAM ROLLING
Complete 1 round through the moves.
- 30 seconds to 1 minute (per side) **foam rolling move #1**
- 30 seconds to 1 minute (per side) **foam rolling move #2**
- 30 seconds to 1 minute (per side) **foam rolling move #3**
- 30 seconds to 1 minute (per side) **foam rolling move #4**

NOTE: *For a whole library of additional moves and options, visit redefiningstrength.com/extras.*

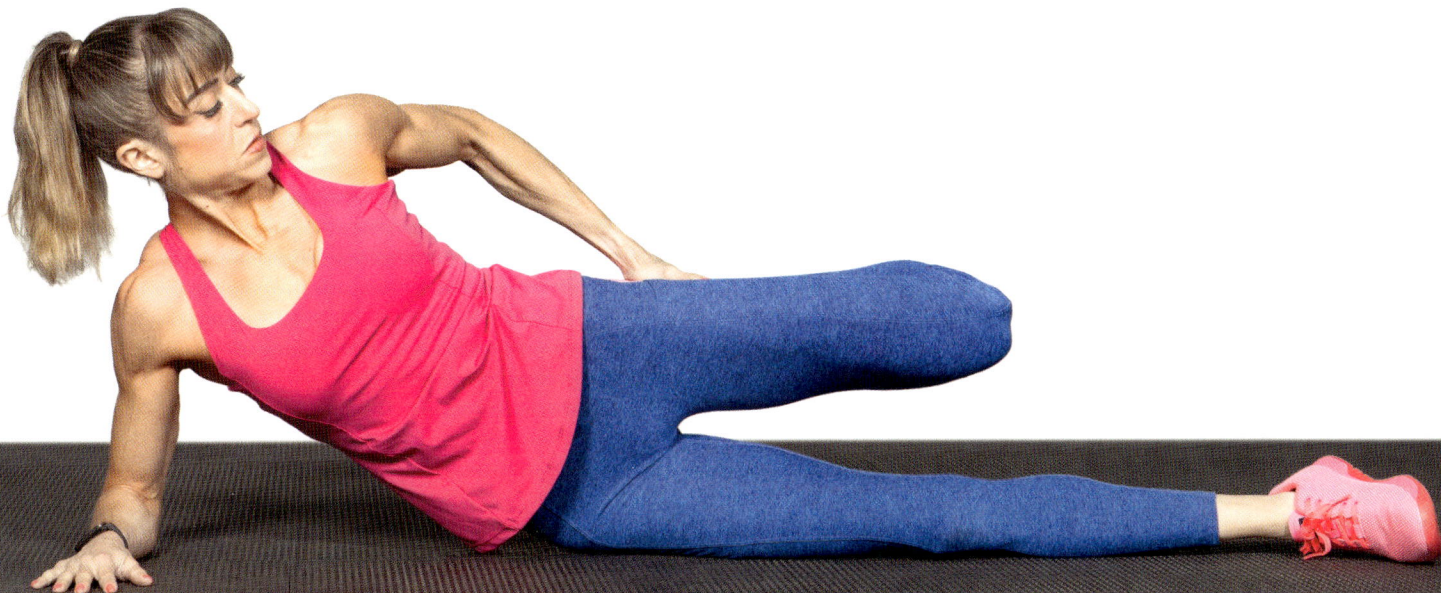

LOWER BODY COOLDOWN #1

This lower body cooldown is perfect for a session focused on the posterior chain or glutes and hamstrings.

STRETCHING
Complete 1 round through the stretches.
- 30 seconds to 1 minute standing **forward bend**
- 30 seconds to 1 minute (per side) **figure 4 wall stretch**

FOAM ROLLING
Complete 1 round through the moves.
- 30 seconds to 1 minute (per side) **piriformis foam rolling**
- 30 seconds to 1 minute (per side) **hamstring foam rolling**

LOWER BODY COOLDOWN #2

This lower body cooldown is perfect for a session focused on the anterior chain or quads and adductors.

STRETCHING
Complete 1 round through the stretches.
- 30 seconds to 1 minute **frog stretch**
- 30 seconds to 1 minute (per side) **side-lying quad stretch**

FOAM ROLLING
Complete 1 round through the moves.
- 30 seconds to 1 minute (per side) **quad foam rolling**
- 30 seconds to 1 minute (per side) **calf foam rolling**

UPPER BODY COOLDOWN #1

This upper body cooldown is perfect for a session focused on the anterior chain or chest, shoulders, and triceps.

STRETCHING
Complete 1 round through the stretches.
- 30 seconds to 1 minute (per side) **standing chest stretch**
- 30 seconds to 1 minute (per side) **overhead triceps stretch**

FOAM ROLLING
Complete 1 round through the moves.
- 30 seconds to 1 minute (per side) **teres minor foam rolling**
- 30 seconds to 1 minute (per side) **triceps foam rolling**

UPPER BODY COOLDOWN #2

This upper body cooldown is perfect for a session focused on the posterior chain or back, lats, and biceps.

STRETCHING
Complete 1 round through the stretches.
- 30 seconds to 1 minute **thread-the-needle stretch**
- 30 seconds to 1 minute (per side) **child's pose with reach—external rotation**

FOAM ROLLING
Complete 1 round through the moves.
- 30 seconds to 1 minute (per side) **lat foam rolling**
- 30 seconds to 1 minute **thoracic extension/ upper back peanut foam rolling**

FULL-BODY COOLDOWN #1

This full-body cooldown touches on key joints and muscles from head to toe.

STRETCHING

Complete 1 round through the stretches.

- 30 seconds to 1 minute (per side) **standing chest stretch**
- 30 seconds to 1 minute (per side) **half-kneeling TFL stretch**
- 30 seconds to 1 minute **thread-the-needle stretch**

FOAM ROLLING

Complete 1 round through the moves.

- 30 seconds to 1 minute (per side) **quad foam rolling**
- 30 seconds to 1 minute (per side) **QL foam rolling**
- 30 seconds to 1 minute (per side) **levator scapulae foam rolling**

FULL-BODY COOLDOWN #2

This full-body cooldown touches on key joints and muscles from head to toe.

STRETCHING

Complete 1 round through the stretches.

- 30 seconds to 1 minute **half wall hang**
- 30 seconds to 1 minute (per side) **lying QL stretch**
- 30 seconds to 1 minute **frog stretch**

FOAM ROLLING

Complete 1 round through the moves.

- 30 seconds to 1 minute (per side) **piriformis foam rolling**
- 30 seconds to 1 minute **thoracic extension/ upper back peanut foam rolling**
- 30 seconds to 1 minute (per side) **chest foam rolling**

ANTERIOR COOLDOWN #1

This anterior cooldown is perfect for a session focused on building strength in your chest, shoulders, triceps, quads, and adductors.

STRETCHING

Complete 1 round through the stretches.

- 30 seconds to 1 minute (per side) **standing chest stretch**
- 30 seconds to 1 minute (per side) **half-kneeling TFL stretch**

FOAM ROLLING

Complete 1 round through the moves.

- 30 seconds to 1 minute (per side) **quad foam rolling**
- 30 seconds to 1 minute (per side) **triceps foam rolling**

ANTERIOR COOLDOWN #2

This anterior cooldown is perfect for a session focused on building strength in your chest, shoulders, triceps, quads, and adductors.

STRETCHING

Complete 1 round through the stretches.

- 30 seconds to 1 minute (per side) **overhead triceps stretch**
- 30 seconds to 1 minute **foam roller snow angels**
- 30 seconds to 1 minute (per side) **side-lying quad stretch**

FOAM ROLLING

Complete 1 round through the moves.

- 30 seconds to 1 minute (per side) **TFL foam rolling**
- 30 seconds to 1 minute (per side) **adductor foam rolling**
- 30 seconds to 1 minute (per side) **chest foam rolling**

POSTERIOR COOLDOWN #1

This posterior cooldown is perfect for a session focused on building strength in your back, biceps, lats, glutes, and hamstrings.

STRETCHING
Complete 1 round through the stretches.

- 30 seconds to 1 minute **thread-the-needle stretch**
- 30 seconds to 1 minute (per side) **figure 4 wall stretch**

FOAM ROLLING
Complete 1 round through the moves.

- 30 seconds to 1 minute (per side) **lat foam rolling**
- 30 seconds to 1 minute (per side) **hamstring foam rolling**

POSTERIOR COOLDOWN #2

This posterior cooldown is perfect for a session focused on building strength in your back, biceps, lats, glutes, and hamstrings.

STRETCHING
Complete 1 round through the stretches.

- 30 seconds to 1 minute **standing forward bend**
- 30 seconds to 1 minute **child's pose with reach—external rotation**
- 30 seconds to 1 minute (per side) **star stretch**

FOAM ROLLING
Complete 1 round through the moves.

- 30 seconds to 1 minute (per side) **lat foam rolling**
- 30 seconds to 1 minute (per side) **QL foam rolling**
- 30 seconds to 1 minute (per side) **hamstring foam rolling**

QUICK PREHAB COOLDOWN #1

This full-body cooldown touches on key joints and muscles from head to toe, focusing a bit more on the posterior chain.

STRETCHING
Complete 1 round through the stretches.

- 20 to 30 seconds per move in the series (per side) **seated hamstring and spinal twist complex**

FOAM ROLLING
Complete 1 round through the moves.

- 30 seconds to 1 minute **thoracic extension/upper back peanut foam rolling**
- 30 seconds to 1 minute (per side) **TFL foam rolling**

QUICK PREHAB COOLDOWN #2

This full-body cooldown touches on key joints and muscles from head to toe, focusing a bit more on the anterior chain.

STRETCHING
Complete 1 round through the stretches.

- 30 seconds to 1 minute (per side) **star stretch with quad stretch**

FOAM ROLLING
Complete 1 round through the moves.

- 30 seconds to 1 minute (per side) **quad foam rolling**
- 30 seconds to 1 minute (per side) **chest foam rolling**

30 DON'T SKIP THE RECOVERY

Rest doesn't mean doing nothing. An object in motion stays in motion, so taking time to "actively" recover can be key to maintaining your forward momentum while addressing the culprits that could lead to overload and injury.

Full rest—aka doing nothing—is sometimes needed, but it doesn't truly correct the compensations or imbalances you have. Compensations happen when muscles try to "take over" the work of performing a move when they shouldn't. For example, you might feel your hamstrings compensating for your glutes in a glute bridge. I don't want to demonize taking a day on the couch, because that form of rest can be needed mentally and physically. But the recovery weeks and days I discuss in this chapter can help you train harder and see better results faster. They prep your body for work and keep you in a positive success mindset.

Over the course of your weekly schedule, you'll normally see one or two recovery workouts listed. If you can't get to them, substitute with a prehab workout on page 288 or use one of the bonus mobility workouts at redefiningstrength.com/extras. But when possible, use the full sessions, including walks, longer runs, or SIT after.

Cycling the intensity levels and areas worked throughout your weekly schedule is key to maximizing every moment you spend training. But even if you're consistent with your weekly prehab work, you may still need a week off.

Changing your workout progression every three to six weeks can be a way to step back and recover. During the first week with a new progression, you'll find you do lower intensity to get comfortable with the new series and moves. You can also use the bodyweight timed strength progressions for a week as a break after intensive heavy lifting in the gym. Don't be afraid to include one of the recovery week schedules every six to twelve weeks as needed or after an "accelerator" phase where you've used an extra-intensive progression for three or four weeks.

Life is messy, so you can time the recovery weeks to coincide with vacations or stressful, busy times at work or in your personal life. Allowing yourself to back off when you're facing burnout is just as important as being flexible and pushing hard when you feel good. Don't stress about having to include a recovery week at set points. Listen to what your body and lifestyle demand. Own when you need to recover mentally more than physically!

In the next section, I give you schedules for recovery weeks with three to five days of training. All of these individual recovery workouts can be used in your weekly schedule once you've selected your progression. Remember that these workouts aren't necessarily "easy"; they're challenging in a way that enables you to focus on mobility, stability, and flexibility with an emphasis on the mind-body connection and recruitment patterns.

RECOVERY WEEK SCHEDULES

With all of these schedules, going on casual walks and upping your steps—even on days "off"—can be amazingly beneficial for results, overall stress management, and hormonal balance. Also consider other fun activities you may not normally do that get you out and active!

Next, I'll share some builders so you can design your own recovery routine and workouts to use with these schedules. Each builder includes the full prehab process, with activation often being isometric holds.

If you're taking a break from a muscle-building phase, don't be afraid to add some SIT sessions, but don't start adding a ton of long-distance training. In a fat-loss phase, walk frequently while also including some SIT.

The isometrics, or holds done for activation, are as close to yoga as many of us non-yoga people get. However, if you enjoy yoga, it can be a great option for recovery weeks! The isometric moves are yoga-esque, but they may have different cues and a different focus than when you've previously done them in routines. When you read the exercise descriptions, note the emphasis on activation and pay attention to that mind-body connection as you hold. (In this way, holds can help people who aren't very zen!) You'll see other activation exercises included as well.

3 DAYS A WEEK	4 DAYS A WEEK	5 DAYS A WEEK
DAY 1	**DAY 1**	**DAY 1**
Isos circuit	Isos circuit	Isos circuit
DAY 2	**DAY 2**	**DAY 2**
Off	Recovery trisets	Recovery trisets
DAY 3	**DAY 3**	**DAY 3**
Strength isos	Off	Isos +
DAY 4	**DAY 4**	**DAY 4**
Off	Strength isos	Off
DAY 5	**DAY 5**	**DAY 5**
Recovery +	Recovery +	Strength isos
DAY 6	**DAY 6**	**DAY 6**
Off	Off	Recovery +
DAY 7	**DAY 7**	**DAY 7**
Off	Off	Off

RECOVERY/ISOMETRIC CIRCUIT
WORKOUT BUILDER

With this template, you can create a fundamental recovery workout using activation moves or isometrics. The focus is on getting the correct muscles working as you build stability and strength through a full range of motion. After the activation moves or isometrics—which can be full-body or focused on one area—you can include a quick, optional burner for a stubborn muscle group and/or a SIT session or walk.

FOAM ROLLING

Complete 1 round through the moves. You can include up to six moves; this is your time to prehab!

30 seconds to 1 minute (per side) foam rolling moves #1 through #6

STRETCHING

Complete 1 round through the stretches. You can include up to six stretches; this is your time to prehab!

30 seconds to 1 minute or 8 to 15 reps (per side) dynamic stretches #1 through #6

ACTIVATION/ISOMETRICS CIRCUIT

Complete 2 to 6 rounds through the circuit, resting 20 seconds to 2 minutes between rounds. Use the rest periods to quickly address anything that is tight by doing a little bonus rolling. You can include four to six moves in a circuit to alternate the areas worked. You can do reps, but intervals of work are often best for focusing on the muscles you feel working, even if you're doing activation exercises rather than isometrics.

20 seconds to 1 minute isometric/activation exercises #1 through #6

Optional BURNER

For any recovery or isometric + workout, you can include a more challenging but very quick burner. This may target your glutes, abs, back, arms—any stubborn muscle group. As a rule, it should take you about 5 minutes to complete 1 to 3 rounds through the burner. (I share a killer booty burner on page 299!) Work for 20 to 40 seconds or do 15 to 30 reps per move.

Optional SIT OR WALK

COOLDOWN STRETCHING

Complete 1 round through the stretches. You can include up to four stretches; this is your time to prehab!

30 seconds to 1 minute (per side) static stretches #1 through #4

COOLDOWN

STRENGTH ISOMETRIC
WORKOUT BUILDER

With this template, you can design a density intervals recovery workout that uses a combination of isometrics and activation moves for reps. Moves for the same area are performed back to back, and you will move through different areas over the series.

FOAM ROLLING
Complete 1 round through the moves. You can include up to six moves; this is your time to prehab!

30 seconds to 1 minute (per side) foam rolling moves #1 through #6

STRETCHING
Complete 1 round through the stretches. You can include up to six stretches; this is your time to prehab!

30 seconds to 1 minute or 8 to 15 reps (per side) dynamic stretches #1 through #6

STRENGTH ISOMETRICS SERIES
Complete 2 to 6 rounds through the series, resting 20 seconds to 2 minutes between rounds. Use the rest periods to quickly address anything that is tight by doing a little bonus rolling. You can include six, eight, or ten moves; two moves will be performed for each area back to back.

- 20 seconds to 1 minute **isometric hold #1**
- 20 seconds to 1 minute **activation reps #1**
- 20 seconds to 1 minute **isometric hold #2 (different muscle group)**
- 20 seconds to 1 minute **activation reps #2**
- 20 seconds to 1 minute **isometric hold #3 (different muscle group)**
- 20 seconds to 1 minute **activation reps #3**
- 20 seconds to 1 minute **isometric hold #4 (different muscle group)**
- 20 seconds to 1 minute **activation reps #4**
- 20 seconds to 1 minute **isometric hold #5 (different muscle group)**
- 20 seconds to 1 minute **activation reps #5**

Optional SIT or WALK

COOLDOWN STRETCHING
Complete 1 round through the stretches. You can include up to four stretches; this is your time to prehab!

30 seconds to 1 minute (per side) static stretches #1 through #4

COOLDOWN FOAM ROLLING
Complete 1 round through the moves. You can include up to four moves; this is your time to prehab!

30 seconds to 1 minute (per side) foam rolling moves #1 through #4

RECOVERY/ISOMETRIC TRISETS
WORKOUT BUILDER

With this template, you can design a trisets recovery workout. You may use a combination of isometrics and activation moves for reps.

FOAM ROLLING

Complete 1 round through the moves. You can include up to six moves; this is your time to prehab!

30 seconds to 1 minute (per side) foam rolling moves #1 through #6

STRETCHING

Complete 1 round through the stretches. You can include up to six stretches; this is your time to prehab!

30 seconds to 1 minute or 8 to 15 reps (per side) dynamic stretches #1 through #6

ACTIVATION

Complete 2 to 6 rounds through each triset, resting 20 seconds to 2 minutes between rounds and trisets. Use the rest periods to quickly address anything that's tight by doing a little bonus rolling. You can include 1 to 4 trisets with three moves each.

TRISET #1
30 seconds isometric/activation exercises #1 through #3

TRISET #2
30 seconds isometric/activation exercises #1 through #3

TRISET #3
30 seconds isometric/activation exercises #1 through #3

TRISET #4
30 seconds isometric/activation exercises #1 through #3

Optional SIT or WALK

COOLDOWN STRETCHING

Complete 1 round through the stretches. You can include up to four stretches; this is your time to prehab!

30 seconds to 1 minute (per side) static stretches #1 through #4

COOLDOWN FOAM ROLLING

Complete 1 round through the moves. You can include up to four moves; this is your time to prehab!

30 seconds to 1 minute (per side) foam rolling moves #1 through #4

ISOS **CIRCUIT**

FOAM ROLLING
Complete 1 round through the moves.

- 30 seconds to 1 minute (per side) **chest foam rolling**
- 30 seconds to 1 minute (per side) **TFL foam rolling**
- 30 seconds to 1 minute (per side) **QL foam rolling**

STRETCHING
Complete 1 round through the stretches.

- 10 to 15 reps **wrist extension stretches**
- 10 to 15 reps **bear squats to foot stretches**
- 8 to 15 reps (per side) **world's greatest stretches**

ISOMETRICS CIRCUIT
Complete 3 to 5 rounds through the circuit, resting up to 90 seconds between rounds. Use the rest periods to quickly address anything that's tight by doing a little bonus rolling.

- 30 seconds (per side) **single-leg deadlift hold**
- 30 seconds **scapular wall hold**
- 30 seconds (per side) **extended twisting triangle**
- 30 seconds (per side) **side plank hold**
- 30 seconds **glute bridge hold**
- 30 seconds **banana**

Optional SIT or WALK

COOLDOWN STRETCHING
Complete 1 round through the stretches.

- 30 seconds to 1 minute **thread-the-needle stretches**
- 30 seconds to 1 minute (per side) **figure 4 wall stretch**

COOLDOWN FOAM ROLLING
Complete 1 round through the moves.

- 30 seconds to 1 minute (per side) **piriformis foam rolling**
- 30 seconds to 1 minute **thoracic extensions/ upper back peanut foam rolling**

STRENGTH ISOS

FOAM ROLLING
Complete 1 round through the moves.

- 30 seconds to 1 minute (per side) **lat foam rolling**
- 30 seconds to 1 minute (per side) **hamstring foam rolling**
- 30 seconds to 1 minute (per side) **calf foam rolling**

STRETCHING
Complete 1 round through the stretches.

- 10 to 15 reps (per side) **wrist flexion stretches**
- 10 to 15 reps (per side) **ankle mobility and groin stretches**
- 10 to 15 reps **dynamic squat stretches**
- 10 to 15 reps **wings chest stretches**

STRENGTH ISOMETRICS SERIES
Complete 3 to 5 rounds through the series, resting up to 90 seconds between rounds. Use the rest periods to quickly address anything that's tight by doing a little bonus rolling. For the lunge holds and rock lunges, you can make things more challenging by completing both on one side before switching.

- 30 seconds **wall sit**
- 30 seconds **squat pulses**
- 30 seconds **push-up holds**
- 30 seconds **push-ups plus**
- 30 seconds (per side) **lunge hold**
- 30 seconds (per side) **rock lunges**
- 30 seconds **seated hinge hold**
- 30 seconds **hinge and twists**

Optional SIT or WALK

COOLDOWN STRETCHING
Complete 1 round through the stretches.

- 30 seconds to 1 minute (per side) **standing chest stretch**
- 30 seconds to 1 minute (per side) **side-lying quad stretch**

COOLDOWN FOAM ROLLING
Complete 1 round through the moves.

- 30 seconds to 1 minute (per side) **TFL foam rolling**
- 30 seconds to 1 minute (per side) **chest foam rolling**

RECOVERY +

FOAM ROLLING
Complete 1 round through the moves.

- 30 seconds to 1 minute (per side) **levator scapulae foam rolling**
- 30 seconds to 1 minute (per side) **teres minor foam rolling**
- 30 seconds to 1 minute (per side) **quad foam rolling**

STRETCHING
Complete 1 round through the stretches.

- 30 seconds **standing hamstring and calf stretches**
- 30 seconds **standing quad stretches with reach**
- 30 seconds **side lunges with rotational reach**
- 30 seconds **downward dogs to upward dogs**

ACTIVATION CIRCUIT
Complete 2 to 4 rounds through the circuit, resting up to 90 seconds between rounds. Use the rest periods to quickly address anything that's tight by doing a little bonus rolling. Focus on the muscles you feel working rather than rushing through these moves. After you complete all rounds of the circuit, use the bonus booty burner for that little extra before any cardio you choose to include.

- 30 seconds (per side) **standing 3-way hip circles**
- 30 seconds (per side) **single-arm scapular push-ups**
- 30 seconds **camel bridges**
- 30 seconds **downward dog scapular presses**
- 30 seconds (per side) **side plank clams**
- 30 seconds **cobra wings**

BONUS BOOTY BURNER
Complete a ladder through these two moves, doing them back to back and resting only as needed. Start with 15 reps of each move; then do 14, 13, and so on until you get to 1 rep of each. You will need to pause occasionally, but try to complete the burner as quickly as you can.

- 15 to 1 reps **mini band glute bridges**
- 15 to 1 reps **mini band bridge hold with abductions**

Optional SIT or WALK

COOLDOWN STRETCHING
Complete 1 round through the stretches.

- 20 to 30 seconds per move (per side) **seated hamstring and spinal twist complex**

COOLDOWN FOAM ROLLING
Complete 1 round through the moves.

- 30 seconds to 1 minute (per side) **piriformis foam rolling**
- 30 seconds to 1 minute **thoracic extensions/upper back peanut foam rolling**

RECOVERY TRISETS

FOAM ROLLING
Complete 1 round through the moves.

- 30 seconds to 1 minute (per side) **lat foam rolling**
- 30 seconds to 1 minute (per side) **hamstring foam rolling**
- 30 seconds to 1 minute (per side) **calf foam rolling**

STRETCHING
Complete 1 round through the stretches.

- 10 to 15 reps (per side) **wrist flexion stretches**
- 10 to 15 reps (per side) **ankle mobility and groin stretches**
- 10 to 15 reps **dynamic squat stretches**
- 10 to 15 reps **wings chest stretches**

ACTIVATION
Complete 2 to 4 rounds through each triset, resting 30 seconds to 1 minute between rounds and trisets. Rest may be longer to quickly address anything that's tight by doing a little bonus rolling.

TRISET #1
- 30 seconds **sumo squat hold**
- 30 seconds **dip hold**
- 30 seconds **extended plank hold**

TRISET #2
- 30 seconds **halos**
- 30 seconds **bulldog shoulder taps**
- 30 seconds **seated leg rainbows**

TRISET #3
- 30 seconds **2-way reach skater lunges**
- 30 seconds **prone snow angels**
- 30 seconds **glute bridges with squeeze**

Optional SIT or WALK

COOLDOWN STRETCHING
Complete 1 round through the stretches.

- 30 seconds to 1 minute (per side) **overhead triceps stretch**
- 30 seconds to 1 minute (per side) **lying QL stretch**

COOLDOWN FOAM ROLLING
Complete 1 round through the moves.

- 30 seconds to 1 minute (per side) **adductor foam rolling**
- 30 seconds to 1 minute (per side) **levator scapulae foam rolling**

ISOS +

FOAM ROLLING
Complete 1 round through the moves.

- 30 seconds to 1 minute (per side) **levator scapulae foam rolling**
- 30 seconds to 1 minute (per side) **teres minor foam rolling**
- 30 seconds to 1 minute (per side) **quad foam rolling**

STRETCHING
Complete 1 round through the stretches.

- 30 seconds **standing hamstring and calf stretches**
- 30 seconds **standing quad stretches with reach**
- 30 seconds **side lunges with rotational reach**
- 30 seconds **downward dogs to upward dogs**

ISOMETRICS CIRCUIT
Complete 3 to 5 rounds through the circuit, resting up to 90 seconds between rounds. Use the rest periods to quickly address anything that's tight by doing a little bonus rolling. After you complete all rounds of the circuit, use the bonus core burner for that little extra before any cardio you choose to include.

- 30 seconds (per side) **side lunge hold**
- 30 seconds **lying scapular hold**
- 30 seconds (per side) **80/20 hip thrust hold**
- 30 seconds (per side) **side plank hold**
- 30 seconds **cobra hold**

BONUS CORE BURNER
Complete 2 or 3 rounds through the burner without resting.

- 20 to 30 seconds **plange plank**
- 20 to 30 seconds (per side) **side plank oblique twists**
- 20 to 30 seconds **full-body crunches**
- 20 to 30 seconds **frog bridges**

Optional SIT or WALK

COOLDOWN STRETCHING
Complete 1 round through the stretches.

- 30 seconds to 1 minute (per side) **star stretch with quad stretch**

COOLDOWN FOAM ROLLING
Complete 1 round through the moves.

- 30 seconds to 1 minute (per side) **piriformis foam rolling**
- 30 seconds to 1 minute (per side) **teres minor foam rolling**

EXERCISE LIBRARY

This exercise library includes cues and instructions for each move as well as tips to help you modify the movements. In some places, I also offer exercise swaps. These are moves that can be substituted for each other because they have a similar focus. You can use them for areas you need to target more or to modify around aches and pains. I list some static stretches to substitute for dynamic stretches if you want to work on extra flexibility.

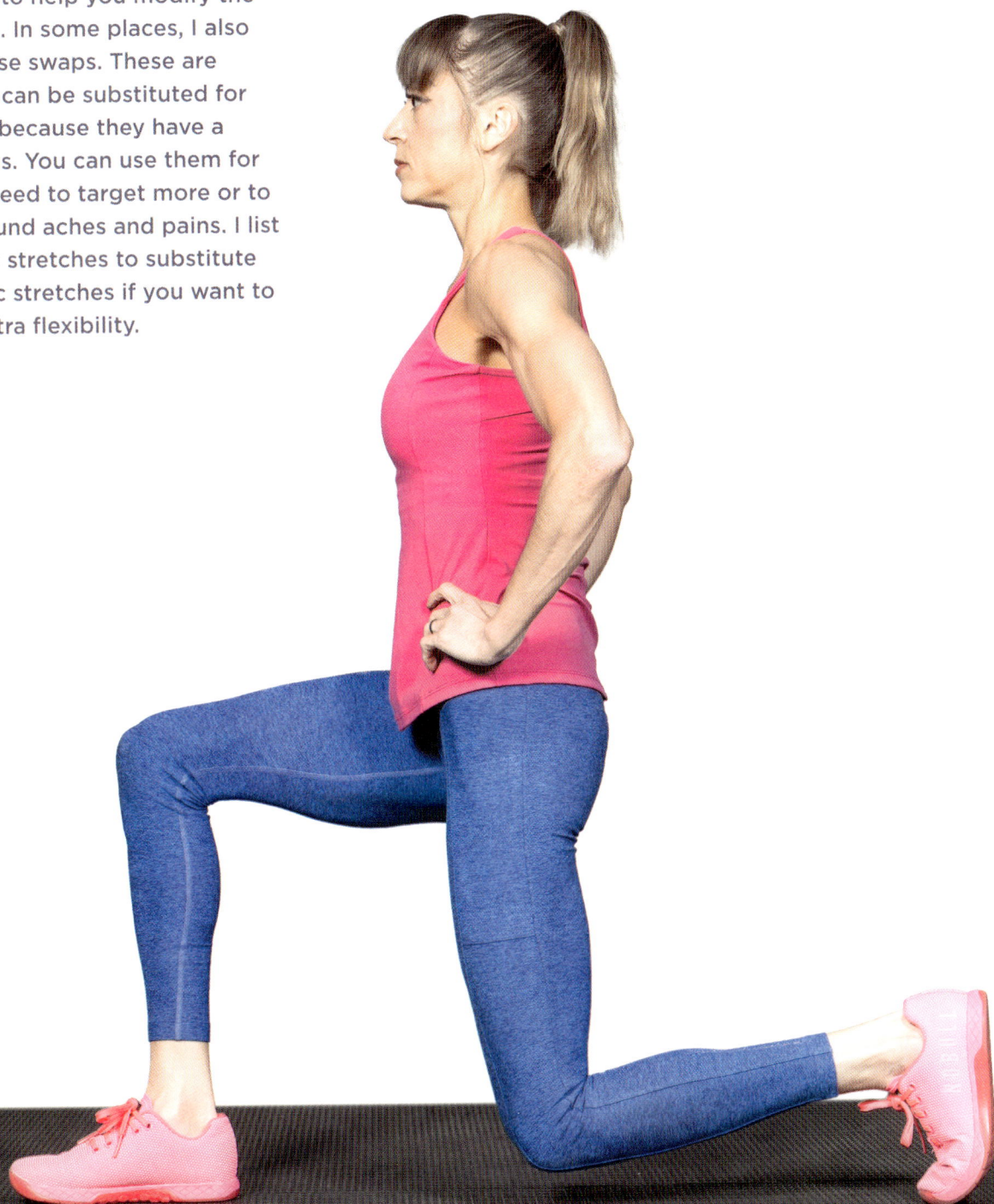

FOAM ROLLING

I recommend a specific rolling tool for each of the moves in this section: ball, roller, peanut, or hand-held roller. Each of these tools applies a different amount of pressure. The harder and smaller the object, the more pressure you can apply. Using a softer or larger ball applies less pressure. One tool for lighter pressure is a foam posture ball, which is about 6 to 8 inches in diameter. The same guidelines about pressure go for rollers: A harder roller with more knobs applies more pressure, whereas a softer, smooth roller applies less.

A hand-held roller also gives you more control over pressure and can be great if you can't get down to the ground to roll. Another tool is a peanut, which you can create by tying two balls in a sock or taping them together. With a peanut, you can roll the muscles on either side of your spine. Unless otherwise noted, you can decide which tool you want to use for any of these techniques.

Aside from using different tools to change the pressure level, you can adjust by placing the tool between your body and a bench or wall instead of on the floor.

As you're rolling, you'll be able to identify where especially tight spots are. Don't roll back and forth quickly over those locations. Instead, pause on those spots and deeply exhale; pausing and focusing on the tight area can help the muscle relax and release. Also try rocking slightly side to side on the spot. Tense the muscle with an inhale, hold, and then exhale as you relax the muscle. Do 3 to 5 breaths while at a tight spot and then find another spot and hold.

QUAD

Lie over a roller with it under the front of your thighs. Prop yourself on your forearms and shift your weight left or right to focus on one leg. Roll until the roller is just above your knee and then roll the opposite direction to the top of your thigh.

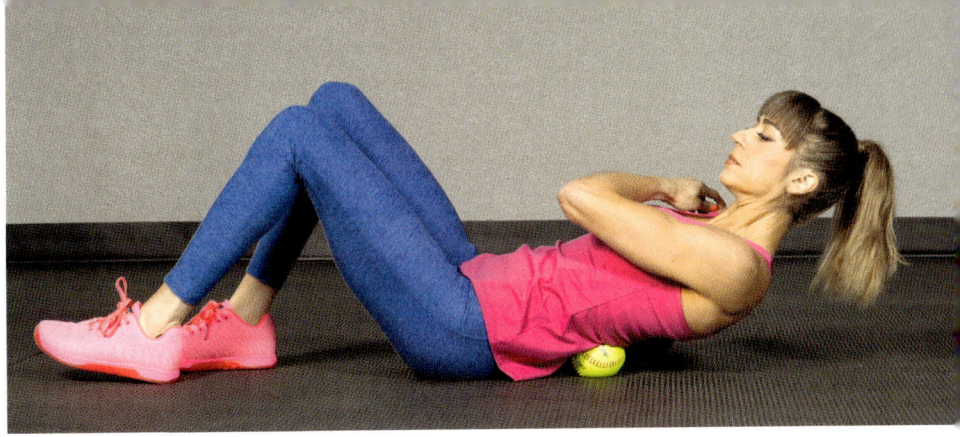

QL

Locate the bottom of your rib cage on your back, just to the side of your spine and at the top of your ilium (the back of your pelvic bone). Between these two points is your quadratus lumborum—what we in the biz call the QL. Hold a ball under your rib cage and then lie back with the ball underneath you. Relax over the ball and breathe. Then move the ball down a bit toward your pelvis and relax again. Take 3 to 5 slow, deep breaths as you relax over the ball before moving it to another spot.

NOTE: *A roller is not recommended. You can also swap in a peanut to cradle your spine and roll out your lower back at the same time.*

HAMSTRING

Sit on a ball on a bench or chair with the ball at the top of your hamstring, right under your butt. Rock very slightly side to side on the ball. Then extend your leg out straight and bring your foot back toward the floor. As you relax your leg back down, exhale to help the muscle relax and release.

You can roll down the entire back of your leg from your inner thigh toward your iliotibial (IT) band to find any tight spots. Don't roll the back of your knee.

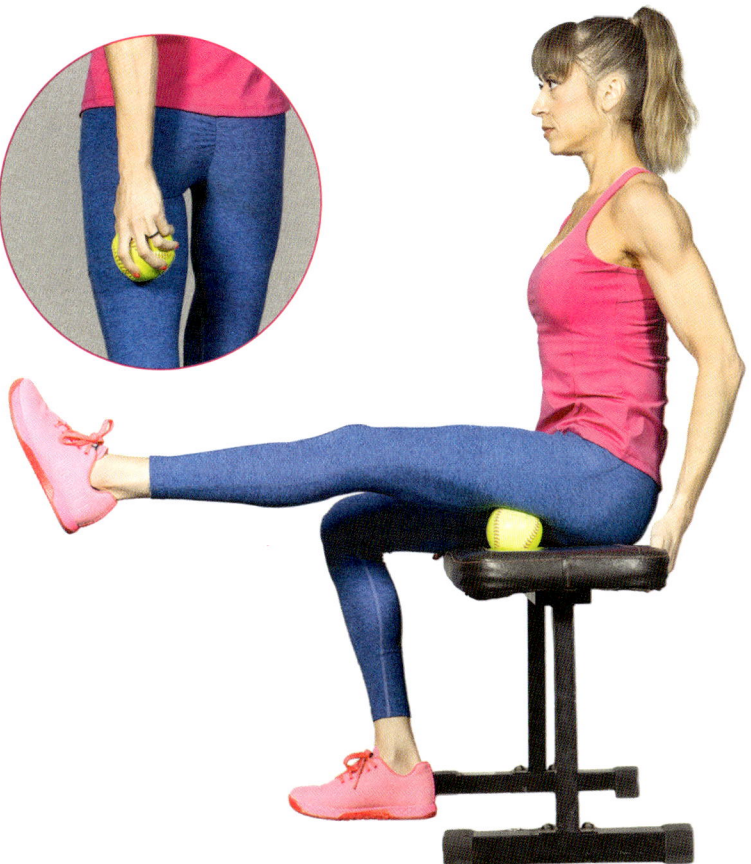

PIRIFORMIS

Find where the top of your back jeans pocket would be on your butt and place a ball at that spot. Stretch out on your side on the ground, with your hand or forearm propping you on the ball. Relax and move to roll the ball toward your tailbone and then out toward the side of your hip. (You can also explore the full glute muscle.)

When you find a tight spot, bend your knee toward your chest and then restraighten your leg. You can also lift and lower your leg when the ball is on a tender area to tense and relax the muscle. Breathe and relax into the pressure of the ball. Repeat about 5 to 10 movements of your leg; then hold on another spot.

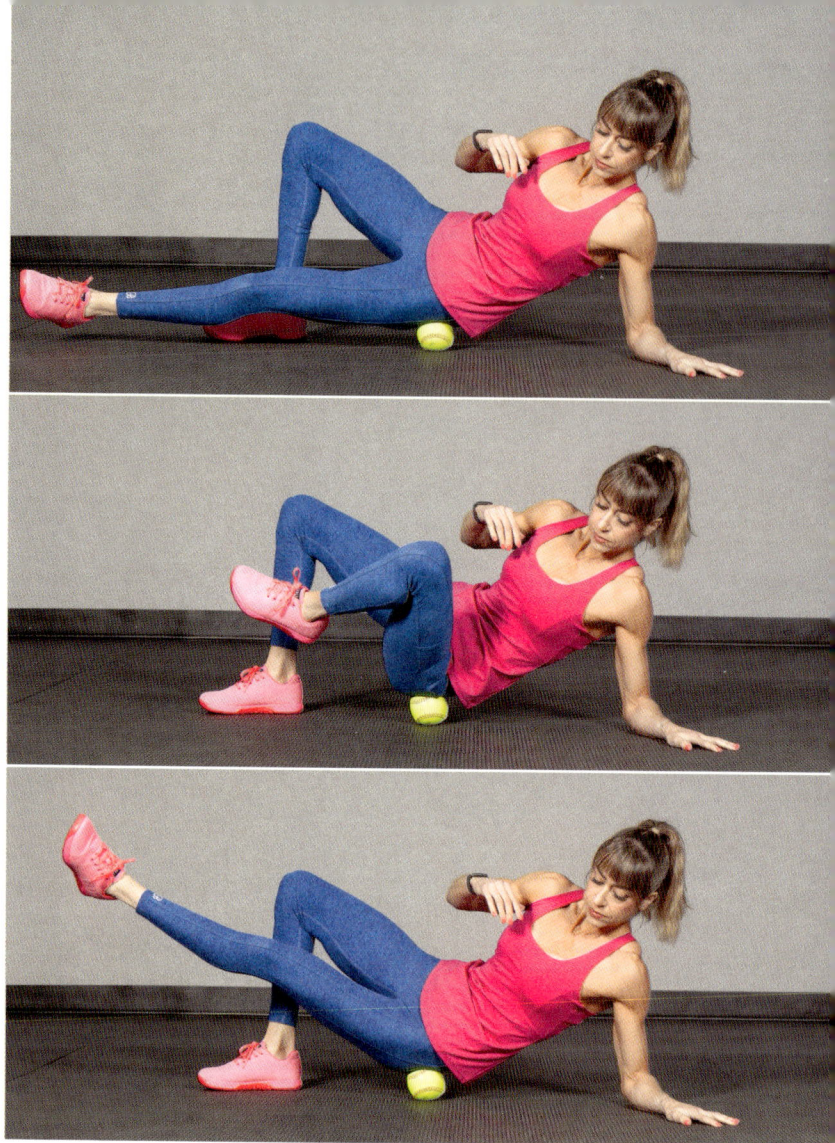

CALF

Place the back of your lower leg (right below the knee) on the roller. Cross your other leg over it to apply a bit more pressure. Rock side to side and roll toward your ankle and then back toward your knee to pinpoint any tight spots. As you breathe, flex and relax (or circle) your foot to tense and release the muscle as you hold. Do 5 to 10 circles or flexes and then move to a different spot and hold, working from the inside of your lower leg to the outside.

MODIFICATIONS: Set a ball on the floor or on top of a yoga block, to dig in more. If you prefer, you can place both legs on the roller to hit both at the same time.

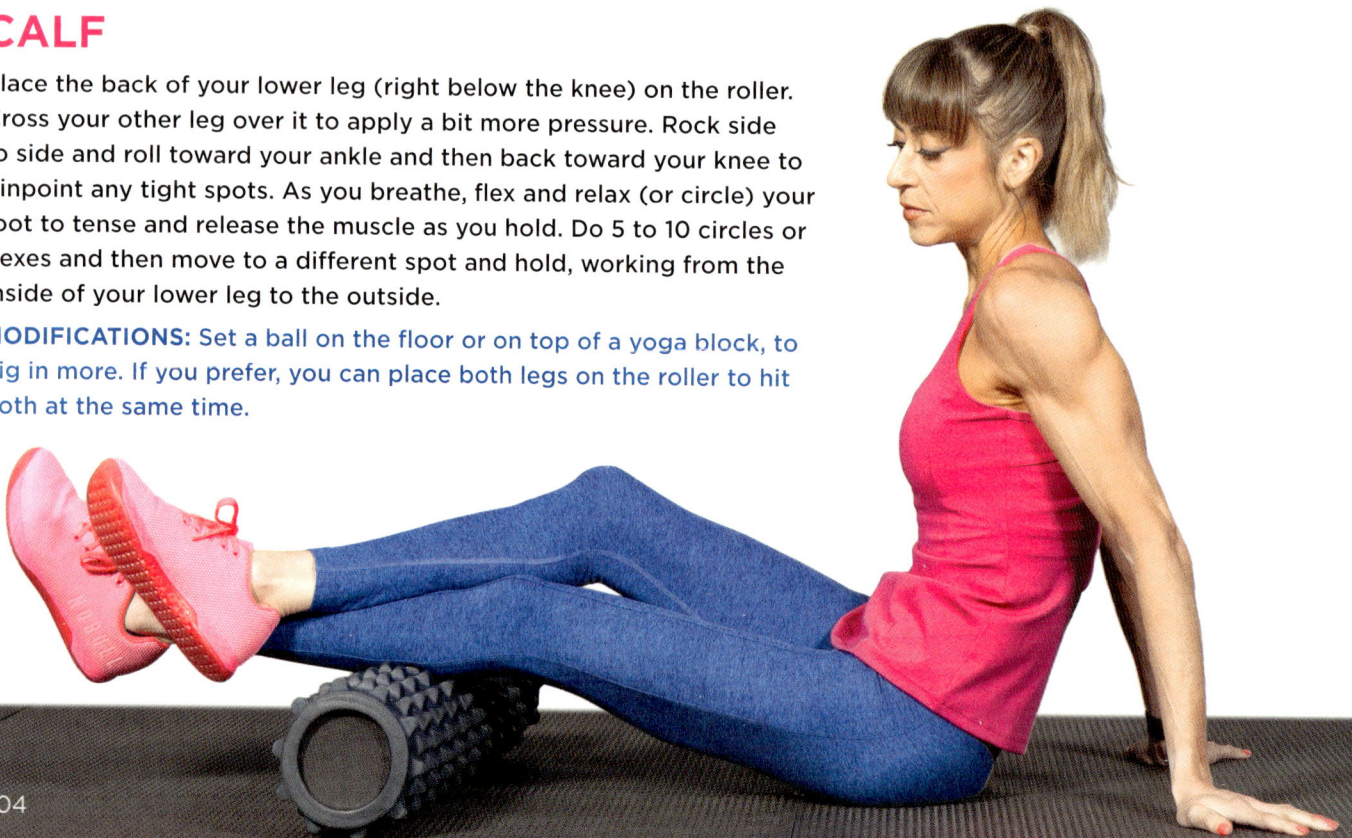

LEVATOR SCAPULAE

Find the top middle edge of your shoulder blade and put the ball there as you lie on your back and push into the ball. Bridge up to push down into the ball more as you hold and breathe.

With the ball positioned on a tight spot, reach overhead and then bring your arm down to your side or reach across your chest and open your arm back out to the side.

Lean your head to the side to look toward the hip opposite to the shoulder you're working on; then turn your head straight to look at the ceiling as you hold. Do 5 to 10 movements before moving the ball slightly up toward the base of your neck.

LAT

Lie on your side, angled slightly so the roller is under one armpit and your arm on that side is reaching overhead. Rock forward and backward on the roller, rotating your chest toward the ground and then up toward the ceiling. Hold here and then lower your arm to sweep it in front of you before moving it back overhead. Breathe and relax.

Then move the roller down the side of your back. Be careful; as you move lower, rock more toward your back than toward the front of your rib cage. Hold, breathe, and relax on any tight spots for 3 to 5 breaths.

MODIFICATIONS: Use a ball on the ground to apply more pressure or roll against the wall with a ball to apply less pressure.

THORACIC EXTENSIONS/UPPER BACK WITH PEANUT

Hold a peanut along your spine so a ball rests on either side of your spine. Lie back on the peanut, with your arms overhead and your feet flat on the ground. Breathe and hold as you relax over the peanut. Slowly sweep your arms down and to the sides, feeling a stretch in your chest as you relax open over the peanut; then cross your arms over your chest.

Crunch up, pushing into the balls as you lift your head and shoulder blades. Then relax back down, exhaling as you go, and extend your arms overhead again. Do this a few times and then move the peanut higher on your back. Work all the way up, even going to the base of your neck and down to the bottom of your rib cage as needed.

CHEST

Hold a ball pressed into your chest just inside your shoulder joint and lean into a doorway or wall edge so that your arm can move freely. Push into the ball and reach your hand out in front of you; then move it overhead before lowering it back toward the ground. Hold and breathe as you do this movement 5 to 10 times.

Move the ball up or down slightly to be in the side of your chest around the front of your shoulder, slightly toward your sternum. Be very careful to go light with pressure if you work under your collarbone toward your sternum. This is very sensitive tissue and needs gentle treatment. You can also open your arm out to the side at or just below shoulder height to stretch your chest; then relax your arm back to your side to help the muscle release.

TERES MINOR

Hold a ball at the back of your armpit where your arm and back connect and lie on your side, tilted slightly so the ball is pressed behind your armpit. Find a tight spot and then hold. Breathe and relax into the pressure.

Bring your arm in front of your chest with your palm facing toward the ceiling; then reach your arm overhead and bring it back down in front of you. Perform 5 to 10 arm raises and adjust the ball as needed. You can roll the ball up just slightly toward your shoulder or down slightly on the side of your back. You can also move it back below your shoulder onto the edge of your shoulder blade.

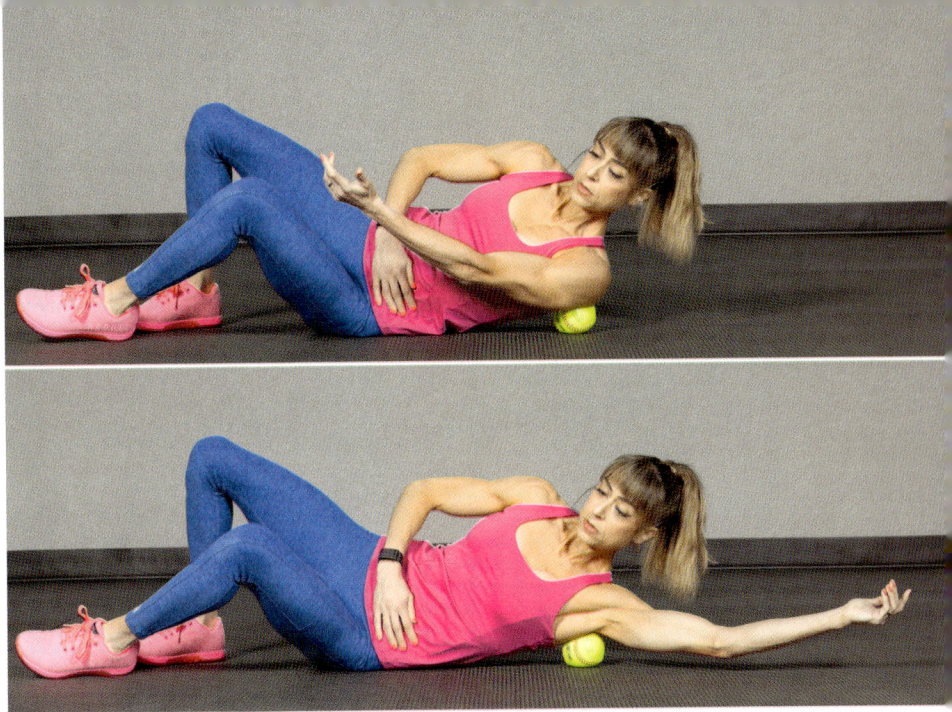

MODIFICATIONS: Rolling against a wall can also reduce pressure and help you adjust more easily.

TFL FOAM ROLLING

MODIFICATIONS: If you use a ball against the wall, make sure you aren't tensing to push the ball into the wall. Just lean into the ball. Using a bigger ball can help.

To find your tensor fasciae latae (TFL), lie on your back and find the bony prominence on the outside of one hip, then move your hand slightly down and to the side. Rotate your toe down toward the ground, turning your leg all the way up toward your hip. Feel the TFL flex under your hand as you do this movement. Put the ball where you feel the muscle flex; then turn onto your side to lie on the ball. You can roll it back toward your glute or slightly down the side of your leg in front of your hip bone.

Find a tight spot and then lift and lower your leg to tense and relax 5 to 10 times. Then move the ball slightly to another tight spot. You can also bend your knee toward your chest and extend your leg to hit this hip flexor.

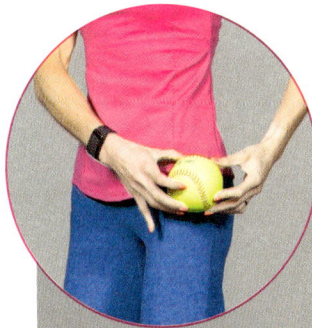

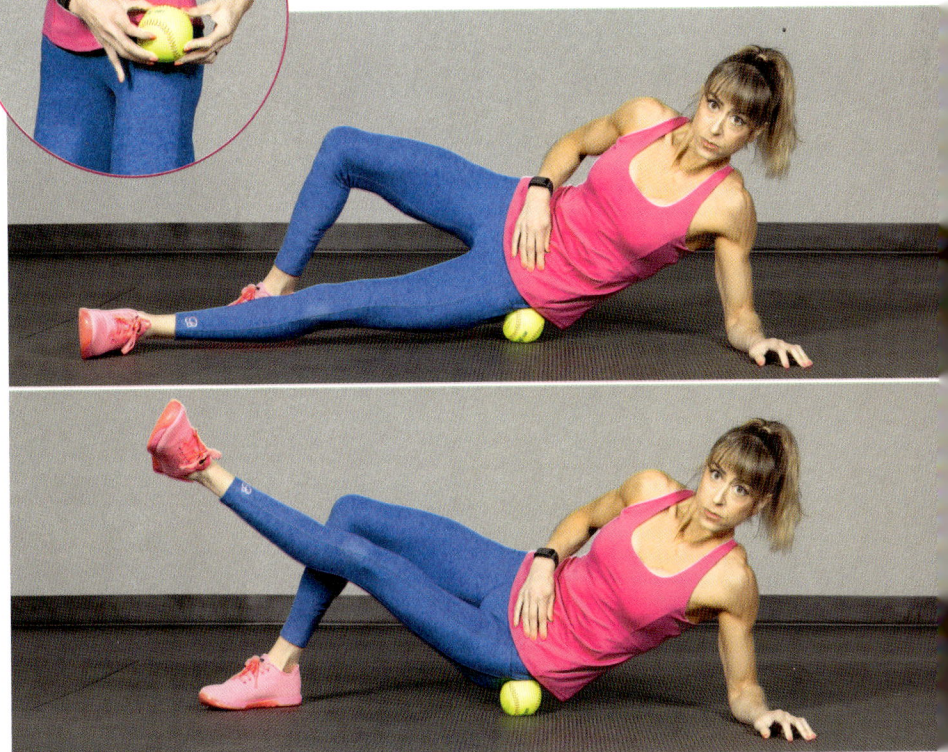

POSTERIOR ADDUCTOR

Hold a ball under your butt toward your inner thigh and sit on top of the ball on a bench. Roll along the bottom of your butt, going all the way out toward your hip to hit your hamstring if you'd like. Roll slightly down the back of your leg a few inches on the inner part of your thigh.

When you find a tight spot, lift and lower your leg, exhaling every time you lower to help the muscle relax and release. Do about 5 to 10 reps before moving to another spot. You may even want to push the ball up under your glute slightly to really get to the origin of the muscle.

PERONEAL

Sit on the floor. Hold a ball at the side of your lower leg just below your knee. It should be to the outside of the meatier part of your calf. Bend your leg and lower it in front of you to press your leg down into the ball. Roll the ball down the outside of your lower leg, stopping a couple of inches above your anklebone.

Hold on any tight spots and circle your foot as you breathe. Make 5 to 10 circles. Adjust the angle of the ball slightly to be toward your calf or shin and work up and down the outside of your lower leg.

MODIFICATIONS: You can also have your knee bent in front of you and use both hands to press the ball into the muscle, or you can use a handheld roller.

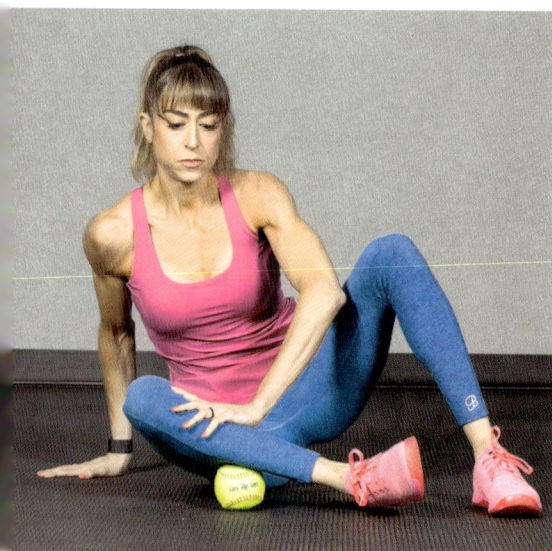

TRICEPS

Place the backside of your upper arm (your triceps) on the ball or roller right above your elbow then rest the ball or roller on a bench or box. Press down into the ball while relaxing the muscle. To apply more pressure, use your other hand to press your arm down into the ball.

Roll all the way up to the back of your armpit. To help the muscle relax, extend and bend at your elbow and rock side to side. Breathe as you hold on one tight spot and then move to the next spot.

NOTE: *The smaller and harder the ball, the more it will dig in.*

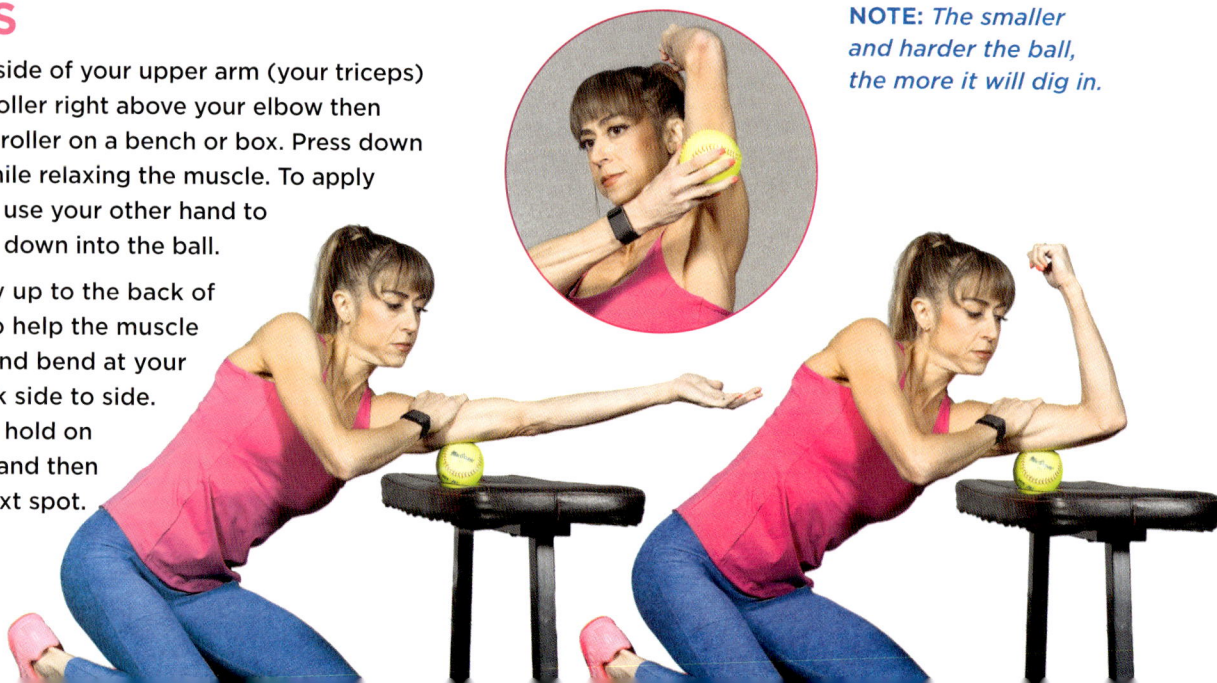

STRETCHING

Don't rush through the reps of the dynamic stretches. Focus on not only the muscles stretching but the opposing muscle group that's driving the stretch. For all static stretches, hold 30 to 90 seconds.

BEAR SQUAT TO FOOT STRETCH

Kneel on the ground with your feet flexed. Feel a stretch through your big toes and along the sole of your foot as you sit back on your heels. Gently rock side to side.

Sit forward, place your hands on the ground, and push your butt up in the air as you drive back and lower your heels toward the ground. (Drive your heels down only as far as you comfortably can.) Feel a nice stretch down your calves and up into your hamstrings. Breathe.

Lower your knees back to the ground and sit back on your heels and then repeat the stretch. Walk your hands closer to your feet for more of a stretch.

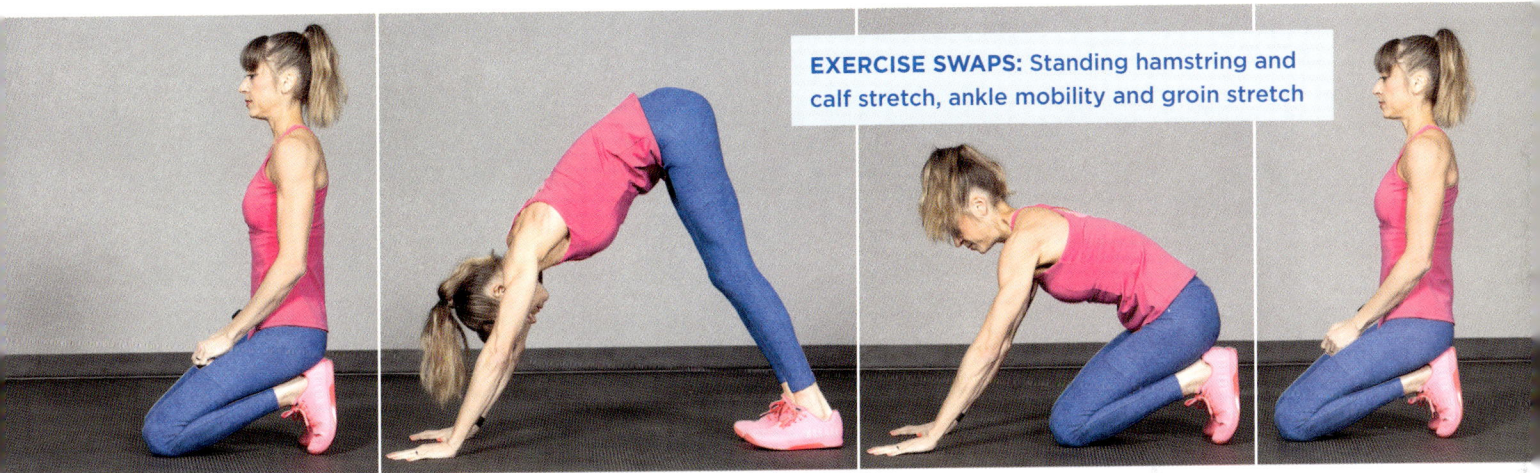

EXERCISE SWAPS: Standing hamstring and calf stretch, ankle mobility and groin stretch

MODIFICATIONS: Set a bench in front of you and place your hands on it instead of touching the ground. If you have knee pain, do a standing single-leg stretch, elevating the ball of your foot on a dumbbell as you push your knee forward.

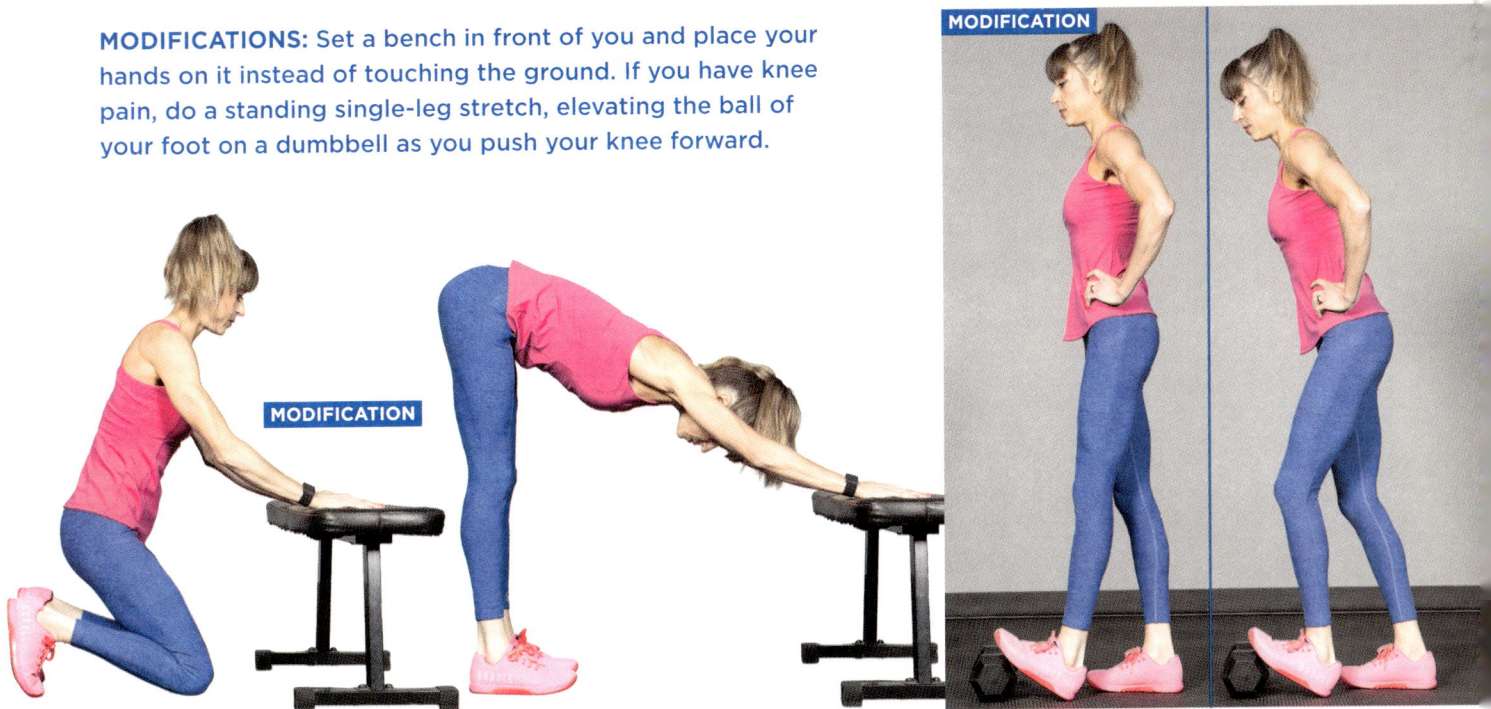

MODIFICATION

MODIFICATION

CRESCENT TO HAMSTRING STRETCH

Step one foot back into a nice wide stance with both legs straight and feet pointing straight ahead. Bend your front knee and sink into a lunge, keeping your back leg straight. Drive back through the heel of your back leg without pressing it into the ground and raise your arms overhead to be in a crescent lunge. Squeeze your back glute to keep your rear leg straight and don't let your front knee cave in.

Pause and then place your hands on the ground on either side of your front foot. Straighten your front leg to stretch your hamstring as you hang over. Drive your back heel toward the ground (as close as it will reach) to stretch that calf into your hamstring. Repeat moving into the crescent position.

MODIFICATIONS: Don't sink as low into the lunge. If you can't touch the ground while keeping your leg straight, you can also place your hands on your shin, a bench, or a block. Just focus on straightening your front leg.

EXERCISE SWAPS: Half-kneeling hip to hamstring stretch, dynamic squat stretch, standing quad stretch with reach, downward dog to runner's lunge

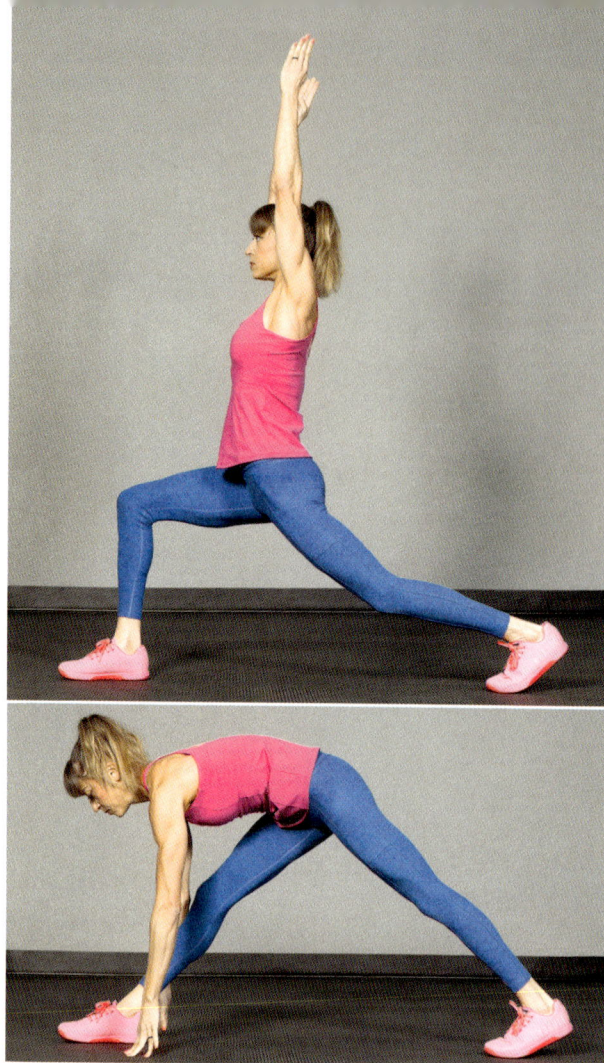

ANKLE MOBILITY AND GROIN STRETCH

Start half-kneeling and open your knee out to the side so your foot and leg are perpendicular to your back kneeling leg. Your front foot is turned out and in line with your back knee. Walk that foot out so your knee is behind your ankle on that side. Engage your glute and then shift your weight, rocking that knee forward over the ball of your foot.

EXERCISE SWAPS: Bear squat to foot stretch, 3-way leg swing, side lunge with rotation

Don't hinge or lean forward. Squeeze your glute to keep your knee open as you drive that knee forward over your toes, keeping your heel down. Then shift back and repeat.

Adjust how far out your foot is from your supporting knee, shifting it closer for more focus on ankle mobility or further out for more stretch in your groin.

MODIFICATIONS: If your knee hurts, perform the move while standing or with a wider stance so your knee doesn't drive past your toe.

ALTERNATING PIGEON POSE

Set up on all fours with your feet flexed and then walk your hands toward one side as you straighten the opposite leg out behind you. In other words, if you're moving your hands to the left then straighten your right leg and slide it behind you. Your left knee will be bent in front of you to move into pigeon pose. Sit into your front glute (on the left, in this example) as you walk your hands out in front of you and reach the other leg straight back.

Then bend your right knee to bring it back in as you walk your hands back around front to come back to your hands and knees. Repeat the move on the other side, walking over to the right to feel that stretch in your right glute and down the front of your hip on your left leg as you reach it straight behind you.

EXERCISE SWAPS: Active foam roller star stretch, half-kneeling thoracic rotations

MODIFICATION

MODIFICATIONS: Instead of alternating sides, stay in pigeon on one side and walk your hands out in front of you from right to left. Alternatively, you can do a seated glute stretch off a bench and alternate sides.

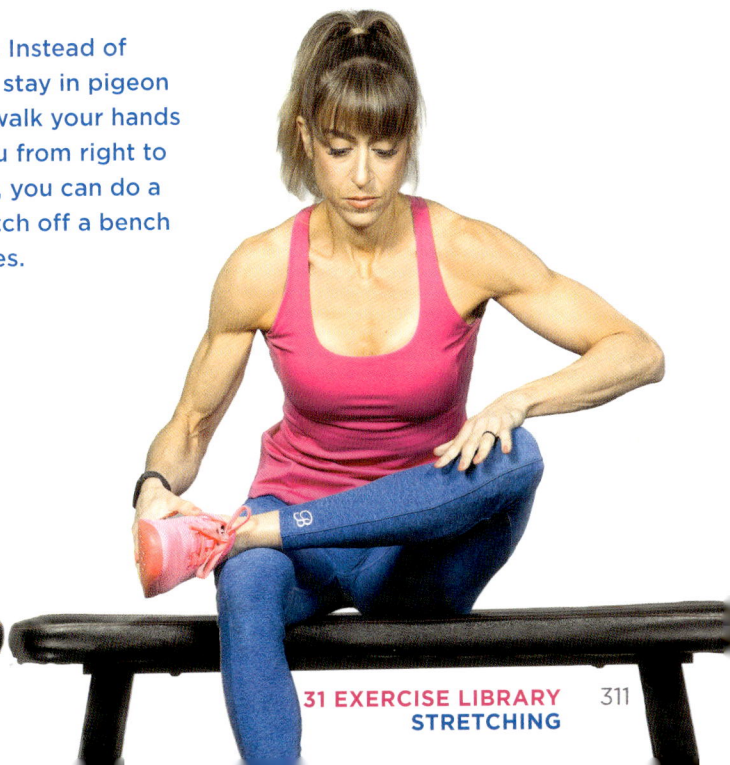

BENCH HIP STRETCH

Lie back on a bench with your butt right at the edge of the bench. Wrap your hands around your shin below one knee and hug that knee to your chest. Drive the heel of your other leg down toward the ground with your knee bent to around 90 degrees. Feel your glute engage on that side.

Then bring the knee of the second leg up to your chest where it's about even with the first leg before driving the heel back down toward the ground. As you extend your hip, really squeeze that glute. Repeat.

MODIFICATIONS: You can hold behind your thigh instead of your shin if needed.

EXERCISE SWAPS: Half-kneeling hip to hamstring stretch, side-lying quad stretch, half-kneeling TFL stretch, standing quad stretch with reach

DYNAMIC SQUAT STRETCH

Stand tall with your feet about hip-width apart and then hinge at your hips, pushing your butt back as you keep your legs straight and reach to place your hands on your feet or on the ground between them.

With your hands at your feet, sink your butt toward the ground to sit in a deep squat, as low as you can go while keeping your heels down. Also keep your chest lifted at the bottom of the squat. Pause, pressing your elbows into your knees for an added inner thigh stretch. Straighten your legs and lift your butt back up toward the ceiling to stand back up. Repeat the stretch.

MODIFICATIONS: You can sit on a bench or box, only squat as far as you can control, place your hands on your shins, or stabilize using a chair or bench instead of the ground.

EXERCISE SWAPS: Half-kneeling hip to hamstring stretch, downward dog to runner's lunge, camel bridge

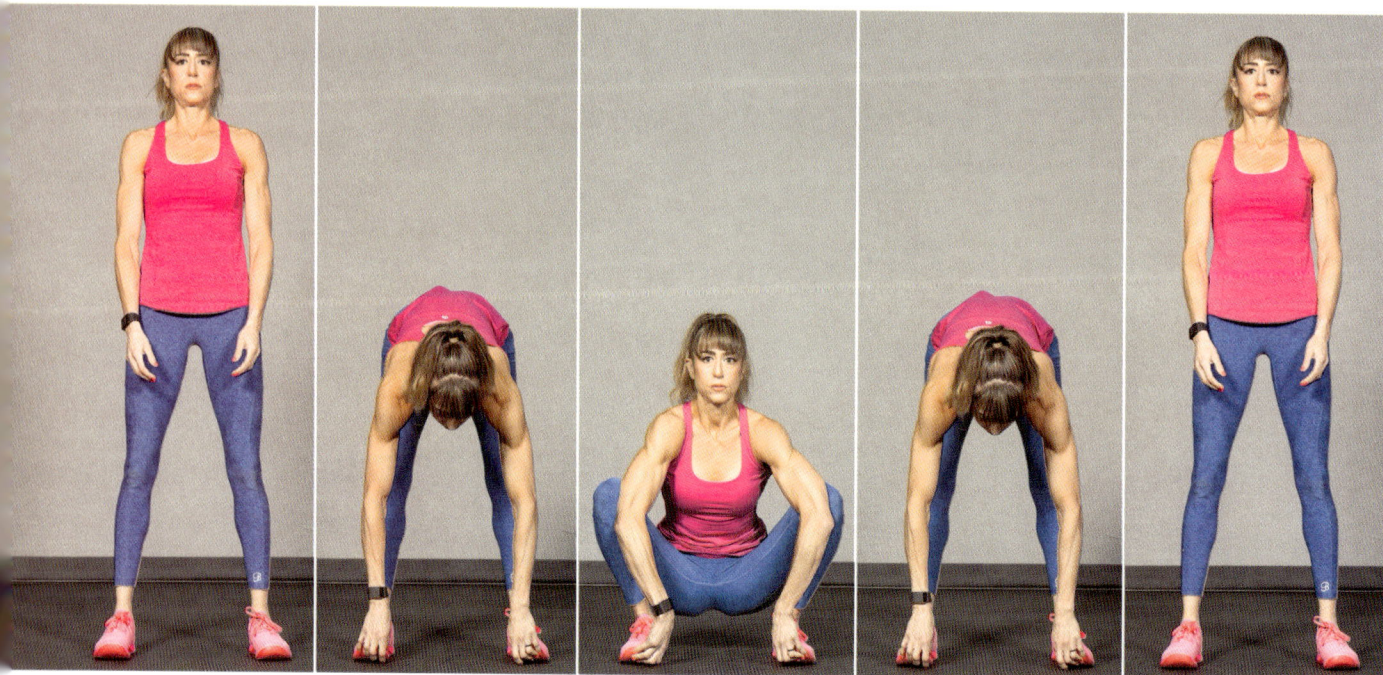

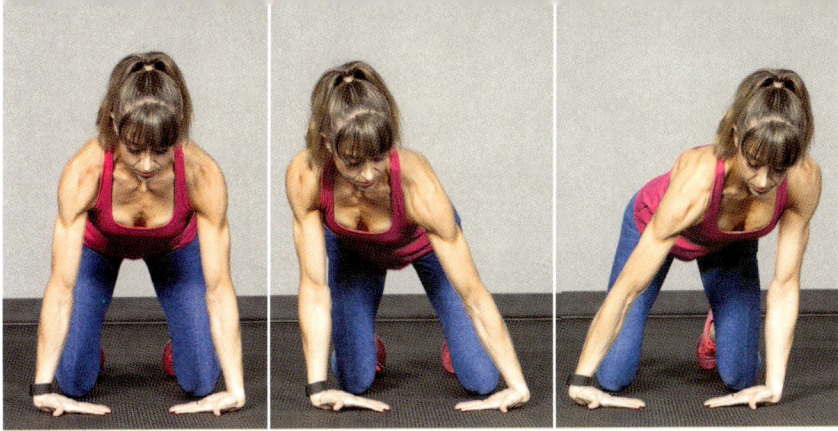

WRIST FLEXION STRETCH

While kneeling on the ground, place the backs of your hands on the ground in front of you with your fingertips pointing toward each other. Your wrists should be aligned under your shoulders. Shift your weight slightly forward onto your hands to feel a stretch down the outside of your forearms.

Gently rock to the right and left, keeping the backs of your hands on the ground and pausing for a second on each side. Do not bend your elbows.

EXERCISE SWAPS: Wrist extension stretch

MODIFICATIONS: You can do one side at a time while you're seated or standing. Use one hand to press against the back of your opposite hand rather than pushing the back of your hand into the ground. You can also do this standing with your hands on a bench or desk.

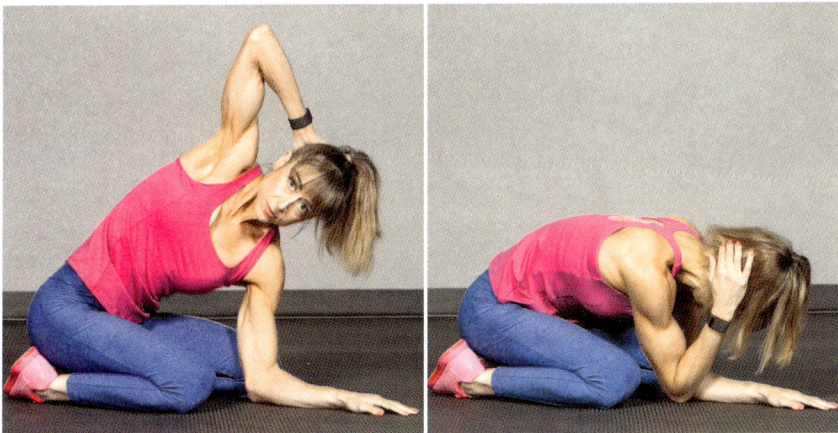

QUADRUPED THORACIC ROTATION

Kneel on the ground and then sit back on your heels as you lean over and place one forearm on the ground with your elbow right inside your knee. This position really isolates your thoracic spine as you rotate. Place your other hand behind your head and bring that elbow down to meet the elbow of your support arm.

Rotate through your spine to open that elbow up toward the ceiling as much as you can, pushing your forearm on the ground down and into your knee to help you twist through your spine. Don't just flap your elbow; rotate your chest open and feel the stretch through your upper back. Rotate back to the closed position and repeat.

EXERCISE SWAPS: Active foam roller star stretch, half-kneeling thoracic rotation, thread-the-needle stretch, star stretch

MODIFICATIONS: You can also do this seated on a bench.

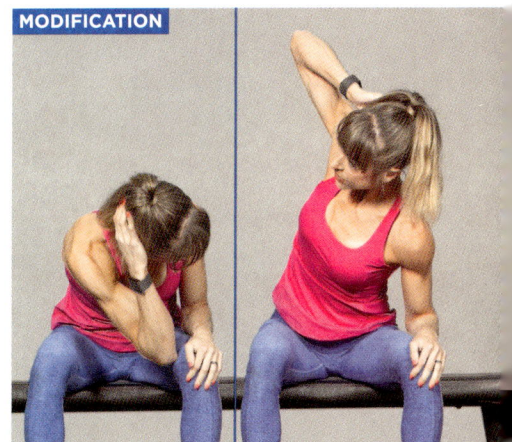

SUSPENSION TRAINER SNOW ANGEL

Stand facing away from the suspension trainer's anchor point and hold a handle in each hand. Walk out so the suspension trainer is pulling back slightly on your arms when you have them straight down by your sides.

Stand with your feet pointing straight ahead and engage your upper back. Feel your chest open and stretch as you swing your arms straight out to the side and then overhead as if you're making a snow angel. (You may need to adjust where you're standing so there's tension while you do the movement.) Move slowly and keep your palms facing forward; focus on engaging your upper back to drive the stretch. Pause for a second in any specific part of the movement where you feel extra tightness.

MODIFICATIONS: You can use a towel or rings and do one side at a time.

EXERCISE SWAPS: Wings chest stretch, foam roller snow angel

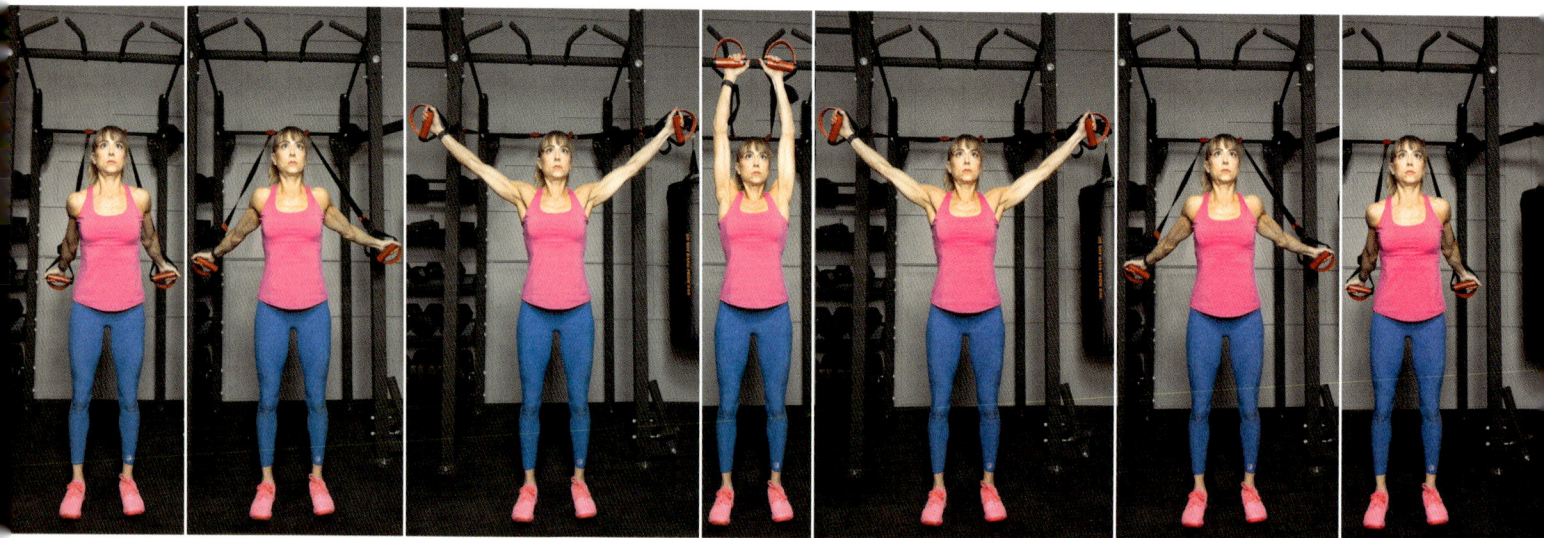

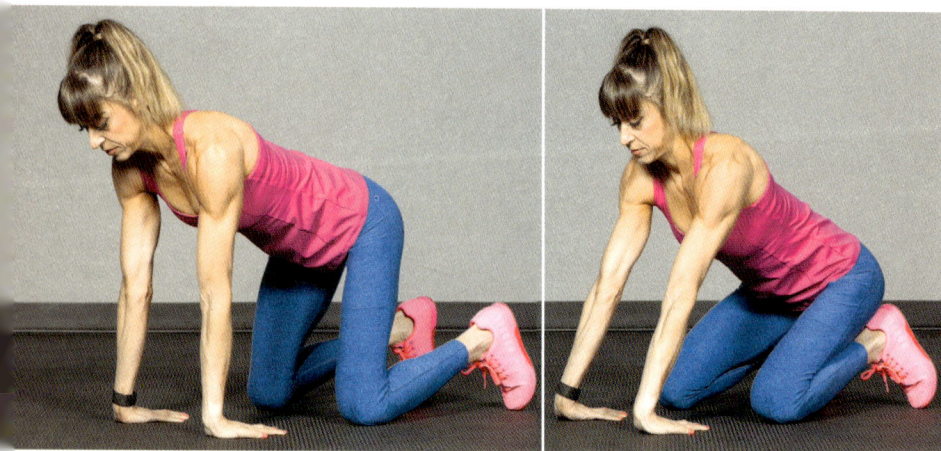

WRIST EXTENSION STRETCH

Kneel on the ground and place your palms on the ground with your fingertips pointing back toward your knees. Sit back toward your heels and feel a stretch up the inside of your forearms. Avoid shrugging your shoulders, keep the heels of your palms down, and do not bend your elbows as you sit back.

Release as you come back forward. The more you sit back, the bigger the stretch in your wrists. Breathe and relax as you stretch; do not tense against it.

MODIFICATIONS: You can do one side at a time while seated or standing. Stretch one arm in front of you with your palm facing up. Use the opposite hand to press your fingertips toward the ground and back toward your forearm. You can also do this standing with your hands on a bench or desk.

EXERCISE SWAPS: Wrist flexion stretch

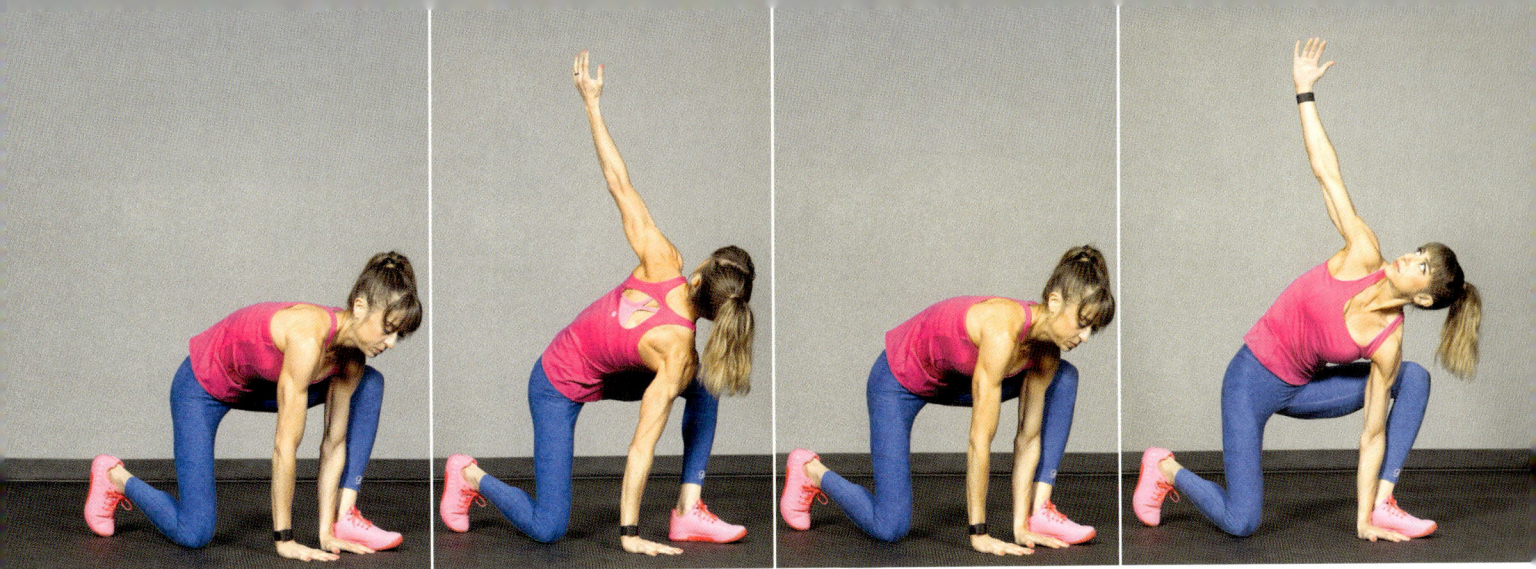

HALF-KNEELING THORACIC ROTATION

Get in a half-kneeling position and lean forward to place both palms on the ground right inside your front foot. Keep your outside hand flat on the ground and lift your inside arm toward the ceiling, rotating your torso toward your front leg. As much as possible, avoid letting your knee bow open or rocking out on your foot. Feel the stretch through your glute and spine.

Place your inside hand back on the floor and then lift your outside hand as you rotate away from your front leg to reach toward the ceiling. As you rotate, make sure to twist through your spine; don't just raise your arm.

MODIFICATIONS: Do this in a standing position with one foot up on a bench or place your hands on a yoga block.

EXERCISE SWAPS: Active foam roller star stretch, side lunges with rotation, quadruped thoracic rotation

KNEELING THORACIC EXTENSION AND LAT STRETCH

Kneel in front of a bench and place your elbows on the bench about shoulder-width apart. Kneel so you can sit back on your heels and drop your head toward the ground between your arms to stretch through your lats and triceps.

EXERCISE SWAPS: Half wall hang, child's pose with reach—external rotation

Extend your upper back and press your chest toward the ground as you sit back on your heels. Feel the stretch through your upper back, down the sides of your back, and down the backs of your arms. Pause and then come back up off your heels to release the stretch.

Repeat, feeling yourself engage your upper back to drive the extension of your spine. Be conscious not to arch your lower back. (Sitting back can help you avoid this.) Exhale as you really drive into the stretch.

MODIFICATIONS: You can do this stretch with your hands on the wall

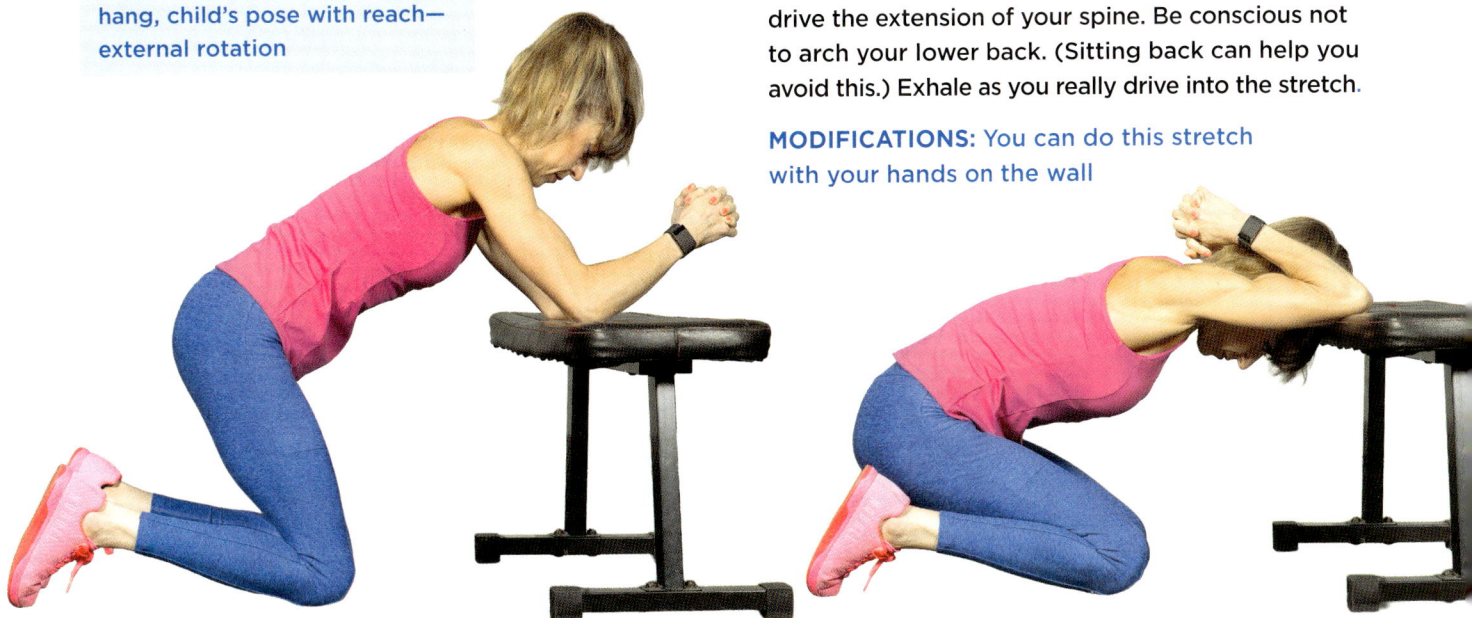

INCHWORM

Stand tall with your feet together then hinge at your hips and push your butt back as you reach for the ground. Keep your legs as straight as you can. Walk your hands in front of you, keeping your legs straight as you lower into the plank position.

Drop your hips as you push the ground away with your hands and arch your back to open your chest toward the wall in front of you. Squeeze your glutes to drive your hips toward the ground and protect your back. Breathe and then bring your hips back up to the plank before walking your hands back toward your feet, still keeping your legs straight.

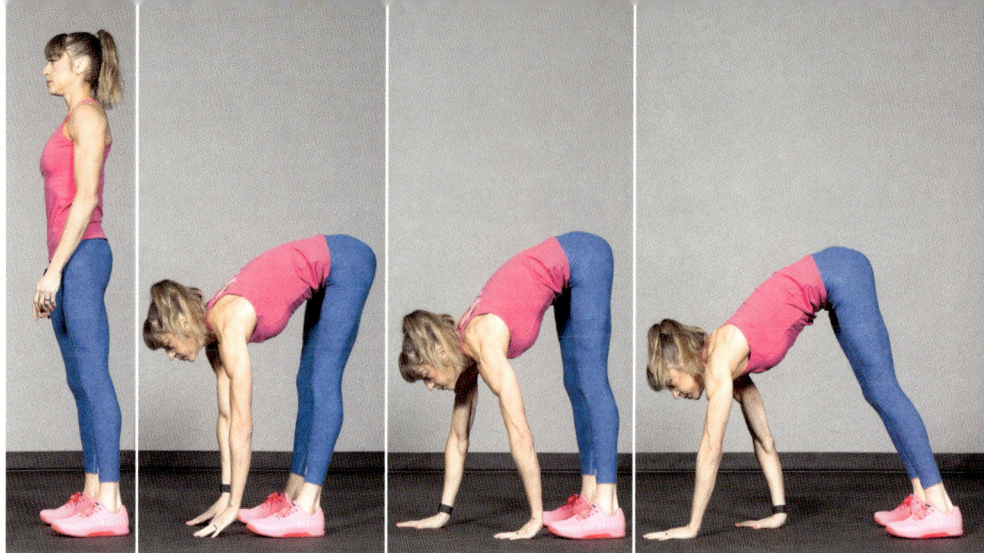

Return to standing and repeat. To start, you may find your knees bend slightly as you walk out or that you can't perform the upward facing dog when you drop your hips.

WORLD'S GREATEST STRETCH

Start in a high plank position with your hands under your shoulders and your feet together. Your body should be in a nice straight line from your head to your heels.

Bring one foot forward to be outside the hand on the same side so you're in a nice lunge. If necessary, adjust your foot so it's flat on the ground. Squeeze your back glute.

Drop the elbow on that side down to the ground near the instep of your foot and rotate your chest away from your front leg to reach under your support arm (not shown). Don't worry if you can't touch the ground. Focus on not rocking outward on your foot.

Now reach that arm toward the ceiling, opening your chest toward your front leg. Focus on your back opening your chest as you rotate.

Place your hand back on the ground and also drop your back knee to the ground. Then sit back on your heel with your front leg straightened. Feel a stretch down your hamstring as you hinge to lean over your front leg and push your butt back.

Come off your back knee and shift back into a lunge; then repeat the elbow-drop and rotation. If you're short on time, immediately switch to the foot on the other side.

MODIFICATIONS: Place your hands on a bench or box to modify the movement.

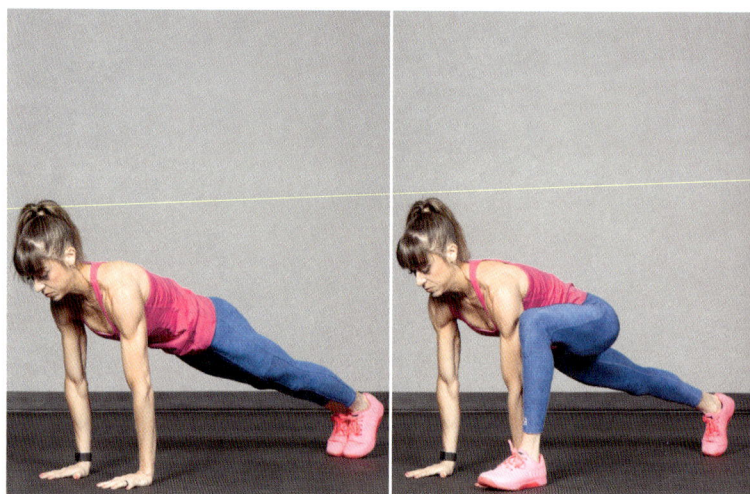

MODIFICATION

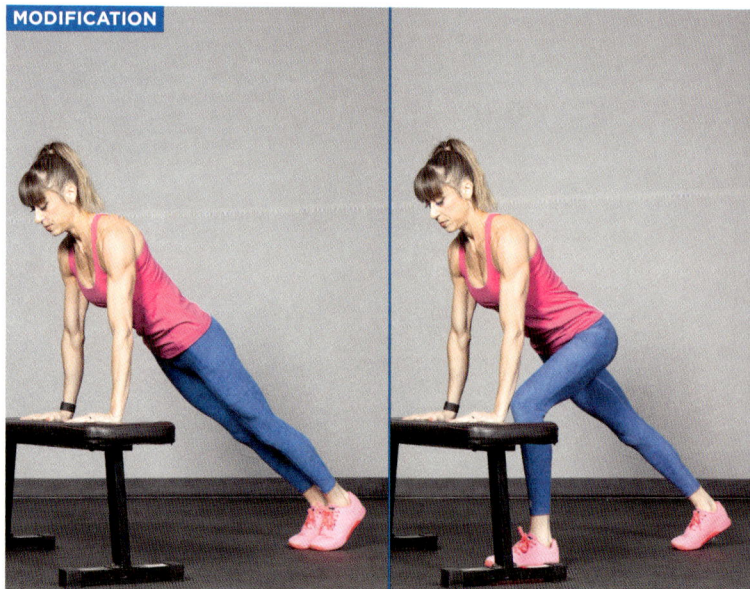

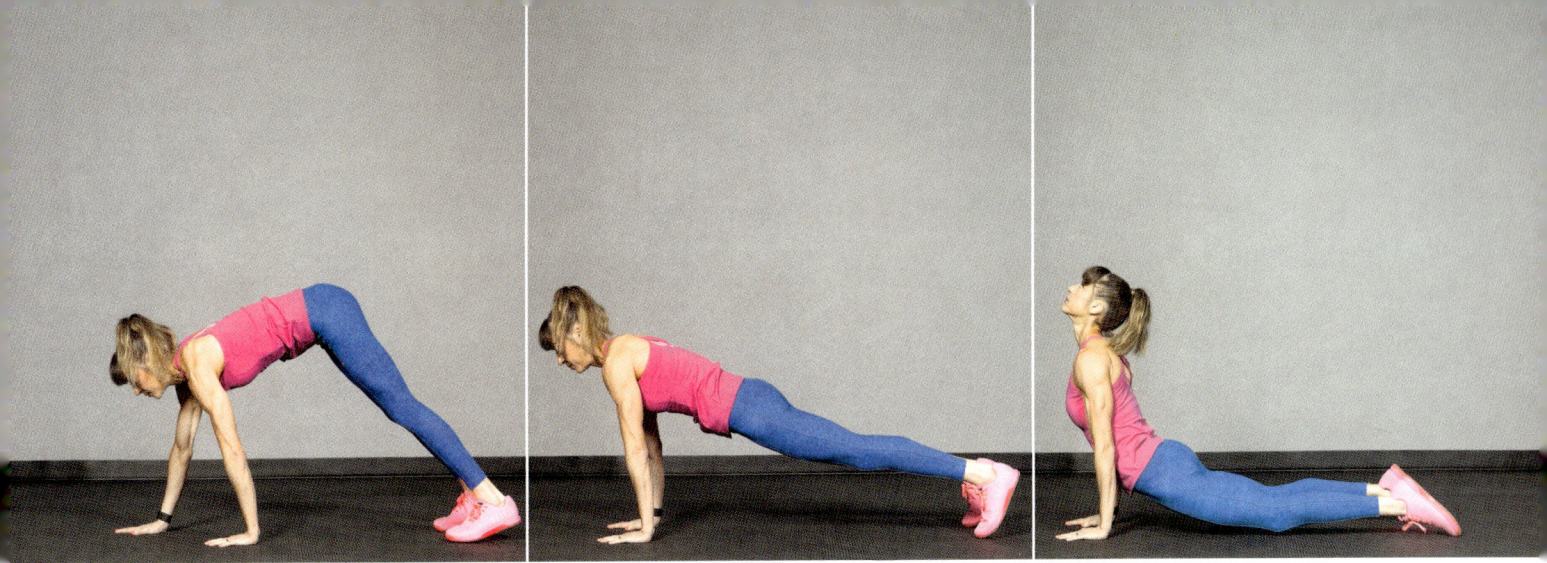

MODIFICATIONS: Perform the inchworm without the hip drop. Or you can place your hands on a bench/low box and reverse the direction so you walk your feet back into a plank. Do not use the upward facing dog with this version.

EXERCISE SWAPS: Downward dog to upward dog, standing hamstring and calf stretch, downward dog to runner's lunge, camel bridge

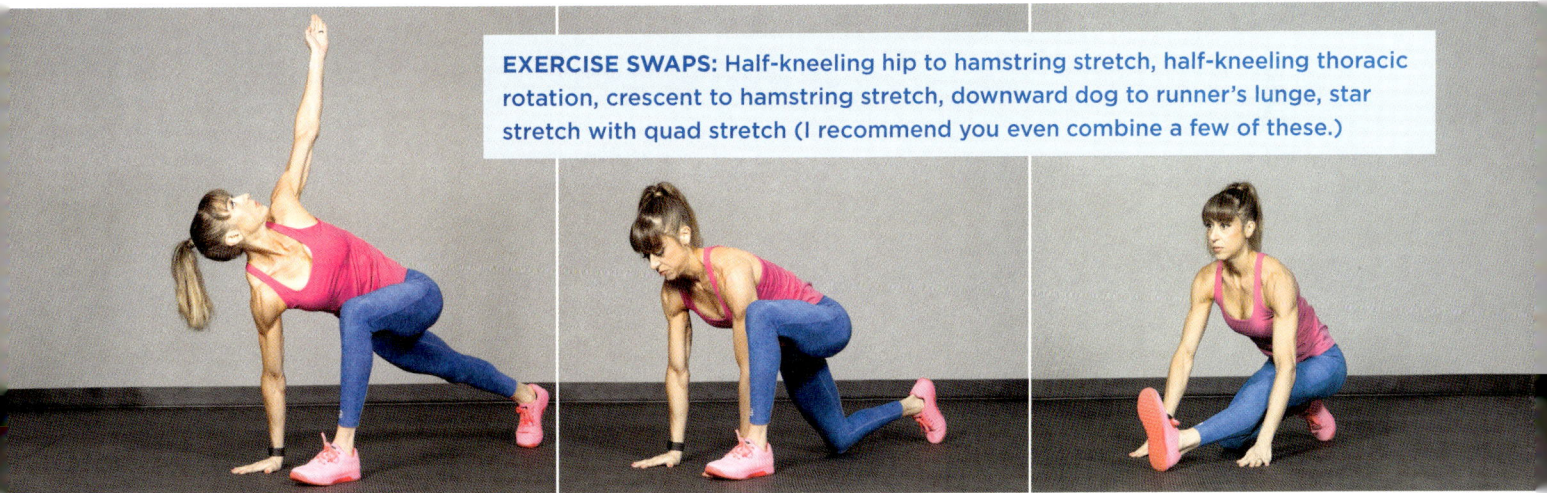

EXERCISE SWAPS: Half-kneeling hip to hamstring stretch, half-kneeling thoracic rotation, crescent to hamstring stretch, downward dog to runner's lunge, star stretch with quad stretch (I recommend you even combine a few of these.)

STANDING HAMSTRING AND CALF STRETCH

Stand tall with your feet together. Hinge at your hips, pushing your butt back while you step one foot forward with its heel on the ground. Keep your front leg straight as you hinge and reach your opposite hand toward the outside of your front foot. Feel the stretch down your hamstrings and calves. Don't round your back to reach further.

Stand up and bring your feet back together; repeat on the other side. Only reach as far as you can. Focus on hinging and sitting back rather than just leaning forward.

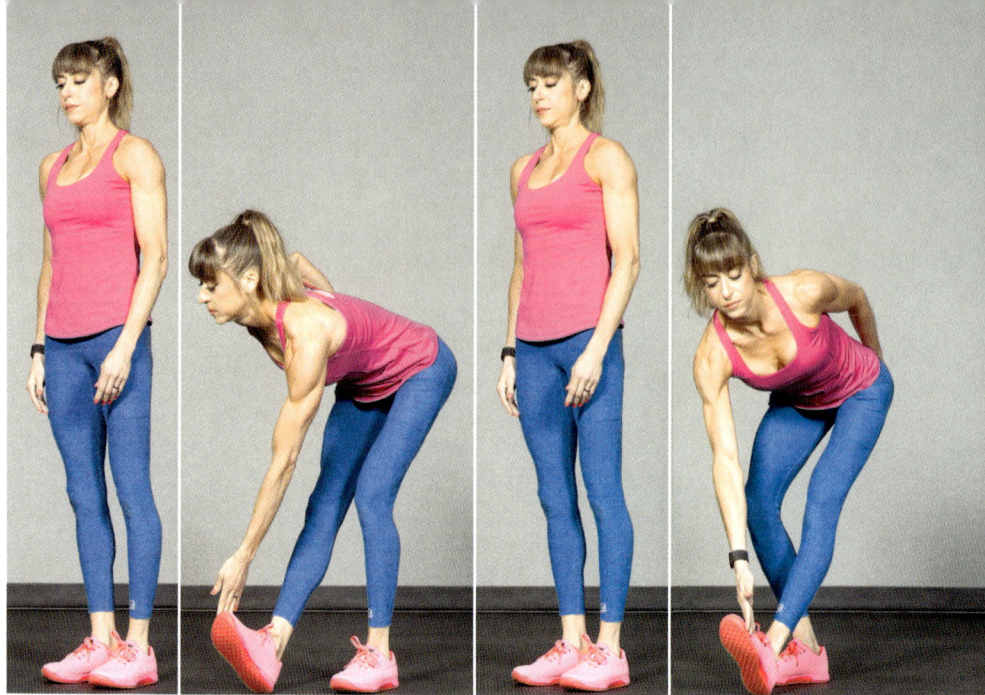

MODIFICATIONS: Don't alternate sides. Place your hand on a wall for balance, if needed. Reach down to your knee or shin to help you focus on the hinge.

EXERCISE SWAPS: Half-kneeling hip to hamstring stretch, crescent to hamstring stretch, standing forward bend, standing calf stretch

STANDING QUAD STRETCH WITH REACH

Stand tall and then raise your heel up behind you as you reach with the same-side hand to grab your ankle. Pull your foot toward your butt while you squeeze your glute. Focus on keeping your bent leg aligned with your standing leg by really engaging the glute to extend your hip.

Reach your opposite arm overhead and feel a stretch down the front of your leg. Release your foot and repeat on the other side. Pause in each quad stretch for a breath or two, feeling your glute driving the hip extension. You can even take a few steps in between to reset and rebalance.

MODIFICATIONS: Don't alternate sides. Place your hand on a wall for balance, if needed. If you're not alternating sides, you can loop a towel around your ankle to help you reach, in which case you don't fully release between reps. You can also do this while side lying on a bench.

EXERCISE SWAPS: Bench hip stretch, crescent to hamstring stretch, half-kneeling hip to hamstring stretch, side-lying quad stretch

SIDE LUNGE WITH ROTATION

Extend your arms out to the sides at shoulder height and set your feet in a wide stance (feet aligned under your hands) and your toes pointed straight ahead. Bend one knee and sit your butt back, hinging at your hips as you sink into a side lunge. Reach one hand across your body toward the opposite foot, placing it on the ground by your toes. Reach the other arm toward the ceiling, twisting through your spine to rotate your chest open toward your supporting leg.

Pause and then bring your raised hand back to the ground. Stay low as you shift into a side lunge on the other side. Each time you lunge, focus on feeling your glutes work as you stay low and your upper back work as you rotate to reach toward the ceiling.

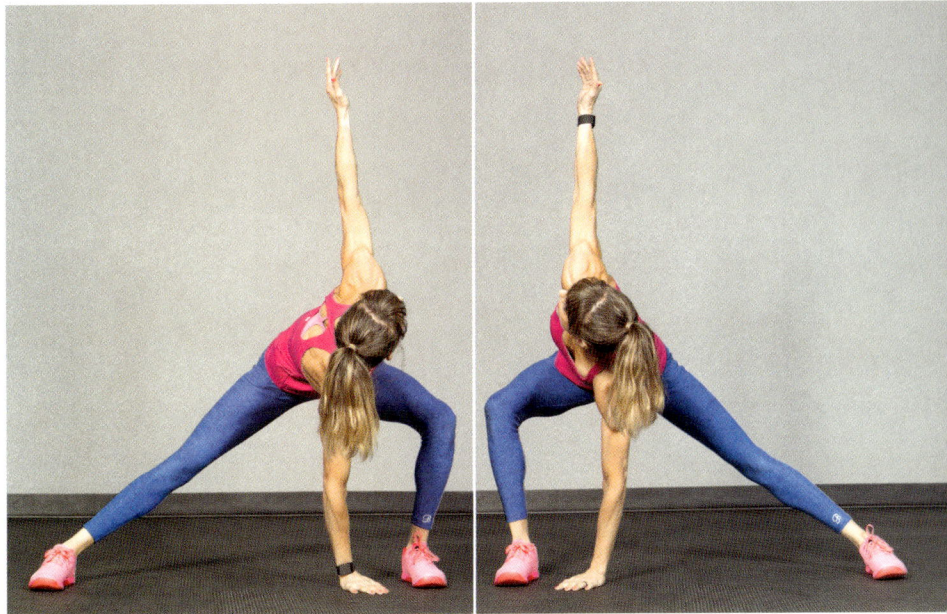

MODIFICATIONS: Do not sink as low in the lunge and place your hand on your knee instead of the floor to help you rotate open. You can also place your hand on a bench in front of you.

EXERCISE SWAPS: World's greatest stretch, half-kneeling thoracic rotation, frog stretch

WINGS CHEST STRETCH

While standing, place your hands behind your head with your elbows open out wide. You can lace your fingers together. Pinch your shoulder blades together to pull your elbows open as you stand tall to stretch your chest.

Bring your elbows together in front of your face, stretching through your upper back. Then open your elbows again, drawing your shoulder blades together as you try to press your chest out wide. Pause in each position but don't move your hands from your head.

MODIFICATIONS: You can modify by placing your hands on the sides of your head.

EXERCISE SWAPS: Suspension trainer snow angel, foam roller snow angel, standing chest stretch

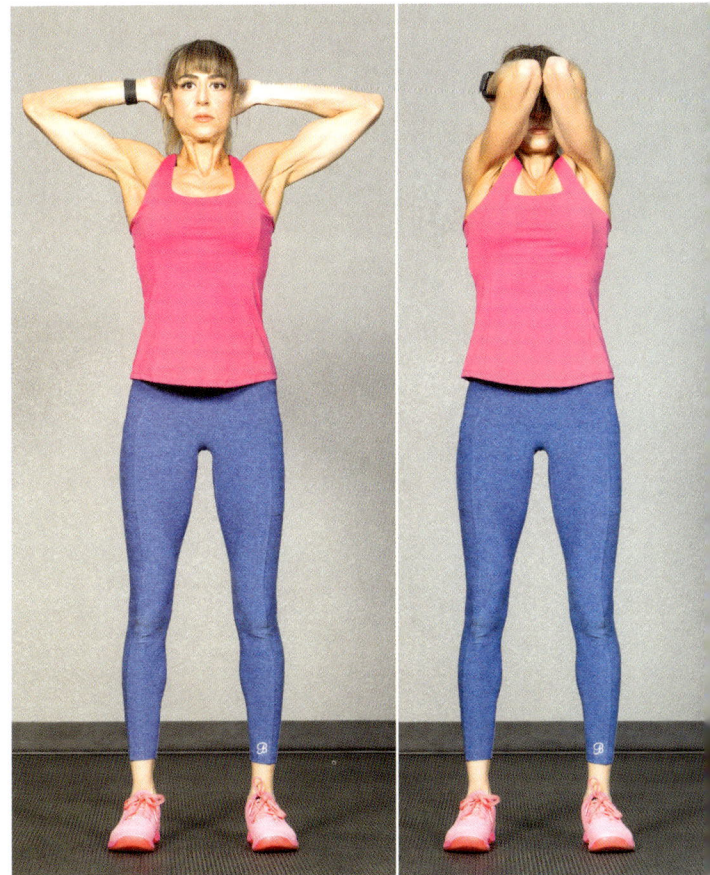

3-WAY LEG SWING

Stand on one leg. Engage the glute of your supporting leg and create tension down into the ground through the two points in the ball of your foot and single point in your heel. Then swing your free leg forward and backward, moving at the hip at a steady pace. Make the swings as big as you can control. Engage your hip flexors to lift forward and your glute to swing backward as you stand tall and stable.

After you've completed the forward/backward reps, move to lateral swings. Keeping your free leg straight, use your adductor to lift your leg across your body and your glute to pull it open out to the side.

After completing all the reps, bend your knee in front of your body to about 90 degrees. Use your glute to pull your knee open to the side. With your knee still bent, move it back front. Do not relax your foot toward the floor as you open and close from your hip.

After all reps on one side are complete, switch sides. Focus on your stability as you feel your hip opening up through your swinging leg.

MODIFICATIONS: Perform smaller swings or use a wall to balance. Ideally, though, you won't use anything to stabilize.

EXERCISE SWAPS: Standing hamstring and calf stretch, ankle mobility and groin stretch

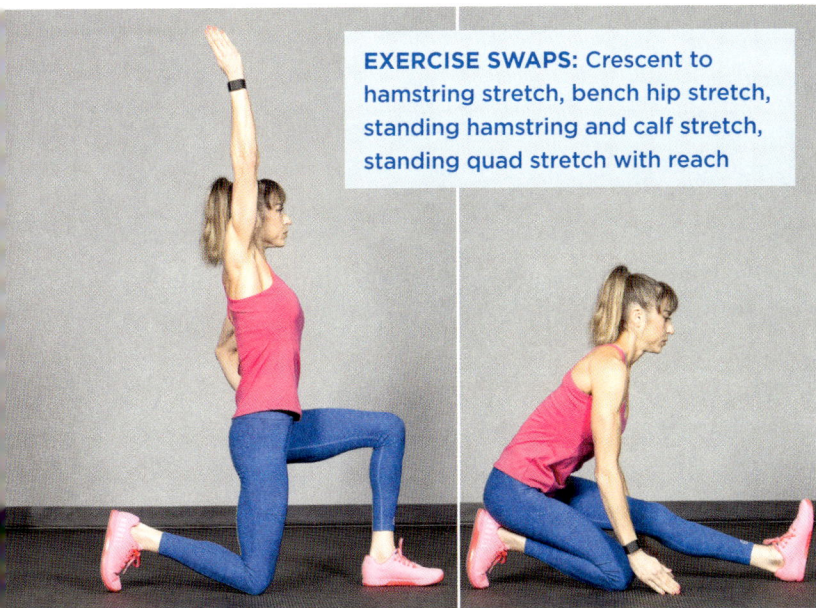

EXERCISE SWAPS: Crescent to hamstring stretch, bench hip stretch, standing hamstring and calf stretch, standing quad stretch with reach

HALF-KNEELING HIP TO HAMSTRING STRETCH

Get in a half-kneeling position with your back knee aligned under your hip. Squeeze your glute on that side to drive your hip forward as you reach overhead with the arm on that side.

Pause for a second as you squeeze your glute and fully extend your hip but be conscious not to lean and arch your back.

Sit back and lower your arm, extending your front leg as you hinge at your hips to stretch your hamstring. Push your butt back as you sit back; don't just round over. Then come back up to half-kneeling and repeat.

MODIFICATIONS: You can do this standing from a lunged position as well.

DOWNWARD DOG TO UPWARD DOG

Set up in the high plank position with your hands under your shoulders and feet about hip-width apart. Push back into downward dog, driving your chest back toward your knees as you straighten your arms to push your butt toward the ceiling. Drive your heels down, feeling a stretch up your calves and hamstrings.

Focus on driving through your palms (and even your thumb and index finger) instead of rocking out on your hand. Return to the plank position; as you do, drop your hips toward the ground with your legs extended behind you. Squeeze your glutes to drive your hips down at the same time you push the ground away with your hands to open your chest toward the wall in front of you. Avoid shrugging.

Pause for a breath and then move back into downward dog. To advance the move, you can shift from downward dog to upward dog by lowering toward the ground as if you're sneaking under a fence as you come forward and up rather than first shifting forward into the plank position.

MODIFICATIONS: Perform this move with your hands on a bench or box.

EXERCISE SWAPS: Camel bridge, inchworm, wings chest stretch

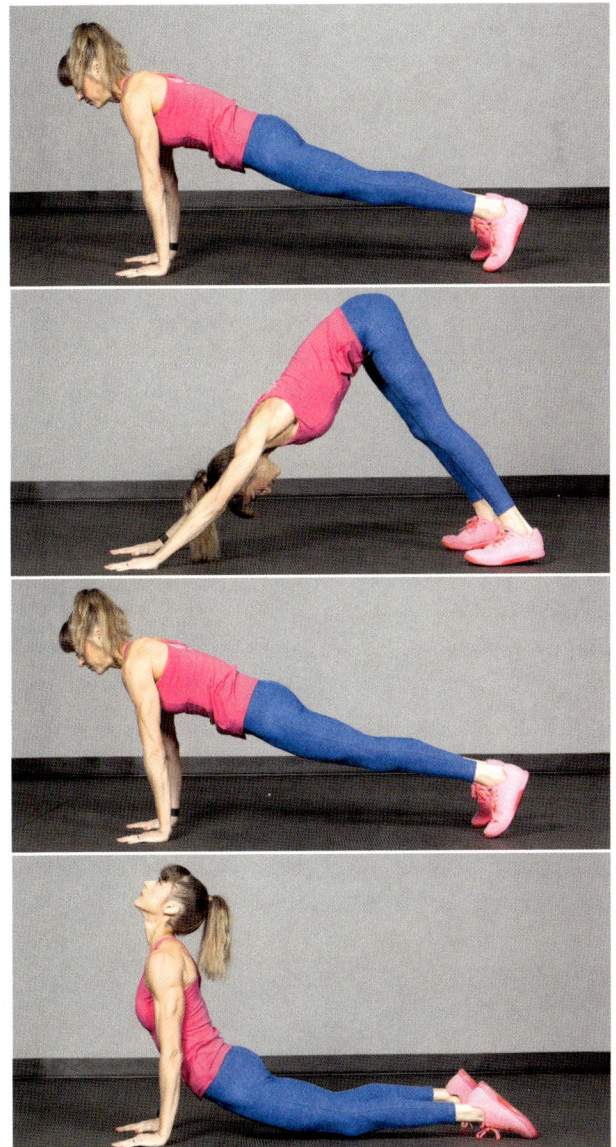

DOWNWARD DOG TO RUNNER'S LUNGE

Set up in a plank position with your feet about hip-width apart and your hands under your shoulders. Push back into downward dog, driving your chest back toward your knees as you straighten your arms to push your butt toward the ceiling. Drive your heels down, feeling a stretch up your calves and hamstrings. Focus on driving through your palms (and even your thumb and index finger) instead of rocking out on your hand.

Take a breath and then move forward into the plank position before stepping one foot up and outside your arms. Squeeze your back glute to drive your hip into extension as you pause in the runner's lunge with your back leg straight. If necessary, adjust your foot forward a bit to get it outside your hand.

Step your front foot back into the plank position before moving back into downward dog. Then do a runner's lunge on the other side.

MODIFICATIONS: Place your hands on a bench.

EXERCISE SWAPS: Crescent to hamstring stretch, kneeling thoracic extension and lat stretch, half-kneeling TFL stretch

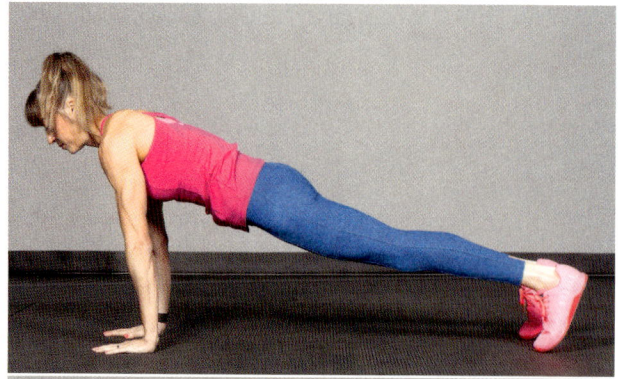

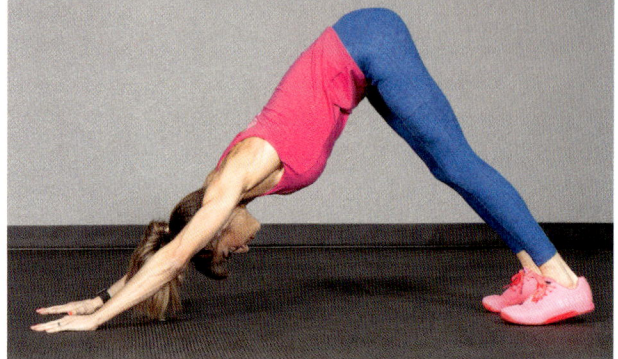

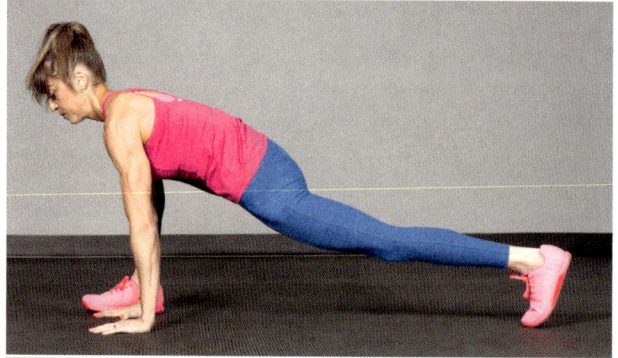

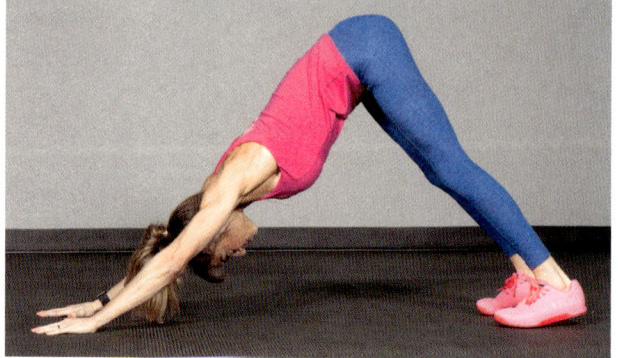

ACTIVE FOAM ROLLER STAR STRETCH

Lie on your back with a foam roller (or yoga block) running parallel to your body on one side. Pull your opposite knee across your body and place it on the roller at about hip height. With your knee and hip bent to about 90 degrees and resting on the roller, use your hand on the same side as the roller to press your knee down into the roller. You may already feel a stretch in your glute.

While holding your knee on the roller, straighten your bottom leg out and turn your shoulders so your back is flat against the ground. Place the hand opposite the roller behind your head so your elbow is open and as close to the ground as possible without your knee coming off the roller.

Rotate through your spine to bring your elbow across your body toward the ground on the side with the roller. Don't just flap your arm; actually rotate your spine. Then rotate open again and engage your back to stretch through your chest as you try to pull your elbow back to the ground while keeping your knee on the roller. Complete all the reps on one side before switching to the other side.

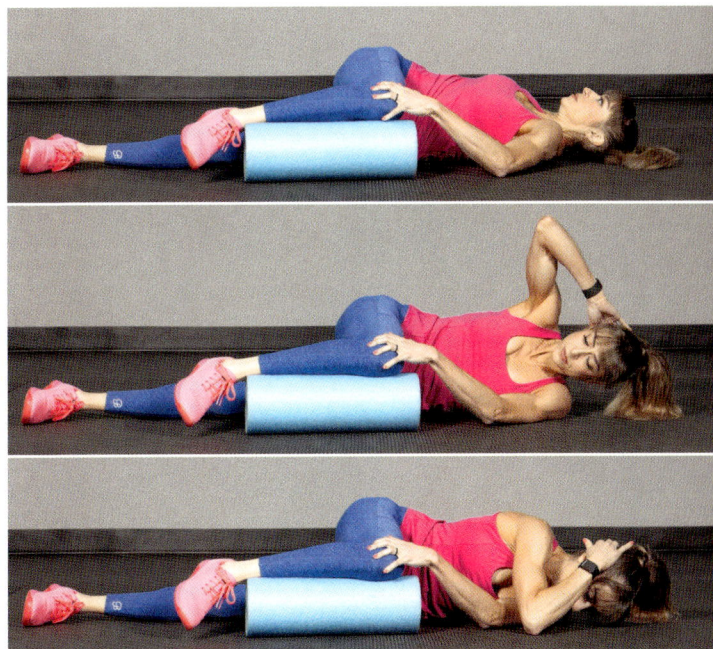

MODIFICATIONS: Only rotate as far open as you can while keeping your knee on the roller. You can use a bigger block if needed.

EXERCISE SWAPS: Quadruped thoracic rotation, star stretch, thread-the-needle, half-kneeling thoracic rotation

---

STANDING FORWARD BEND

Stand with your feet slightly wider than shoulder width (although you can adjust your stance wider for more of a stretch). Fold your forearms over each other. Push your butt back to hinge at the hips, dropping your forearms toward the ground. Keep your legs straight as you relax and hang, feeling a stretch up your hamstrings. Breathe and rock your torso toward one leg and then recenter yourself. Then move to the other side. Pause in each position. You can hold longer in one position as needed.

MODIFICATIONS: You can do the forward bend while seated.

EXERCISE SWAPS: Half wall hang, seated hamstring and spinal twist complex, child's pose with reach—external rotation

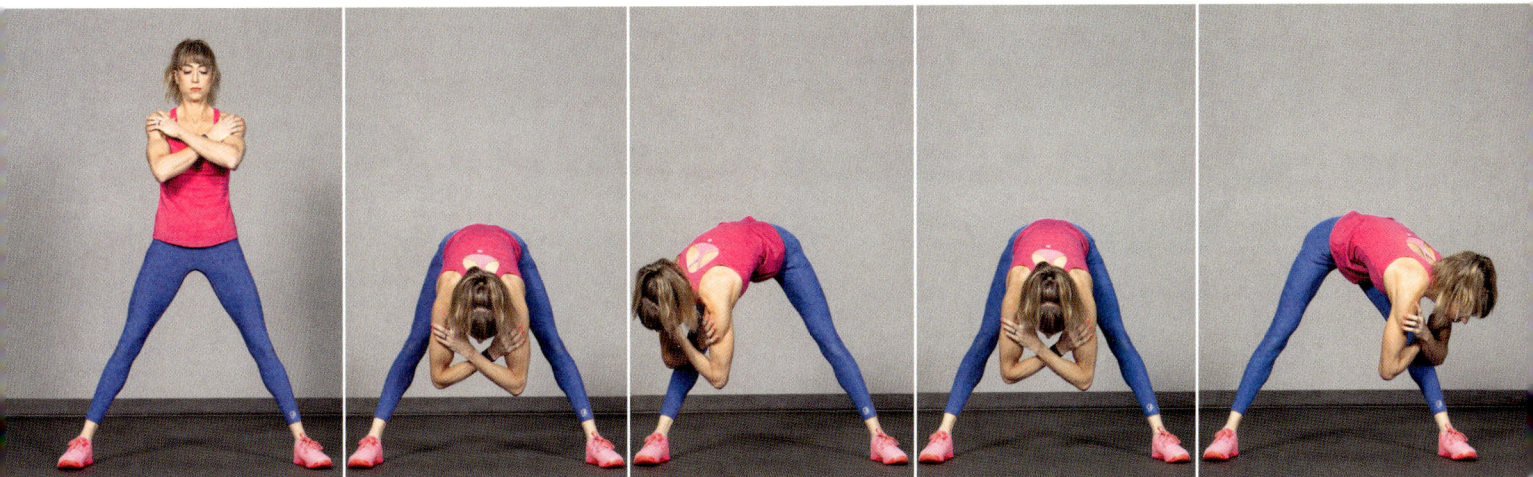

FIGURE 4 HEEL ON WALL

Lie on the ground so that you can place one foot on the wall with your knee bent to 90 degrees. Cross your other ankle over your thigh just above your knee. Press your lower back into the ground. Flex the foot of the crossed-over leg to protect your knee as you press it toward the wall. Feel the stretch in the outside of your glute. Breathe and relax into the stretch.

EXERCISE SWAPS: Extended twisting triangle, star stretch, alternating pigeon pose, seated hamstring and spinal twist complex

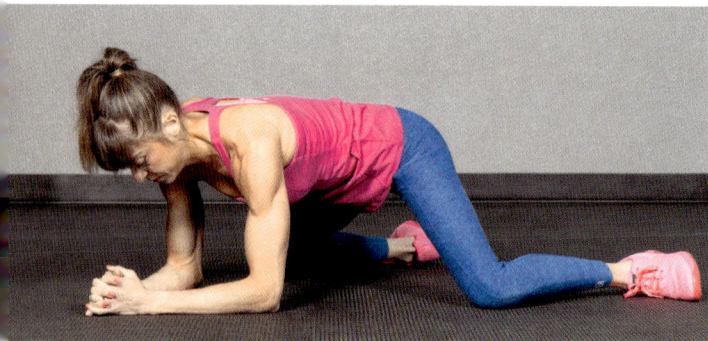

MODIFICATIONS: Perform this seated on a bench, hinging forward to increase the stretch as you hold.

EXERCISE SWAPS: Side lunge hold, standing forward bend, side lunge with rotation, ankle mobility and groin stretch

MODIFICATIONS: You can perform a standing variation, stretching one side at a time by placing a heel on a bench as you take a wide stance with the leg on the bench outstretched.

MODIFICATION

FROG STRETCH

Kneel on the ground and lean on your forearms as you spread your knees apart as wide as possible, slowly sliding or adjusting them open. Turn your feet out as you open your knees to lay the inside of your feet against the ground. Keep your ankles in line with your knees because bringing your heels together behind you reduces the stretch.

Sit your butt back toward your heels as much as possible while keeping your knees wide. Feel the stretch through your inner thighs. This may be a small movement but relax into it. Adjust your knees wider as you breathe into the stretch. You may even rock slightly out of the stretch and then move back into it to help yourself release tension.

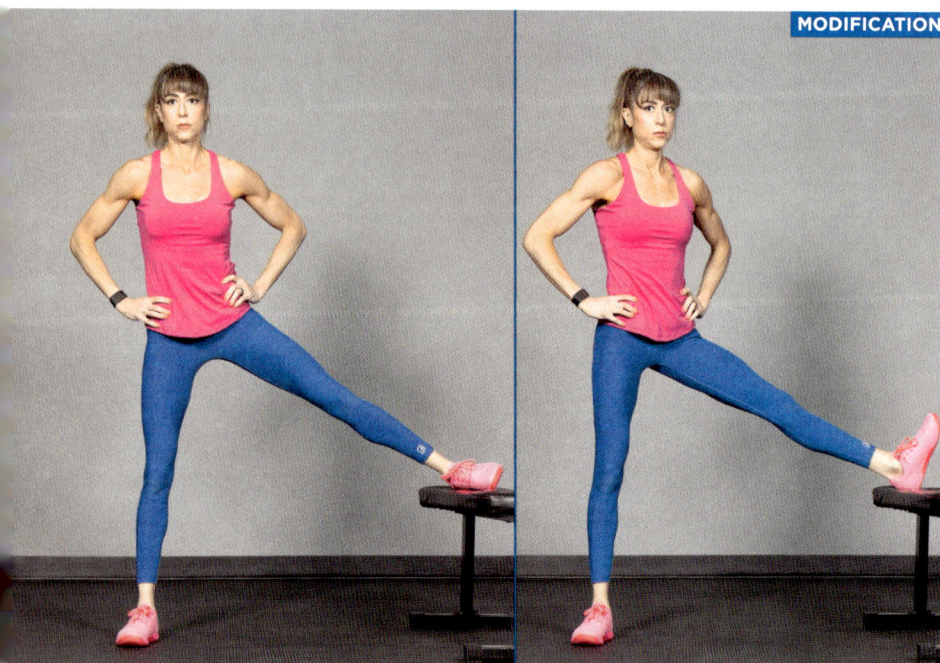

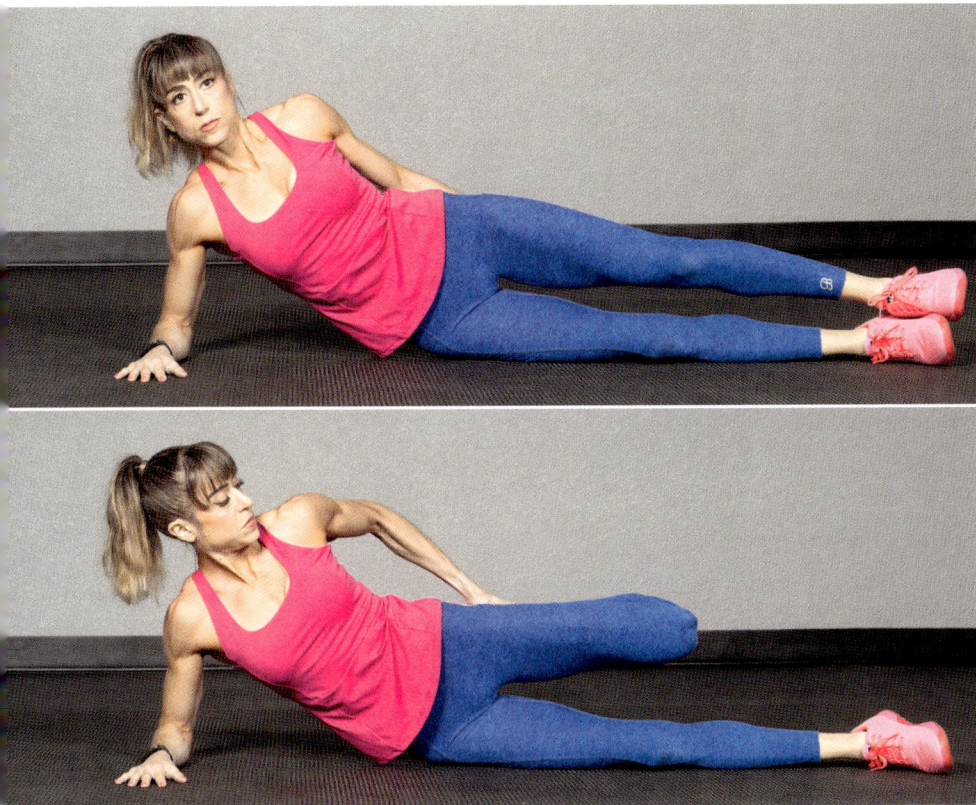

SIDE-LYING QUAD STRETCH

Lie on your side on the ground or on a bench. Prop yourself on your forearm and extend your legs. Grab your top foot and pull your heel toward your butt. Keep your thigh in line with your bottom leg as you engage your glute to extend your hip. Feel the stretch down the front of your thigh. Hold and then roll over and switch sides.

MODIFICATIONS: You can loop a towel around your ankle to help you pull your heel in if needed.

EXERCISE SWAPS: Star stretch with quad stretch, half-kneeling TFL stretch, hip to hamstring stretch, bench hip stretch, standing quad stretch with reach

STANDING CHEST STRETCH

Place one hand on a wall or doorway edge behind you so that your arm is outstretched at shoulder height or a little lower. Make sure you aren't shrugging. Turn away from the hand on the wall, using your back to rotate your chest away. Relax and breathe. Feel a nice stretch in your chest and shoulder. Really engage your back to open up your chest. You don't want all of the stretch to come from the shoulder joint.

Rotate your palm toward the ceiling so your thumb is pointing back behind you to give your shoulder slight external rotation. This helps if you find you're really rounded forward from long hours at the computer.

MODIFICATIONS: You can do both arms at the same time by standing in the doorway and positioning your arms more like goal posts.

EXERCISE SWAPS: Foam roller snow angel, star stretch with quad stretch, wings chest stretch, downward dog to upward dog

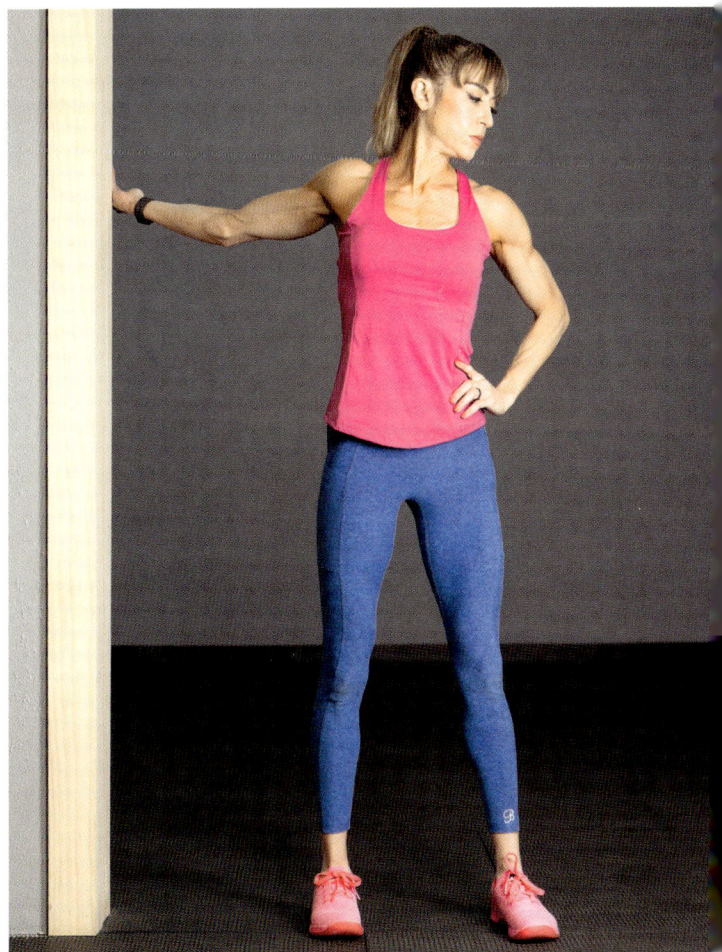

OVERHEAD TRICEPS STRETCH

Reach one hand overhead, bending your elbow to drop your palm behind your back as you reach for your shoulder blades. Place the opposite hand on your bent elbow to push down while also pulling your elbow toward your head. Feel a stretch down the back of your arm as you do this but be conscious not to round forward. Stay up nice and tall.

MODIFICATIONS: You can also do this by using a wall to apply pressure, or you can do a cross-body version if going overhead causes neck or shoulder pain.

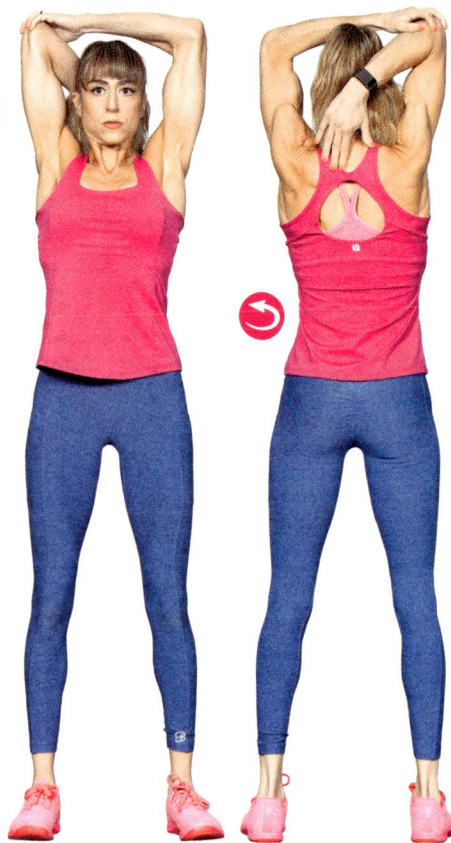

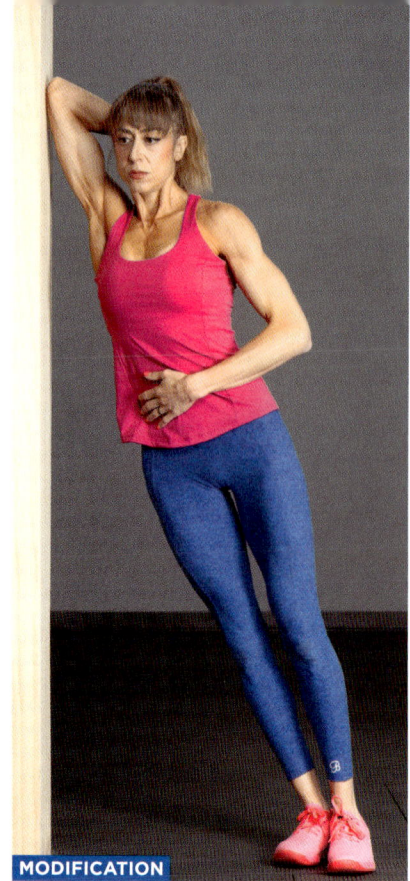

MODIFICATION

EXERCISE SWAPS: Kneeling thoracic extension and stretch, child's pose with reach—external rotation

THREAD-THE-NEEDLE STRETCH

As you kneel on the ground, walk your hands out in front of you and sit your butt slightly back toward your heels (but not all the way on your heels) to feel a stretch up the sides of your back and backs of your arms. You may even feel a slight stretch in your lower back.

Reach one hand (with your palm toward the ceiling) under your body to the other side, twisting through your spine to reach as far as you can. Relax the side of your head and your bottom shoulder down. Breathe and relax into the stretch so that you feel it down your neck and across your shoulder blades. Focus on trying to rotate your chest up as you reach through. You can walk the hand above your head back slightly behind you to increase the stretch.

Recenter yourself and then thread the other arm under and through. Focus on engaging your back to power the twist.

MODIFICATIONS: Modify by standing with your hands on a wall or on a bench.

EXERCISE SWAPS: Seated hamstring and spinal twist complex, half wall hang, half-kneeling thoracic rotation, quadruped thoracic rotation, active foam roller star stretch, star stretch

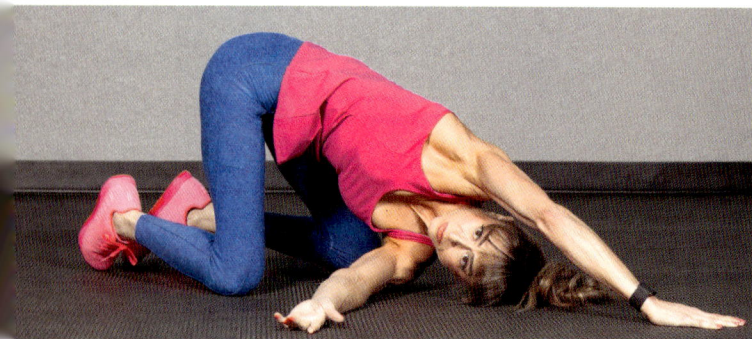

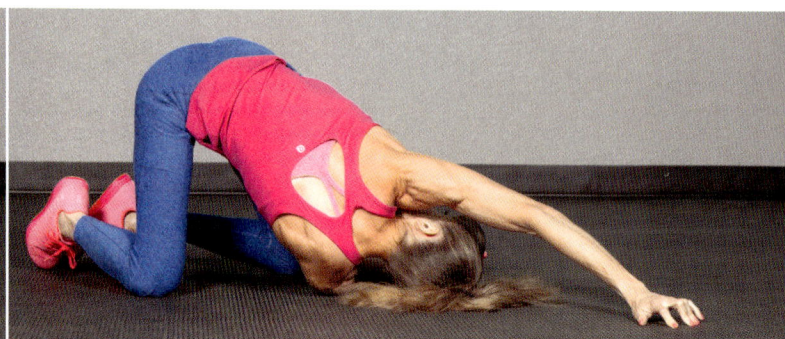

CHILD'S POSE WITH REACH—EXTERNAL ROTATION

Kneel on the ground, sit back on your heels, and walk your arms out in front of you. Rotate your palms toward the ceiling so your thumbs point out to the sides. (Opening your palms toward the ceiling externally rotates your shoulders to increase the stretch on the lats. You can place your palms down if needed.) Reach as far as you can on the ground to feel a nice stretch down the sides of your back. Walk your hands to one side to give the opposite side a deeper stretch. Pause and then walk to the other side.

MODIFICATIONS: Modify with your hands up on a bench or wall, if needed.

EXERCISE SWAPS: Half wall hang, kneeling thoracic extension and lat stretch, half-kneeling TFL stretch, standing forward bend

HALF-KNEELING TFL STRETCH

Position yourself in a half-kneel with your front toes right at a wall and your back knee under your hip. Reach overhead and place your hands on the wall. Walk your hands along the wall past your front leg to feel the stretch down your opposite side. Squeeze the glute of your supporting leg and drive that hip into extension.

While you're leaning forward, don't flex your supporting hip. Squeeze your butt as you reach across and relax into the stretch down your lat and front of your hip.

MODIFICATIONS: Perform this as a standing lunge at the wall.

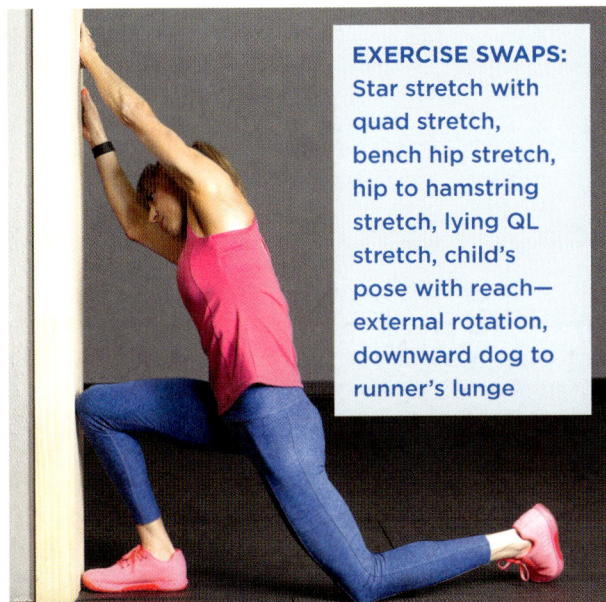

EXERCISE SWAPS: Star stretch with quad stretch, bench hip stretch, hip to hamstring stretch, lying QL stretch, child's pose with reach—external rotation, downward dog to runner's lunge

HALF WALL HANG

Place your hands on a wall at about shoulder height and walk your feet back slightly as you hinge at the hips to drop your chest toward the ground and extend your spine. Keep your arms straight, pushing back off the wall as you use your upper back to drive your spine into extension. Your head and biceps should be in line with your arms. Don't just lean over, though. Push your butt back as you hinge to get a bonus stretch up your hamstrings.

Hold here and breathe. Adjust your hands higher or lower as needed to feel the spinal extension and stretch down your arms and back.

MODIFICATIONS: Place your hands up higher on the wall as needed based on your mobility.

EXERCISE SWAPS: Child's pose with reach—external rotation, kneeling thoracic extension and lat stretch, standing forward bend

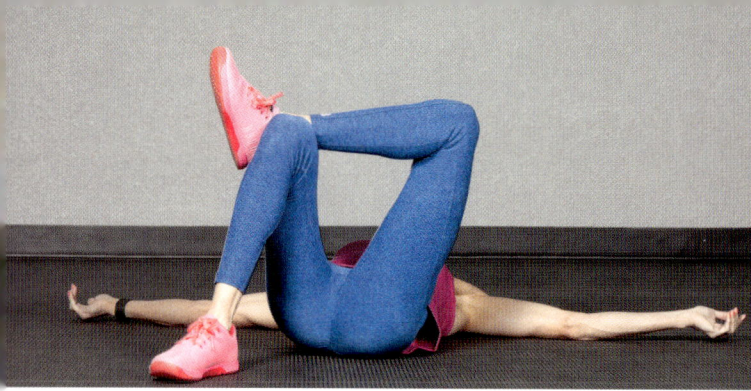

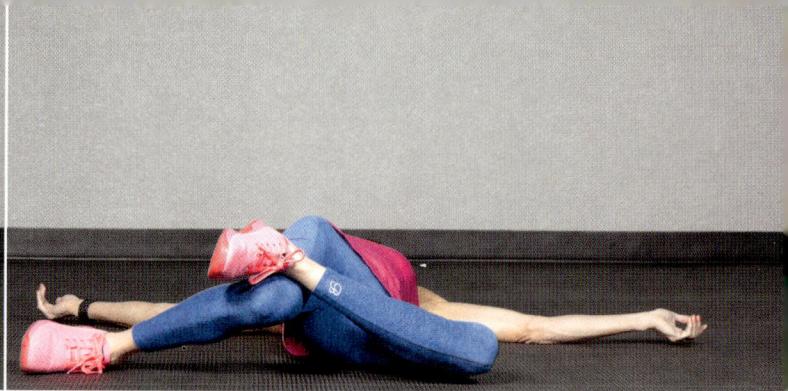

LYING QL STRETCH

Lie on your back with your arms reaching out on the ground at about shoulder height. Bend one knee and place your foot flat on the ground. Cross your other ankle over your thigh right above your bent knee.

Use the crossed-over leg to pull the other knee down to the side and push it toward the ground. If your knee shifted forward as you twisted, you may have to adjust your support leg to keep your hip in extension and your knee in line with it.

Keep your upper back and arms flat against the ground as you twist your legs. Feel a nice stretch through the side of your lower back and the side of your hip and IT band. Breathe and relax your knees toward the ground. Hold and then switch sides.

MODIFICATIONS: You can do a standing side bend or use the standing version of the TFL stretch to modify.

EXERCISE SWAPS: Half-kneeling TFL stretch, child's pose with reach—external rotation, standing forward bend

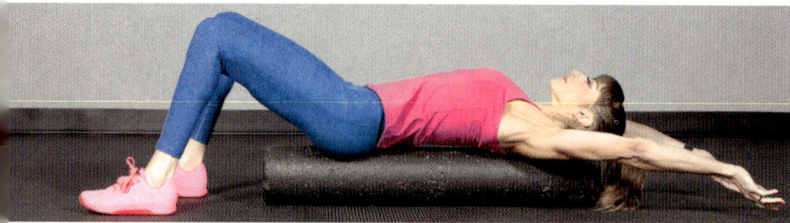

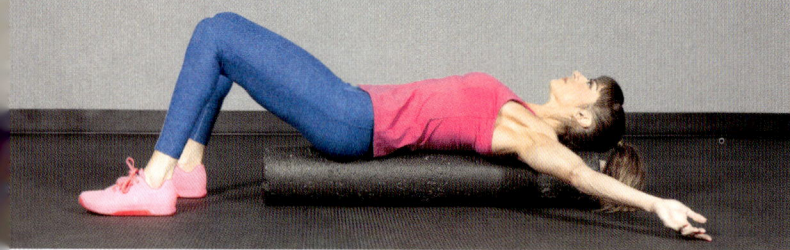

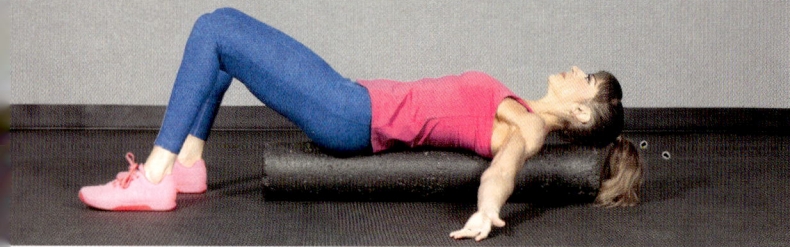

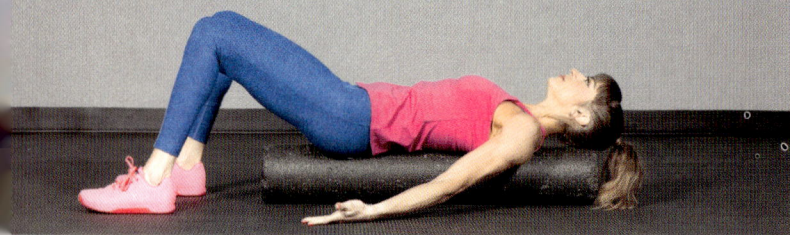

FOAM ROLLER SNOW ANGEL

Lie with a long foam roller aligned under your spine and with your head supported. Bend your knees and place your feet flat on the ground to help you balance. Let your arms open at shoulder height with your palms facing up so you feel a stretch through your chest. Sweep your arms overhead toward the wall behind you and then sweep them back toward your feet. Relax your arms open as you make the snow angel move, pausing to hold in any specifically tight spot. Focus on engaging your back, almost pinching the roller with your shoulder blades to feel an extra stretch in your chest.

MODIFICATIONS: You can lie on a bench and let your arms hang off the sides.

EXERCISE SWAPS: Wings chest stretch, suspension trainer snow angel, star stretch, downward dog to upward dog, prone snow angel, cobra wings

SEATED HAMSTRING AND SPINAL TWIST COMPLEX

There are three stretches within this series (hamstring, glute, and spinal twist).

HAMSTRING: Sit on the ground with one leg out straight in front of you and the bottom of your other foot against the inner thigh of the outstretched leg so your knee is falling open. Hinge at your hips to reach for your foot by folding over your straight front leg. Don't simply round over; focus on feeling the stretch through your hamstrings. Hold and breathe and try to relax further into the stretch.

GLUTE: Cross the ankle of the bent leg over your straight leg right above your knee. Place your hands on the ground behind your butt and bend the straight leg, bringing your heel in toward your butt so you're in a figure 4, glute-stretch position. Sit up nice and tall and press your leg and chest closer together to feel a stretch in the outside of your glute. Focus on pushing the knee of your crossed-over leg open as you hold. Walk your hands toward your butt to help push yourself taller. You can also move the foot on the ground closer to your glutes to bring your leg in closer. Flex the foot of your crossed-over leg to protect your knee. Hold in this position.

SPINAL TWIST: Twist and drop the bottom of your crossed-over foot to the ground. As you twist, let your bottom leg fall open onto its side. Sit nice and tall and reach across your top leg with your opposite arm to push your elbow into your thigh as you twist your chest toward that leg. Use your arm to help you twist open as your other hand supports you. Breathe and feel the stretch through your spine, glute, and chest by engaging your upper back to help you twist.

MODIFICATIONS: Use a towel to help you reach your foot for the hamstring stretch and do not bring your heel in as close with the glute stretch. You may find sitting on a bench or against a wall helps for that move. For the spinal twist, you can straighten your bottom leg or sit on a bench.

EXERCISE SWAPS: Standing forward bend, thread-the-needle stretch, star stretch, figure 4 heel on wall, world's greatest stretch

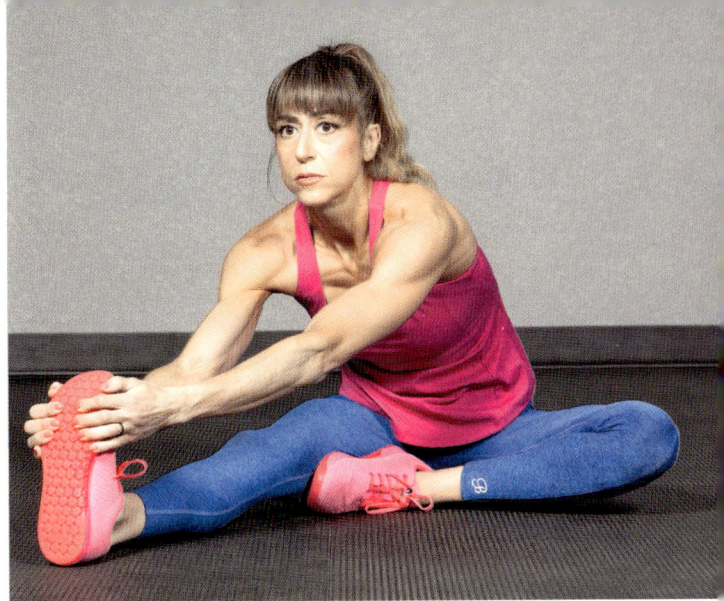

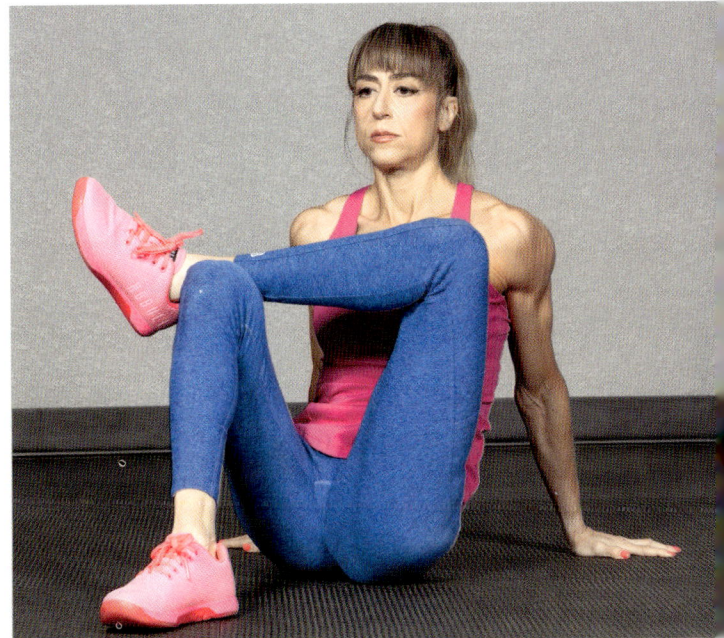

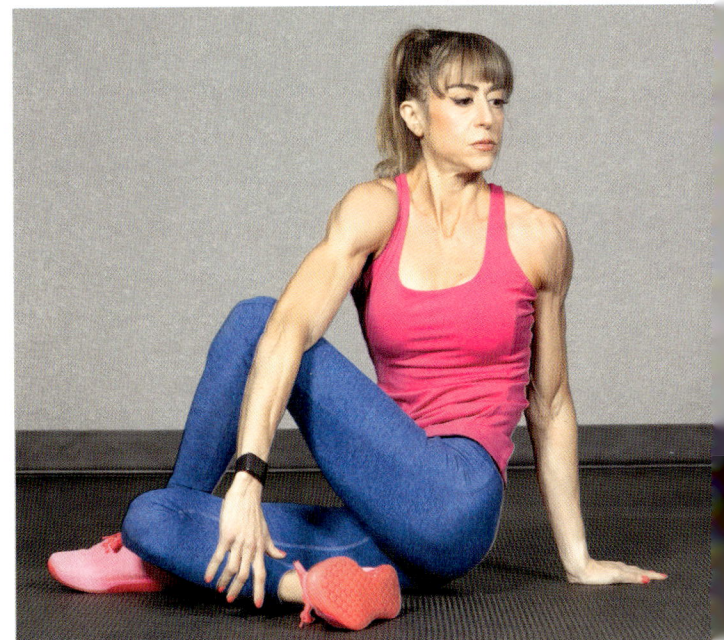

EXERCISE SWAPS: Star stretch with quad stretch, seated hamstring and spinal twist complex, active foam roller star stretch, thread-the-needle stretch, half-kneeling thoracic rotation, alternating pigeon pose, figure 4 heel on wall

STAR STRETCH

Lie on your back with your legs out straight and your arms stretched on the ground at about shoulder height. Bend one knee to about 90 degrees and pull it across your body with your opposite hand while keeping your other leg fairly straight on the ground. Use your hand to press your knee toward the ground so you feel a stretch through your glute and up into your spine.

Keep your other arm outstretched and your upper back fully pressed down. Do not let that shoulder lift with the rotation of your hips. Only push the knee down as close to the ground as you can while keeping your back down. Relax and feel a stretch through your chest, spine, and butt.

MODIFICATIONS: Place a block under the knee you've pulled across to support the stretch.

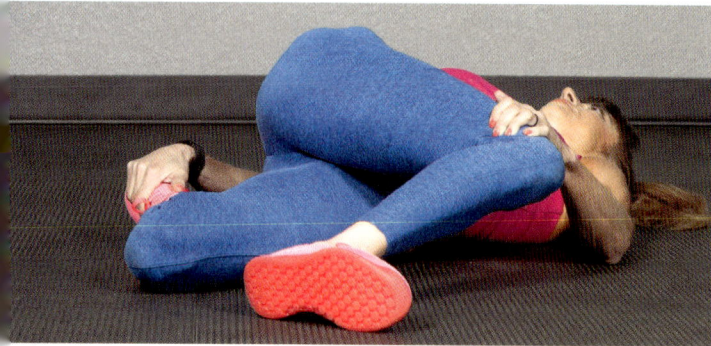

STAR STRETCH WITH QUAD STRETCH

Lie on your back with your legs straight and your arms out on the ground at about shoulder height. Bend one knee to about 90 degrees and pull it across your body with your opposite hand. Use your hand on top of your knee to press it toward the ground so you feel a stretch through your glute and up into your spine.

Then bend your bottom leg and grab your ankle to pull your heel in toward your butt. Extend your hip and make sure your knee is in line with your hip to feel a stretch down the front of your thigh.

As you pull that heel toward your butt and press your other knee down, breathe and relax as you press your upper back into the ground. Keep your shoulder blades down to help you open your chest and get a full stretch through your spine. If you can't keep your back on the ground, do not push down as much on the crossed-over knee. Breathe and relax into it as you feel your chest, spine, glute, and quad stretching.

MODIFICATIONS: Place a block under the crossed-over knee to support it and control the range of motion of the stretch. Use a towel to reach your ankle and pull into the quad stretch.

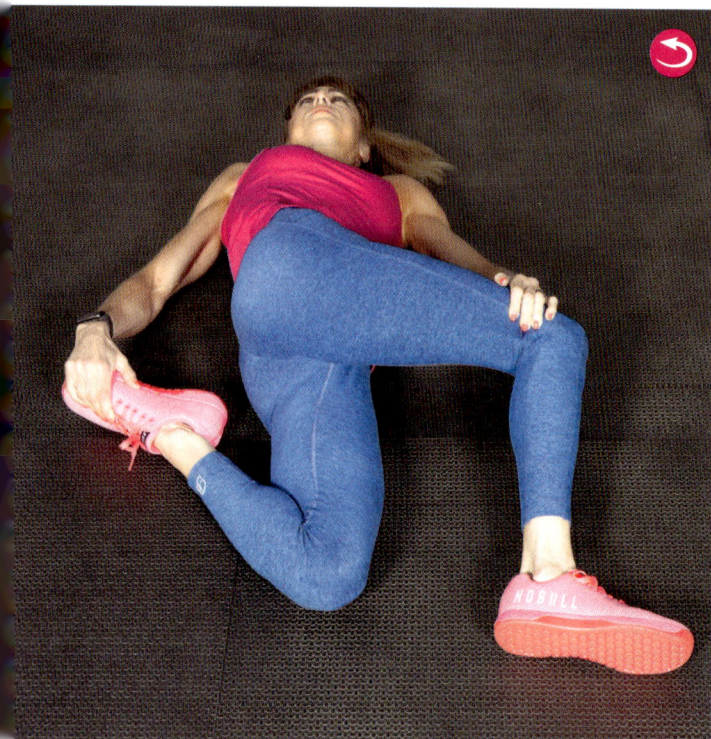

EXERCISE SWAPS: Star stretch, side-lying quad stretch, half-kneeling TFL stretch, standing quad stretch with reach

ACTIVATION/ISOMETRICS

WALL SIT

Sink into a squat with your back pressed into the wall behind you as you try to get your quads as close to parallel to the ground as possible. Keep your ankles aligned under your knees and drive back into the wall through your entire foot. Do not rock forward onto your toes. Hold parallel to the ground and focus on feeling the front of your thighs work. Do not round or lean forward.

MODIFICATIONS: Do not sink as low in the squat or consider stabilizing yourself with a chair or suspension trainer.

EXERCISE SWAPS: Rock lunge, lunge hold, sumo squat hold

SIDE PLANK CLAM

Set up on your side with your forearm on the ground, your elbow underneath your shoulder, and your legs stacked. Bend your knees so that your feet and lower legs are just slightly behind you. Turn your top foot so the toe is pointing toward the ground over your bottom foot to prevent your top hip from rotating open as you lift.

With your top hand on your hip, lift your bottom hip, driving through your knee and forearm to come into a side plank position. As you lift, drive your hips forward to make sure you engage your glutes and extend your hips while using your top glute to open your top knee in the clam movement.

Do not let your feet come apart. Really feel your bottom oblique and glute working to hold the side plank as the side of your top glute works to lift your leg open laterally. Do not rotate. Lower to the floor and repeat the side plank and clam. Focus on engaging your glutes to keep your hips extended and lift your knee. Don't let your elbow get out in front of your shoulder and make sure to engage your back to support your shoulder as you plank up.

MODIFICATIONS: Place your elbow on a low box or do a basic clam or knee side plank hold.

EXERCISE SWAPS: Fire hydrant, side plank hold, mini band glute bridge, mini band bridge hold with abduction

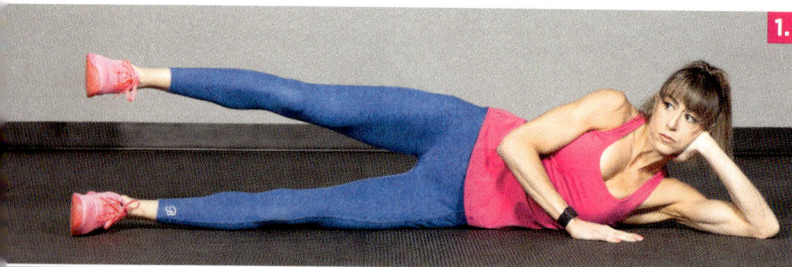

SIDE-LYING SERIES

There are five movements to this series. Set up by lying on your side with your head propped up in one hand and the other hand down on the ground in front of you to help you stabilize. Make sure your body is in a nice straight line with your glutes engaged to extend your hips so you aren't slightly hinged forward. You can slightly turn your bottom foot down to push through the ball of your foot a bit to stabilize. Raise your top leg up about 8 inches from your bottom leg and do not let it lower from here through all the movements.

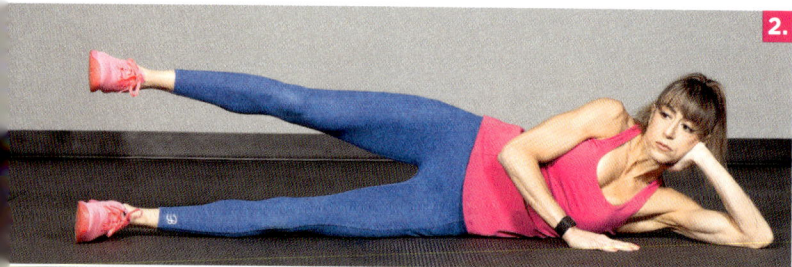

1. LYING LEG RAISES: Lift your top leg without rotating your toe open. You can slightly kick back to engage that glute maximus. Feel the side of your butt engage to try to stop the lift from going higher and to prevent you from rotating your toe open. Don't just swing your leg; use your glute to lift. Lower your leg until it's again 8 inches above your bottom leg and complete all reps of this movement before moving to the next.

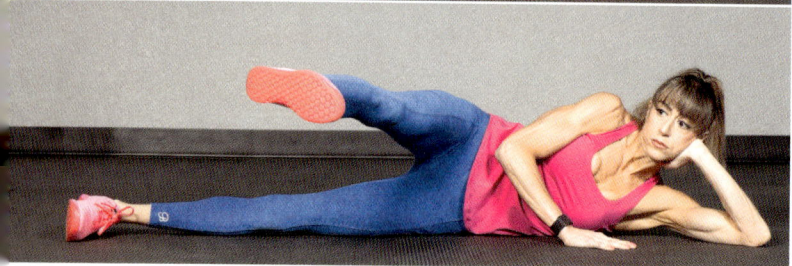

2. LYING FRONT KICKS: With your leg still raised, kick forward. Do not let your leg drop closer to the ground. You're doing small kicks forward and then moving back to the starting position over your bottom leg. Move at a controlled pace so your torso stays stable.

3. LYING BACK KICKS: With your leg still raised, kick your leg back. Feel your glute work to extend your hip; don't just swing your leg back. Bring it back above your bottom leg and repeat.

MODIFICATIONS: Do fewer reps or pause between moves. You may include just the raises and front to back kicks if needed.

EXERCISE SWAPS: 3-way hip circle, fire hydrant, standing 3-way hip circle, mini band glute bridge, mini band bridge hold with abduction

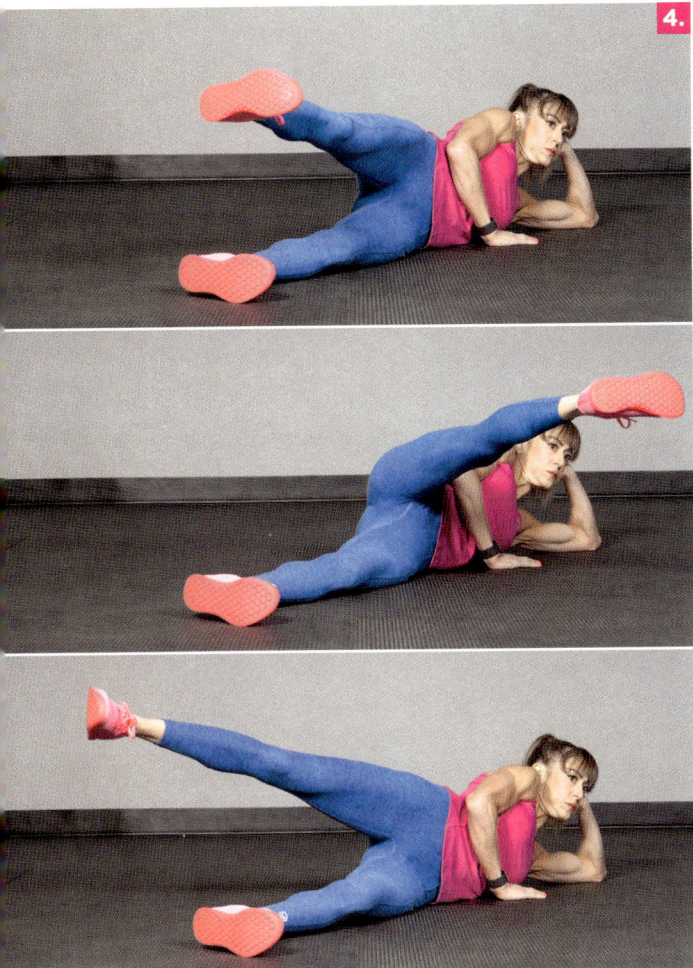

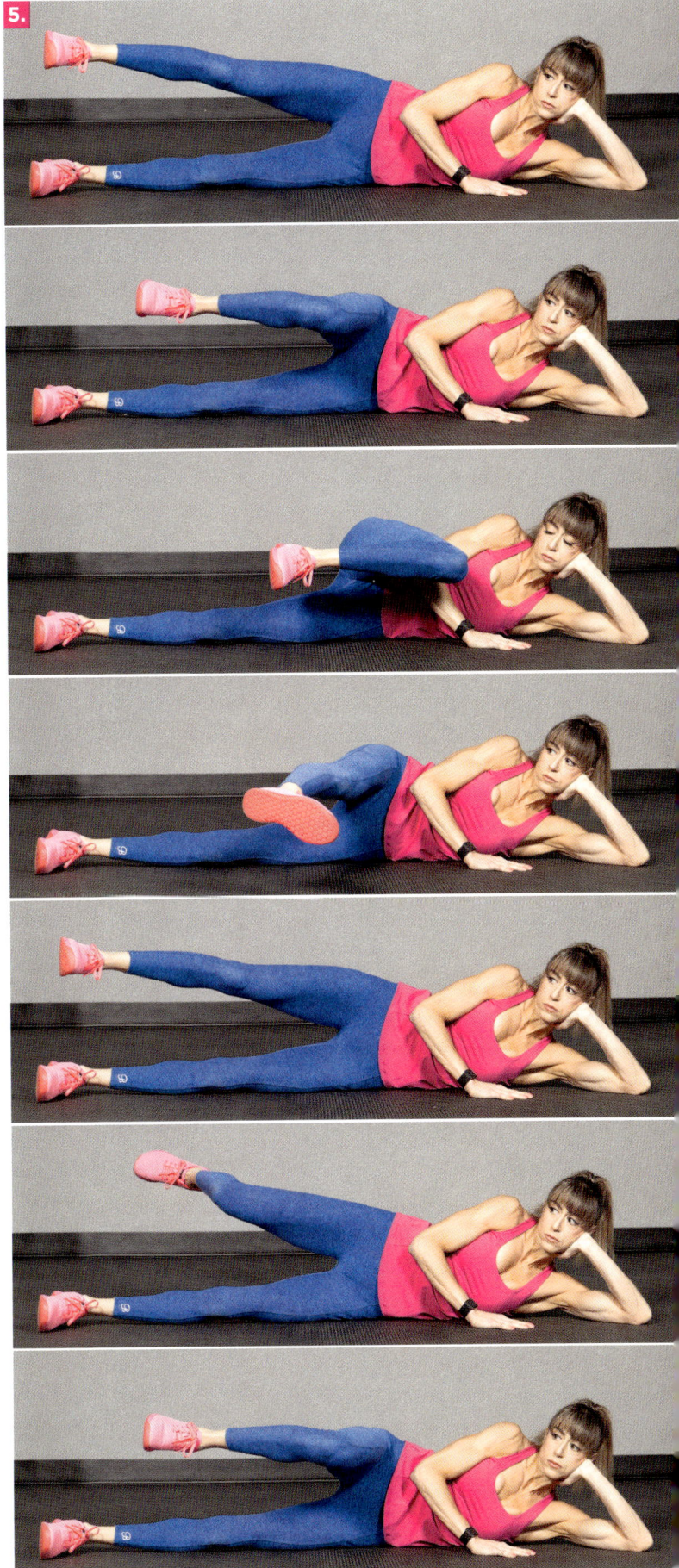

4. LYING FRONT TO BACK KICKS: Combine the front to back kicks into one motion. Perform a full range of motion, kicking forward then all the way back behind you. Do not swing or let your leg come closer than 8 inches from the ground. Keep your body still as you kick your leg forward and back. Make sure to avoid arching your lower back as you kick behind you.

5. LYING BICYCLES: Keeping your leg raised, move your leg as if you're pedaling on a bicycle. Draw your knee up to your chest then circle your foot down in front of you before pulling it back up to your chest.

Feel the outside of your hip and glute working through all of these movements with your hip flexors also engaging in the front kicks and lying bicycles.

GLUTE BRIDGE WITH SQUEEZE

Place a block or ball between your knees and lie on your back with your knees bent and your feet flat on the floor. Bend your elbows and drive your upper arms down into the ground as you squeeze the block. Tuck your hips just slightly toward your ribs to engage the posterior pelvic tilt and brace your abs.

Bridge up, driving your knees toward your toes as you push through your upper back, arms, and full foot. Squeeze your glutes to extend your hips as you squeeze the block. If necessary, you can raise your toes to help engage your glutes but watch that your hamstrings don't take over. Lower and repeat.

ROLLER SERRATUS ANTERIOR EXTENSION

Stand facing the wall with a roller or sliders under your wrists; your palms are facing each other. The roller should be at about eye height to start, and your arms should be about shoulder-width or just slightly wider apart. Walk your feet backward so you're angled into the wall and resting a bit of your weight against the roller so you can push into it as you extend your arms.

Brace your abs as you roll your arms until they're extended. Lean into the wall as you extend. Do not arch your lower back. Think of pulling your shoulder blades "out and around" as you slide up. Pull with your back to roll your arms back down. You may feel your upper traps slightly, but do not allow them to compensate as you keep consistent pressure on the roller. If you feel your lower back taking over, stagger your feet to help maintain a neutral spine.

MODIFICATIONS: Do a single arm with sliders if you're struggling to control the move or have an imbalance.

EXERCISE SWAPS: Downward dog scapular press, plange plank, side plank oblique twist

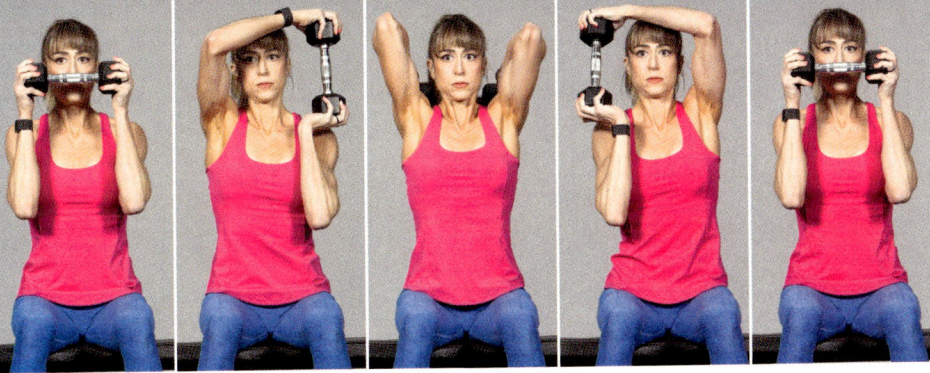

MODIFICATIONS: If it's too much of a challenge to do this move while seated, you can stand with your feet hip-width apart. You can use a kettlebell or plate weight in place of the dumbbell. To create even more of a core challenge, do this while kneeling.

SEATED HALO

Sit on a bench with your legs hip-width apart. Hold a dumbbell in both hands with one hand on each head of the weight. Position the dumbbell in front of your face with your elbows close to your body and pointing down toward the ground. Sit straight with your chest tall and your shoulders down and back. Squeeze your glutes and brace your core as you begin to move the weight.

EXERCISE SWAPS: Prone snow angel, cobra wings, bulldog shoulder tap, plank with toe touch, dip hold

Circle the weight back toward one side of your head and then continue moving it to drop it down behind your head. When the weight is behind your neck, your elbows are rotated to point toward the ceiling. Keep your core tight as you isolate your upper body. Avoid tucking your chin or moving your head. Continue to circle the weight to the other side of your head before bringing it back in front of your face. Reverse the direction of your circle. Keep alternating directions until all reps are complete.

PRONE SNOW ANGEL

Lie face down on the ground with your legs out straight. Place your hands behind your head. Engage your glutes and upper back to lift your chest slightly off the ground so your elbows are hovering. Your head is in line with your spine. Straighten your arms overhead and then slowly move them out to the side with your palms facing down as if you're creating a snow angel.

Swing your arms out to the sides while flipping your hands over; then rotate your shoulders as you bend your elbows to bring the backs of your hands to your lower back. Reverse the motion, bringing your hands back out to the sides and then back up overhead and behind your head. Feel the muscles of your upper back and the backs of your shoulders working to keep your arms elevated off the ground through the movement.

MODIFICATIONS: Place a towel under your forehead for support or perform this move standing and hinged over.

EXERCISE SWAPS: Cobra wing, scapular wings, halo, bulldog shoulder tap, plank with toe touch, dip hold

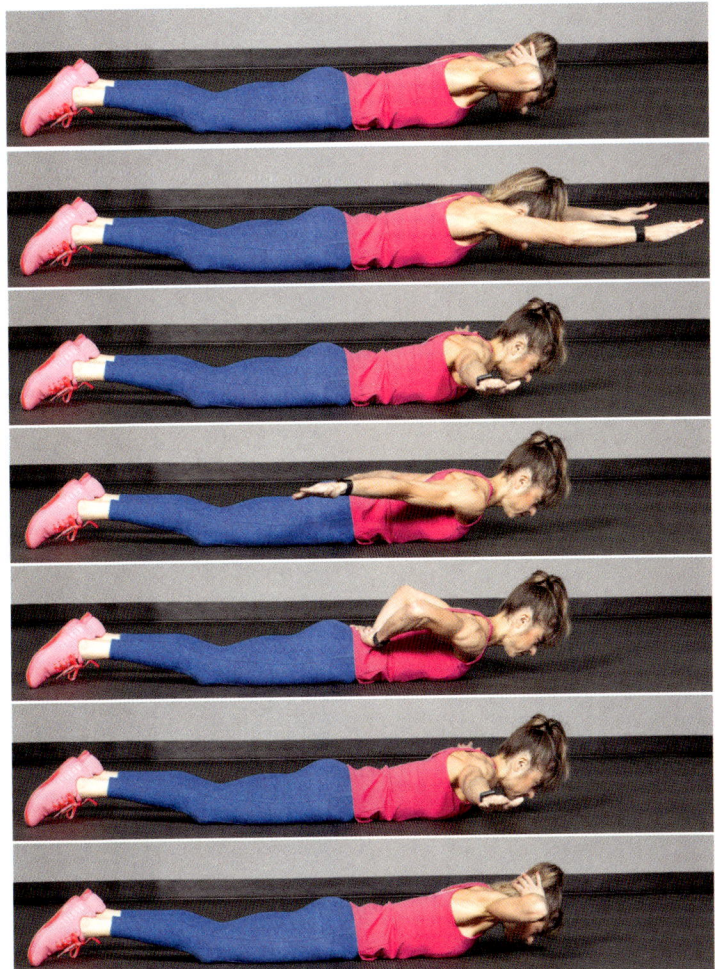

SINGLE-ARM SCAPULAR PUSH-UP

Place one hand on a wall at about shoulder height or just slightly below with your arm straight. Stand so you're slightly leaning into the wall and engage your back to make sure your shoulders aren't shrugged. You can put your other hand across your chest or let it hang.

Keeping your elbow straight while pressing into the wall, pinch your shoulder blade toward your spine. Do not shrug; instead, perform a small movement to draw your shoulder blade toward your spine as you press your chest out. Then push the wall away to move your shoulder blade back forward around your rib cage. Do not round your back. This is a small movement. Do not rotate or swing or bend your arm to make it bigger. Focus just on that pinch of the shoulder blade toward your spine.

MODIFICATIONS: You can do this without the wall if you find the push into it prevents you from feeling the shoulder blade movement.

EXERCISE SWAPS: Scapular push-up, scapular wall hold, lying scapular hold, scapular wings

PLANK WITH TOE TOUCH

Start in a high plank position with your feet about shoulder-width apart and your hands under your shoulders. Spread your fingers wide to grip the ground. Lift one hand and push back into downward dog as you reach toward the toes of the opposite foot. Extend your spine as you lift your butt toward the ceiling. Also drive your heels toward the ground as you push off with your hand to press your chest back and rotate to reach. Then move back into the plank while bracing your abs so you don't drop your hips. Lift the other hand to repeat on the other side.

Focus on feeling your back support the shoulder of the hand on the ground as you extend your spine. You should also feel your abs and obliques working to perform the reach while your hamstrings and calves feel a stretch from driving your heels down as you touch your toe.

MODIFICATIONS: Place your hands on a bench or box or remove the toe touch.

EXERCISE SWAPS: Prone snow angel, cobra wings, bulldog shoulder tap, halo, extended plank hold, downward dog scapular press, plank with reach back and out

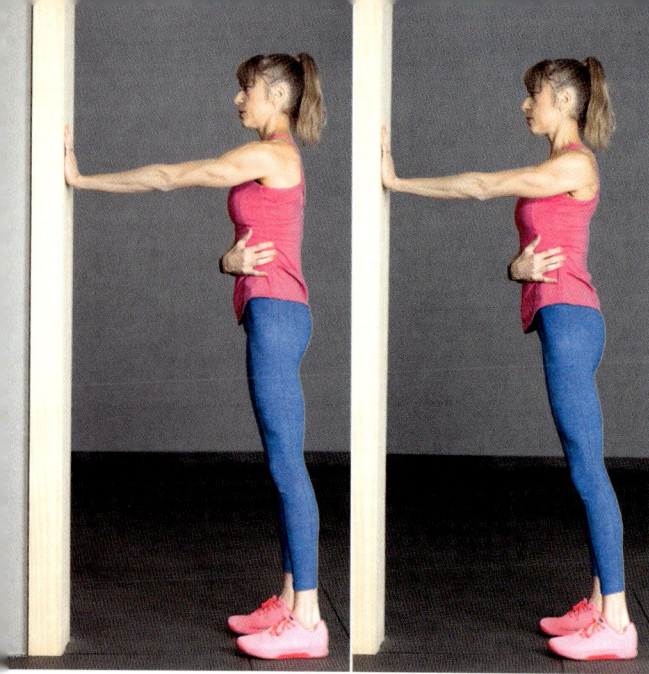

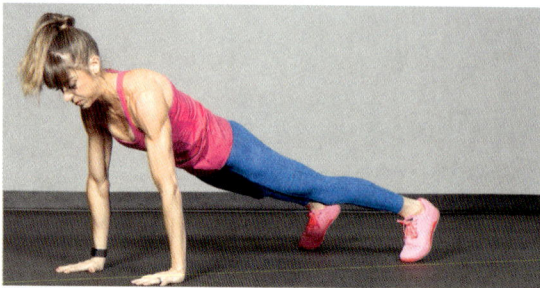

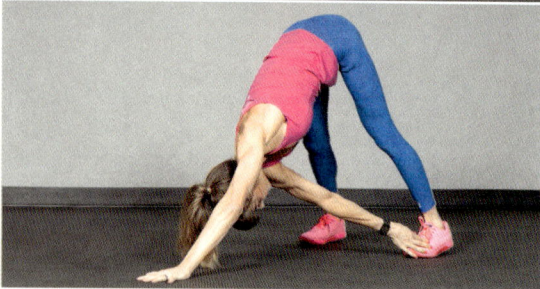

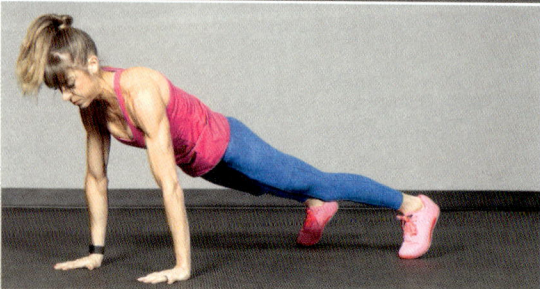

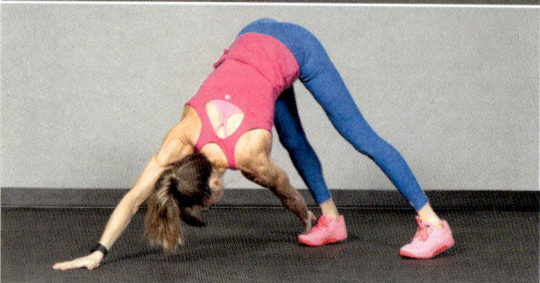

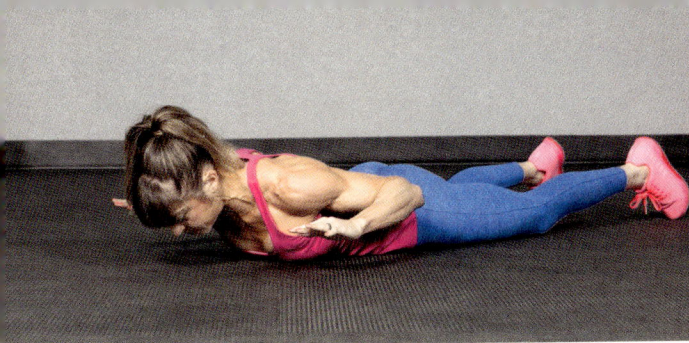

LYING W PULLDOWN

Lie face down on the ground with your hands hovering above the ground by your shoulders and your elbows in by your body. Actively pull your elbows down and in toward your sides, feeling the sides of your back and the backs of your shoulders engage to keep your arms off the ground.

Keep your hands off the ground as you extend your arms straight out toward the wall beyond your head. Then bring your hands back down. Focus on that active pull to bring your hands in line with your shoulders as if you're performing a pull-up or lat pulldown.

MODIFICATIONS: Place a towel under your forehead for support or perform this move while standing and hinged at your hips.

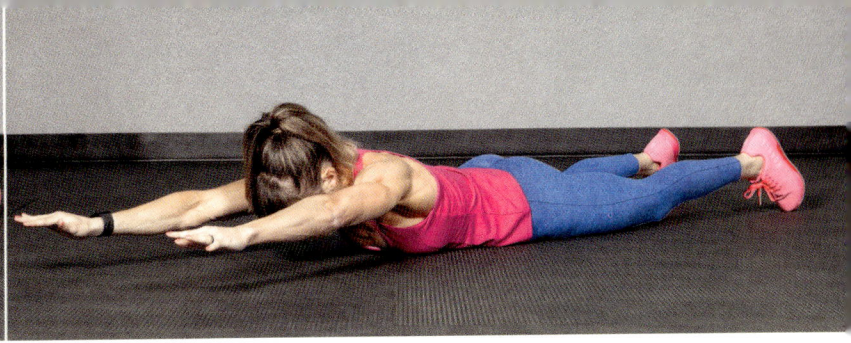

EXERCISE SWAPS: Dip hold, cobra hold, cobra wings, scapular push-up, single-arm scapular push-up

CAMEL BRIDGE

Kneel on the ground with your knees about hip-width apart; sit back on your heels with your feet flexed. Pointing your toes will make the move harder and require more flexibility. Place your hands on your heels. While holding onto your feet, bridge up, pressing your chest out as you drive your hips up. Really concentrate on opening your chest and extending your hips by engaging your back and glutes. Focusing on these areas will prevent you from arching only your lower back. Pause in the bridge and relax your head back as needed. Then sit back down.

EXERCISE SWAPS: Tabletop bridge, plank with reach back and out, glute bridge hold, scapular wall hold, single-leg reverse hyper, sit-thru to thoracic bridge, mini band glute bridge

MODIFICATIONS: Place your hands on a bench or chair behind you instead of placing them on your feet.

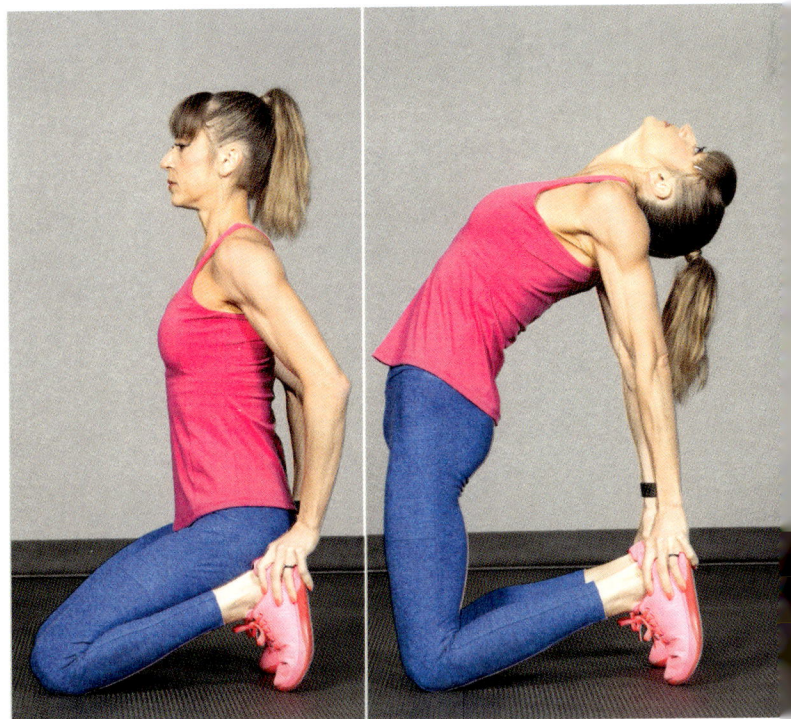

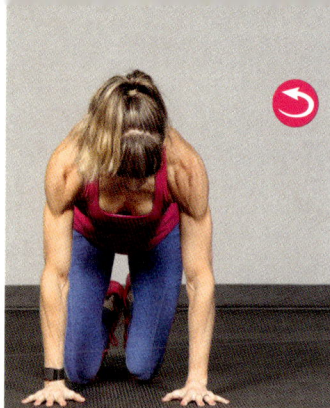

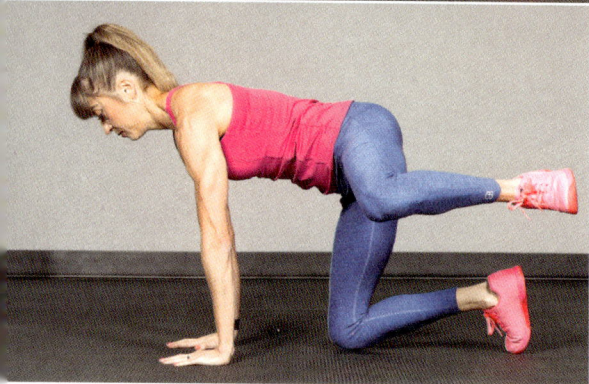

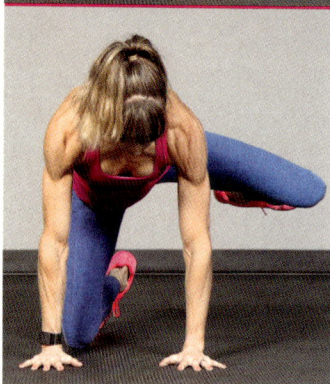

FIRE HYDRANT

Set up on all fours with your hands under your shoulders and your knees under your hips. Flex your feet. Keeping your arms straight, knees bent, and feet flexed, raise one leg out to the side. Focus on keeping your raised knee in line with your hip. Also keep your lower leg parallel to the ground rather than having your knee way higher than your ankle or your ankle way above your knee. Pause then lower your leg. Focus on feeling your glute lift your leg to the side. It's tempting to swing, rotate, lean, or bend your arms to lift your leg higher, but don't.

MODIFICATIONS: Do this off a bench or use a smaller range of motion. To progress, straighten your leg or add a band.

EXERCISE SWAPS: Side plank clam, side-lying series, 3-way hip circle, standing 3-way hip circle, mini band bridge hold with abduction

SCAPULAR WINGS

Lie face down on the ground with your legs out straight and hands behind your head. Lift your chest slightly off the ground, engaging your glutes and upper back so just your elbows are touching the ground. Your head should be in line with your spine. Pinch your shoulder blades together, lifting your elbows off the ground. Feel the muscles between your shoulder blades and the backs of your shoulders working.

Pause and then lower your elbows. Don't arch your back or move your hands from your head. Just focus on your shoulder blades moving toward your spine to lift your elbows as you feel a stretch in your chest.

MODIFICATIONS: Place a towel under your forehead if needed for support or perform this move standing and hinged at your hips.

EXERCISE SWAPS: Single-arm scapular push-up, scapular push-up, scapular wall hold, lying scapular hold

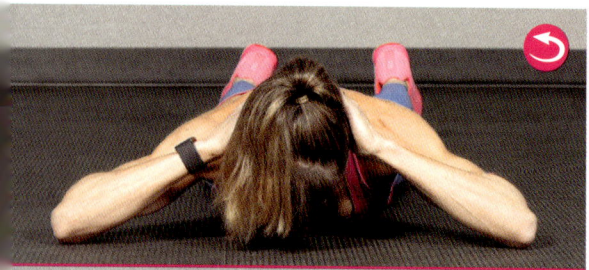

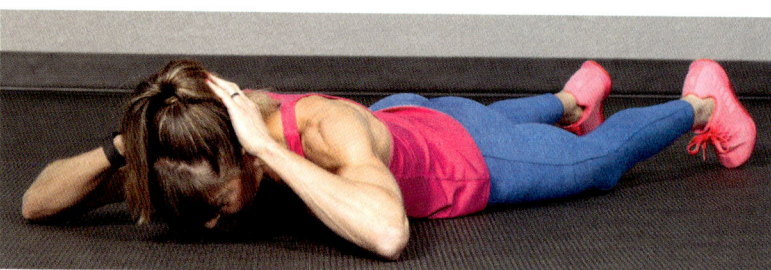

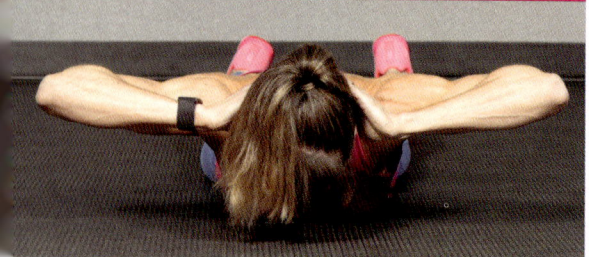

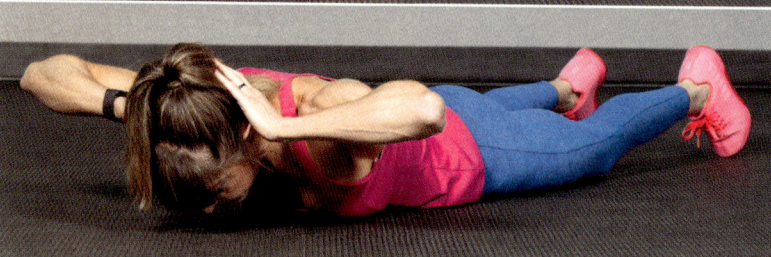

3-WAY HIP CIRCLE

Set up on all fours with your hands under your shoulders and your knees under your hips. Flex your feet. Kick one leg back to drive your heel up (like a donkey kick, with your knee bent at about 90 degrees). Feel your glute work to drive your heel toward the ceiling but stop the movement before you arch your lower back. Your hips should stay level to the ground. Pause here to feel your glutes.

With your knee still bent, circle your knee out to the side in the fire hydrant position. Do not lower your leg as you move from the donkey kick to the fire hydrant. Keep your knee and ankle in line as you pause and feel the side of your glute working.

Without touching your knee down, drive it forward and toward your elbow. Feel your abs engage as you hold and curl your knee in. Pause and then repeat the kick back. Don't bend your elbows as you do this and focus on really keeping your core braced and your body still.

MODIFICATIONS: Perform this off a bench. Pausing between each move can also help.

EXERCISE SWAPS: Standing 3-way hip circle, fire hydrant, plank with reach back and out, 2-way reach skater lunge, mini band glute bridge, mini band bridge hold with abduction

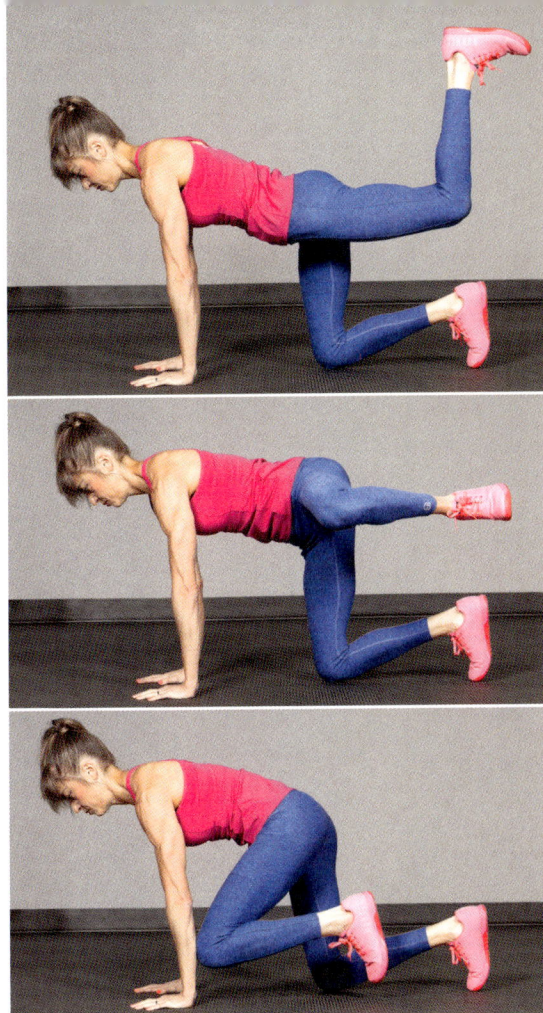

SIT-THRU TO THORACIC BRIDGE

Start on all fours with your hands under your shoulders and your knees under your hips. Flex your feet and lift up onto your hands and the balls of your feet. Then lift one hand up as you tuck the opposite knee under your body toward the side of your lifted hand so you flip over and end with your foot flat on the ground. As you rotate your hips toward the ceiling, squeeze your glutes to lift them up as high as you can. Reach your raised hand down toward the ground, rotating your chest back toward the floor.

Then drop your hips and step your foot back under your body while placing your hand back on the ground. Then rotate the other direction.

MODIFICATIONS: Place your hands on a bench or box to reduce the mobility and strength demands.

EXERCISE SWAPS: Tabletop bridge, 3-way hip circle, standing 3-way hip circle, side plank oblique twist

COBRA WINGS

Lie face down on the ground with your legs straight and your arms along your sides with your palms facing the ceiling. Engage your upper back to lift your chest and arms off the ground. Focus on opening your chest as you keep your head in line with your spine. Sweep your arms out to the sides as you rotate your palms to face toward the ground; then continue to sweep them overhead.

Reverse the movement, sweeping your arms back down as you rotate your shoulders so your palms are facing up as your arms return to your sides. With your arms back by your sides, lower your chest to the ground. Repeat the movement. Make sure to engage your glutes and focus on lifting your chest by extending your upper back, not by arching your lower back. Also, feel the muscles working in the backs of your shoulders and between your shoulder blades.

MODIFICATIONS: Place a towel under your forehead for support and keep constant tension throughout the lift. Perform this move standing while hinged at your hips, if needed.

EXERCISE SWAPS: Prone snow angel, scapular wings, halo, bulldog shoulder tap, plank with toe touch, cobra hold

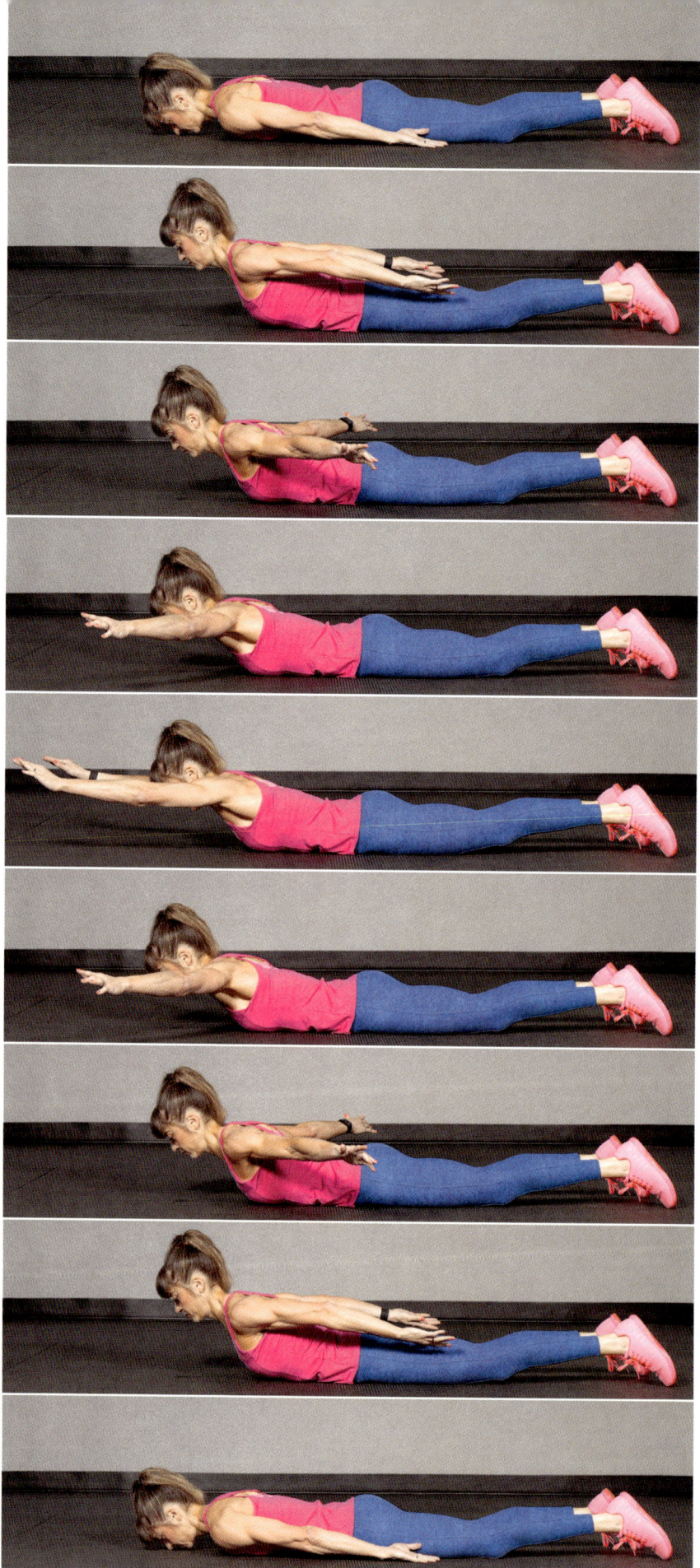

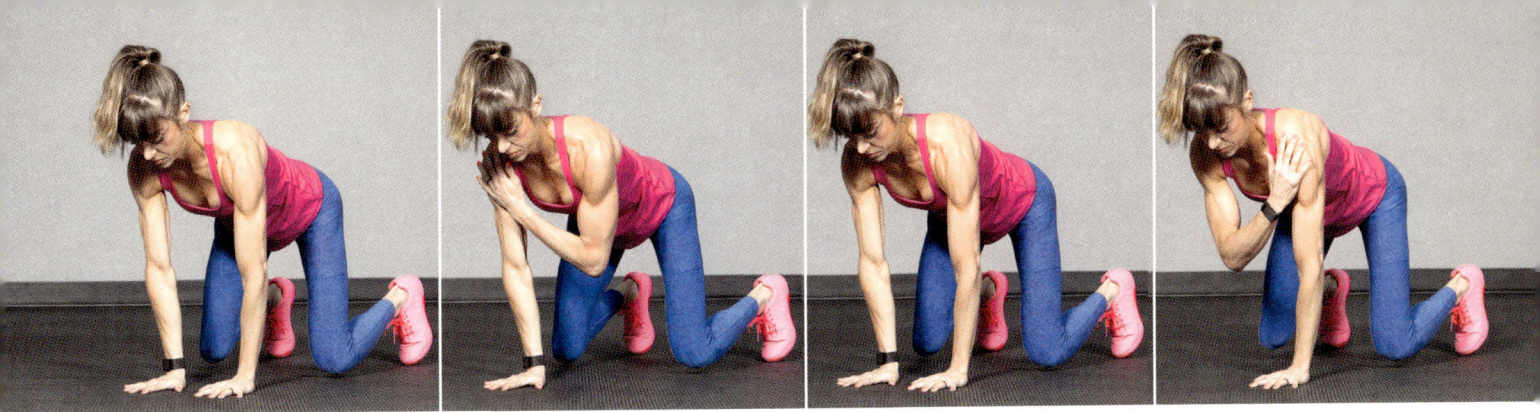

BULLDOG SHOULDER TAP

Start on all fours with your knees under your hips and hands under your chest. This tripod position will help you stabilize as you do the shoulder taps. Lift up onto your feet and hands with your fingers spread for even pressure.

Lift one hand and tap your opposite shoulder. Place the hand back down and raise the other hand to touch the other shoulder. Fight the desire to rush or rotate; keep your abs engaged and your knees hovering just off the ground. Do not let your butt go up in the air.

MODIFICATION

EXERCISE SWAPS: Plank with toe touch, plank with reach back and out, plange plank, extended plank

MODIFICATIONS: Place your hands on a bench or box. You can also start by doing just the bulldog hold (raising your knees off the floor) as an isometric exercise.

TABLETOP BRIDGE

Sit on the ground with your knees bent, your feet flat in front of you, and your hands behind you. You can adjust how your fingers are pointing according to your wrist mobility, but out to the side is a good place to start.

Drive through your hands and feet to bridge your hips. Squeeze your glutes and tuck your pelvis toward your ribs as you extend your hips to protect your lower back. You can lean your head back at the top. Focus on your glute and upper back engagement to open your chest as you pause in the tabletop position. Do not arch your lower back. Lower and repeat.

MODIFICATIONS: Place your hands on a bench behind you. To progress, add a mini band around your upper legs for added glute medius engagement.

EXERCISE SWAPS: Camel bridge, glute bridge hold, frog bridge, scapular wall hold

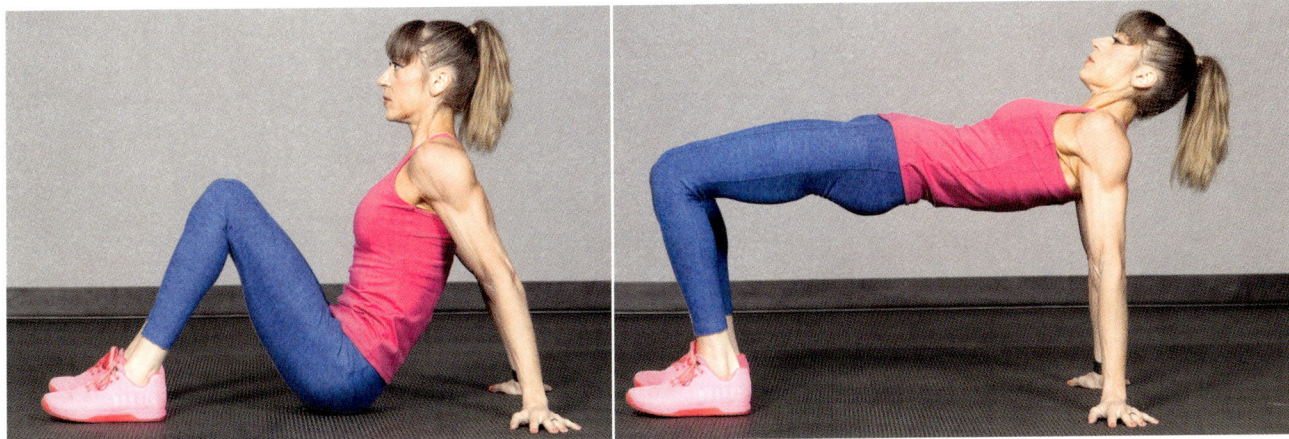

SEATED LEG RAINBOW

Sit on the ground with your legs extended but positioned slightly to the right of your shoulders. Lift your hands to your chest and then raise your left leg, as if you're lifting it over something on the ground, moving it in an arc like a rainbow. Place it down slightly to the left of your left shoulder. You'll feel your abs brace to keep you seated nice and tall as your hips and quads work to lift your leg up and over.

ROCK LUNGE

From a standing position, step back into a wide stance as if you're going to do a reverse lunge, but lunge back further than you normally would. Sink down, bending your front knee to about 90 degrees with your back leg straight. Adjust as needed so your front knee is behind your front ankle.

Staying low, push off your back foot to rock forward in the lunge. Your knee may move over your toes or even past your toes if you can keep your heel down. Then shift back. Do not lean your torso or lift your front heel. Feel like you're gliding in this low lunge.

MODIFICATIONS: Do not sink as low or perform as big a rock forward. You may even start with more of an isometric hold.

EXERCISE SWAPS: Lunge hold, wall sit, sumo squat, seated leg rainbow, standing quad kickout

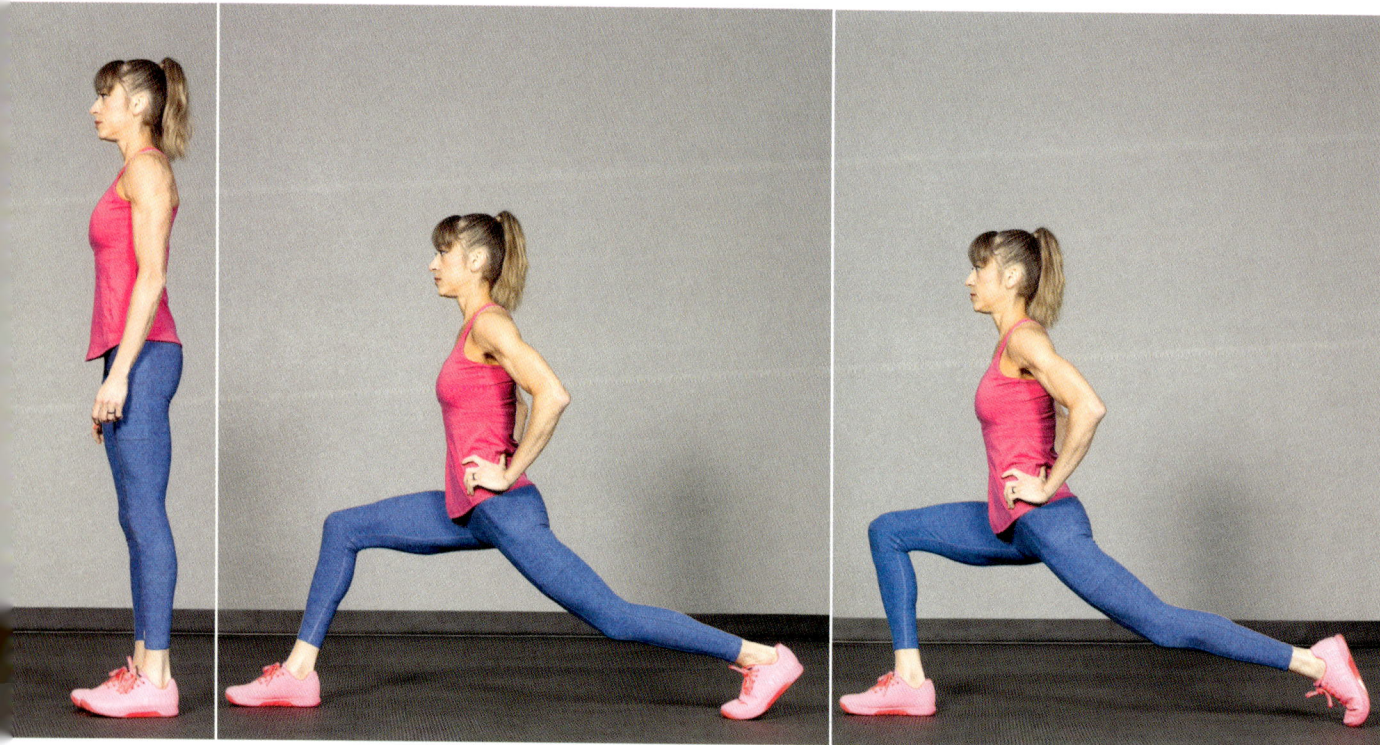

Repeat the rainbow lift with your right leg so you end up with both legs back together on the left side.

Repeat, starting with the leg you just moved and going back the other direction.

MODIFICATIONS: Bend your knees more or sit on a bench to help reduce the mobility and strength demands of this move.

EXERCISE SWAPS: Rock lunge, wall sit, lunge hold, sumo squat

DOWNWARD DOG SCAPULAR PRESS

Set up in a high plank position with your hands under your shoulders and your feet about hip-width apart. Drive through your hands to push your chest back toward your knees as you lift your butt toward the ceiling. Extend your spine and keep your legs straight as you drive your heels down.

Then push the ground away with your hands, shrugging your shoulders toward your ears. Feel your shoulder blades shrug up and the muscles around your rib cage working. Then relax. This is a very small press, as if you're shrugging your shoulders. When you relax, make sure to stay in the downward dog position. Bend your knees slightly if needed to focus on the spinal extension and this shrugging movement.

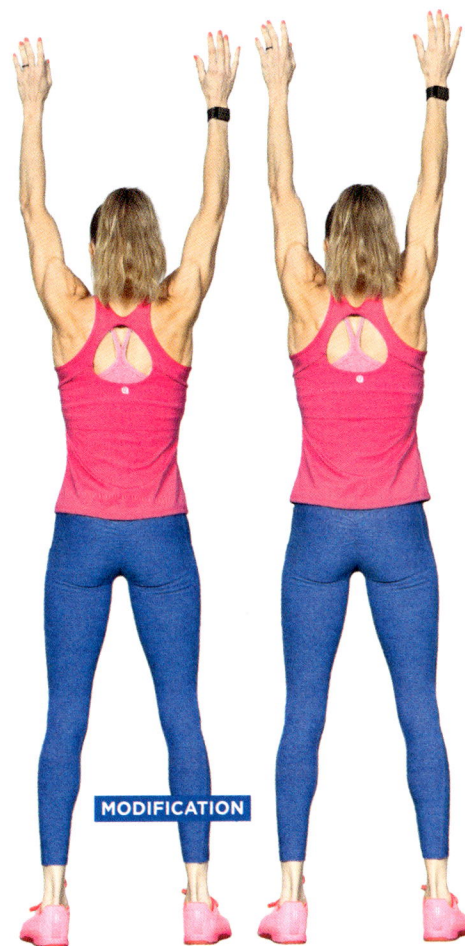

MODIFICATION

MODIFICATIONS: You perform this shrug while standing and reaching your hands overhead. You also can place your hands on a bench or box.

EXERCISE SWAPS: Roller serratus anterior extension, plange plank, side plank oblique twist

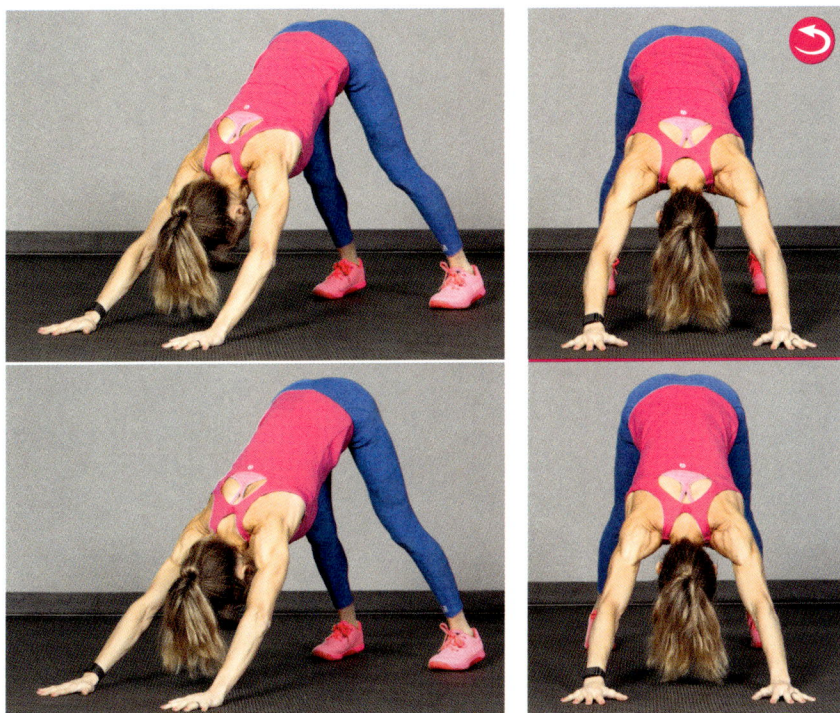

PLANK WITH REACH BACK AND OUT

Set up in a high plank with your hands closer together under your chest and your feet about hip-width to shoulder-width apart. The wider your feet, the more stable your base. Reach one hand toward the opposite ankle, pushing your butt back and toward the ceiling as you reach.

Then come back forward into the plank and reach your raised hand in front of you toward the wall beyond your head. Do not drop your hips or arch your lower back. Keep your hips level and engage your glutes as you reach out. Then repeat by reaching back and across to your ankle. Make sure to engage your back on the side of your supporting arm to support that shoulder and avoid shrugging. This is a deceptively hard move to do while moving slowly and avoiding rotation or your hips dropping as you come forward.

EXERCISE SWAPS: Plank with toe touch, extended plank hold, camel bridge, tabletop bridge, bulldog shoulder tap

MODIFICATIONS: Do a plank from your knees or place your hands on a bench or box.

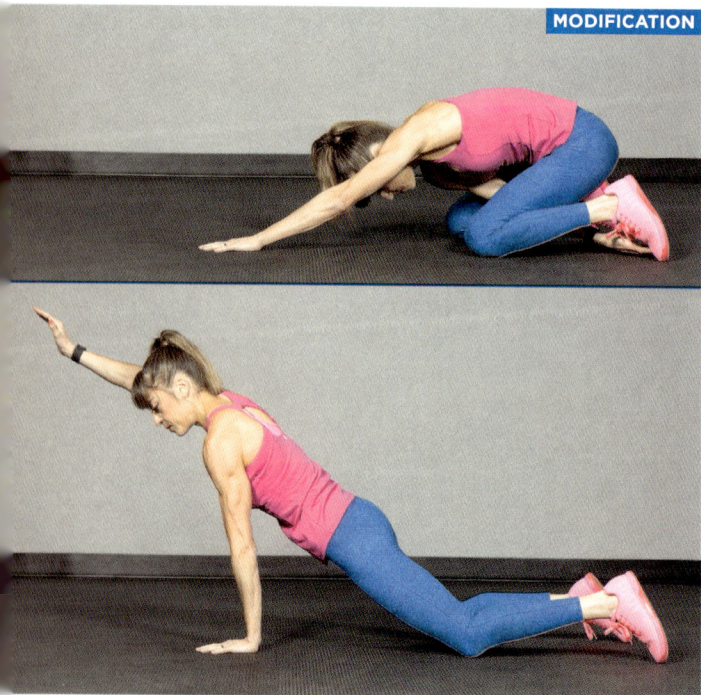

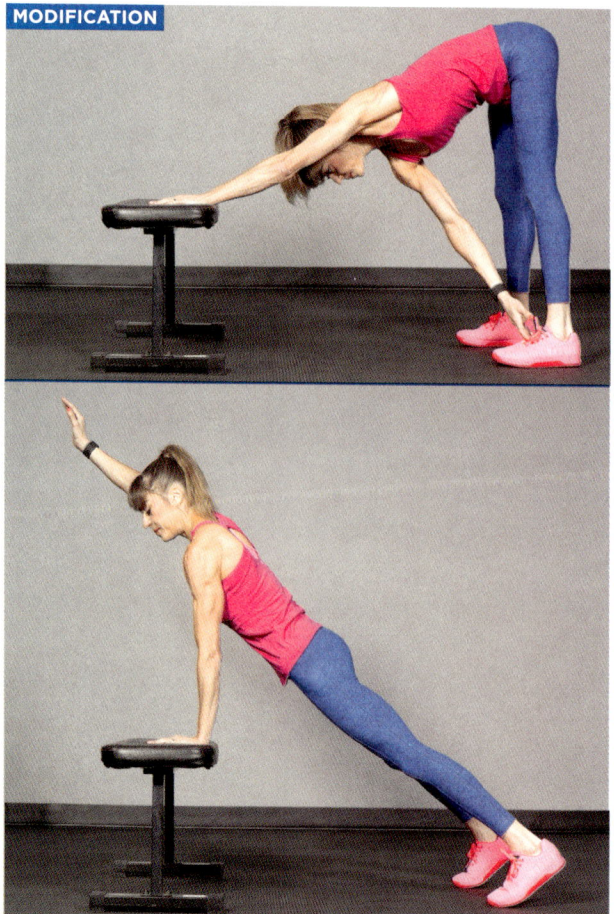

MODIFICATION

MODIFICATION

FROG BRIDGE

Lie back on the ground and place the bottom of your feet together, letting your knees fall open as in a butterfly stretch. Bend your elbows to 90 degrees and drive your upper arms into the ground. Tuck your pelvis slightly toward your ribs for a posterior pelvic tilt to help you avoid arching your lower back as you bridge.

Push through the outsides of your feet and your upper arms to bridge up while keeping your knees open. Feel your glutes work to lift your hips but try pulling your knees slightly more open as you bridge. Pause to feel your glutes engage; then lower your hips and repeat.

MODIFICATIONS: You can do this as a hip thrust variation with your back on a bench or modify to the basic glute bridge if you have ankle issues.

EXERCISE SWAPS: Single-leg reverse hyper, glute bridge hold, mini band glute bridge, mini band bridge hold with abduction, 80/20 hip thrust hold

SCAPULAR PUSH-UP

Set up in a high plank position with your hands under your shoulders and your feet together so your body is in a nice straight line from your head to your heels. Keeping your arms straight and hips stable, pinch your shoulder blades toward your spine. Do not jut your head forward or try to make the movement bigger.

Draw your shoulder blades toward your spine and then push the ground away to pull your shoulder blades back apart. Don't round your upper back at the top, and make sure not to bend your elbows or shrug your shoulders as you pinch your shoulder blades together. Feel the sides of your back working to keep your shoulders down and press your chest out as you pinch.

MODIFICATIONS: Perform the plank from your knees or place your hands on a bench or box.

EXERCISE SWAPS: Single-arm scapular push-up, scapular wing, scapular wall hold, lying scapular hold

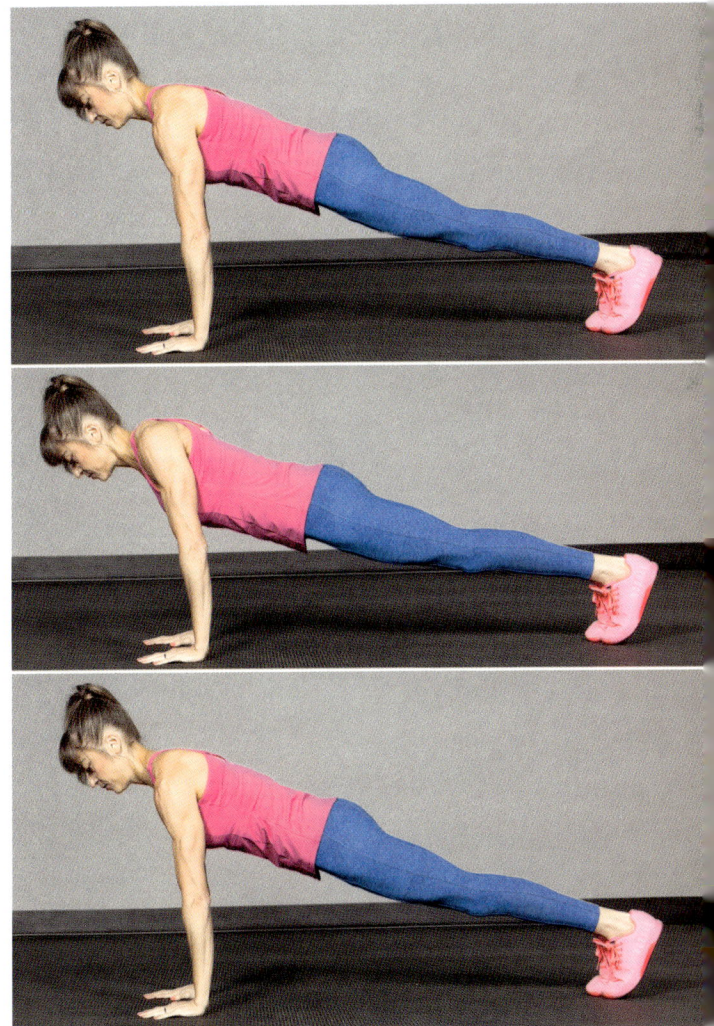

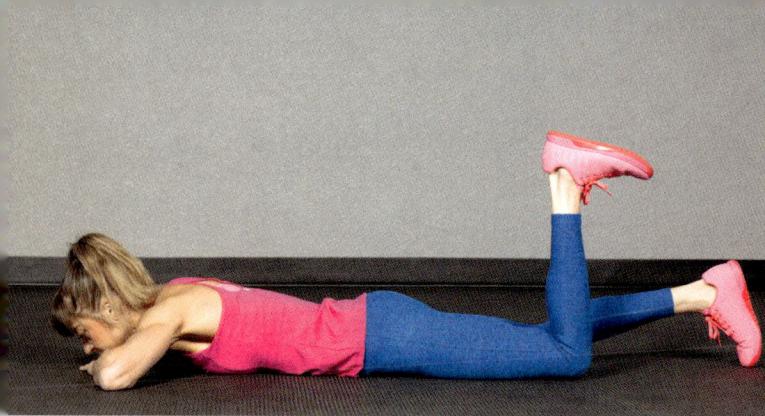

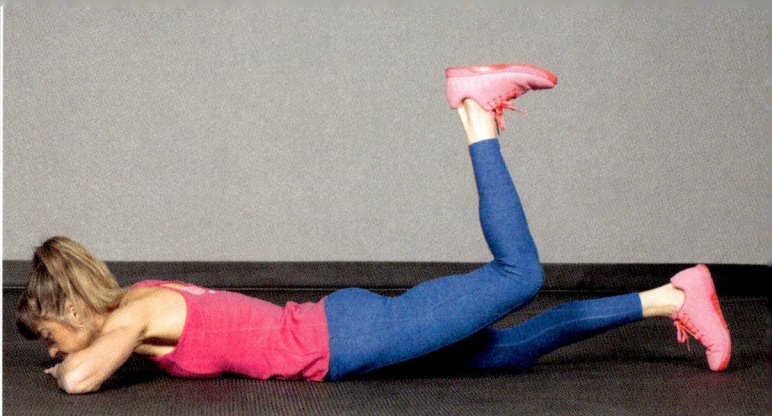

SINGLE-LEG REVERSE HYPER

Lie face down on the ground and relax your chin on your hands. Bend one knee to about 90 degrees so your foot is up toward the ceiling. Engage your glute to kick that heel toward the ceiling, lifting your thigh up off the ground. Do not rotate to lift higher than you can control with your glute or arch your lower back. Think about pushing your pelvis into the ground as you lift with your glute to avoid rotating. Pause and then lower your leg.

If you feel your engagement in your hamstring rather than your glute, relax your foot or even kick slightly back instead of bending your knee as much. If you're struggling to engage your glute, you can move your knee slightly out to the side rather than keeping it straight in line with your hip.

MODIFICATIONS: Perform this off a bench. For progression, add a mini band or ankle weight.

EXERCISE SWAPS: 3-way hip circle, frog bridge, glute bridge hold, mini band glute bridge, 80/20 hip thrust hold

---

SINGLE-LEG DEADLIFT HOLD

MODIFICATIONS: Touch the toe of your lifted leg to the wall behind you or place your hand on a chair or the wall to help slightly with balance.

EXERCISE SWAPS: 2-way reach skater lunge, extended twisting triangle, single-leg reverse hyper, standing 3-way hip circle, 80/20 hip thrust hold, side lunge hold

Stand tall and shift your weight to one foot, focusing on the two points in the ball of your foot and one point in your heel pushing down into the ground. Raise your other leg off the ground, hinging at your hips as you lean your torso over to counterbalance the leg that's lifting toward the wall behind you.

Focus on leveling your pelvis so it's square to the ground as you create a straight line from your head to your raised heel. Reach your hands toward the ground or out in front of your head. Push through your standing leg without locking your knee and hold.

SCAPULAR WALL HOLD

Bend your elbows to about 90 degrees and place them on the wall. Press off your elbows, engaging your upper back as you press your chest out. Walk your feet out from the wall, leaning into your elbow to apply more resistance. Do not shrug your shoulders or walk out so far you can't engage your upper back.

Stand with your feet together and flex your feet, engaging your glutes and quads so you have a nice straight line from your shoulders to your heels. Your head may be slightly limited by your angle and the wall, but try to relax it back rather than tucking your chin. Breathe and focus on really engaging your back to press out. Think about lifting your chest open toward the ceiling, and don't shrug.

MODIFICATIONS: Do not walk your feet out more than a few inches from the wall. You can do this anywhere; you don't have to be in front of a wall. Just stand and drive your elbows back.

EXERCISE SWAPS: Lying scapular hold, scapular push-up, single-arm scapular push-up, scapular wall rep

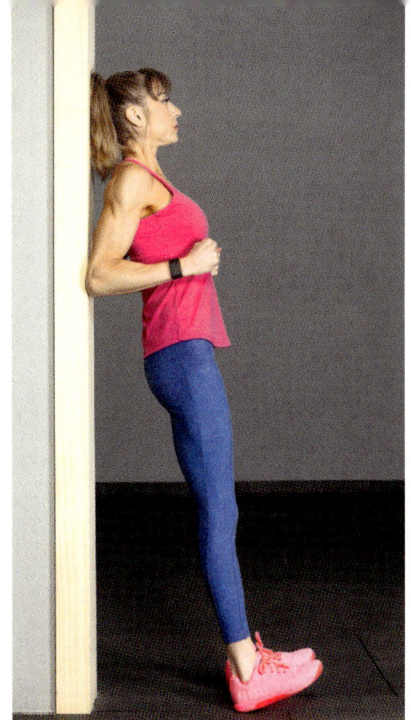

SIDE LUNGE HOLD

Stretch your arms out to your sides at shoulder height and set your feet about as wide as your fingertips are apart. You can adjust exact positioning as you sink. With your toes pointing straight ahead and your feet parallel, sit to one side, bending that side's knee as you hinge at your hips to sit your butt back. Slightly lean forward but don't round over.

Hold here with your thigh about parallel to the ground and feel your glute. Keep your other leg straight and feel a stretch in that leg's hamstrings and adductors.

MODIFICATIONS: Do not sink as low in the lunge or stabilize yourself with a chair or suspension trainer.

EXERCISE SWAPS: Single-leg deadlift hold, sumo squat hold, fire hydrant, extended twisting triangle, 80/20 hip thrust hold, single-leg reverse hyper

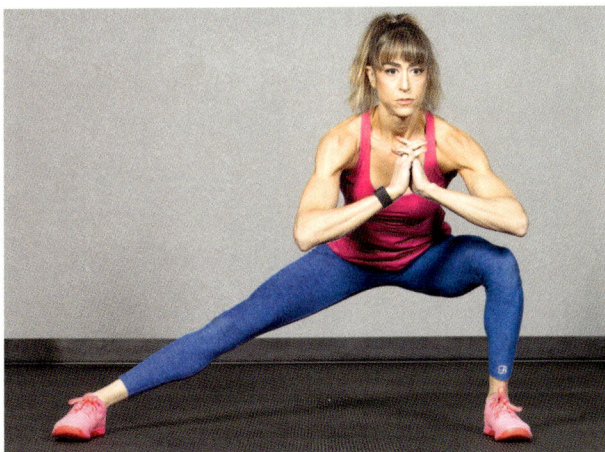

EXTENDED PLANK HOLD

Start in a high plank position with your hands under your shoulders and your feet no wider than hip-width apart. Putting them closer together makes this move harder.

With your body in a nice straight line from your head to your heels, walk your feet back so your hands end up beyond your shoulders and up by your head—even beyond your forehead. The more extended you are, the harder the move is. Hold and breathe. Focus on bracing your core with a slight posterior pelvic tilt so that you're tucking your pelvis toward your ribs. Flex your quads and focus on feeling your upper back and lats support your shoulders. Do not drop your hips or push your butt up in the air.

MODIFICATIONS: Perform this off a bench or box or do not walk back as far so you're less extended. You can also do the plank from your knees.

EXERCISE SWAPS: Basic plank hold, seated hinge hold, banana, plange plank, plank with toe touch

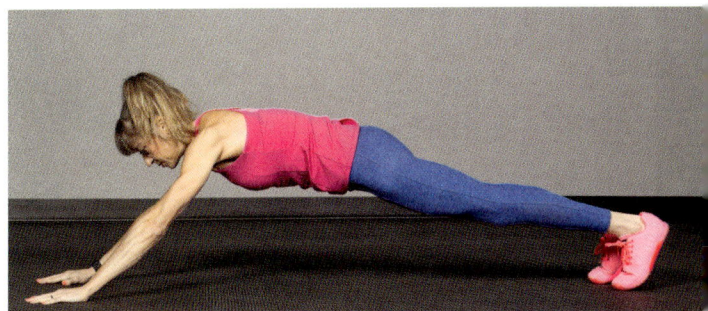

EXTENDED TWISTING TRIANGLE

Set up with your feet just a few inches wider than shoulder-width apart. Pick a "front leg" and turn your torso that direction, pointing that leg's toes toward the wall in front of you. Turn out your back toe just slightly. With your legs straight, hinge at your hips to push your butt back, rotating to reach the opposite hand toward the ground at about the instep of your front leg. Reach your other hand toward the ceiling and rotate your chest open toward the front leg. Engage your back to really twist your chest open as you push your butt back, keeping your legs straight and your weight evenly loaded between both legs.

Breathe and hold while focusing on the stretch as you load your glutes and use your back to rotate your spine. Make sure that you aren't locking your knees as you stretch.

MODIFICATIONS: Place a block or bench by your front leg for your hand if you can't yet reach the ground.

EXERCISE SWAPS: Single-leg deadlift hold, figure 4 heel on wall, seated hamstring and spinal twist complex, active foam roller star stretch, side lunge hold, standing 3-way hip circle

SIDE PLANK HOLD

Set up on your side on your forearm with your elbow right below your shoulder. Your legs should be out straight and stacked. Flex your feet and make sure your shoulder isn't shrugged. Feel the side of your back engage to lock that shoulder down.

Lift your hips. Feel the bottom oblique holding your side up as you engage your glutes to push your hips forward in alignment but also feel the side of your bottom glute lifting your hips. Flexing your foot should help you feel tension through your lower leg to support everything. Really focus on pushing the ground away with your forearm and outside of your bottom foot. Hold here and breathe. Do not let yourself rotate your chest toward the ground.

MODIFICATIONS: You can unstack your feet, staggering your top foot in front. You can also plank off your knees or with your forearm on a bench. You can also progress this move, doing it from your hand instead of your forearm.

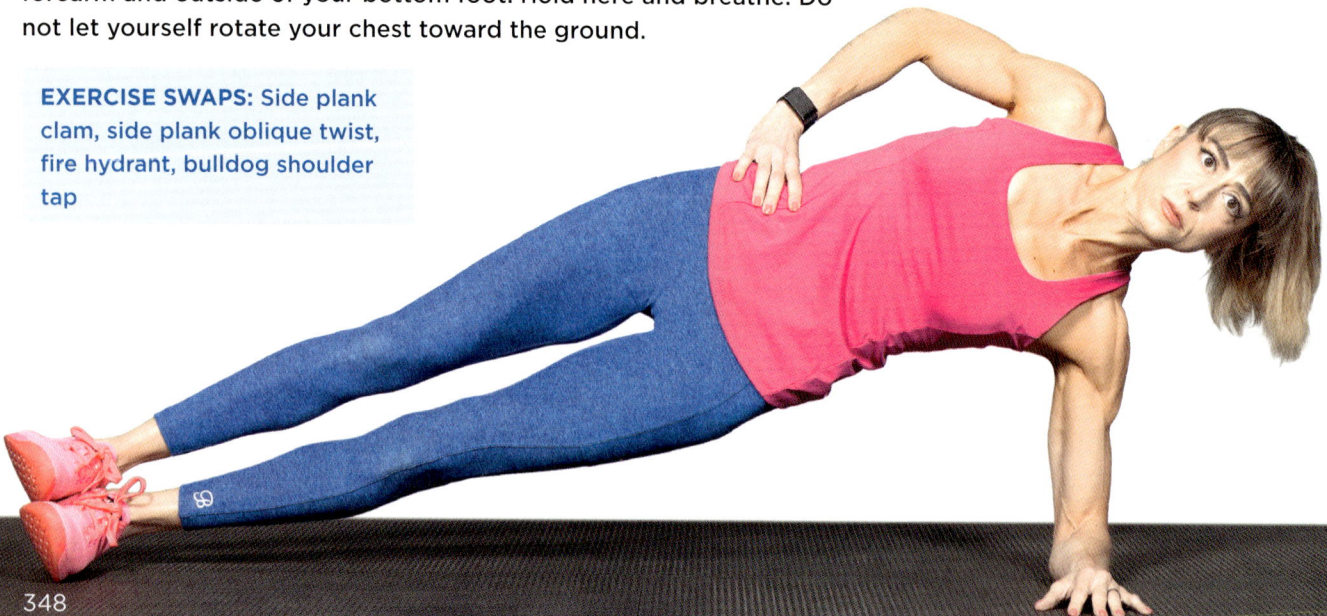

EXERCISE SWAPS: Side plank clam, side plank oblique twist, fire hydrant, bulldog shoulder tap

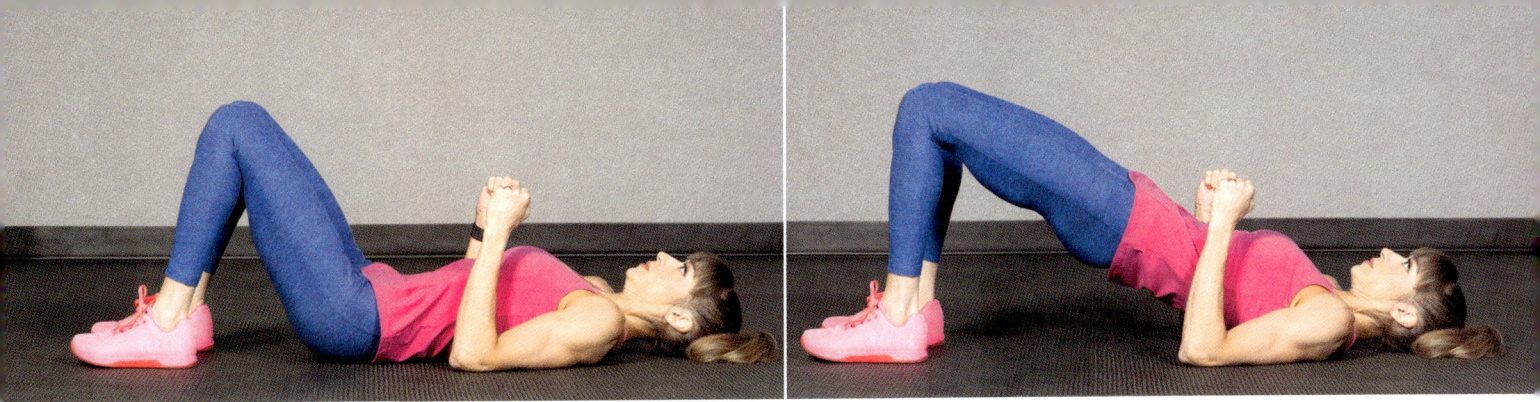

GLUTE BRIDGE HOLD

Lie on your back and put your feet flat on the ground so your knees are bent. Your feet should be about hip-width apart. Bend your elbows to 90 degrees and drive through your upper arms and back. Tuck your pelvis slightly toward your ribs to get that posterior pelvic tilt and avoid arching your lower back as you bridge.

Lift into the bridge, pushing through your entire foot and your upper back and arms. Think about driving your knees toward your toes as you lift. Don't let your lower back arch. Focus on your glutes driving the hip extension to hold. Focus on engaging them as hard as you can as you maintain the bridge.

If you struggle with your hamstrings taking over, make sure you have the pelvic tilt engaged. You can adjust the distance between your feet and your butt; move them a bit closer or further away based on hip mobility. It may help to drive more through your heels. However you do it, actively hold in the bridge; don't just go through the motions.

MODIFICATIONS: You can do a hip thrust hold off a bench or add a mini band to progress.

EXERCISE SWAPS: Frog bridge, single-leg reverse hyper, mini band glute bridge, single-leg deadlift hold, 80/20 hip thrust hold, 2-way reach skater lunge

BANANA

Lie on your back with your legs together and out straight. Reach your arms overhead along the ground so your biceps are by your ears. Tuck your pelvis toward your ribs and press your low back toward the ground for that posterior pelvic tilt. As you do, lift your legs by engaging your glutes as you also curl your shoulder blades up off the floor. Squeeze your legs together as you reach your toes toward the wall beyond them. Also reach your arms out overhead as you crunch your upper body up. Don't tuck your chin. Focus on feeling your abs, adductors, glutes, and quads working to hold as you press your lower back toward the ground and stay crunched up.

MODIFICATIONS: Do not lower your legs as close to the ground. For the setup, you may find it easier to tuck your knees in toward your chest, extend your legs up toward the ceiling, and then lower them to hover a few inches off the ground. For some people, this is preferable to raising them from the ground.

EXERCISE SWAPS: Seated hinge hold, plange plank, basic front plank, extended plank hold

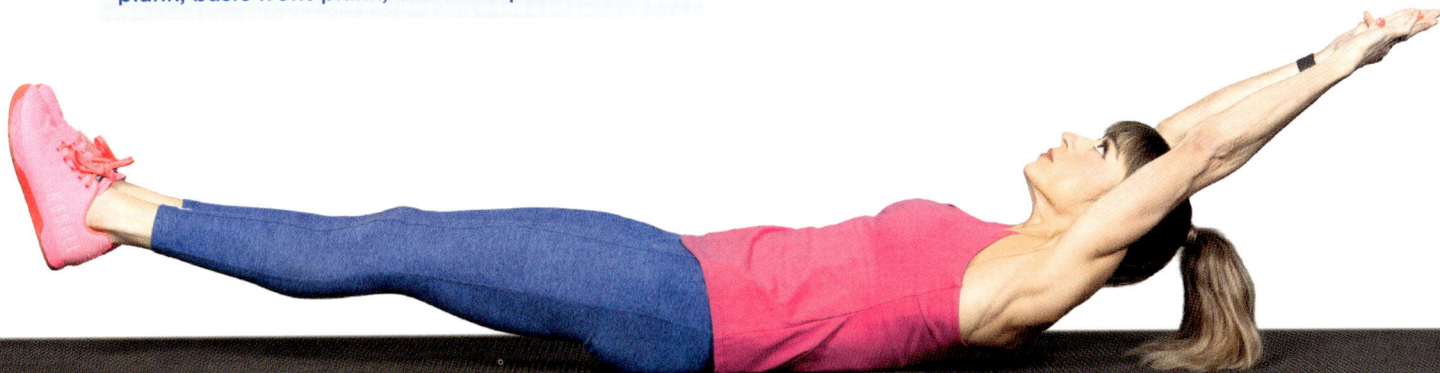

PUSH-UP HOLD

There are three main holds you can focus on, choosing to use one or all of them based on your needs and goals. If you cycle through the holds, hold each position 3 to 5 seconds.

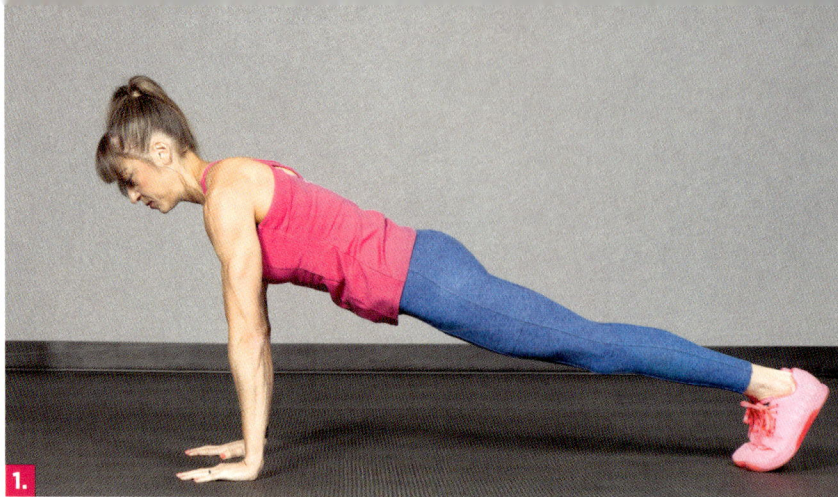

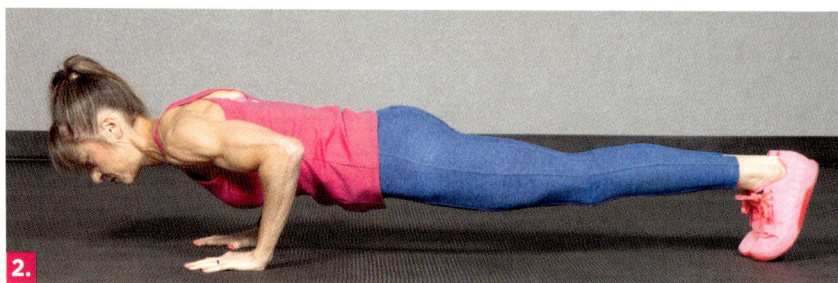

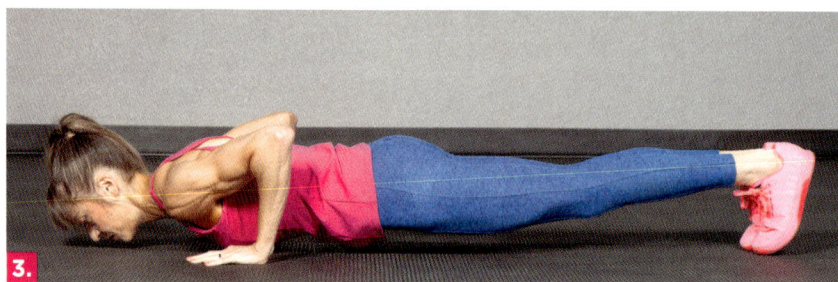

1. HIGH PUSH-UP HOLD: Set up at the top of a push-up with your feet together and your hands outside your chest. With your body in a nice straight line from your head to your heels, engage your abs, tucking your pelvis slightly toward your ribs. Focus on pulling your shoulders down slightly so they aren't shrugged. Drive back through your heels to flex your quads.

MODIFICATIONS: Perform the holds from your knees or with your hands on a bench or box.

2. MID PUSH-UP HOLD: With your body in a nice straight line from your head to your heels, bend your elbows to about 90 degrees and lower into the push-up and hold. Do not let your hips sink or your butt go up toward the ceiling as you hold at this midpoint. Do not tuck your chin or let your elbows flare way out. You want your arms and body to create an arrow shape. Drive back through your heels. Feel the sides of your back supporting your shoulders as your shoulder blades draw toward your spine. Push the ground away with your hands and feet to keep tension. You can vary the exact positioning to address any push-up "sticking points" you have.

3. BOTTOM PUSH-UP HOLD: Lower until your chest is an inch off the ground. Make sure to engage your glutes and quads to keep your body in a nice straight line as you drive back through your heels. Do not tuck your chin, let your hips sag toward the ground, or your butt go up in the air. Do not let your elbows flare way out as you hold and focus on your shoulders not shrugging. Feel your shoulder blades draw toward your spine to support your shoulders and load your chest.

EXERCISE SWAPS: High front plank hold, push-up plus, plange plank, dip hold, side plank hold, halo, plank with toe touch, scapular push-up, downward dog scapular press

LUNGE HOLD

Get in the half-kneeling position with your back knee about under your hip and your front knee positioned over your ankle. Flex your back foot and make sure your feet are basically in line with your hips. Drive evenly through your front heel and the ball of your back foot to lift up and hover your back knee an inch or two above the ground in a low lunge. Keep your chest up nice and tall and squeeze the glute of your back leg to drive your hip into extension. Hold.

MODIFICATIONS: You can start from a standing position and sink into a lunge instead of starting from the half-kneeling position and hold higher in the lunge, or you can place your hand on a wall or chair to help with balance.

EXERCISE SWAPS: Rock lunge, wall sit, sumo squat hold, 2-way reach skater lunge, seated leg rainbow

SEATED HINGE HOLD

Sit on the ground with your legs out in front of you and your knees bent to almost 90 degrees. Drive your heels into the ground and lean your torso back, rounding through your lower back to tuck your ribs slightly toward your pelvis. You should be hinged to about a 45-degree angle from the floor, but you may hinge more or less based on what you can do for a challenge without engaging your lower back. The C curve to your spine should engage your abs as you hinge back. Hold and focus on feeling your abs working to prevent you from rolling back further.

MODIFICATIONS: Only hinge back as far as you can control. You can do this while seated on a bench.

EXERCISE SWAPS: Plange plank, banana, full body crunch

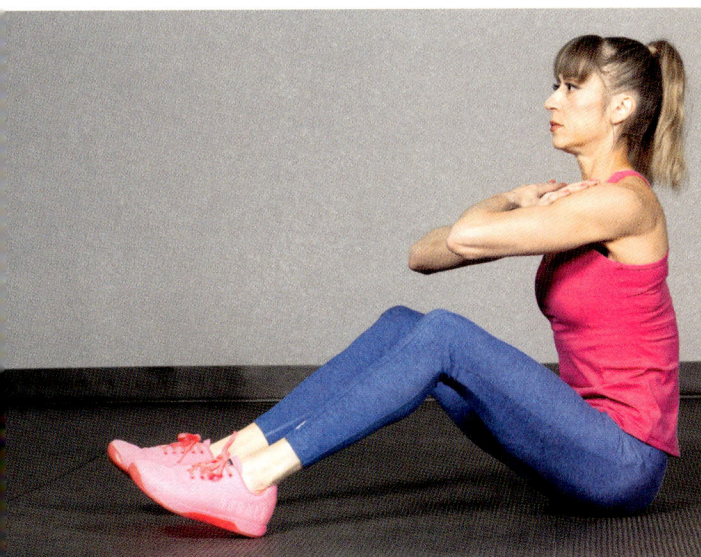

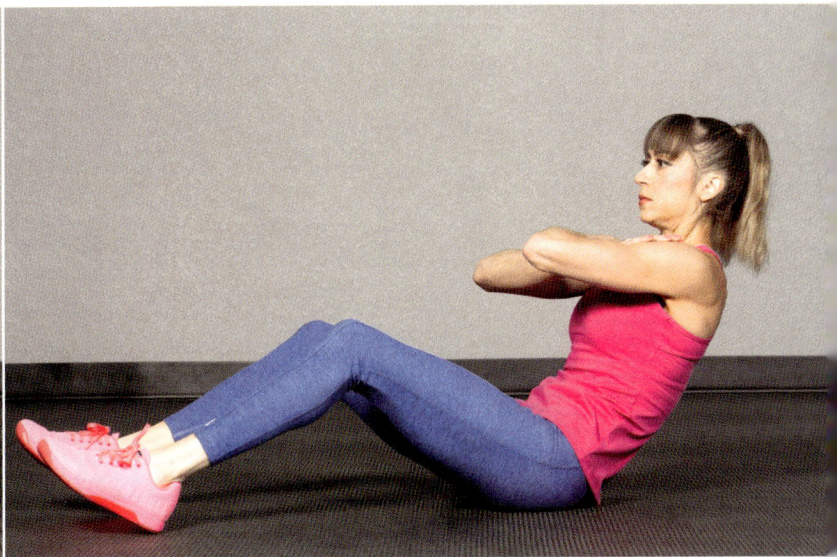

STANDING 3-WAY HIP CIRCLE

Place your hands or forearms on a box or chair in front of you as you hinge over so your chest is about parallel to the ground. Sit back to load your glutes, shifting your weight onto one leg. Brace your abs and kick one leg straight back toward the wall behind you. Do not arch your back as you kick. Pause and focus on engaging your glute to lift your leg until it's about parallel to the ground.

Then tuck your knee up and out to the side with your knee about even with your hip. You want your knee and ankle to stay in line so you feel the side of your glute working in this "fire hydrant"–like position. Pause and then tuck your knee in toward your chest between your arms, curling through your spine to engage your abs. Kick back out and repeat the series.

Focus on keeping your standing leg straight and feel its glute working to balance as you push your entire foot into the ground. Don't rotate your torso or arch your lower back; instead, focus on the glute of your active leg for the kick back and lateral raise. Take time to focus on what you feel working in each position and don't touch your foot down between each move.

MODIFICATIONS: Touch down between each movement and perform a smaller range of motion on each lift.

EXERCISE SWAPS: 3-way hip circle, fire hydrant, single-leg deadlift hold, 2-way reach skater lunges, mini band bridge hold with abduction

SUMO SQUAT HOLD

Set your feet wider than shoulder-width apart (although you can adjust your stance based on your mobility). Turn your toes out to about a 45-degree angle. Make sure that your ankles, knees, and hips are in alignment as you sink into a squat. You do not want your knees caving in or bowing way open.

Squat until your thighs are about parallel to the ground and hold. You can have your hands at your chest or reaching out in front of you, but do not round forward. Focus on feeling your legs working—especially your inner thighs and your glutes. Your glutes should feel like they're working to open up your hips as you hold.

MODIFICATIONS: Modify by not sinking as low. Hold onto a suspension trainer or chair to help with balance.

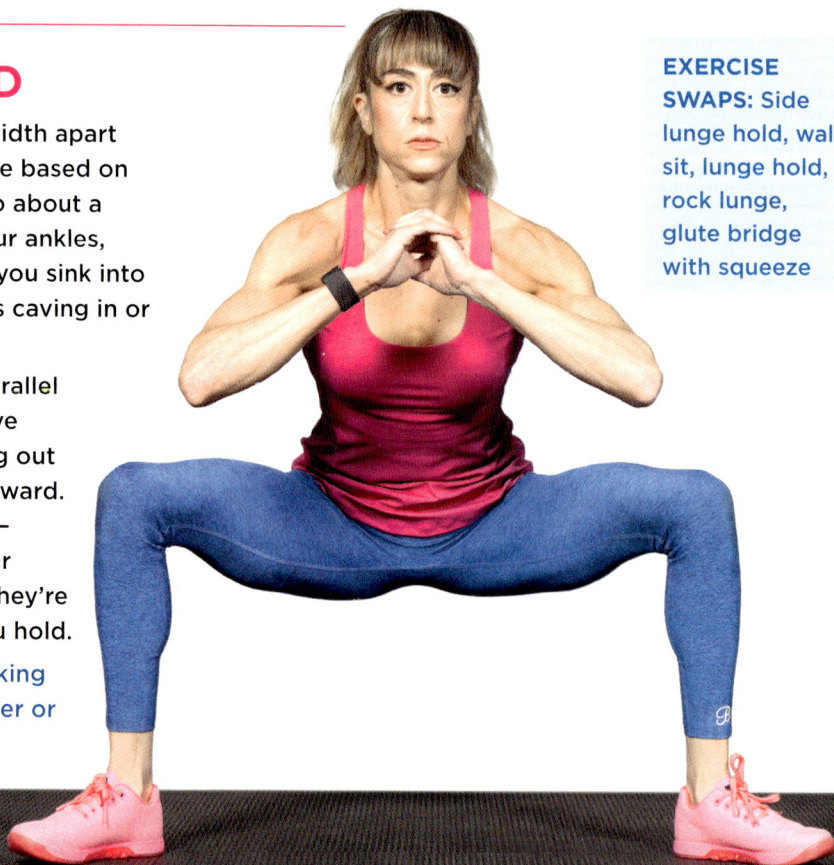

EXERCISE SWAPS: Side lunge hold, wall sit, lunge hold, rock lunge, glute bridge with squeeze

MINI BAND GLUTE BRIDGE

Place a mini band around your legs right above your knees and lie back with your feet flat on the ground about hip-width to shoulder-width apart. Press your knees open against the resistance of the band to keep them in line with your ankles and hips. Push down into the ground through the two points in the balls of your feet and one point in your heel and do not rock out on the edge of your feet as you press out on the band. Bend your elbows to 90 degrees and drive your upper arms and back into the ground. Tuck your pelvis toward your ribs.

Then bridge up as you drive through your feet, upper back, and arms. Think about driving your knees slightly toward your toes as you lift. Engage your glutes and make sure to keep your knees in line as you bridge. Do not let them cave in.

Pause at the top and feel your glutes working to bridge up. Extend your hips as you feel the sides of your butt working to prevent the band from making your knees cave in. Don't arch your lower back. Lower to the starting position and repeat.

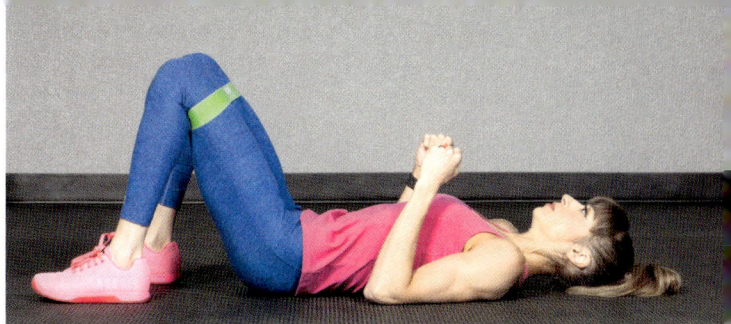

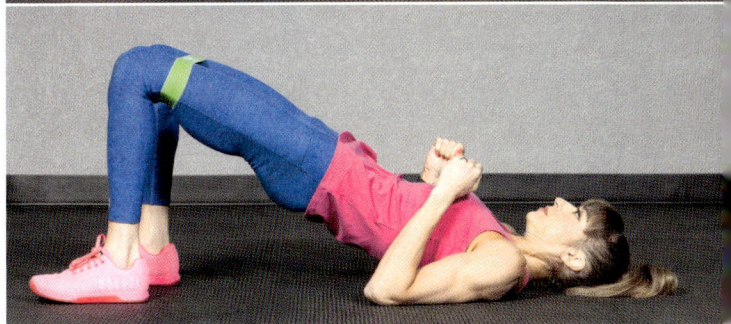

MODIFICATIONS: Use a lighter band, or you can do this as a hip thrust with your back on a bench. You can also swap in a booty band.

EXERCISE SWAPS: Frog bridge, 3-way hip circle, 2-way reach skater lunge, standing 3-way hip circle

MODIFICATIONS: Use a lighter band, or you can do this as a hip thrust with your back on a bench. You can also swap in a booty band.

EXERCISE SWAPS: Fire hydrant, 3-way hip circle, 2-way reach skater lunge, standing 3-way hip circle

MINI BAND BRIDGE HOLD WITH ABDUCTION

Place a mini band around your legs right above your knees and lie back with your feet flat on the ground about hip-width apart. Press your knees open against the resistance of the band to keep them in line with your ankles and hips. Push down into the ground through the two points in the balls of your feet and one point in your heel and do not rock out on the edges of your feet as you press out on the band. Bend your elbows to 90 degrees and drive your upper arms and back into the ground. Tuck your pelvis toward your ribs.

Bridge up as you drive through your feet, upper back, and arms. Think about driving your knees slightly toward your toes as you lift. Engage your glutes and make sure to keep your knees in line as you bridge. Do not let them cave in.

As you hold this bridged position, press your knees open farther. Then bring your knees back to hip-width apart. Control the movement (it will be small). Do not let your knees cave in, allow the band to pull you back, or let your hips sink. Engage your glutes to maintain the bridge. Be conscious that you don't start to arch as you fatigue.

DIP HOLD

Sit on the edge of a bench, box, or chair with your hands just outside your butt and turned so your fingertips hang over the front edge of the support. Press through your hands to lift yourself off the bench as you walk your feet away from you. Your butt is hovering just in front of the bench or support. Your legs should be straight out in front of you as you press your hands down hard into the bench to keep yourself lifted. Focus on engaging the sides of your back as you press your chest out and avoid shrugging your shoulders as you hold.

MODIFICATIONS: Bend your knees to modify the move. To progress, consider doing the hold off of dip bars or parallel bars.

EXERCISE SWAPS: Cobra wings, scapular wings, halo, bulldog shoulder tap, plank with toe touch, prone snow angel

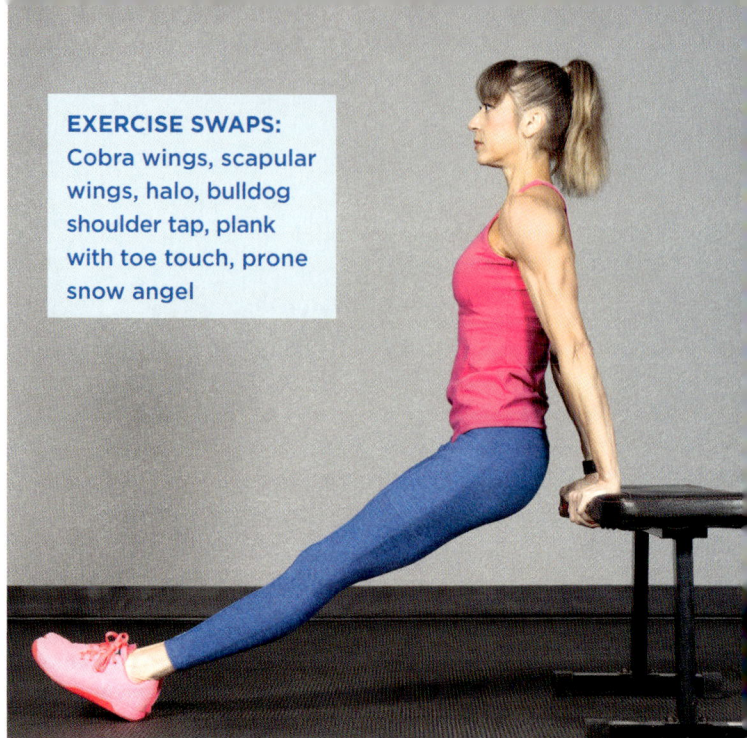

2-WAY REACH SKATER LUNGE

Stand with your feet no more than a couple of inches apart as you sink into a small squat, sitting your butt back as you lean your torso forward to counterbalance. You can think of it like a squat with a hinge to help you load your glutes. Shift your weight onto one leg and reach the other leg behind you.

Tap your toe down as you extend your leg back, keeping your weight on your support leg. Bring the foot back in and lightly tap the ground next to your support leg before extending that same leg out to the side. Your focus is on working the support leg, especially the glute, as you challenge your balance with the movement. Complete all reps on one side, focusing on fatiguing just the support leg through reps, or you can alternate sides. Regardless, do not shift your weight from your support leg during the taps.

MODIFICATIONS: Modify by making the squat more shallow or use a chair or wall to help you balance.

EXERCISE SWAPS: Standing 3-way hip circle, fire hydrant, mini band glute bridge, mini band bridge hold with abduction, single-leg deadlift hold, side lunge hold

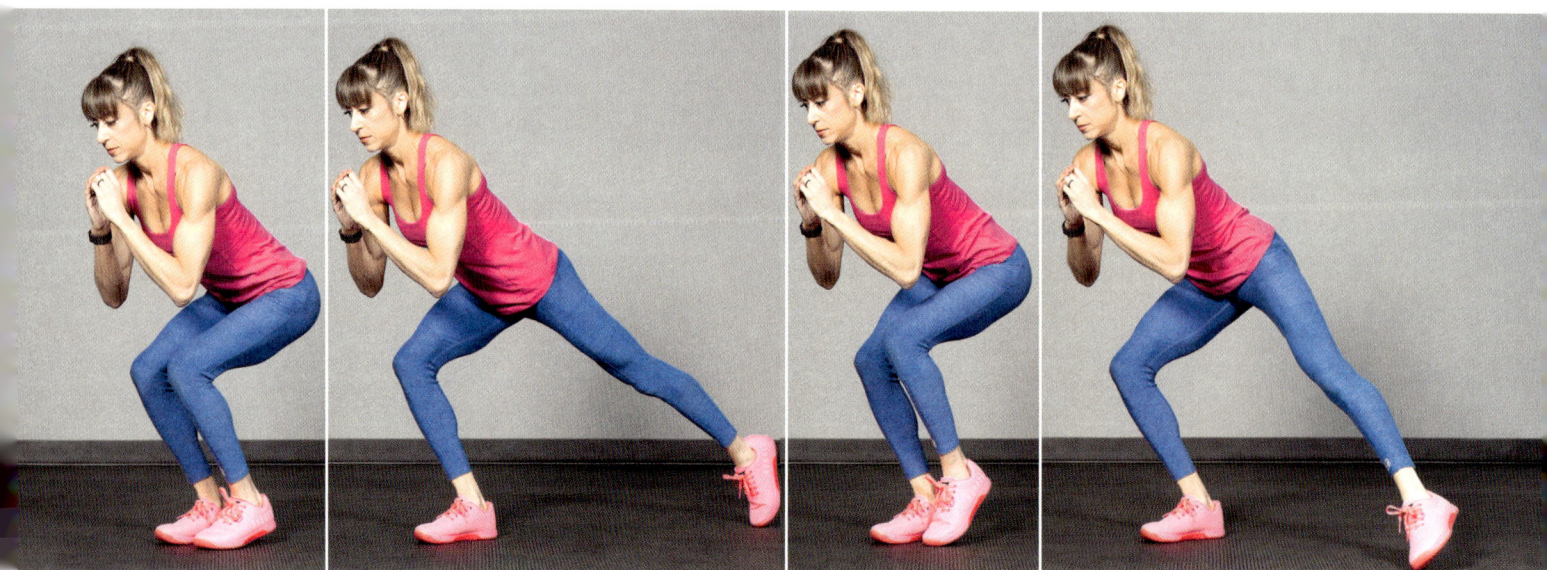

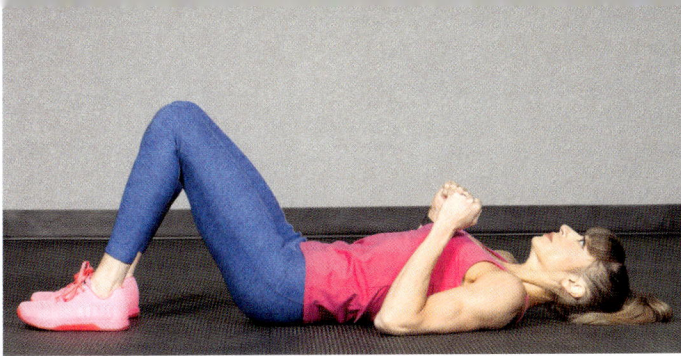

LYING SCAPULAR HOLD

Lie on your back with your knees bent and feet flat on the ground. Bend your elbows to 90 degrees and place your arms at your sides. Engage your abs and drive your elbows down into the ground to lift your back up off the ground as you press your chest out. Keep your head in line with your spine as you lift, but you can just slightly tuck your chin to look forward if it helps alleviate tension on your neck. Focus on pressing your chest out as you pull your shoulder blades toward your spine to engage your back and shoulders. Really drive through your elbows to push up and hold.

MODIFICATIONS: Swap this hold for the scapular wall hold to reduce strain.

EXERCISE SWAPS: Scapular wall hold, scapular push-up, single-arm scapular push-up, scapular wing, lying W pull-down

80/20 HIP THRUST HOLD

Sit on the ground with your back against a bench or box so that the edge of the support hits at about the bottom of your shoulder blades. Your arms can rest out to the side along the bench. With one foot flat on the ground, walk the other foot out to stagger your stance with that forward foot's heel about even with the ball of your back flat foot. Flex your forward foot so it's rocked back on its heel. Eighty percent of the work will be done by your back (support) leg with a 20 percent assist from your forward foot.

Drive through your support foot with an assist from the heel of your forward leg to bridge up. As you lift to the top, tuck your pelvis slightly toward your ribs; you may slightly tuck your head as you look toward your knees. Feel your glutes working to lift your pelvis, especially that glute of the support leg.

Hold at the top, really focusing on actively engaging the support side. At the end of the hold, lower to the ground and switch your legs to focus on the other side.

MODIFICATIONS: You can do this as a glute bridge or a basic hip thrust instead of having a more unilateral (one-sided) focus.

EXERCISE SWAPS: Frog bridge, glute bridge hold, 3-way hip circle, 2-way reach skater lunge, single-leg deadlift hold, single-leg reverse hyper

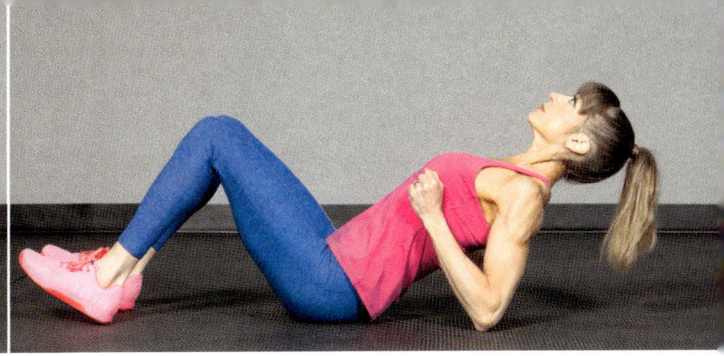

COBRA HOLD

Lie face down on the ground with your legs straight behind you and your arms by your sides with your palms turned to the ceiling. Engage your upper back to lift your chest and arms off the ground. Focus on opening your chest as you keep your head in line with your spine. Really work to extend your spine. Actively reach your hands toward the wall at your feet to try to pull yourself up higher.

Pause, making sure you're engaging your glutes and not just arching your lower back to lift and hold.

MODIFICATIONS: You can do this standing facing a wall or even carefully off a bench. Using sliders to provide hand support can also help.

EXERCISE SWAPS: Dip hold, cobra wings, scapular push-up, single-arm scapular push-up, lying W pull-down

---

PLANGE PLANK

This plank is an amazing way to improve your shoulder health and prevent lower back pain. Because of the spinal flexion (rounding), it works your serratus anterior more and utilizes the spinal C-curve position for greater ab engagement.

Set up in a plank position on your forearms and toes with your feet together and elbows under your shoulders. Make sure your body is in a nice straight line from your head to your heels and focus on driving back through your heels as you engage the sides of your back to support your shoulders.

Slowly round your upper back as you tuck your hips under, drawing your belly button in toward your spine. (The gross cue I like is, "as if you're trying to 'vomit up a hairball.'") Tuck your pelvis toward your ribs as you round your upper back and feel your shoulder blades move forward around your spine. Focus on pushing the ground away with your forearms as your head slightly tucks forward with the rounding. Don't let your butt go up in the air as you hold.

MODIFICATIONS: Place your forearms on a bench or box to modify. You can also do this plank from your knees or the quadruped position.

EXERCISE SWAPS: Roller serratus anterior extension, downward dog scapular press, banana, seated hinge hold

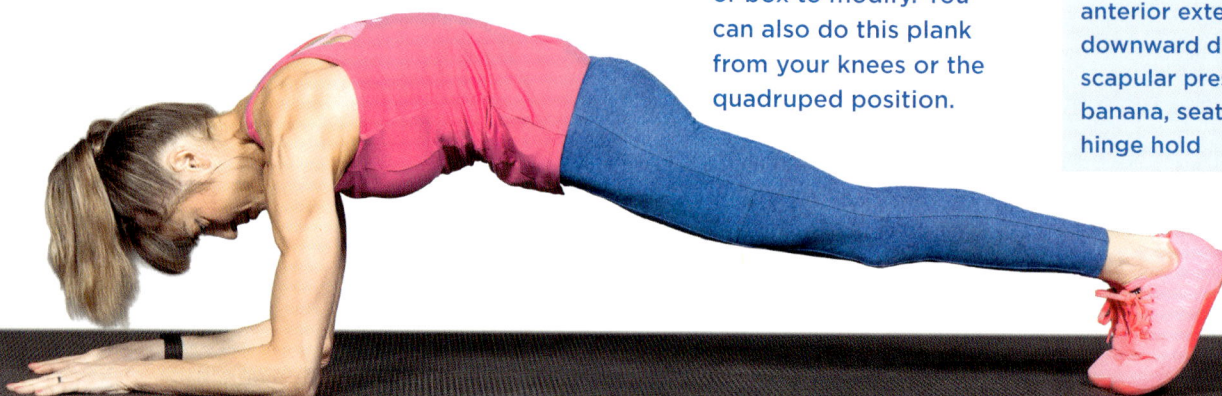

STRENGTH

Some of the exercise swaps I include here are for inspiration. You'll find common moves you can include that go beyond the options I share in the workouts—moves that are based on other tools or are progression moves.

PUSH-UP PLUS

Set up at the top of a push-up with your hands outside your chest, your feet together, and your body in a nice straight line down to your heels. Brace your core and lower your body to an inch above the ground to perform a standard push-up, driving back through your heels. Feel your shoulder blades move toward your spine as you lower. Your upper arms should make an arrow shape with your body for this standard push-up.

Press back up, and as you reach the top of the push-up, round your upper back toward the ceiling, tucking your pelvis toward your ribs. Really push the ground away as you try to pull your shoulder blades forward around your ribs. Move back into the plank position and repeat the push-up.

MODIFICATIONS: Perform the push-up with your hands on a bench or box or do it from your knees.

EXERCISE SWAPS: Push-up, roller serratus anterior extension, bench press, single-arm rotational chest press

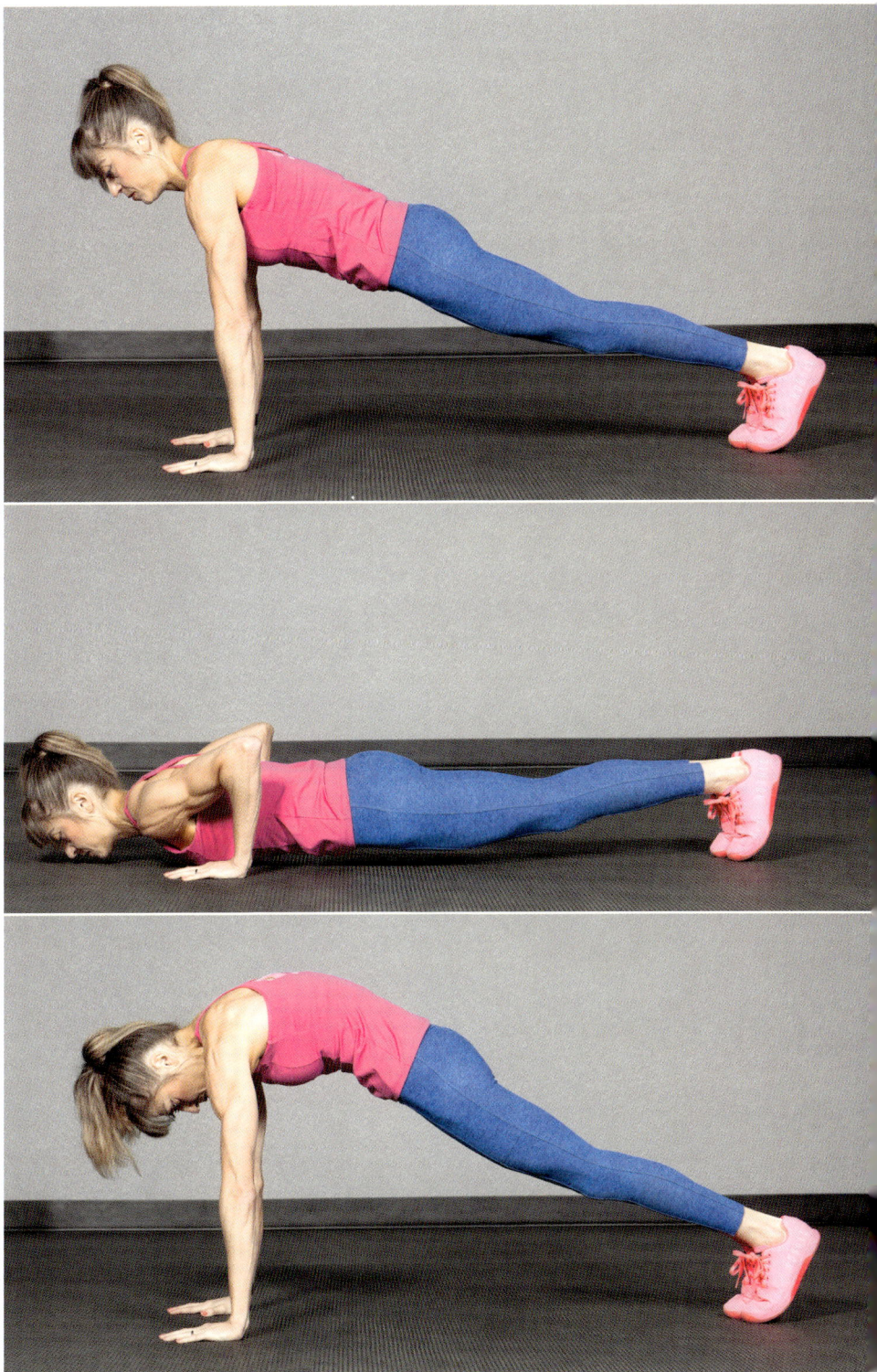

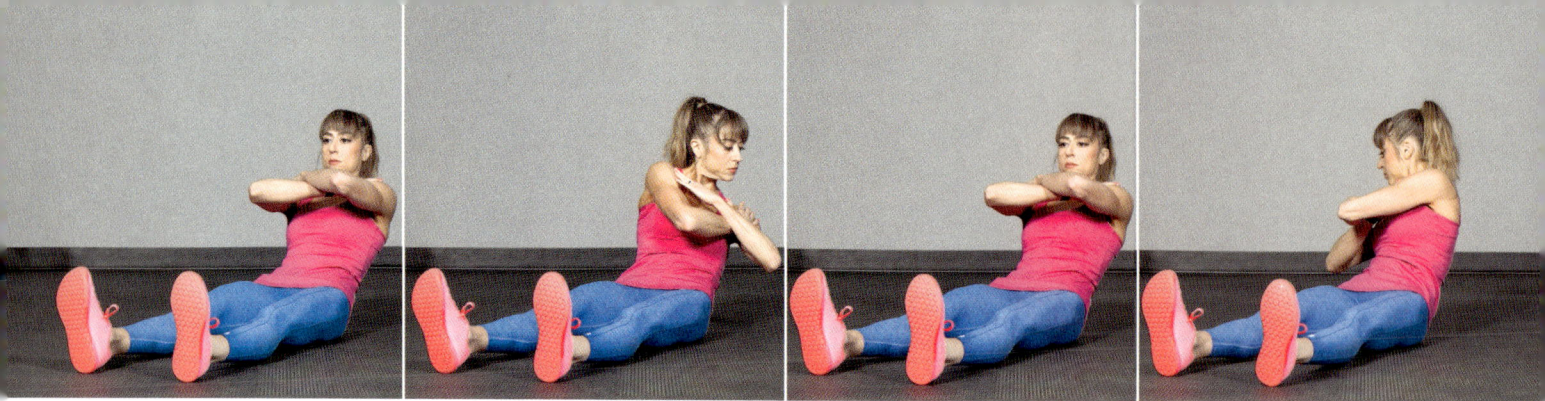

HINGE AND TWIST

Sit on the ground with your legs straight in front of you about hip-width apart. Cross your arms over your chest with your hands on your shoulders and lean back. As you lean back and engage your abs, tuck your ribs slightly down toward your hips to create that C curve of your spine. Then twist toward one side, rotating your elbow close to the ground. Pause and feel the muscles working down the sides of your torso and around your rib cage. Twist back to center and rotate toward the other side. Do not sit up as you rotate back and forth; stay in the hinged position. If you feel discomfort in your lower back, do not lean back as far and make sure you're rounding your spine.

MODIFICATIONS: Don't hinge back as far. You also can perform this seated on a bench.

EXERCISE SWAPS: Seated hinge hold, side plank hold, side plank oblique twist, Russian twist, cable twist

SIDE PLANK OBLIQUE TWIST

Set up on your side on your forearm with your elbow right below your shoulder. Your legs should be out straight and unstacked with your top foot in front. Flex your feet and engage the side of your back to support your shoulder; make sure you don't shrug.

Lift your hips, squeezing your glutes and keeping your chest open as you drive your bottom hip up. Place your free hand behind your head with your elbow pointing toward the ceiling. Then, keeping your bottom hip up, rotate your top elbow toward the ground—perhaps even aiming toward your supporting elbow.

Your butt may hike up a bit as you rotate, but don't consciously lift it up higher to reduce the work your obliques are doing. Truly twist through your spine to reach toward the ground and then rotate back open and up. Control the movement and don't just flap your arm. Move slowly and don't let your side drop toward the ground. Switch sides after all reps are complete.

MODIFICATIONS: Place your forearm on a bench or box or perform this side plank from your knees.

EXERCISE SWAPS: Hinge and twist, sit-thru to thoracic bridge, side plank hold, side plank clam, downward dog scapular press, cable hip rotation

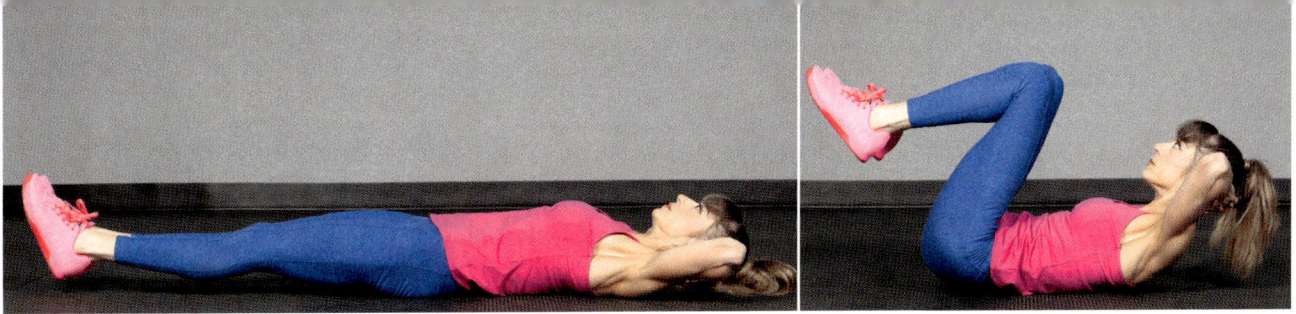

FULL-BODY CRUNCH

Lie on your back with your legs out straight and place your hands behind your head. Tuck your knees in toward your chest and crunch your upper body up, lifting your shoulder blades off the ground. Think about rolling up one vertebrae at a time to lift. Keep your elbows open and push your head back into your hands to keep space between your chin and your chest. Press your lower back into the ground and tuck your pelvis toward your ribs to engage your abs.

Then kick your legs out as you relax your upper body down to the ground. Engage your glutes as you extend your legs and keep that posterior pelvic tilt, pressing your lower back toward the ground with that pelvis tuck. Then crunch your upper body back up as you tuck your knees in again.

Focus on curling your knees in, not just moving at the hips.

MODIFICATIONS: Kick your legs out higher from the ground or perform a bent knee variation, touching your feet down between reps instead of kicking out.

EXERCISE SWAPS: Incline reverse crunch, banana, extended plank hold, seated hinge hold, lying knees, plank knee tuck, body saw, bench V-up, hanging knees to elbow

HIP THRUST

Set up a bench that won't move as you push back into it. It should hit your back at about the bottom of your shoulder blades. Place a pad on the center of a barbell, preferably loaded with bumper plates so you can roll it over your legs while you're seated against the bench. Bend your knees so your feet are flat on the floor. When you lift your hips, you want your knees to be aligned over your ankles.

Rest the bar at the top of your thighs and grip it just outside hip width; then drive through your back on the bench and your feet to bridge up. Focus on feeling your glutes to extend your hips. To guard against hyperextending your back, tuck your pelvis slightly toward your ribs as you reach the top. Pause and then lower back down.

Tuck your chin slightly to look toward your knees to help avoid pushing yourself backward. This can help with glute engagement. As you lift, push the bar toward your knees to engage your lats and stabilize the weight.

Lower your hips to touch the bar to the ground and repeat.

MODIFICATIONS: Use a slightly lower bench to decrease the range of motion or a dumbbell to decrease the weight. Adjust your foot positioning but be conscious that you don't let your feet get so far out that your hamstrings end up taking over.

EXERCISE SWAPS: Weighted glute bridge, hip thrust machine, kneeling cable pull-through/band hip hinge, banded hip thrust, feet-raised hip thrust, single-leg hip thrust, 80/20 hip thrust, Smith machine hip thrust

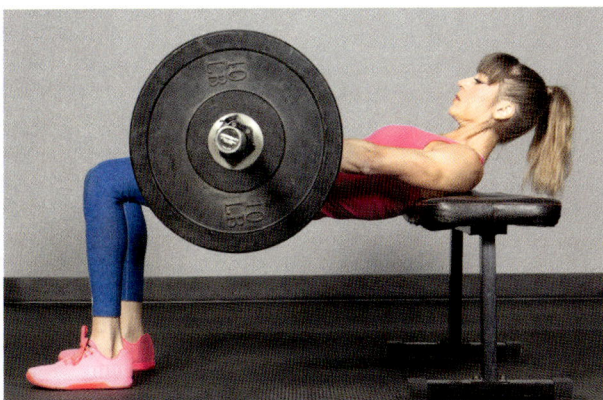

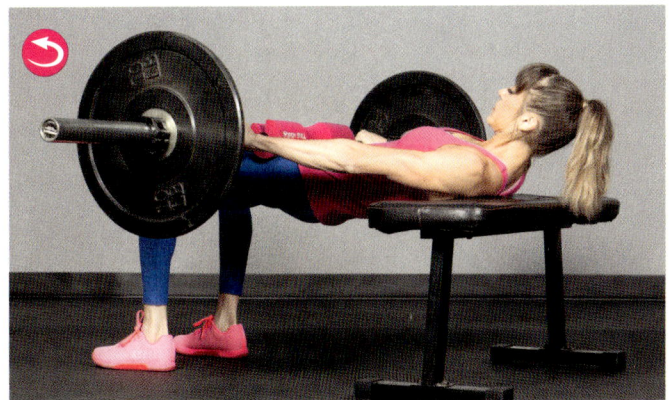

SINGLE-LEG DEADLIFT

Stand up nice and tall, shifting your weight to one leg with the knee of your "free" leg slightly bent and its toes lightly touching the ground. Focus on pushing the two points in the ball of your foot and one point in your heel of your support leg down into the ground to create tension and stability. If you're using weights, hold one in each hand with your arms down by your sides and engage your lats to stabilize them.

Then, hinge at your hips, pushing your butt back as you lean your chest toward the ground and lift your free leg toward the wall behind you. Do not reach the weights toward the ground. They're lowering in response to your hip hinge. Think about dropping the weights toward the instep or heel of your support foot to help you keep your lats engaged. Avoid reaching out or shifting your weight forward.

Sit your butt back as you hinge and feel a stretch up your hamstring. Once your chest is about parallel to the ground, or if you feel your lower back starting to round, drive through your foot to push back up to standing. Think about pushing the ground away. Engage your glute at the top to extend your hip, touching the toe of your free foot down lightly to maintain balance. Then repeat the hinge, focusing on the loading of your support leg.

EXERCISE SWAPS: Bench single-leg deadlift, 80/20 deadlift, slider single-leg deadlift, kettlebell single-leg deadlift, barbell single-leg deadlift, cable single-leg deadlift, unilaterally loaded single-leg deadlift, mini band deadlift, Romanian deadlift

MODIFICATIONS: Do not add weight. Use a wall or chair to help you balance.

CABLE SEATED HAMSTRING CURL

Place a bench a bit back from a cable machine so you can sit on it and extend your leg out in front with tension still in the cable. Sit on the bench facing the cable machine and attach the cable's ankle strap to one leg.

Extend your leg in front of you, flex your foot, and then flex your knee to curl your heel toward your butt. Focus on feeling your hamstring pull your heel in and then control the movement to extend your leg again.

MODIFICATIONS: Start with light weight to perform the full range of motion.

EXERCISE SWAPS: Seated hamstring machine, band seated hamstring curl, glute bridge and curl, cable lying hamstring curl, posterior plank, mini band hamstring curl, standing ankle weight hamstring curl, Nordic hamstring curl, glute-ham hip hinge, RDL pulse

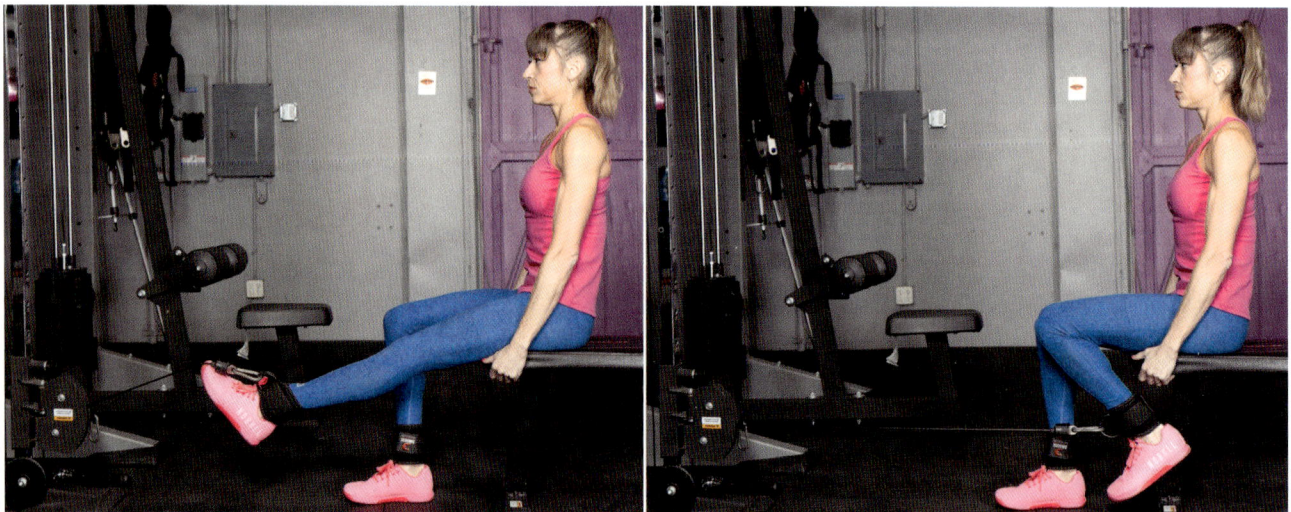

FRONT LUNGE

Stand tall with your feet together. If you're holding weights, hold them by your sides and engage your lats to stabilize the weights. Step forward on one side, dropping your back knee toward the ground as you bend your front knee to 90 degrees. Sink as if moving to half kneel on the ground, but do not come to rest on the ground. The closer to the ground you get, the harder this move will be. You want to work through the fullest range of motion you can control.

Make sure to keep your front heel down and your chest up as you lunge forward. Don't let the weights swing and throw you off balance. Your weight should feel mostly centered with slightly more loaded on your front leg.

Drive off your front foot to move back to standing. You may stay on one side or alternate, depending on the workout.

Keep a more vertical shin angle (your knee right over your ankle) if you have knee pain or limited ankle mobility. Your knee can travel over the ball of your foot if you want to load your front quad more.

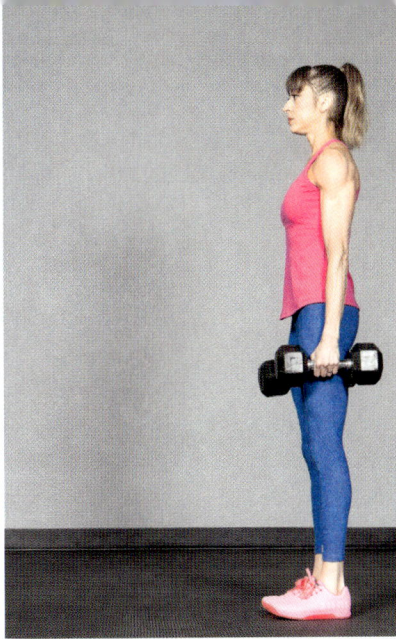

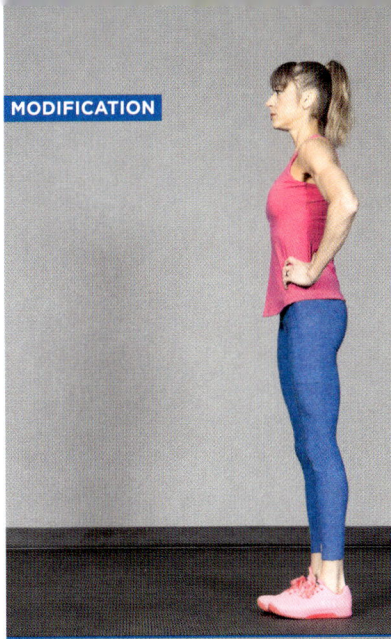

MODIFICATIONS: Do not use weights or lunge as deep to start. You can also modify to a split squat or use an anterior reach lunge, which has a bit more of a hip hinge and a straighter rear leg. You can also adjust load placement—front loading or loading with a barbell on your back.

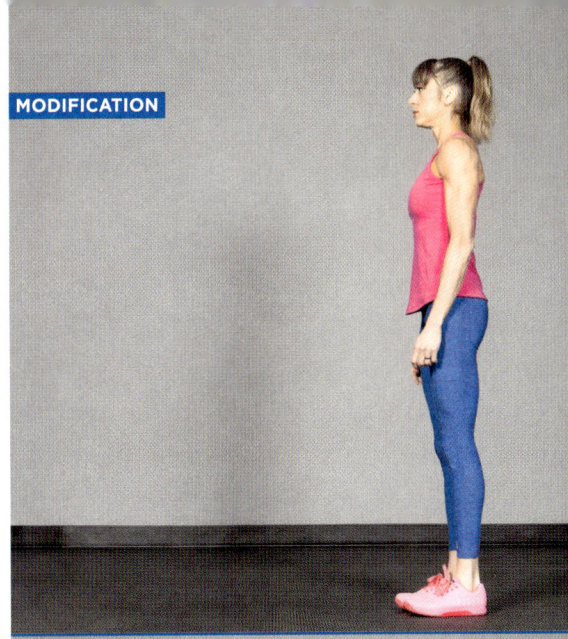

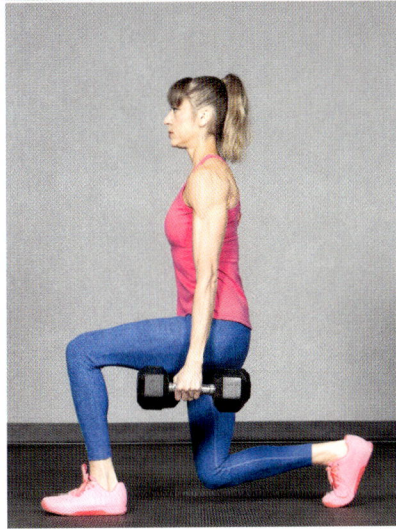

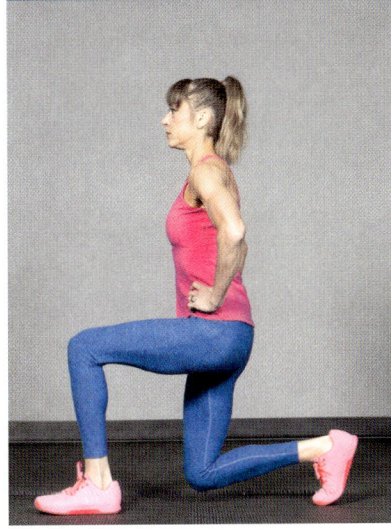

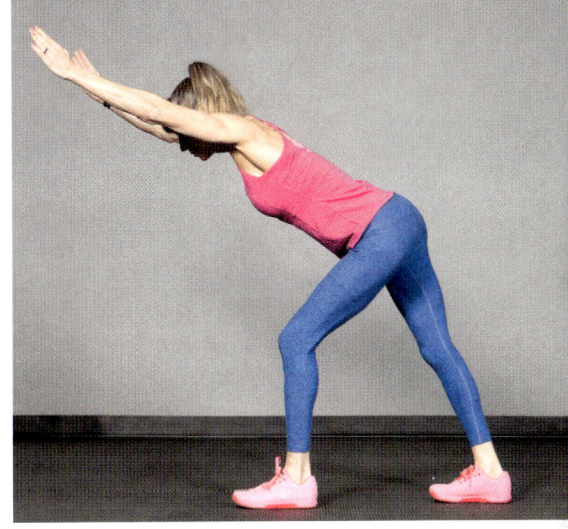

EXERCISE SWAPS: Barbell front lunge, goblet front lunge, anterior reach lunge, unilaterally loaded front lunge, split squat, deficit split squat, get-up lunge, alternating angled front lunge, bodyweight front lunge

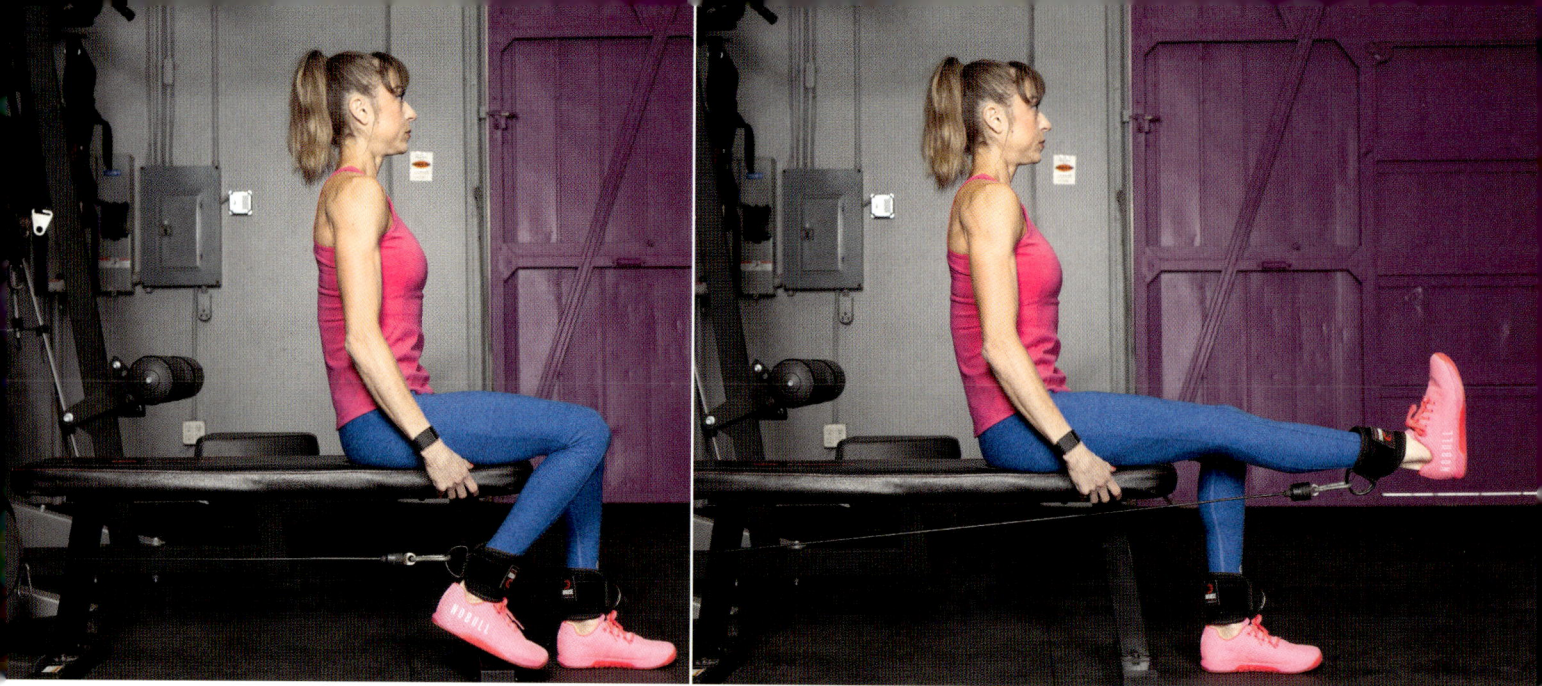

CABLE SEATED QUAD EXTENSION

Place a bench so you can sit with the cable machine behind you. If you have long legs, a taller box may be helpful so you have a full range of motion. Put an ankle strap around one ankle and sit on the bench with your back to the machine. Flex your foot so your heel just touches the ground.

Engage your quad to straighten your knee, lifting your lower leg straight out in front of you. Lower your foot, allowing your heel to move back toward the cable machine and behind you. Try to allow the extra flexion so your knee bends past the 90-degree point rather than stopping when your ankle is just below your knee.

EXERCISE SWAPS: Machine leg extension, ankle weight quad extension, kneeling lean back, quad kickout, band leg extension, squat pulse, rock lunge

MODIFICATIONS: Start with a lighter weight, use an ankle weight, or use a leg extension machine. You can also change your posture to target your quads in different ways, such as by leaning back more to have your rectus femoris work extra.

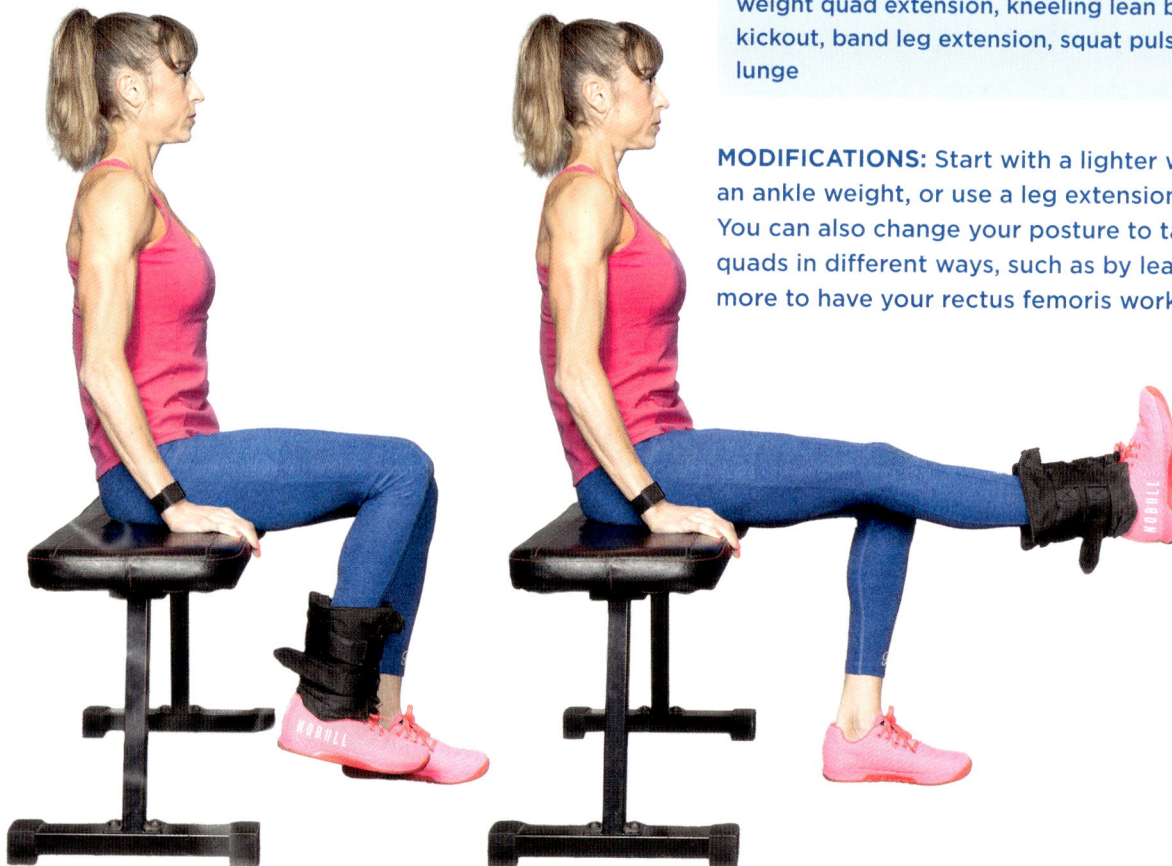

FRONT SQUAT

Set up the rack so the bar is positioned a little lower than your shoulders. Step forward under the bar, bringing it to rest against your shoulders with your arms out straight. Then reach back to grip the bar with your elbows up in front of you. Push the bar back into your collarbone area as you lift and unrack the weight.

Step back from the rack and set your feet about hip-width to shoulder-width apart based on your build and hip mobility. Take a big inhale; then sit down and back to squat. Make sure your weight doesn't shift forward to the balls of your feet and toes. Focus on engaging your upper back to support the bar and keep your chest up. Keep your heels down to sink as low in the squat as your mobility allows.

Exhale as you drive back up to standing and repeat the squat. If you feel yourself leaning forward, your butt rising first, or your heels coming up, you need to regress the range of motion and go lighter.

MODIFICATIONS: Start out with a goblet squat or squat to a box to make it easier to control the range of motion. If you can't get parallel to the ground, consider using a lighter weight to start. If you have limited ankle mobility or want to focus more on your quads, a heel lift (wedge) can help. If you have wrist mobility issues, you can use straps or cross your hands over your chest to secure the bar.

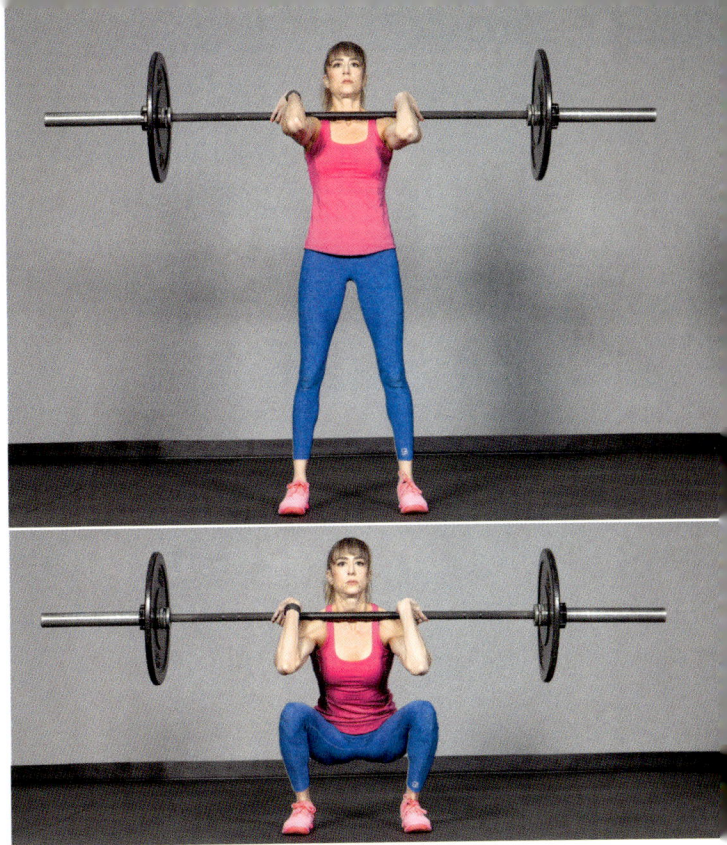

EXERCISE SWAPS: Goblet squat (kettlebell or dumbbell), split squat, get-up lunge, single-leg squat, sumo squat, leg press, back squat, Smith machine squat

BENCH PRESS

Sit on the bench with a dumbbell in each hand, resting an end of each dumbbell on your thighs. As the weights get heavier, you can give them a slight bump off your legs to set up at the top of the bench on the first rep. Engage your back, pressing your chest out just slightly to support your shoulders and make sure they aren't shrugged.

Lower the weights to your chest with your upper arms creating an arrow shape with your body. At your chest, press back up, exhaling to help you power the press. You can do a wider grip, more overhand position if you want, but make sure not to shrug your shoulders as you press straight up from your chest.

Really feel yourself engaging your back to support your shoulders and help power the press as you drive your feet down into the ground.

MODIFICATIONS: You can do a barbell bench press with a variety of grips; however, the dumbbell variation is a great go-to for not only strength but shoulder health. Go lighter to start. Modify by using a band or cable press.

EXERCISE SWAPS: Barbell bench press, Smith machine bench press, machine chest press, cable/band chest press, single-arm bench press, alternating arm bench press, push-up, band push-up, floor press

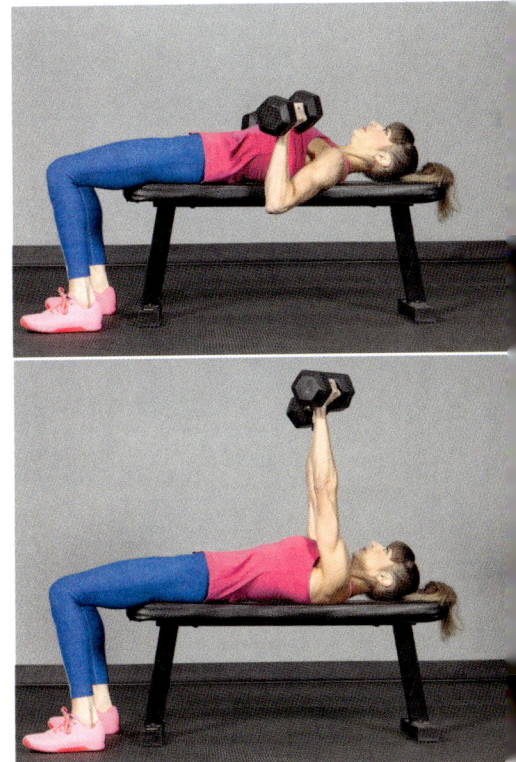

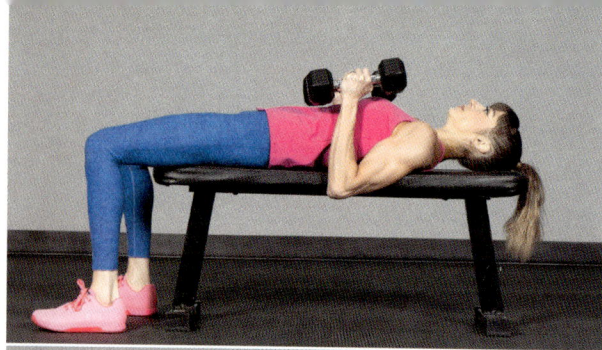

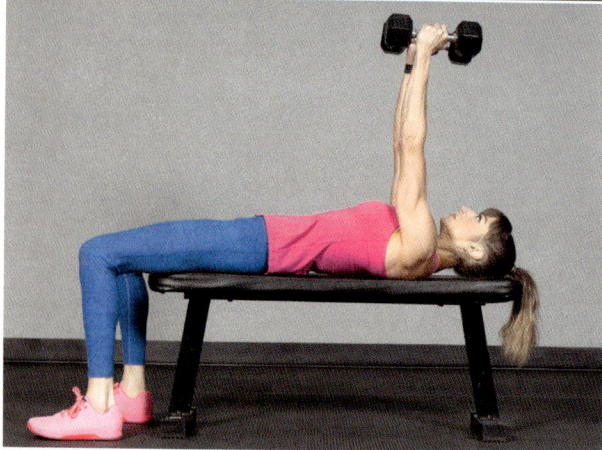

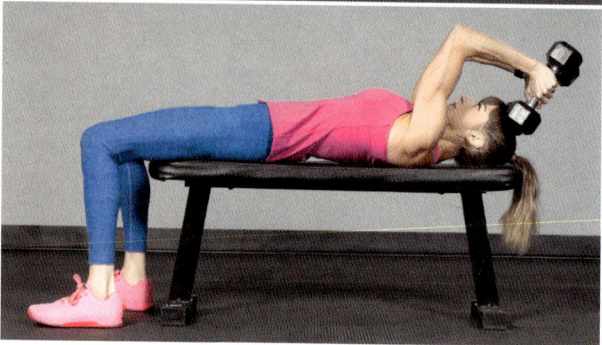

CHEST PRESS TO SKULL CRUSHER

Lie back on a bench with your feet flat on the ground. Hold a dumbbell in each hand at your chest with your palms facing in toward each other. Engage your back to avoid shrugging your shoulders. Press the weights up from your chest while keeping your arms in tight to your side.

Fully extend your arms and then bend only at the elbows to lower the weights toward the top of your head. You can allow your upper arms to move backward slightly for an extra stretch on your triceps, but you want the movement to mainly be due to the bending of your elbows. Then feel your triceps work to extend your elbows and bring the weights back up over your chest before you lower them for another chest press, keeping your arms tight to your body as you do.

MODIFICATIONS: Start with a light weight so you can really control the movement. You also can hold a single dumbbell in both hands. You can progress the move with an EZ curl bar and get an extra stretch on your triceps by reaching a bit beyond your head with the skull crusher.

EXERCISE SWAPS: Floor press to skull crusher, EZ bar press to skull crusher, narrow grip bench press, narrow grip push-up, skull crusher, overhead triceps extension, push-up to dip

TRICEPS PUSHDOWN

Connect the rope attachment to a cable anchored above head height. With one end in each hand, walk back just a bit from the machine to create tension when your hands are at your chest. Press your chest out and think wide shoulders. Stand upright with your torso straight or with a very slight hinge forward and your arms tight by your sides; then straighten your arms to push down on the rope. The movement should come only from your elbows straightening as you feel the backs of your arms working. Fully extend your arms and then bring your hands back up in front of your chest. Do not reach higher than chest height by letting your arms come away from your sides.

MODIFICATIONS: Start lighter. Use a band anchored up high.

EXERCISE SWAPS: Band triceps pushdown, bench dip, triceps push-up, overhead triceps extension

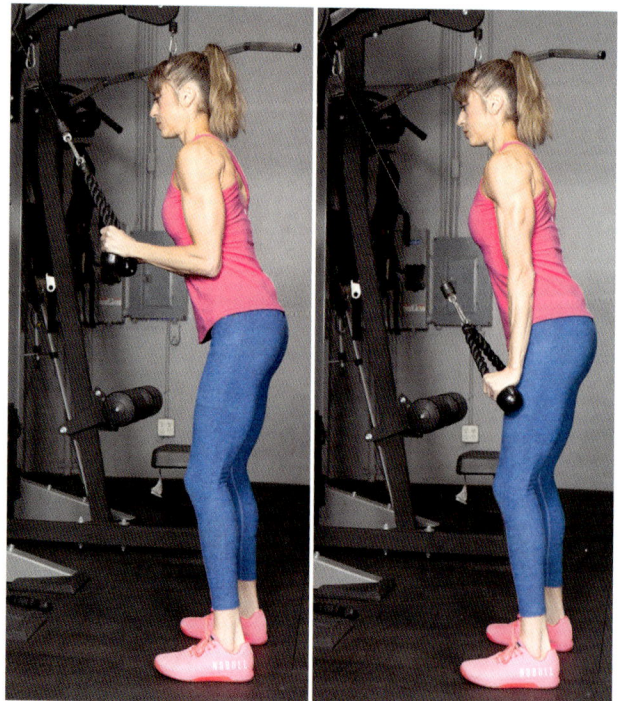

OVERHAND ROW

Grab a barbell in both hands with your hands about shoulder-width apart and your palms facing back toward your legs. Hinge at your hips, pushing your butt back. With a flat back and soft knees, extend your arms down in front of your legs. Making sure your shoulders aren't shrugged, drive your elbows toward your hips and back toward the ceiling, keeping your chest pressed out. Focus on your shoulder blades moving toward your spine as you row the weight up to the bottom of your rib cage. Do not round your spine as you row or round your shoulders at the bottom of the movement. The pull is coming from your back, not your shoulders.

Keep your back flat as you row and think about drawing your shoulder blades together. Then slowly lower the bar. Stay in the hinged position as you perform all reps. Your elbows shouldn't flare up by your shoulders as you do this. If they do, make sure to engage your upper back and avoid shrugging.

MODIFICATIONS: Start with dumbbells. If you feel strain in your lower back, do chest-supported rows or a standing cable variation.

EXERCISE SWAPS: Overhand seated row, overhand T-bar row, overhand cable/band row, overhand dumbbell row, chest-supported row, single-arm row, machine back row

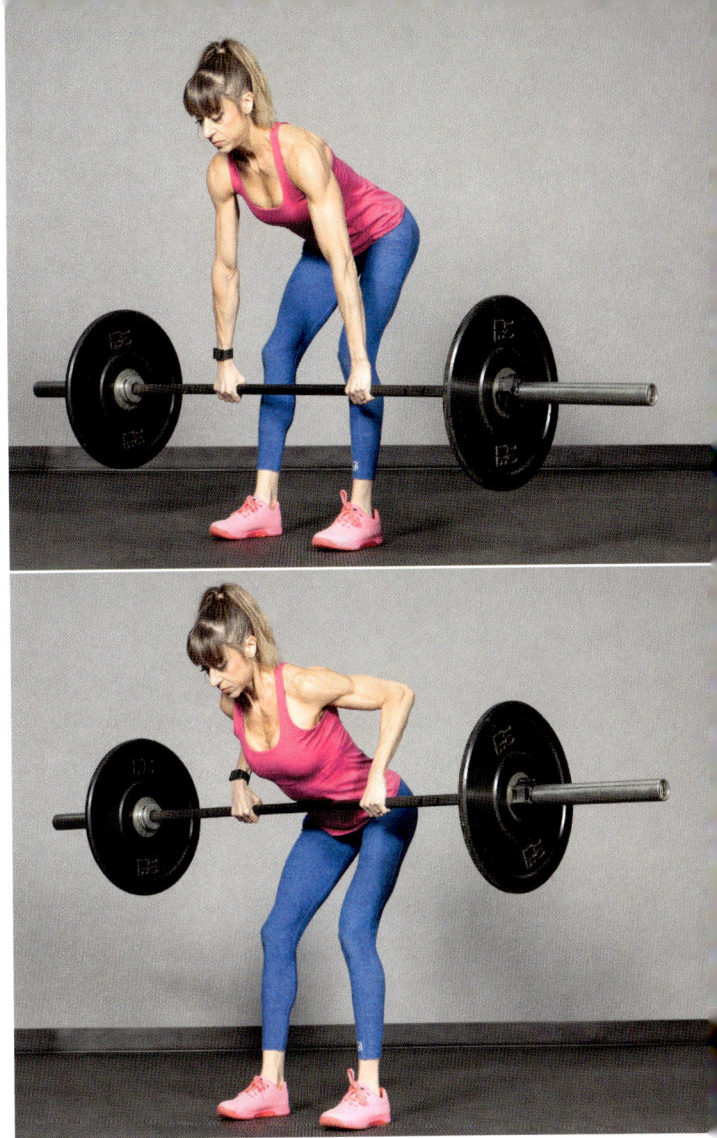

BACK FLY

Hold a light dumbbell in each hand and hinge at your hips, pushing your butt back as you lean your chest forward. Keep your back flat and slightly bend your knees as your arms hang down with a slight bend in your elbows. Fly your arms out to the side, keeping your elbows soft, to lift the backs of your hands toward the ceiling until your arms have reached just below shoulder height. Focus on your shoulder blades pinching together to lift your arms up and open. You'll feel your upper back and the backs of your shoulders working. Then lower your arms.

Do not stand up between reps. Stay hinged over and really focus on the movement of your shoulder blades. Keep your neck in line with your spine and make sure not to shrug or round your shoulders.

MODIFICATIONS: Start light and use a chest-supported or lying variation if you struggle with your lower back engaging. You can perform these from a seated, lying, or standing position.

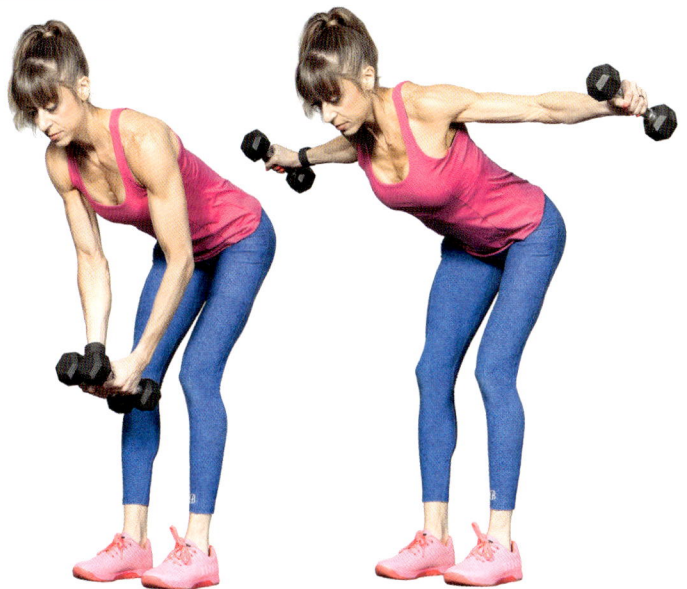

EXERCISE SWAPS: Cable back fly, reverse pec deck, seated back fly, lying back fly, chest-supported back fly, suspension trainer back fly, band back fly, scapular wing, scapular push-up, back shrug

BACK SHRUG

Hold a dumbbell in each hand with your palms facing toward each other and hinge at the waist, pushing your butt back as you lean over with your back flat. Let your arms hang down and engage your lats to make sure your shoulders aren't shrugged. Keep your knees soft and make sure you aren't arching your lower back.

Pinch your shoulder blades together while letting your arms hang down. Do not bend your elbows with this movement or allow your shoulders to hunch up to your ears. Draw your shoulder blades toward your spine. Pause then release and let your back relax. Your shoulder blades can even move slightly forward around your ribs, but don't round over. Repeat the retraction.

MODIFICATIONS: If you struggle with bending your elbows, try doing one side at a time. If your shoulders elevate toward your ears or you're feeling your lower back, try a chest-supported variation or even modify to the single-arm scapular push-up.

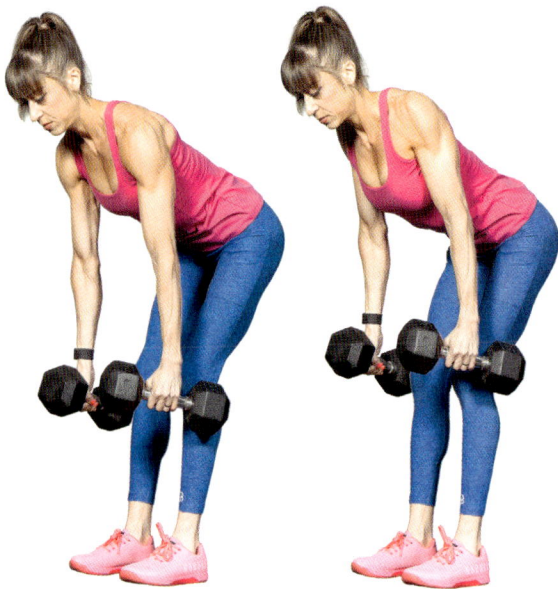

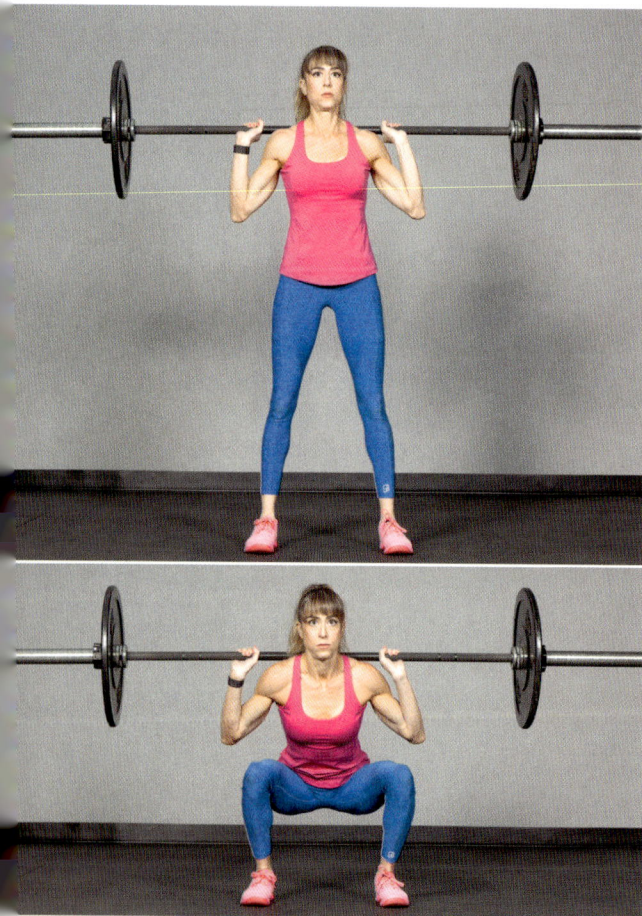

EXERCISE SWAPS: Back fly, cable back shrug, band back shrug, reverse pec deck, chest-supported back shrug, single-arm scapular push-up, scapular wing

BACK SQUAT

Set up the rack so the bar is positioned just lower than your shoulders. Step forward under the bar with your hands shoulder-width apart on the bar. Bring the bar to rest against the backs of your shoulders right at the top of your shoulder blades. The exact placement of the bar will depend on where it's most comfortable, but don't rest it up on your neck. You can position it lower on your shoulder blades, especially for a more glute-dominant squat. Grip the bar to create tension, pulling it in to your back as you step away from the rack to stand with your feet hip-width to shoulder-width apart based on your build.

Sit your butt down and back to squat. You may lean forward a bit as you squat, but do not simply hinge or round forward. Bend your knees to sink as you sit back to balance. Keep your heels down to squat as low as your mobility and build allows. If you can't sink to parallel, reduce the weight.

Drive back up to standing, thinking of your foot as a tripod pushing the ground away. Do not rock forward as you drive up. Squeeze your glutes at the top to stand tall but don't arch or shove them forward. Take a big inhale and brace your abs as if you're preparing to be punched in the gut before you squat; then exhale on the exertion to drive back up.

MODIFICATIONS: Start with a lighter weight or control the range of motion by squatting to a higher box. A goblet squat is also a great modification to build up core strength while loading down the squat. To make this a more glute-dominant move, perform a squat to box. If you prefer more quad-intensive squat, perform a front squat.

EXERCISE SWAPS: Back squat to box, front squat, Smith machine squats, leg press, reverse lunge, goblet squat, trap bar deadlift

STEP-UP

Place one foot on a box or bench as you hold weights down by your sides. Engage your lats to stabilize the dumbbells and shift your weight onto the foot on the box. Drive up through the foot on the box until you're standing on top. Squeeze your supporting glute as you come to standing and lightly touch the other toe on the box. Don't push off the trailing foot; just touch the box. If you need to use that second foot, drop the weights or adjust the height of the box.

Step back down with control, keeping more of your weight on the foot on top of the box to avoid using the momentum of pushing off the ground. Repeat the step-up without removing your foot from the top of the box. You will step off completely only if you're alternating sides.

Keep your chest up as you drive up. Do not round forward or let the heel on top of the box come up. Be careful of shifting forward and arching your lower back; doing so hints that you need a lower box or weight (or both).

MODIFICATIONS: Don't start with any weights and use a low box or step. If you want to target your glutes, start on top of the box to lower down only as far as you can control to barely touch the ground. You can also make this a more glute-dominant move by using more of a hip hinge to step up and down on a higher box. To make it a more quad-intensive move, use a lower box and stay more upright.

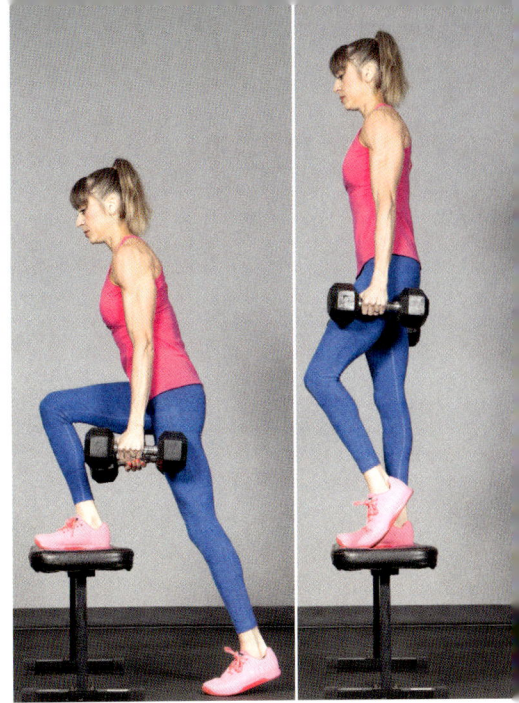

EXERCISE SWAPS: Barbell step-up, goblet step-up, unilaterally loaded step-up, step-up to balance, step-down, cable step-down, high box step-down, Smith machine step-down, single-leg leg press, split squat, balance lunge, deficit split squat, airborne lunge

KNEELING LEAN BACK

Kneel on the ground with your knees no wider than hip-width apart. Flex your feet and squeeze your butt to kneel nice and tall. Reach your hands out in front of you at shoulder height and then lean back, moving from your knees. Go back as far as you can with your body in a nice straight line from your head to your knees.

If you feel yourself starting to arch your lower back or sit your butt back, don't lean back further. You want to lean back as far as you can, feeling your quads stretch and glutes and abs working to brace; then use your quads to power your move back up to kneeling.

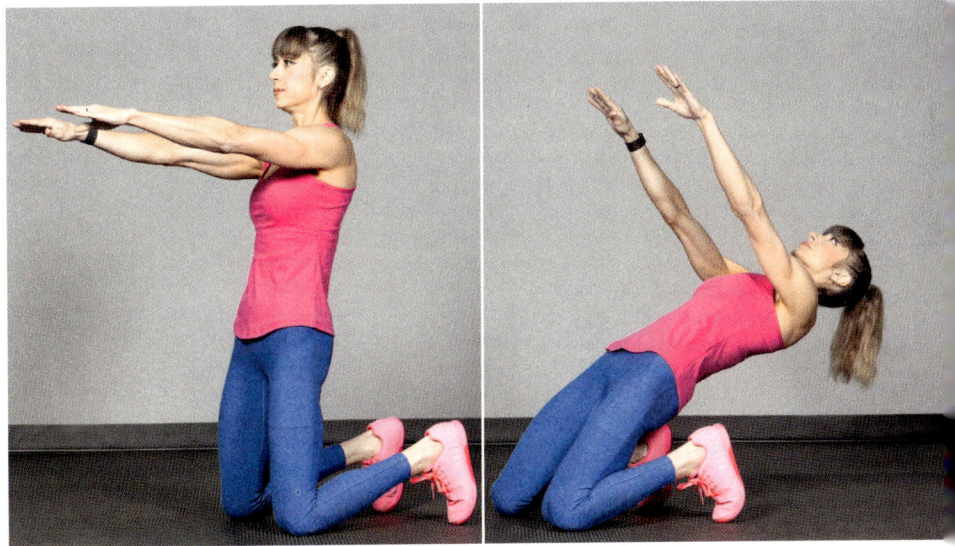

MODIFICATIONS: Anchor a band in front of you and step into it to reduce the resistance as you lean back. You can also hold the band or a pole to help assist you. Progress the move by not counterbalancing with your arms or take it even further by holding a weight at your chest. You can also use a band anchored behind you, looped around you under your chest, to pull back on you to make it harder to move forward again.

EXERCISE SWAPS: Sissy squat, squat pulse, cable lying quad extensions quad kick-out

REVERSE LUNGE

Stand tall with your feet together. If you're holding dumbbells, hold them by your sides and engage your lats to stabilize them. Step back with one foot, bending your front knee to 90 degrees while dropping your back knee down to hover just above the ground. Sit back into that front glute, keeping more weight on your front leg. The deeper you lunge, the harder the move will be. Do not add weight if you can't lower close to the ground yet.

Then drive back up to standing, pushing off that front foot to bring your back foot up and forward. You can slightly hinge to load your glutes more, but do not round over. Keep the knee of your support leg over your ankle with a vertical shin angle to load your glutes as well.

MODIFICATIONS: If you have knee pain, perform a straighter leg lunge or don't sink as deep. A more vertical shin angle can also help if you've had knee pain. To progress this move, you can place your support leg on a plate or box to work through a bigger range of motion.

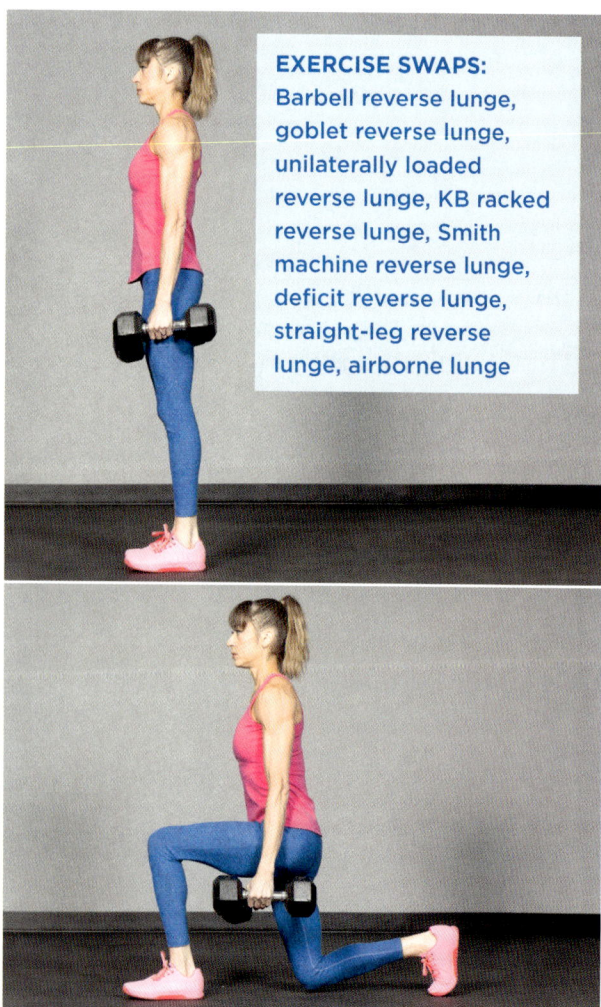

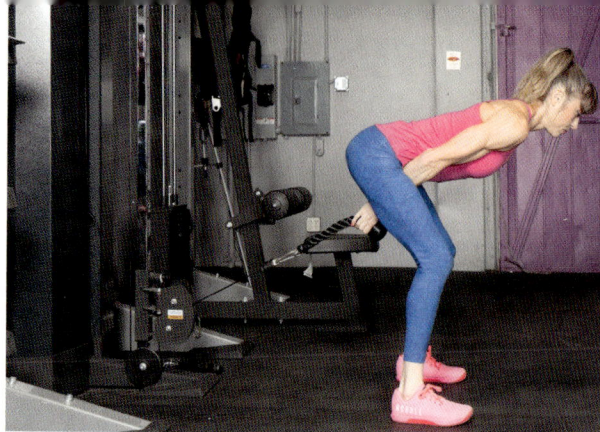

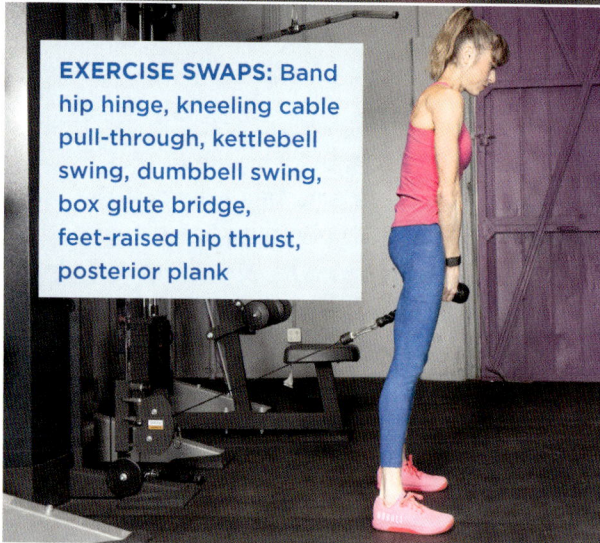

EXERCISE SWAPS: Barbell reverse lunge, goblet reverse lunge, unilaterally loaded reverse lunge, KB racked reverse lunge, Smith machine reverse lunge, deficit reverse lunge, straight-leg reverse lunge, airborne lunge

EXERCISE SWAPS: Band hip hinge, kneeling cable pull-through, kettlebell swing, dumbbell swing, box glute bridge, feet-raised hip thrust, posterior plank

CABLE PULL-THROUGH

Set a cable machine to a low setting (the rope attachment works well) or anchor a band down low. Grab the handles between your legs. Keep your arms straight as you walk away from the anchor point so the cable is pulling you back. With your feet flat on the ground and parallel, hinge at the waist, letting the cable pull you back. Keep your back flat as you reach back through your legs, keeping your knees soft and sitting your butt back.

Squeeze your glutes and push your hips forward to come back up to standing. Keep your arms straight down and lats engaged as you drive your hips forward. You may have a slight lean forward against the resistance but don't arch your back at the top. Squeeze your glutes as you drive up, pushing the ground away with your feet. Do not let your heels come up as you stand up. Then hinge back over, driving your butt back toward the anchor point. Keep your back flat as you hinge and do not round over.

MODIFICATIONS: Use a lighter weight or perform a wall hip hinge without any weight, sitting your butt back to touch a wall and then standing up. You can also use a pull-up assist band around your hips to help you learn that hip-hinge movement.

HYPEREXTENSION

Set the 45-degree hyperextension bench so that the hip pad is just below your anterior iliac crest or about at your hip bones. Set up on the bench with your heels locked in behind the pad.

Relax over the top of the bench so your hips feel support but you don't feel that flexion at your hips is restricted. Cross your hands over your chest and even slightly round your back with a slight posterior pelvic tilt and thoracic rounding. This spinal flexion will help you target your glutes.

Engage your glutes to extend your hips and lift your chest up so your body is in a "line" from your head to your heels. (I put "line" in quotes because with the rounding of your back, it won't be perfectly straight.) Don't arch your lower back or let it take over. Think about this movement not as your torso moving but as the movement coming from your hips extending. Lower and repeat.

MODIFICATIONS: Perform a reverse hyperextension or use a barbell set up in a rig if you don't have a 45-degree hyperextension machine. Hold a weight at your chest to progress the move or do a single-leg variation to isolate each side independently.

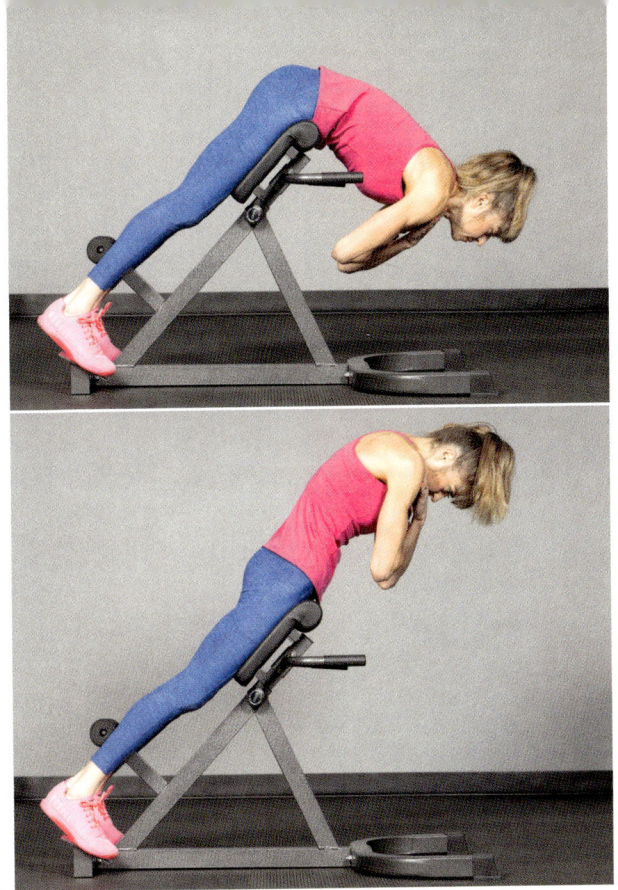

EXERCISE SWAPS: Straight-leg glute bridge, band hip hinge, posterior plank, reverse hyper, single-leg reverse hyper, feet-raised hip thrust, seated hinge

LAT PULL-DOWN

Grab the bar of the cable machine with your grip just wider than shoulder width and sit on the bench, making sure the knee rollers are set so they help anchor you by pushing down into your legs as you put your legs under them. Look up slightly toward the bar with your arms fully extended and slightly open your chest toward the ceiling.

Drive your elbows down to pull the bar to just below your collarbone, as if you were pulling your chest to the bar in a pull-up. Feel your back work and your shoulder blades move down and together. Then extend your arms up, allowing your shoulders to elevate before repeating the pull-down.

An overhand grip targets your lats and back. Adjust your hand positioning to an underhand grip if you want to target your lats and biceps.

MODIFICATIONS: Start with a lighter weight or perform a unilateral variation (one side at a time) with a band or single handle on a cable machine if you struggle with the scapular movement.

EXERCISE SWAPS: Band lat pull-down, pull-up, machine pull-up, cable lat pull-down, single-arm lat pull-down, close-grip lat pull-down, pullover

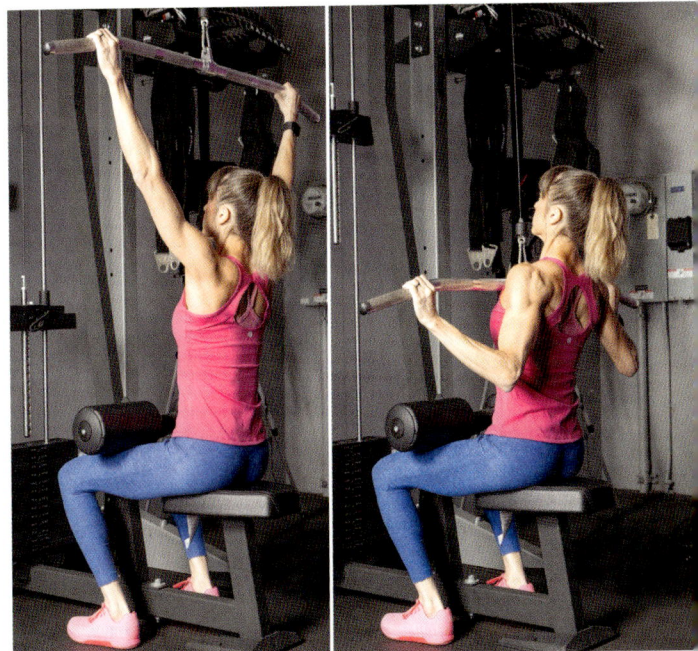

UNDERHAND ROW

Grab a barbell in both hands with an underhand grip and your hands just outside your chest (a narrower grip is good). Hinge at your hips with your arms extended toward the floor, pushing your butt back and keeping your knees soft and your back flat. Make sure your shoulders aren't shrugged and then drive your elbows toward your hips and the ceiling, keeping your chest pressed out. Focus on your shoulder blades moving toward your spine as you row the weight up to the bottom of your rib cage. Don't round your spine or round your shoulders to try to row up higher; keep your back flat and think about drawing your shoulder blades together. The pull is coming from your back.

Slowly lower the bar. Stay hinged at your hips as you perform all reps. Your elbows shouldn't flare up by your shoulders as you do this. If they do, make sure to engage your upper back and avoid shrugging. You will feel your biceps and lats with this version; the overhand row works your upper back more.

MODIFICATIONS: Start with dumbbells. If you feel discomfort in your lower back, use the chest-supported or standing cable variation.

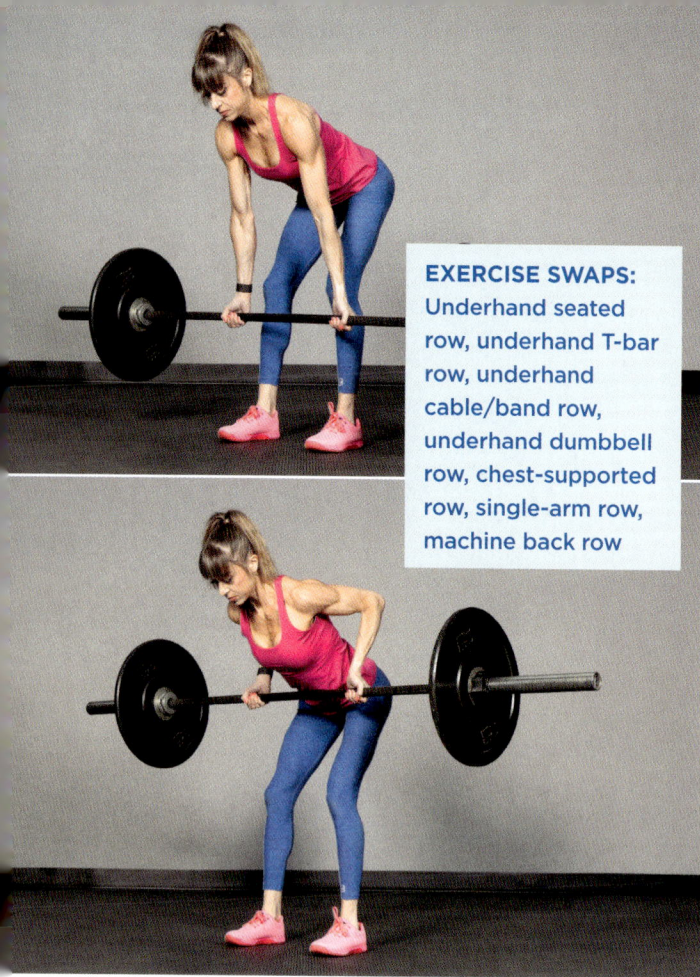

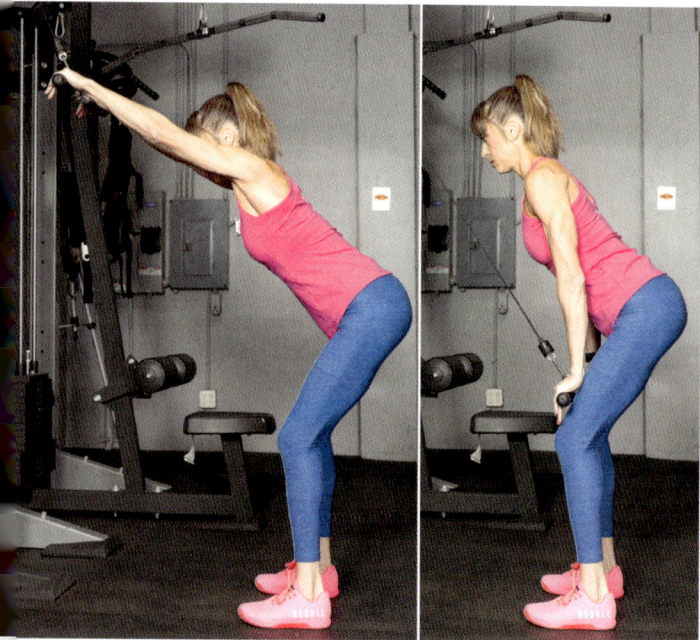

EXERCISE SWAPS:
Underhand seated row, underhand T-bar row, underhand cable/band row, underhand dumbbell row, chest-supported row, single-arm row, machine back row

LAT PUSHDOWN

Anchor a cable pulley or resistance band up high. A straight bar works well, although you can use the rope attachment or handles on a resistance band. Holding the bar in both hands with your palms facing the ground and about shoulder-width apart, walk back a bit from the anchor point, and hinge at your hips as you bring your hands up to about eye height (you can go overhead depending on your cable or band height). Sit back to load your glutes and keep your back flat with your arms straight and chest pressed out.

Push down on the bar, keeping your arms straight to bring your hands toward your legs. Feel your lats working to push the bar down. Then control the extension back up. You don't have to return the bar all the way overhead but extend back up to about eye level and repeat. Do not stand up; stay hinged over as you do this movement. Allow your shoulders to elevate slightly at the top but make sure to pull them down as you bring the bar down; don't round them as you use your lats to push the bar down.

EXERCISE SWAPS: Pullover, single-arm lat pushdown, seated lat pushdowns, lying side slide

MODIFICATIONS: Start with lighter weight. You can do one arm at a time to focus on each side working correctly.

OVERHEAD PRESS

Stand with your feet about hip-width to shoulder-width apart. Hold a dumbbell in each hand at your shoulders with your palms facing in. You can also do an overhand grip with your palms facing forward and away from your body. Squeeze your glutes and brace your abs as if you're preparing to be punched in the gut.

Press the weights overhead toward the ceiling, exhaling as you press. Fully extend your arms, lower the weights to your shoulders, and repeat.

MODIFICATIONS: You can also use a barbell, or if you want to focus on each side independently, do an alternating overhead press. If you struggle with feeling your lower back, perform the move while seated. If your overhead mobility is limited, consider an incline press with a cable, band, or landmine. Start with a lighter weight to modify and build up.

EXERCISE SWAPS: Barbell overhead press, seated overhead press, machine overhead press, Smith machine overhead press, alternating arm overhead press, landmine press, incline bench press, pike push-up, downward dog pike push-up, band overhead press

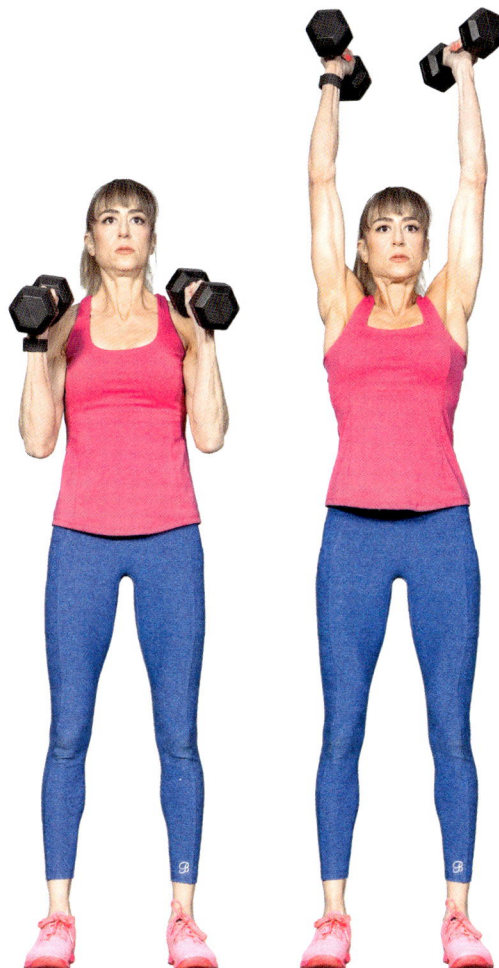

DIP

Place a hand on each bar and grip tightly as you use your foot to assist you in setting up with your arms extended. Press down hard into the bars to engage your lats and avoid shrugging your shoulders. Let your legs hang down, although you can bend them behind you if the bars are low.

Lean forward a bit to target your chest as you bend your elbows to lower yourself. When your upper arms are about parallel to the ground, push back up to the top. Exhale as you drive back up and squeeze your glutes to avoid arching your lower back.

To target your triceps more, don't lean forward as much.

MODIFICATIONS: Use a band for assistance or do a machine-assisted dip variation. You can also swap in triceps push-ups or floor presses to skull crushers to modify based on the tools you have.

EXERCISE SWAPS: Machine dip, chest press to skull crusher, incline cable fly, decline push-up, weighted dip, band assisted dip

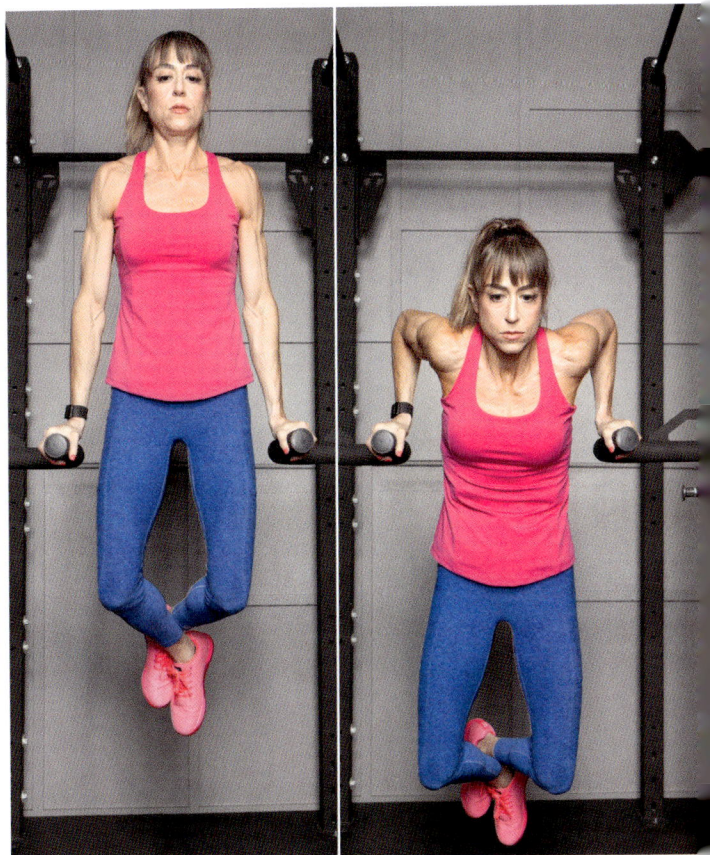

LATERAL RAISE

Hold a dumbbell in each hand down by your sides with your palms facing your legs. Stand tall and press your chest out. With a slight bend to your elbows, lift your arms up and out to the sides to about shoulder height. Make sure not to round forward as you raise your arms.

Lower your arms and repeat. Try not to use momentum by swinging the weights to help you go heavier.

MODIFICATIONS: You can vary your grip. Turning your wrists so your palms face forward engages the back of your shoulders a bit more. Go light to start because this move is very isolated.

EXERCISE SWAPS: Cable lateral raise, band lateral raise, seated lateral raise, lateral raise machine, leaning lateral raise, front to side raise

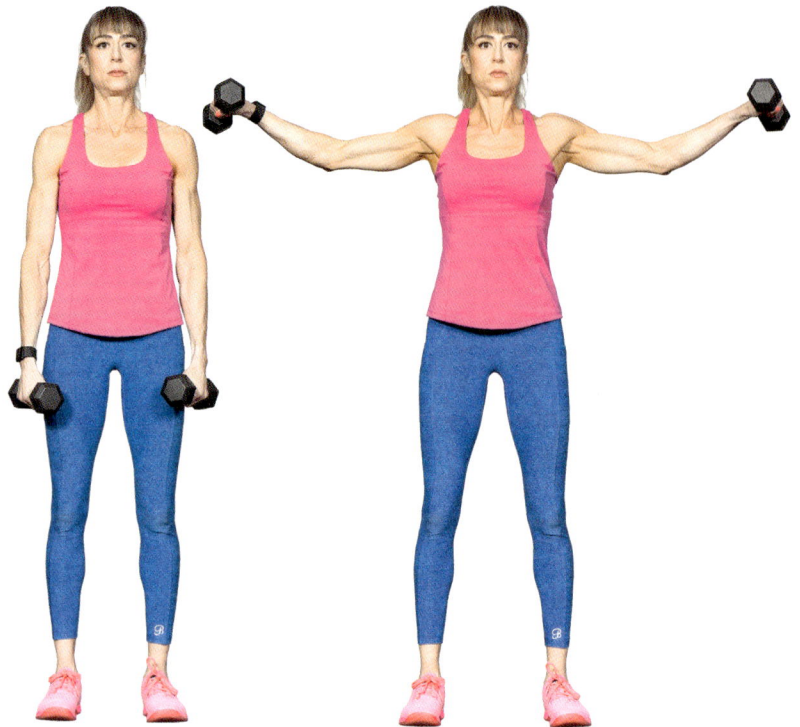

DEADLIFT

Stand at the center of a barbell with your feet parallel and about hip-width to shoulder-width apart. Set up so the bar is over the balls of your feet; the idea is that when you hinge at the hips and grab the bar, the bar will hit your shins. As you lift, you want to keep the bar against you to help load your backside. If the bar drifts forward and away from your body, you risk overloading your lower back.

Push your butt back and reach to grab the bar with your hands just outside your shins. Your knees should be soft as you push your butt back and keep your back flat. Think about engaging your lats and upper back to keep your spine flat.

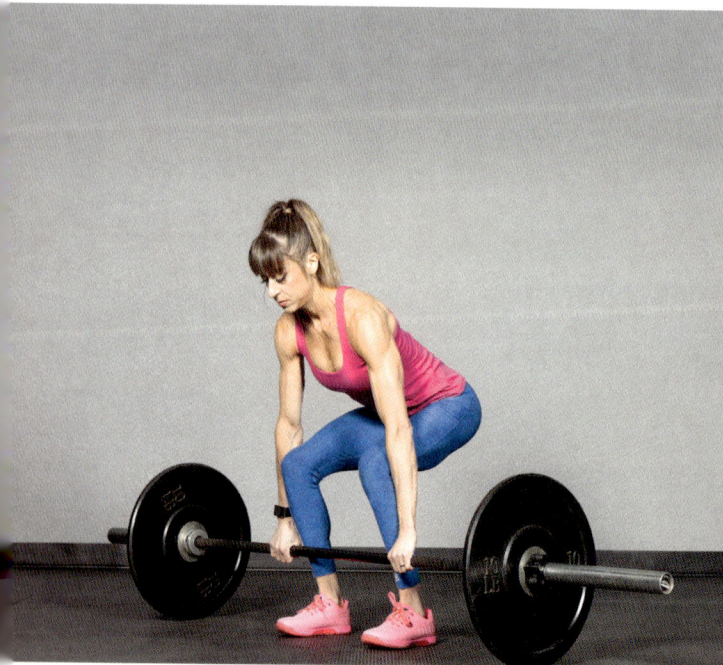

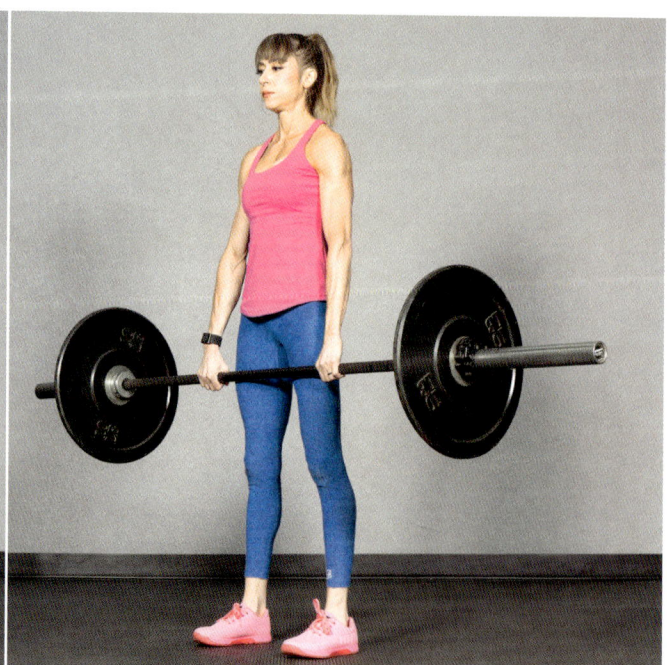

CURTSY LUNGE

Stand tall with your feet together. If you're holding dumbbells, hold them by your sides and engage your lats to stabilize them. Lunge back, stepping your foot across and behind your front leg so you sit back into your front glute. You aren't lunging straight back; you're crossing behind as you keep your chest facing forward, pushing your glute out to the side. Keep your front foot pointing straight ahead.

Sink down into the lunge, hinging slightly to sit into your front glute as you lean your torso slightly forward. Do not round over; just push your butt back as you keep a more vertical shin angle. Slightly more of your weight will be in your front leg. Drop your back knee so it hovers just off the ground to work your legs through a full range of motion. Drive through your front foot to come back up to standing. Squeeze your glute as you come up.

Alternate sides or stay on the same side based on your workout.

MODIFICATIONS: If you've had knee issues, modify by keeping your back leg straighter (side shift skaters) and not sinking as deep. You can also do it with just your bodyweight.

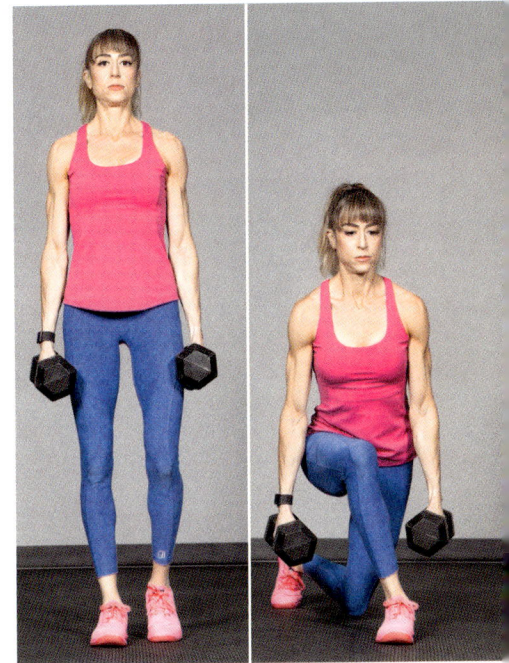

EXERCISE SWAPS: Alternating curtsy lunge, barbell curtsy lunge, goblet curtsy lunge, deficit curtsy lunge, side to curtsy lunge, single-leg deadlift squat, side shift skater, reverse lunge

---

With your arms straight and your core engaged, put tension on the bar to pull up slightly without trying to lift. Set your feet to be ready to push down into the ground and the drive through your feet, pushing the ground away to lift the bar off the ground as you exhale. Feel like you're pulling the bar back into your body as you lift.

At the top, stand tall and squeeze your glutes to extend your hips fully. Don't lean back at the top or arch your back. Hinge your hips, sitting your butt back to lower the bar, keeping it close to your body. Control the descent so you don't drop the bar.

Once you touch the ground, pause but do not fully release tension if you are doing multiple reps. Do not try to squat or lean or round over. Keep tension through your upper back, engage your lats, and sit your butt back while hinging at the hips. Your knees should be soft, but your exact knee bend will be dependent on your mobility and build.

NOTE: *Swap in the deadlift version you're most comfortable with or that addresses what you want to focus on. Sumo deadlift will be more legs, especially glutes and adductors. Conventional deadlifts, which I describe here, will be more back, glutes, and hamstrings. Trap bar deadlifts will work your quads and can be best if you struggle with feeling your lower back becoming overworked.*

MODIFICATIONS: The barbell is a hard version of the deadlift to master. Using dumbbells or kettlebells can be helpful at the start.

EXERCISE SWAPS: Sumo deadlift, trap bar deadlift, dumbbell deadlift, kettlebell deadlift, single-leg deadlift

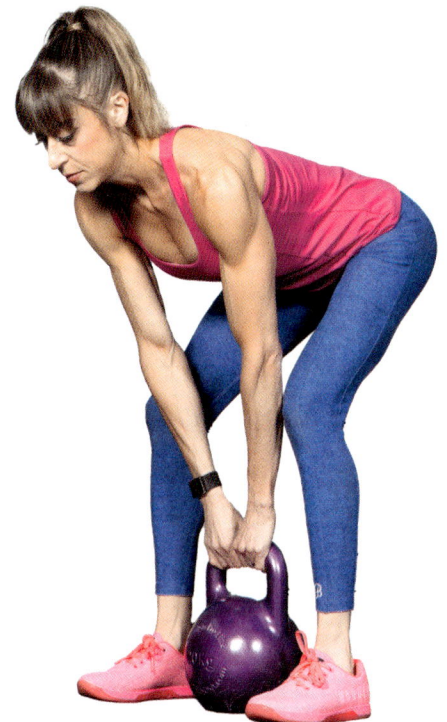

MODIFICATION

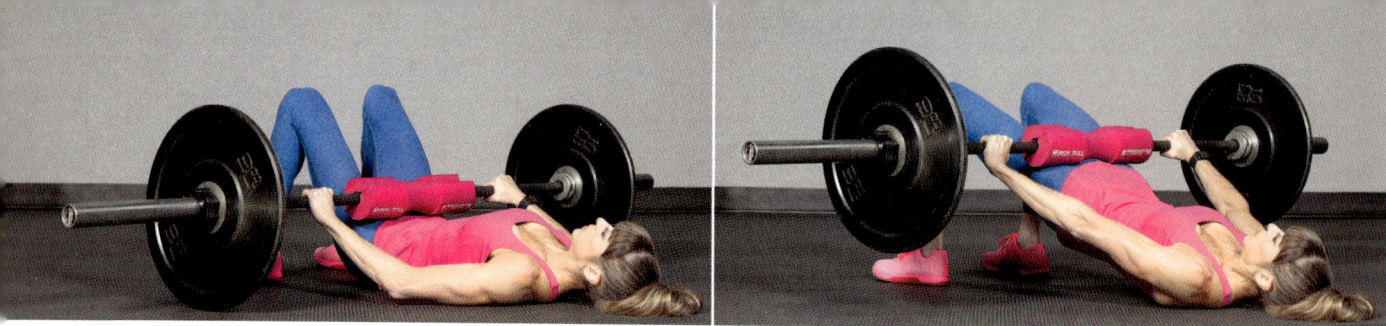

WEIGHTED GLUTE BRIDGE

Set up a barbell with a pad and bumper plates. Sit on the ground with your legs out straight and roll the barbell up your legs. Lie back and bend your knees so your feet are flat on the ground. Hold the bar on either side of your hips and push your arms down straight to press the bar into your body and create tension through your upper back. Tuck your pelvis toward your ribs to engage your abs.

Drive your hips up and squeeze your glutes, pushing your knees slightly toward your toes as you lift. Make sure you drive through your feet and upper back to lift straight up. Do not let your knees fall open or hyperextend your low back as you squeeze your glutes at the top. Hold for a second or two and then lower.

MODIFICATIONS: You can use a dumbbell to start. For progression, if you can't go heavier or don't have weights, do bridges by placing your feet on a bench.

EXERCISE SWAPS: Dumbbell glute bridge, hip thrust, mini band barbell glute bridge, kneeling hip hinge, glute bridge off box, single-leg glute bridge, hip thrust machine, 80/20 glute bridge

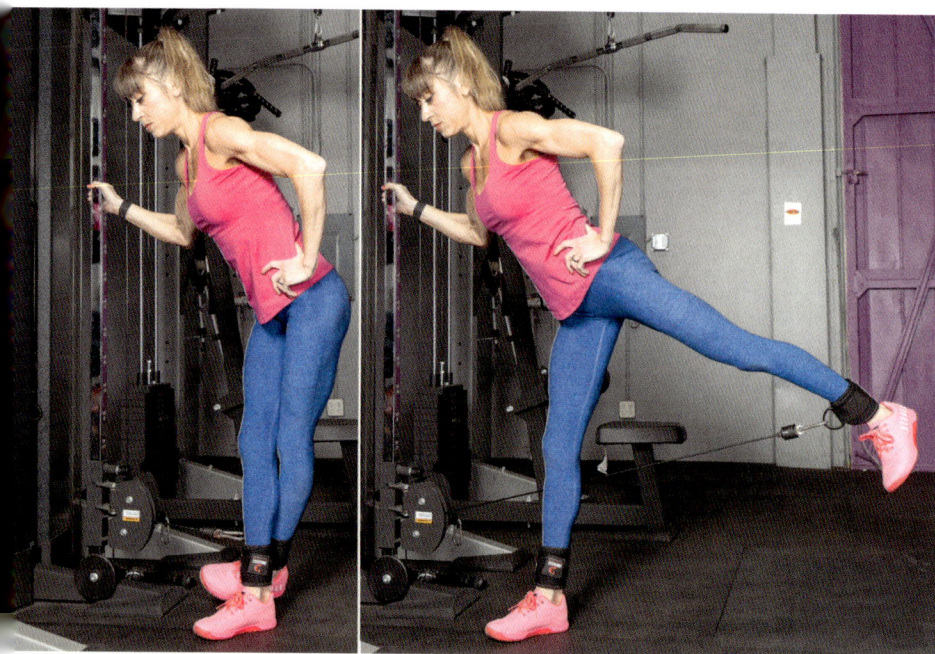

MODIFICATIONS: Start with a smaller range of motion. Use ankle weights or a mini band to start doing lateral raises or abductions without a cable machine.

EXERCISE SWAPS: Abduction machine, band abduction, mini band abduction, side-lying clam, side-lying lateral raise, incline bench abduction, quadruped abduction, standing clam, side plank leg raise

CABLE ABDUCTION

Anchor the cable pulley down low and put on an ankle strap. Stand so you can hold the machine for balance; your working leg (the one with the cable attached to it) will be away from the machine so it can move behind your supporting leg. This positioning will help you better focus on the glute medius and even hit the upper glute max. You can slightly rotate your torso toward the cable machine to balance.

Lift your working leg out to the side away from the machine, kicking back just slightly. Avoid letting your toe rotate open. You can slightly turn your toe down toward the ground if you struggle with feeling the side of your butt. Lift as high as you can control without swinging; then lower your leg, even letting your foot come slightly further back behind your supporting leg toward the anchor point. This extra stretch can make the move more challenging.

PULL-UP

Grab a pull-up bar with your palms facing away from you and about shoulder-width apart. Hang from the bar with your body straight and feel your shoulders shrug slightly. Then pull your shoulders down to begin to pull-up. Feel your shoulder blades moving down as you engage your back and think about leading with your chest. Drive your elbows down as you feel your shoulder blades draw down and together to pull you up.

Once you get your chin above the bar, lower yourself until your arms are fully extended. Try not to swing a ton or kick to pull yourself up.

MODIFICATIONS: Use bands, a machine, or your feet to assist. You can also swap in a lat pull-down. You can vary your grip: A neutral or chin-up grip (palms facing you) works the biceps more, and a wider grip isolates your lats even more.

EXERCISE SWAPS: Chin-up, assisted pull-up, lat pull-down, pullover

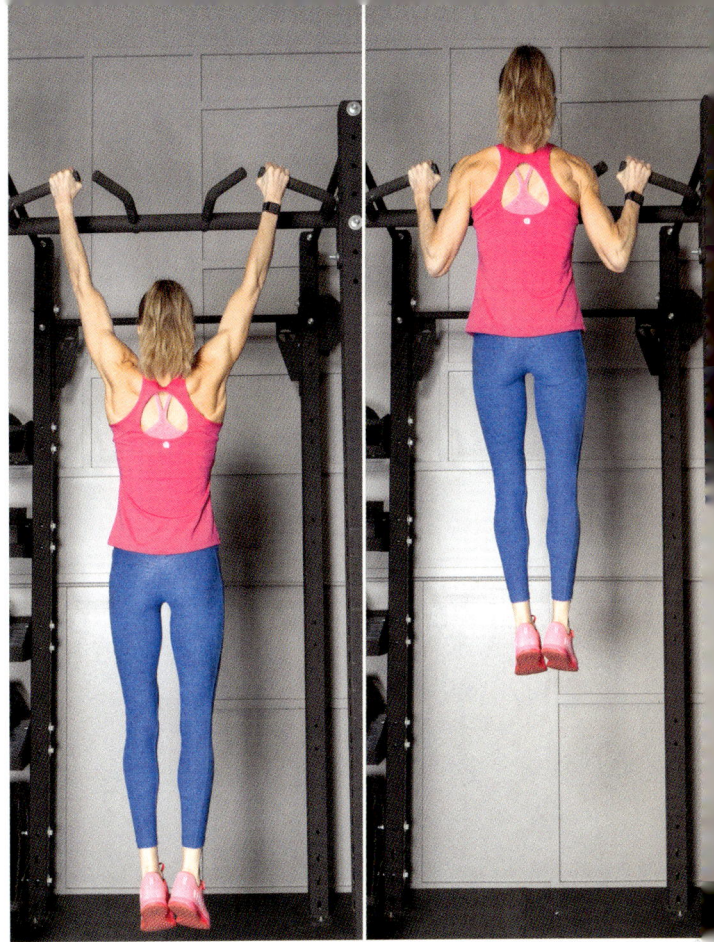

SINGLE-ARM ROW

Hold a dumbbell in one hand and place your opposite knee and hand on a bench or box as you stand with one leg planted on the ground. Maintain a flat back and press your chest out to feel the muscles of your back activate. You want your back to stay nice and flat as you row.

Drive your elbow up and back to row the dumbbell up to your side while keeping your back flat. Do not let your shoulder shrug. Focus on your shoulder blade moving toward your spine to power the row. Don't turn it into a biceps curl.

Extend your arm all the way back down. You can reach out slightly at the bottom if you can control the row without shrugging.

MODIFICATIONS: Start with a lighter weight and really engage your back before you even start the row.

EXERCISE SWAPS: Single-arm band row, single-arm cable row, chest-supported row, single-arm doorway row, single-arm half-kneeling mini band row, machine row, bent-over dumbbell row

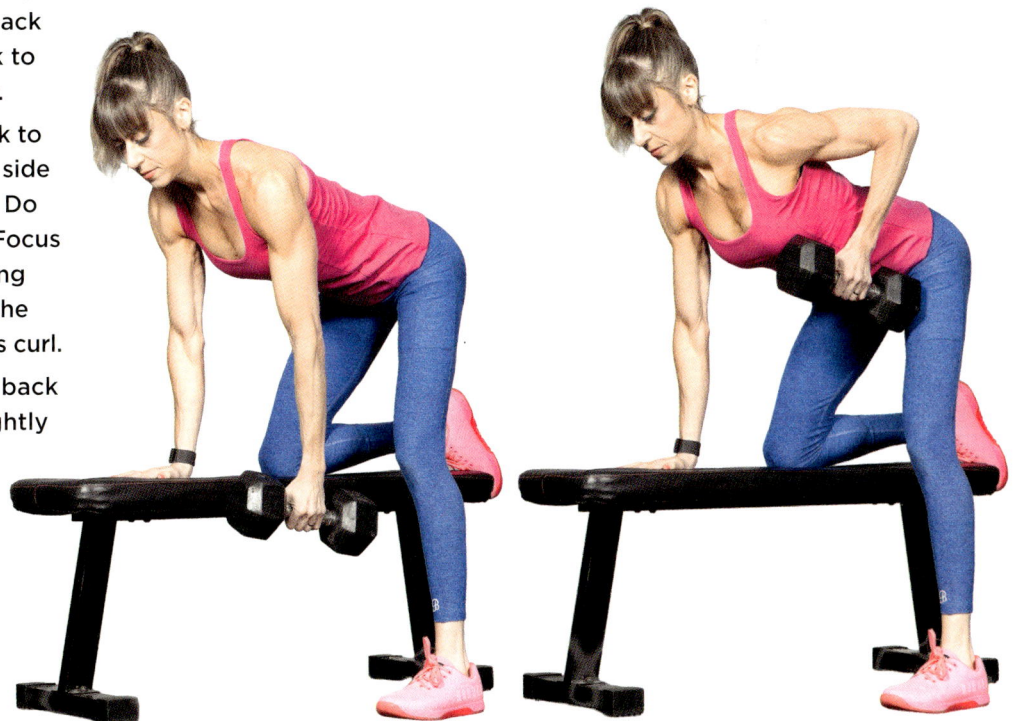

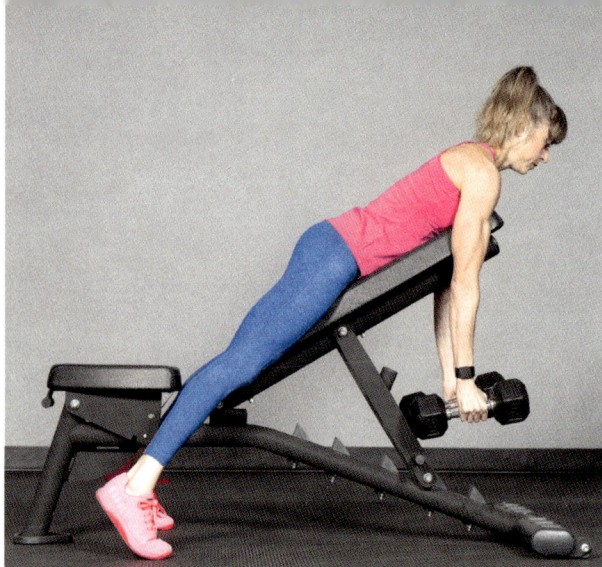

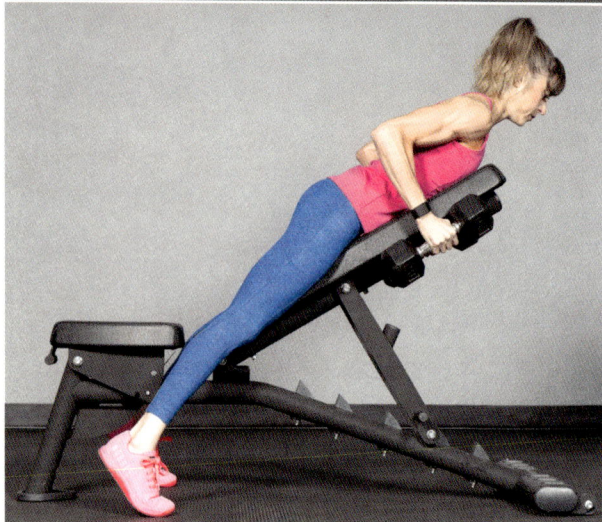

CHEST-SUPPORTED ROW

Set an incline bench to a 45-degree angle. Relax face down into the bench with a dumbbell in each hand and your head just above the top of the bench. Set up so you can firmly plant the balls of your feet but don't feel like your legs are straining to hold you.

Extend your arms toward the ground with a weight in each hand. Make sure you aren't shrugging. Your head should be in line with your spine. Engage your back and then row up by driving your elbows toward your hips and back.

Make sure you don't turn this into a shrug or biceps curl. Feel your shoulder blades draw together toward your spine. Relax your arms back down. Avoid using momentum or arching off the bench.

MODIFICATIONS: Start with lighter weights.

EXERCISE SWAPS: EZ bar chest-supported row, overhand/underhand chest-supported row, bent-over row, machine row, T-bar row, cable row, single-arm row, doorway row, scapular wall reps

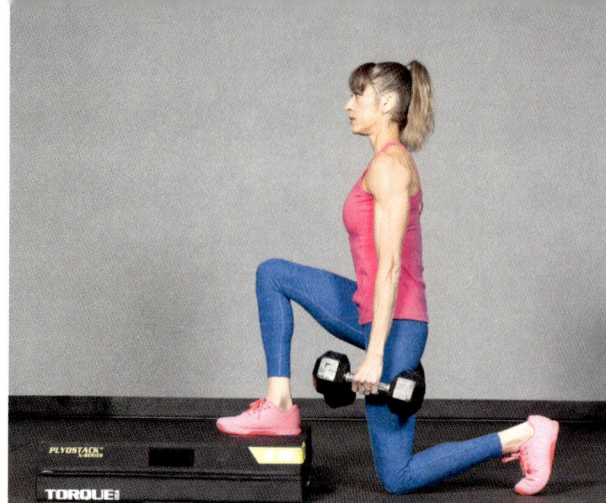

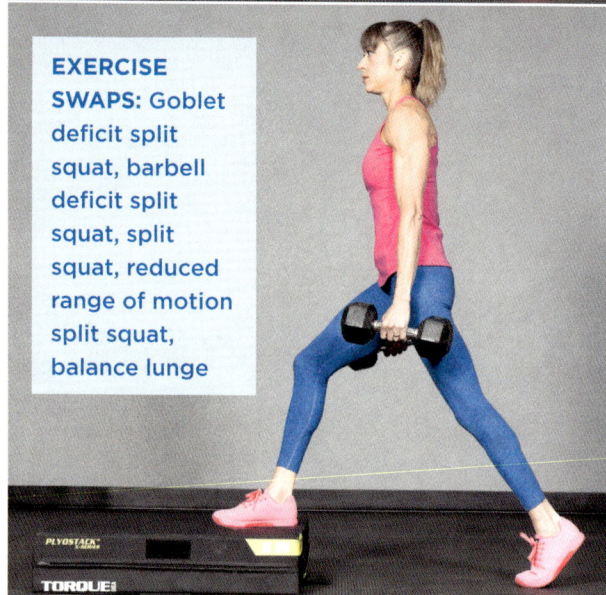

DEFICIT SPLIT SQUAT

EXERCISE SWAPS: Goblet deficit split squat, barbell deficit split squat, split squat, reduced range of motion split squat, balance lunge

Place your front foot on a box or plate weight and step your other foot back. Sink to the bottom of a lunge and place your knee on the ground to check the height of the box and placement of your legs. At the bottom, your front heel should be firmly pushing into the box while your back knee is about under your back hip. You can grab weights at the bottom or start holding them at the top if you're comfortable with your setup.

Drive through the ball of your back foot and your entire front foot to stand up. Drive straight up. Your front leg may be slightly bent at the top of the lunge, but your back leg will be fully extended. Lower into another lunge. Make sure to engage your lats as you hold the weights down by your side.

Touch the ground or hover just above it with each lunge. If you don't work through the increased range of motion this move creates, you aren't getting the full benefit of this move!

MODIFICATIONS: Start with no weights or do the basic split squat off the ground.

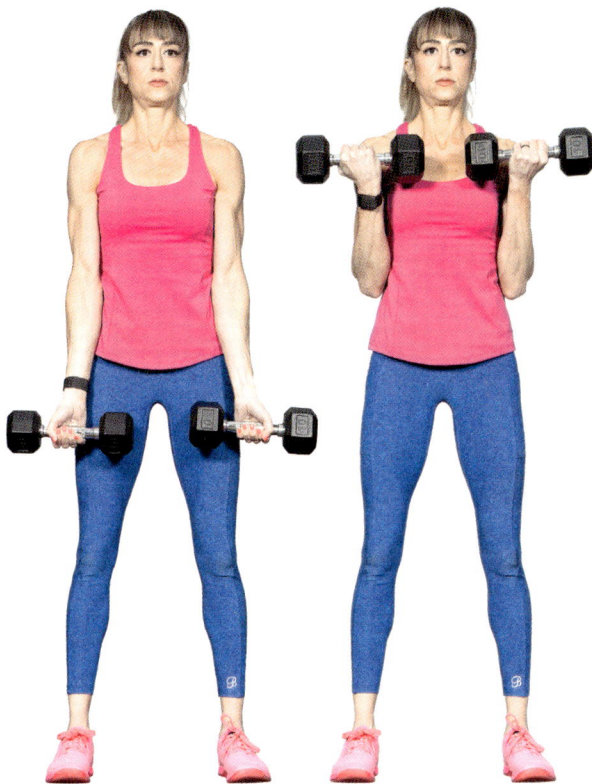

BICEPS CURL

Hold a dumbbell in each hand in front of your legs with your palms facing away from your body. Your arms and elbows should be tucked by your sides. Stand with your feet about hip-width apart or slightly staggered to help you avoid swinging.

Curl the weights up, keeping your elbows in by your sides. Do not swing or let your elbows come forward just so you can use a heavier weight. Bring the weights up to about your shoulders, feeling your biceps work, then lower the weights. Fully extend your elbows before repeating the curl.

MODIFICATIONS: Perform the move one side at a time and go light to start. You can also do hammer curls with your palms facing in if that feels better on your elbows.

EXERCISE SWAPS: Band biceps curl, cable biceps curl, supinated curl, barbell curl, preacher curl, hammer curl, suspension trainer biceps curl

SPLIT SQUAT

Setting up from the bottom of this move can be helpful: Get in a half-kneeling position to make sure your front knee is over your front ankle and your back knee is under your hip. Keep your chest up nice and tall while squeezing your back glute and drive up to standing, pushing through your front foot and the ball of your back foot. Hold dumbbells in each hand down by your sides with your lats engaged to progress this move.

Drop your back knee toward the ground. Do not lean forward as you drop your back knee. Pause at the bottom to do this from a dead stop, if you can.

MODIFICATIONS: Reduce the range of motion, starting with your back knee on a block rather than on the ground. You can use a wall or chair to help you balance.

EXERCISE SWAPS: Goblet split squat, reduced range of motion split squat, barbell split squat, balance lunge, deficit split squat, front lunge, Smith machine split squat, mini band split squat

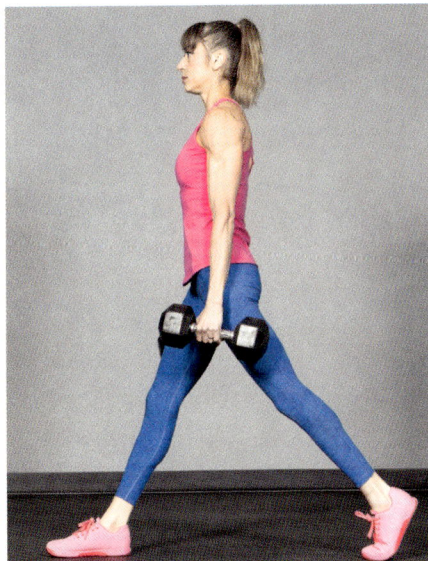

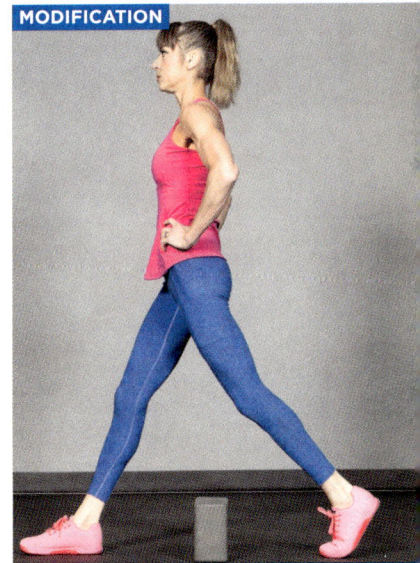

MODIFICATION

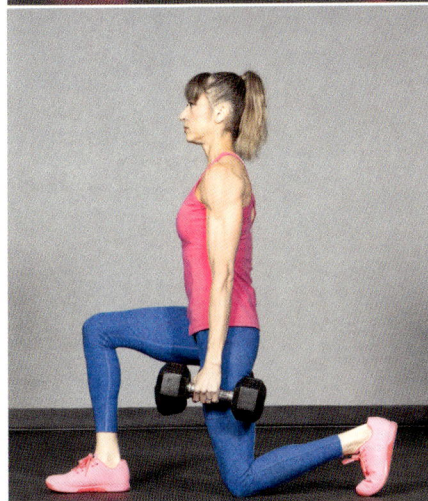

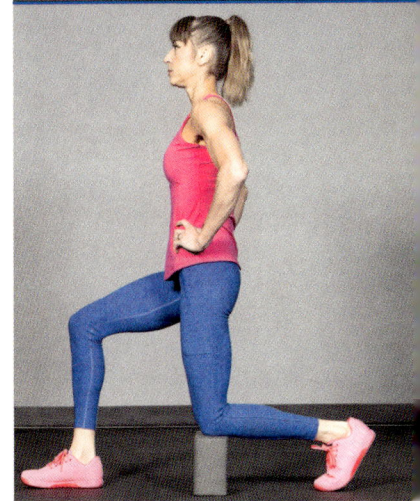

GOBLET SQUAT

Hold a dumbbell or kettlebell in both hands at chest height. Engage your back to pull the weight in and support it; then set your feet between hip-width and shoulder-width apart. Keeping the weight near your chest and your upper back engaged, brace your abs and sit your butt back and down in a squat.

Don't let your back round forward. You may hinge slightly forward as you sink, but focus on the knee bend as you squat. Don't turn this into a hip hinge. Sink to parallel (lighten the load if you can't) and then drive through your feet to push the ground away and come back to standing. Do not lean or rock forward as you stand up.

MODIFICATIONS: Do not hold weight to start. Squat to a bench or box to help you control the range of motion.

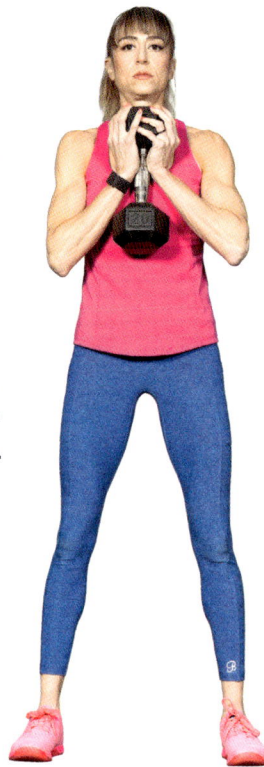

EXERCISE SWAPS: Front squat, Smith machine squat, leg press, single-leg squat, squat to box, heel-raised goblet squat

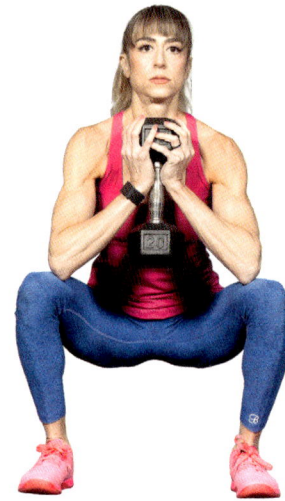

SQUAT PULSE

Stand with your feet between hip-width and shoulder-width apart. Reach your hands out in front of you. If you're holding a weight, hold it in the goblet position. Sit your butt back and sink into a squat. Keep your chest up and your core braced.

At the parallel position of the squat, pulse up and down. Drop a little below parallel and then come a few inches above.

Keep your chest up and your heels down as you pulse. Make sure you continue to sit your butt back as you pulse.

MODIFICATIONS: Perform the pulse squat as a shallower movement, staying up higher and not adding load. You can also hold on to a suspension trainer or chair.

EXERCISE SWAPS: Goblet squat pulse, mini band goblet squat pulse, mini band squat pulse, reduced range of motion squat pulse, kneeling lean back, split squat pulse, rock lunge, wall sit

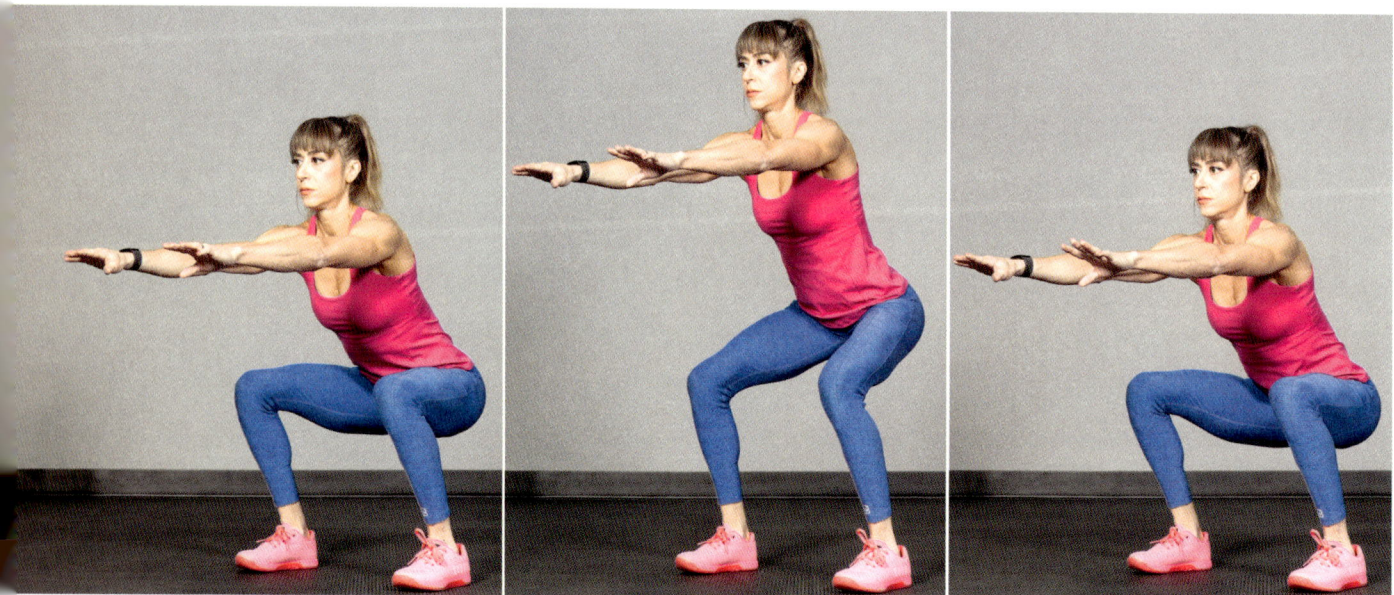

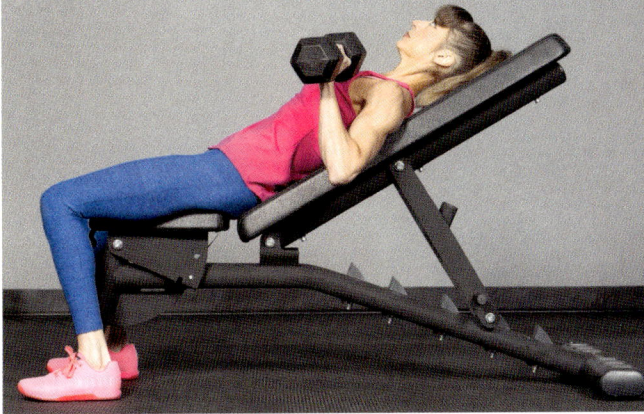

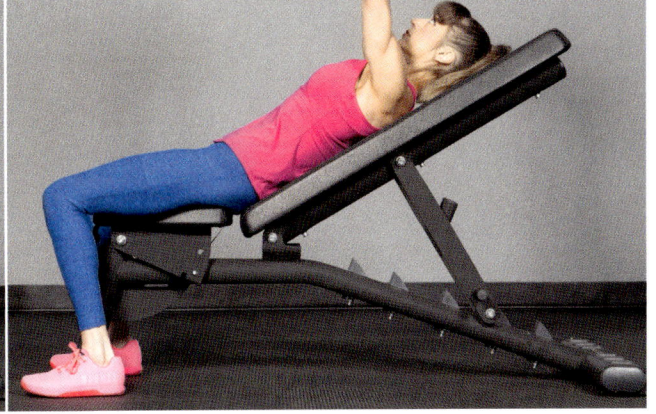

INCLINE BENCH PRESS

Set your incline bench at a 45-degree angle and lie back on the bench. Hold a dumbbell in each hand at your chest with your palms turned toward your feet. Engage the sides of your back to unshrug your shoulders as you set up.

Press the weights straight toward the ceiling, fully extending your arms without allowing your elbows to flare up by your shoulders. Lower the weights back to your chest and repeat.

At the bottom of the press, focus on your upper arms making an arrow shape with your body and feel your back supporting the press.

MODIFICATIONS: Start with lighter weights.

CHEST FLY

Lie on your back on a bench with a dumbbell in each hand at your chest. Extend your arms straight toward the ceiling with your palms facing each other and the weights together. With your elbows slightly bent, fly your arms open, lowering the backs of your hands toward the ground. Open your arms to just below shoulder height.

Feel your chest stretch open as your arms are about parallel to the ground; then focus on using your chest to pull your hands back up and together.

Do not shrug your shoulders as you lower the weights. You want your hands to be about in line with your chest the entire time, and your elbows should be soft. Don't turn this into a bench press. Only lower as far as you can control, and don't use such a heavy weight you can't perform a full range of motion.

MODIFICATIONS: Start light or try a standing cable or band chest fly.

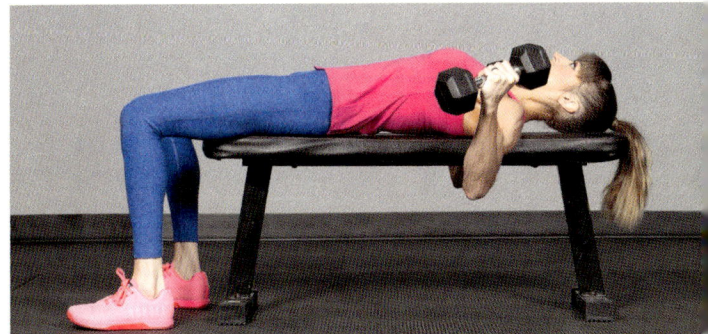

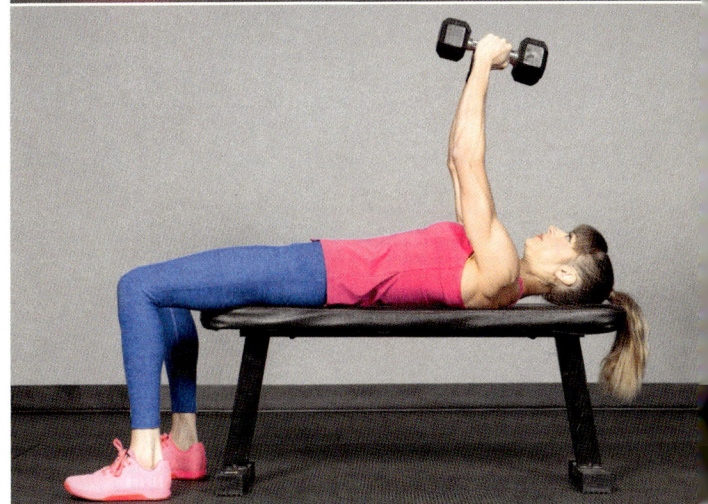

PUSH-UP

Set up in the high plank position with your hands under your shoulders and outside your chest. Don't shrug your shoulders. Place your feet together and set up so your body is in a nice straight line from your head to your heels. Drive back through your heels to engage your legs and brace your abs.

Lower your body as one unit. Your upper arms should make an arrow shape with your body. Be conscious not to rock out on your hands or tuck your chin. Keep pushing back through your heels to keep tension so your hips don't drop and your butt doesn't go up in the air.

Touch your chest to the ground or hover right over it and then push back up with a big exhale. Focus on your body moving as one unit.

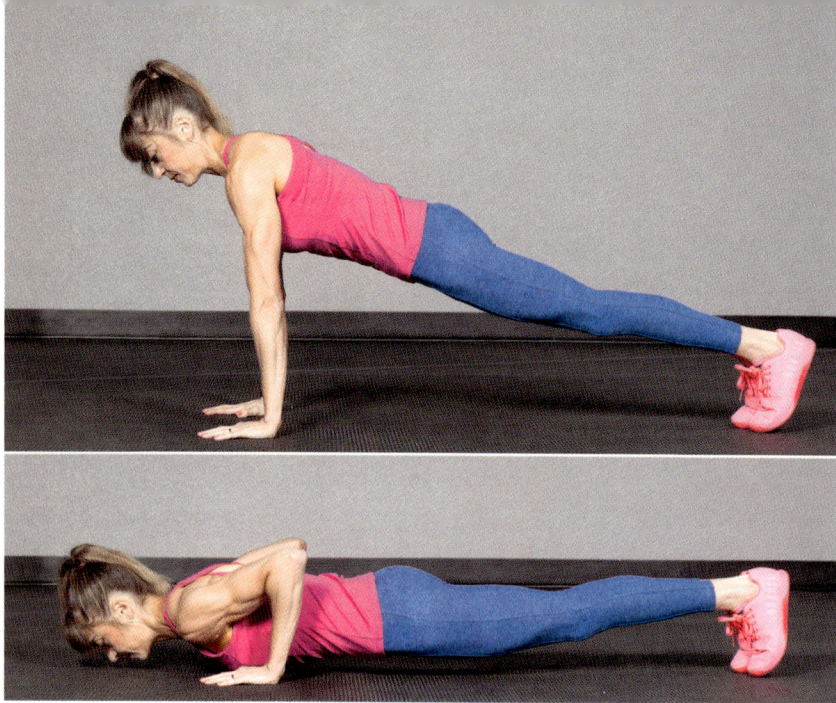

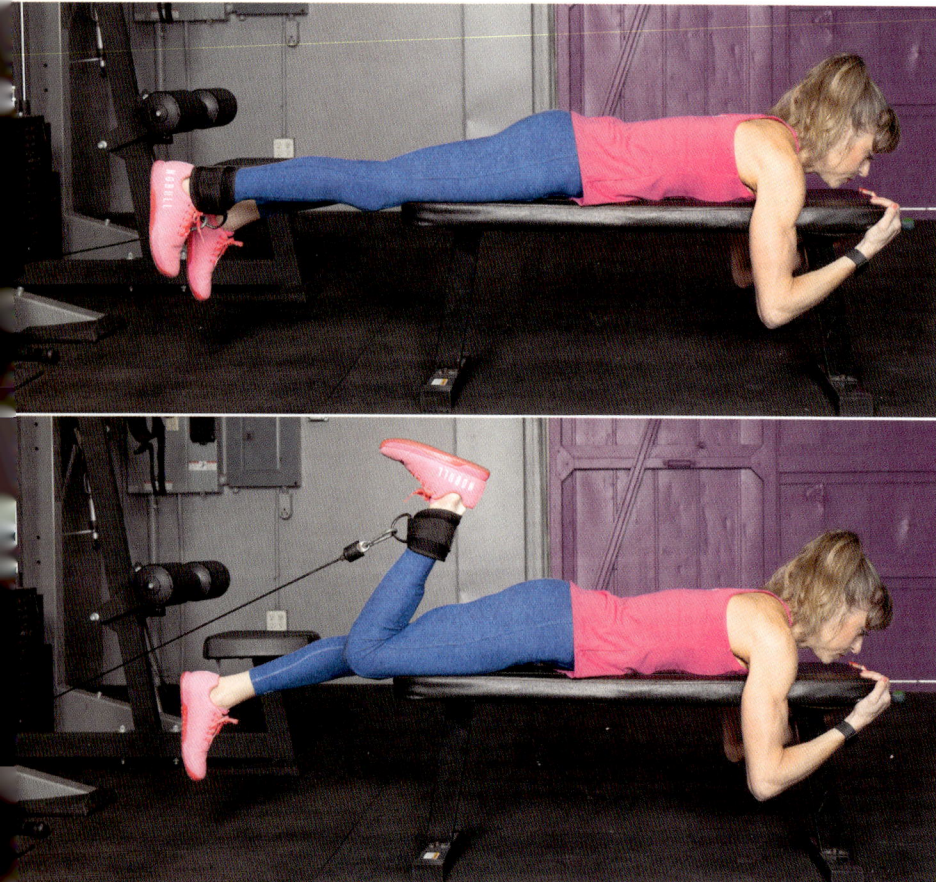

MODIFICATIONS: Place your hands on an incline like a wall, counter, or box, or you can perform knee push-ups.

EXERCISE SWAPS: Incline push-up, knee push-up, band push-up, bench press, machine chest press, Smith machine bench press, push-up plus, wide-grip push-up

CABLE LYING HAMSTRING CURL

Put a bench in front of a cable machine so you can lie along it with your feet toward the anchor point. Anchor the pulley down low and hook the ankle strap around one ankle. Lie face down along the bench so your knees are just off the edge and your legs are extended behind you. Flex the foot of your working leg and curl your heel toward your butt. Feel the back of your thigh work. Extend your leg and repeat. Try not to bounce or use momentum for the curl.

EXERCISE SWAPS: Machine lying hamstring curl, band lying hamstring curl, glute bridge and curl, Nordic hamstring curl, standing ankle weight hamstring curl

MODIFICATIONS: Use a band or start light.

GLUTE BRIDGE AND CURL

This move can be done with sliders, paper plates, towels, a suspension trainer, a rower, a yoga ball, or a power wheel.

Set up in a glute bridge with your knees bent and a slider under each heel (or your heels on one of the other tools). Bridge up, driving your heels down hard into the equipment. Squeeze your glutes and tuck your pelvis toward your ribs to engage your abs so your back doesn't arch.

With your hips up off the ground and your glutes engaged, slide your legs out straight. Do not arch your lower back. Your butt may even graze the ground with some tools.

Curl your heels back in, bringing your hips up again into a glute bridge. Really pull your heels in using your hamstrings. Squeeze your glutes hard, especially during the transition to curl back in, which may be when you want to arch.

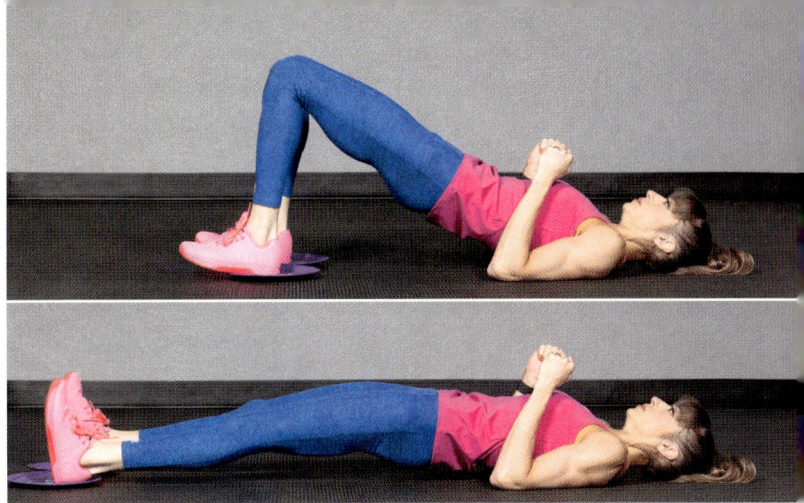

MODIFICATIONS: You can use a single-leg variation to both advance and modify the move. If you raise the nonworking leg, the move is even harder. Sliding one out at a time (alternating glute bridge and curl) will help reduce the strain on your hamstrings. You can also perform a straight-leg glute bridge.

EXERCISE SWAPS: Machine lying hamstring curl, straight-leg glute bridge, cable lying hamstring curl, ball glute bridge and curl, suspension trainer glute bridge and curl, single-leg glute bridge and curl, alternating glute bridge and curl

SIDE LUNGE

Stand tall with your feet together. If you're holding dumbbells, hold them down in front of your legs. Step one foot out to the side in a wide stance. Bend the knee of the leg you stepped out to the side with, keeping the other leg straight. Sit your butt back, hinging slightly at the hips to lean forward as you push your butt back and sink into the side lunge.

Keep your back flat and make sure to keep both heels down with both feet parallel and pointing straight ahead. Don't bend your other straight leg or pivot that foot open to turn the toe up toward the ceiling. Lower the weights toward your heel of your bent leg.

Drive up off the foot of your bent leg to come back to standing. Don't bend the other leg as you push back up center. Really drive off your heel and feel your glute working to push you back to center. Come back to standing and then repeat the lunge on that side.

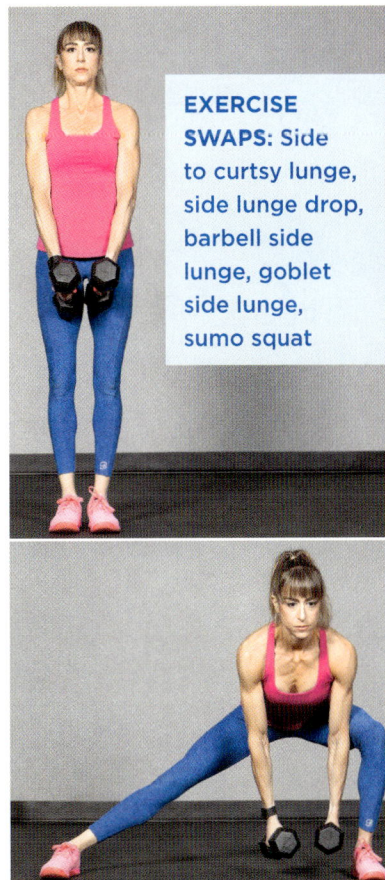

EXERCISE SWAPS: Side to curtsy lunge, side lunge drop, barbell side lunge, goblet side lunge, sumo squat

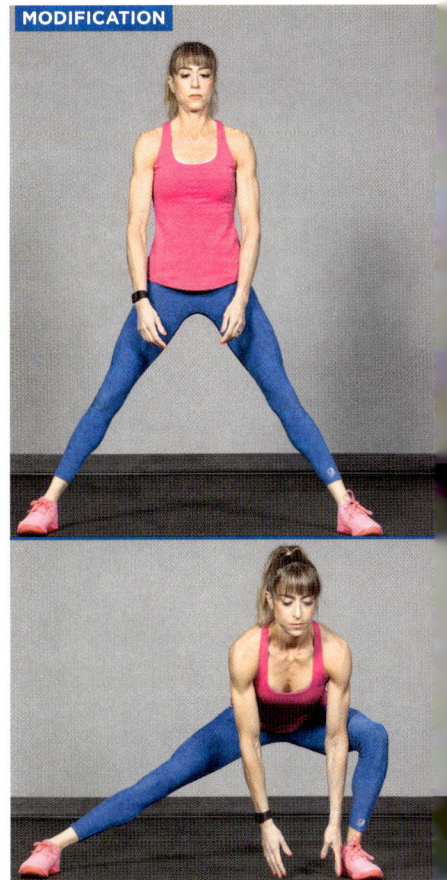

MODIFICATION

MODIFICATIONS: Do not step out as wide. You also can start wide and perform side lunge drops to each side without stepping back to center.

OVERHEAD TRICEPS EXTENSION

Cup one end of a dumbbell in both hands and extend your arms overhead so the weight is slightly behind you. Brace your abs and squeeze your butt to prevent your lower back from becoming overloaded. If you feel your lower back engaging during this movement, try holding a lighter dumbbell in each hand.

Bend your arms at your elbows to lower the weight behind your head. Keep your elbows pointing toward the ceiling and lower the dumbbell as far as you can before extending your elbows to press the weight back overhead. Do not tuck your chin as you lift and lower.

MODIFICATIONS: Perform a single-arm overhead extension if your mobility makes this uncomfortable. You can also use the cable overhead triceps extension.

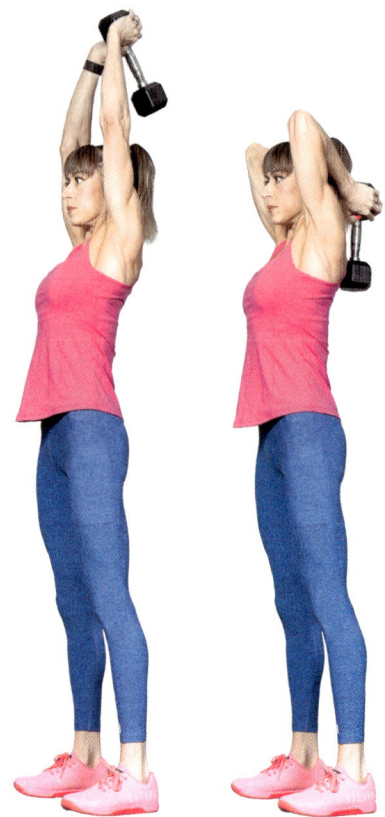

EXERCISE SWAPS: Band overhead triceps extension, cable overhead triceps extension, floor press to skull crusher, body saw, close-grip push-up

DECLINE PUSH-UP

Place your feet on a box or bench and set up in a high plank position with your hands under your shoulders and outside your chest. The higher the support for your feet, the harder this move will be. Engage your core and drive back through your heels to set your body in a nice straight line from your head to your heels.

Keeping your body in that nice straight line, drop your chest down to the ground between your hands. You may feel like your face comes close to the ground. Do not let your hips sag or your butt go up in the air as you lower. Then push the ground away so your body moves as one unit back to the top.

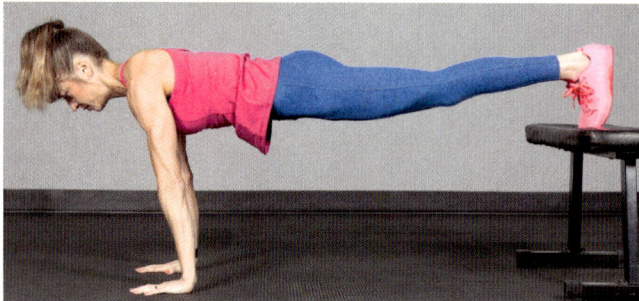

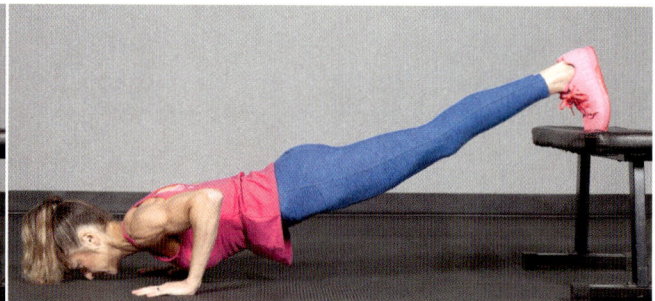

MODIFICATIONS: Place your knees on the bench. Perform an incline push-up or incline bench press if you aren't able to do a decline push-up with proper form.

EXERCISE SWAPS: Incline bench press, knee modified decline push-up, incline chest fly, dip

MODIFICATION

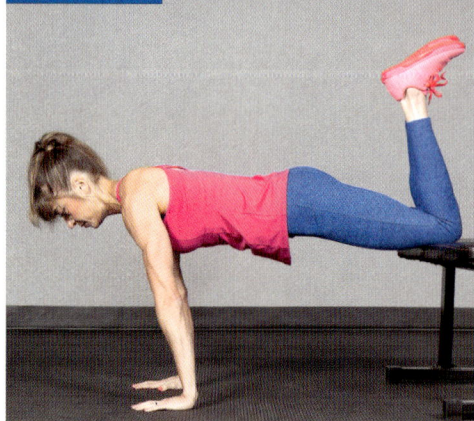

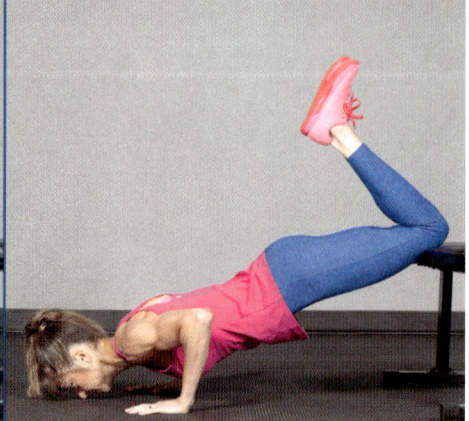

PULLOVER

Lie along the length of a bench with your feet pressed firmly into the ground. Cup one end of a dumbbell in both hands and bring the weight over your chest.

With a slight bend in your elbows, reach back over your head toward the ground behind you. Reach as far as you can and then pull the dumbbell over to bring it forward over your chest. Feel your lats and abs stretch as you control the reach over your head. Then feel your lats and abs work to pull the dumbbell back over your chest.

Do not turn this into a triceps exercise by bending and extending only at the elbows. While there will be a slight flexion in your elbows as you reach, you want to think about this movement coming from your shoulders. If you can't reach very far back, try using a lighter weight. You will also feel this movement around your rib cage and pecs as they work with the sides of your back.

MODIFICATIONS: Perform this with a lighter weight or do a lat pushdown.

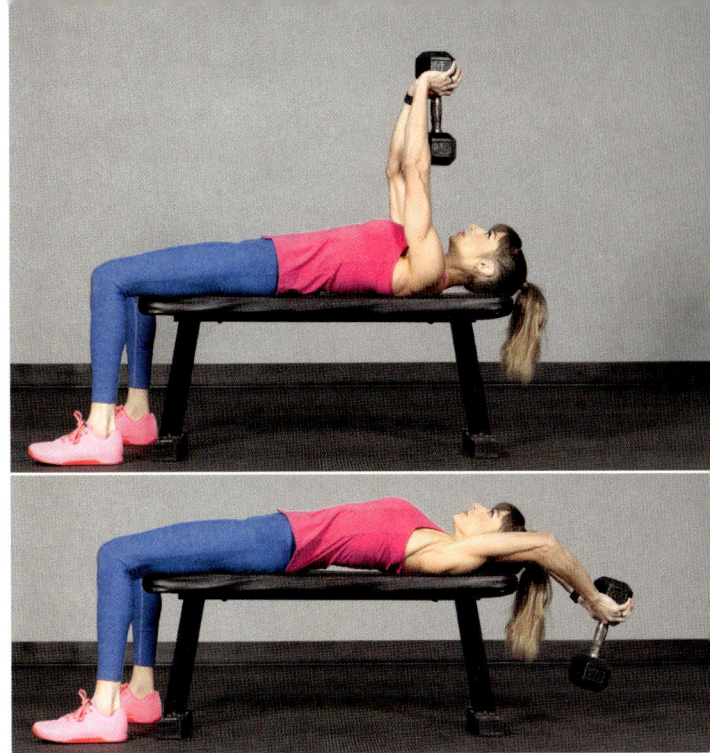

EXERCISE SWAPS: Bridged pullover, cable lat push-down, band lat push-down, slider ab extensions, pull-up, lying side slide

ROMANIAN DEADLIFT (RDL)

Stand behind a barbell with your feet about hip-width apart. Place your hands on the bar so they're right outside your shins. Since the range of motion for this movement is often limited, you can set up the bar in a rack or on a platform so you can start at the top of the move with the bar against your thighs. If you can't start with the bar in an elevated position, you can use a conventional deadlift to get it up and then start the Romanian deadlift at the top.

Push your butt back a little, allowing a slight anterior pelvic tilt or arch in your lower back to put your hamstrings under more stretch—just a little extra "butt stick out." Soften your knees as you hinge so you can really sit back, but don't actively bend them. Keep the bar against your thighs as you hinge more to lower the bar to just below your knees. If you can properly hinge and load your hamstrings, you may go lower—to mid-shin if you're sufficiently flexible. Think about this move as if you're trying to stretch your hamstrings by pushing your butt back rather than trying to take the bar all the way to the ground.

Drive through your heels to come back to standing. You may slow down slightly as you lower the bar to make sure you have full control over the stretch.

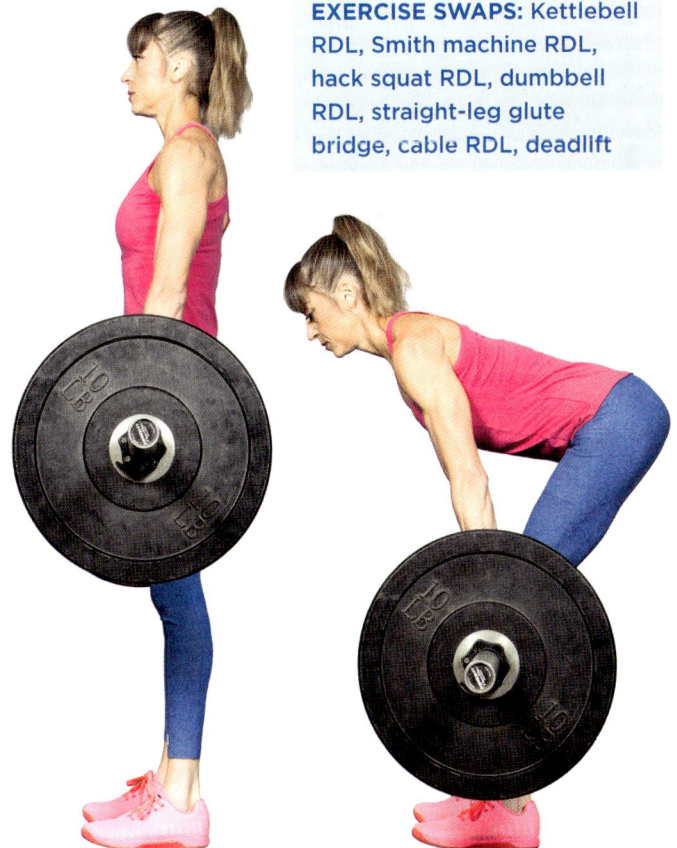

EXERCISE SWAPS: Kettlebell RDL, Smith machine RDL, hack squat RDL, dumbbell RDL, straight-leg glute bridge, cable RDL, deadlift

MODIFICATIONS: Use a kettlebell or dumbbells rather than the barbell.

CABLE LYING QUAD EXTENSION

Place a bench at the cable machine so you can lie on it lengthwise with the machine behind your head. You may find lying on a tall box helpful for allowing a full range of motion, but you need to be able to lie back on it. Put an ankle strap around your ankle and lie on the bench as shown in the photos. The end of the bench should hit right above the back of your knee to allow for an extra stretch back.

Engage your quad to straighten your knee and bring your foot up. Lower your leg and allow your heel to move behind you toward the cable machine. Try to get that extra flexion and stretch rather than stopping when your ankle is directly below your knee. Lying back should help you feel the rectus femoris (one of the muscles on the front of your thigh that extends your knee) or slightly higher up on the front of your thigh rather than just around your knee.

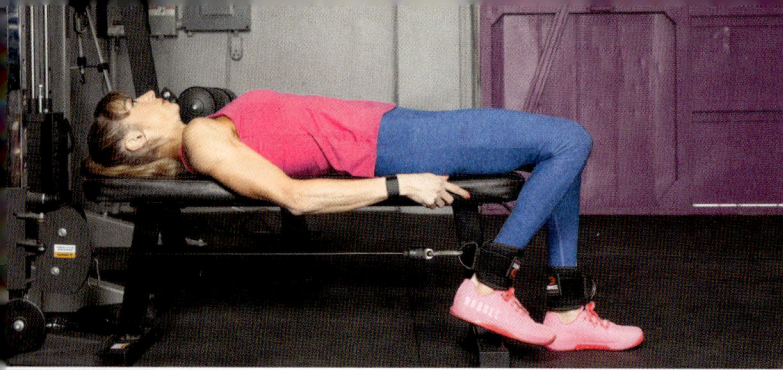

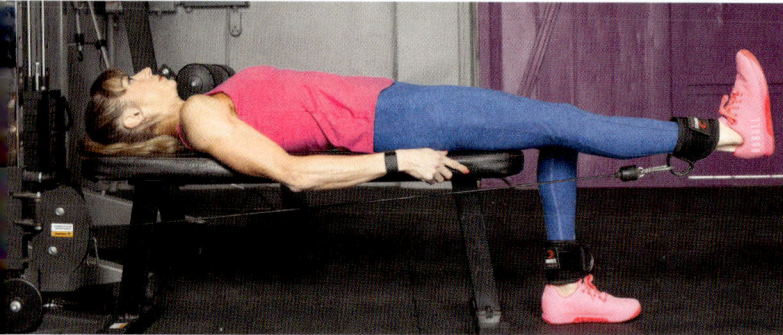

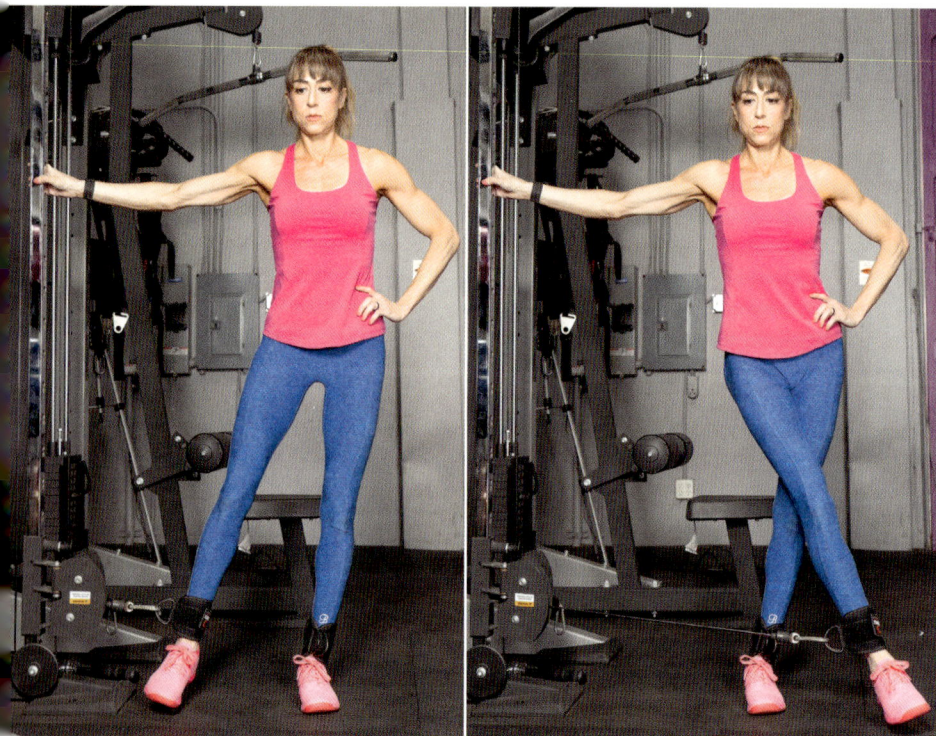

MODIFICATIONS: Start with a lighter weight or use a leg extension machine with the back reclined.

EXERCISE SWAPS: Machine leg extension, ankle weight lying quad extension, band lying quad extension, kneeling lean back, sissy squat

CABLE ADDUCTION

Anchor the cable pulley down low and put on an ankle strap. Stand so you can hold the machine (or a bench) to balance, but make sure you are far enough away so your inside leg can cross in front of you with the cable. Your leg closest to the machine will be the one working.

Pull your leg across your support leg, feeling your inner thigh working. Think about really squeezing your thighs together while pulling your foot past your support leg. Then control the movement as you move your working leg back toward the anchor point.

MODIFICATIONS: Start with a smaller range of motion to bring your working leg to where it just meets the support leg. If you don't have a cable machine, you can use ankle weights or a mini band to do adductions while lying on your side.

EXERCISE SWAPS: Adduction machine, side-lying adductor lift, kneeling adductor slide, band adduction, glute bridge with squeeze

KETTLEBELL SWING

Set the kettlebell on the ground and slightly in front of you so it's centered between your feet. Hinge at your hips, bending your knees slightly and pushing your butt back as you lean forward with your back flat. Place both hands on the kettlebell handle, tilting the bell back toward you. Hike the kettlebell back between your legs like you would a football to pull it back and up between your legs toward your butt.

Drive your hips forward and stand up tall. Think about driving the ground away with your feet as you stand up tall and squeeze your glutes. Pop your hips forward to propel the kettlebell off your hips. Don't worry about how high the bell goes. It shouldn't go higher than your shoulders. Squeeze your glutes as you stand tall.

EXERCISE SWAPS: Single-arm kettlebell swing, skier swing, dumbbell swing, double kettlebell swing, band hip hinge, cable pull-through, glute bridge off box

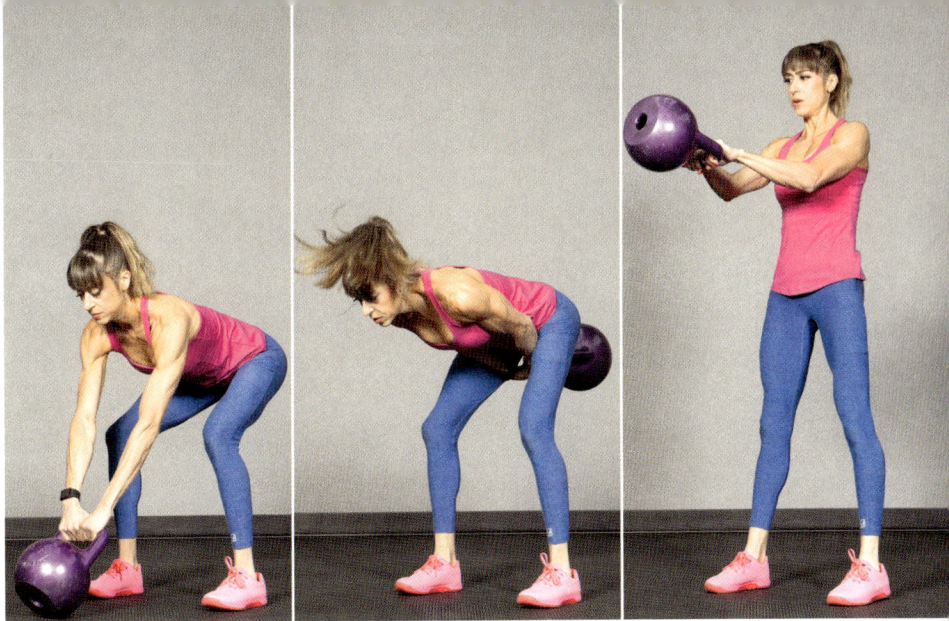

Keep your glutes tight and wait as the kettlebell comes back down so your forearms meet your pelvis; then hinge over again. As your forearms connect and you hinge, sit your butt back. Let the kettlebell pass through your legs toward the wall behind you.

Then squeeze your glutes again and swing the kettlebell back up as you return to standing.

MODIFICATIONS: This is an explosive and technical move, so start light or modify if you feel your lower back; you can use the cable pull-through or band hip hinge.

MED BALL SLAM

Stand with the ball between your feet by your heels. Sit your butt back and hinge over as you bend your knees to grab the ball in both hands. This is very much a conventional deadlift position. Pick up the ball and bring it overhead, almost like you're performing a standing pullover.

Quickly bring your hands down as you slam the ball into the ground between your feet while you sit your butt back so your legs can generate more force. Hinging as you slam the ball allows you to use your glutes and lats better; it also prepares you to pick up the ball safely. Pick up the ball and repeat the movement, exhaling as you slam. Start light and think of being explosive and quick rather than going heavier and slower.

Make sure you throw the ball back between your feet because having to reach out for the ball can cause you to overuse your lower back.

MODIFICATIONS: Start light and move at a controlled pace. If you don't have a med ball, you can do a lat pushdown or pullover.

EXERCISE SWAPS: Pullover, lat pushdown, med ball overhead throw

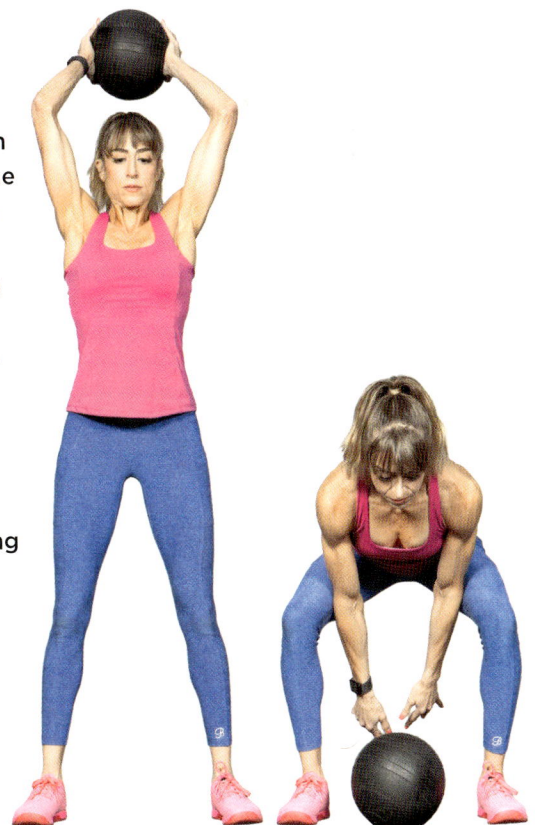

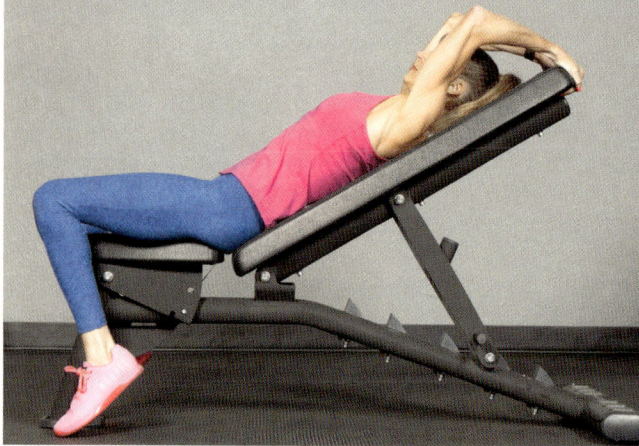

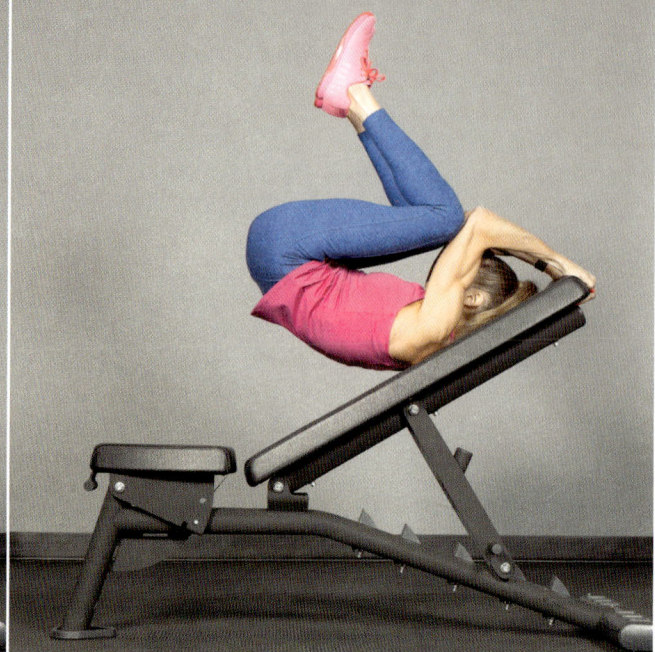

INCLINE REVERSE CRUNCH

Set an incline bench on the second position up from flat (about a 45-degree angle) and sit on the bench. Reach overhead to grab the top of the bench. Bend your knees so your toes or balls of your feet are lightly touching the ground. Pull down hard on the bench as you curl your knees toward your elbows, focusing on your abs working to roll one vertebrae up at a time. Then slowly lower your legs and tap your feet to the ground before repeating. Use your abs to control the movement down so you your legs don't flop.

MODIFICATIONS: Perform just a lower body crunch, on the ground or lying on a flat bench while holding on to the edge near your head.

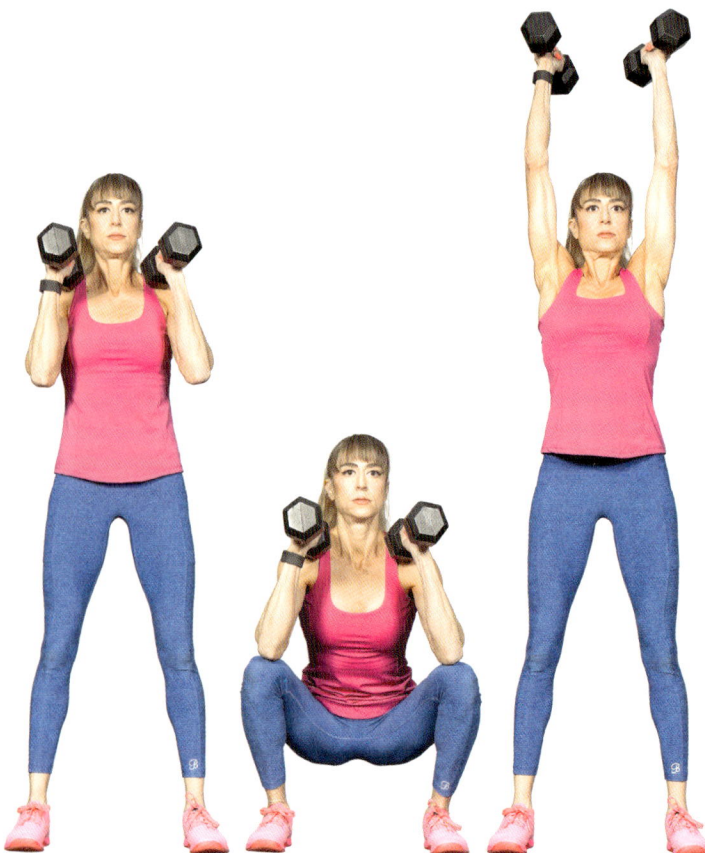

SQUAT TO PRESS

Hold a dumbbell in each hand and bring the weights up to your shoulders with your palms facing each other. With the weights at your shoulders, squat, sinking as low as you can while keeping your heels down and chest up. If you can't sink to parallel, lower the weights or squat to a bench to start.

Then drive back up to standing while pressing the weights straight overhead. Make sure you don't lean forward as you squat or stand up. The more you use your legs to press, the easier it should be on your upper body. If you want to do a stricter press, do it as separate movements: squat, stand up, and then press after you're fully standing.

MODIFICATIONS: Hold a single weight or kettlebell at your chest to start. If you don't have weights, a burpee is always a killer full-body swap.

EXERCISE SWAPS: Burpee, barbell squat to press, kettlebell squat to press

SUMO SQUAT

Stand with your feet wider than shoulder-width apart (adjusting your stance according to your mobility). Turn your toes out to about a 45-degree angle. Make sure that your ankles, knees, and hips are in alignment as you sink into the squat. You do not want your knees caving in or bowing way open. Hold a dumbbell or kettlebell at your chest (as you would for a goblet squat), pulling it in tight to your body as you engage your upper back.

Squat, sitting your butt down and back as you keep your chest up. Feel your glutes almost pulling your knees open to keep your hips, knees, and ankles all in line. Sink to about parallel or slightly lower and then drive back up to standing. Do not let your heels come up or your toes turn forward.

EXERCISE SWAPS: Cossack squat, deficit sumo squat, barbell sumo squat, sumo squat to box

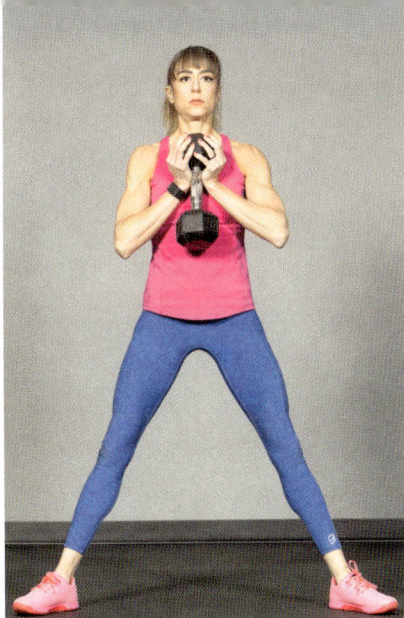

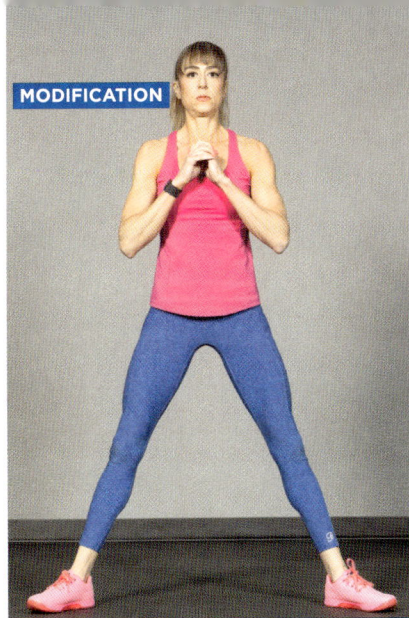

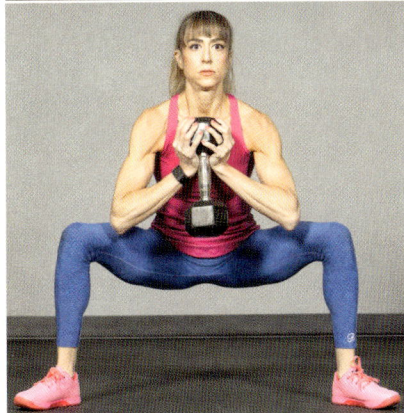

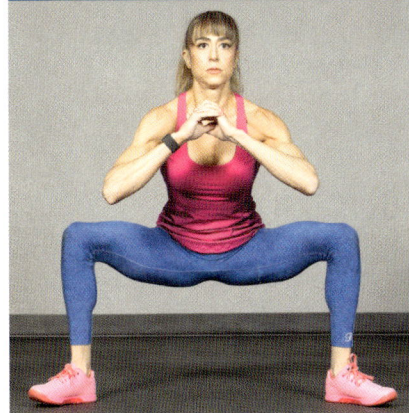

MODIFICATION

MODIFICATIONS: Sit down to a box or do not add weight to start. If this position is hard on your hips, move to a normal squat stance or swap in a side lunge.

BAND PUSH-UP

Pull a band across your back and hold an end in each hand. Set up in the high plank position with your hands outside your chest and your feet together. Press your hands down into the ground as you drive back through your heels, flexing your quads and bracing your abs.

Slowly lower with your body moving as one unit until you're a few inches off the ground, then press back up against the band. Make sure your body moves as one unit; do not let your hips sag. Also, avoid rocking out or bowing your elbows because this is what leads to wrist and elbow issues. Make sure your back is engaged to help power this resisted press!

MODIFICATIONS: Do not use the band until you can perform push-ups from your toes. Modify the push-up off an incline.

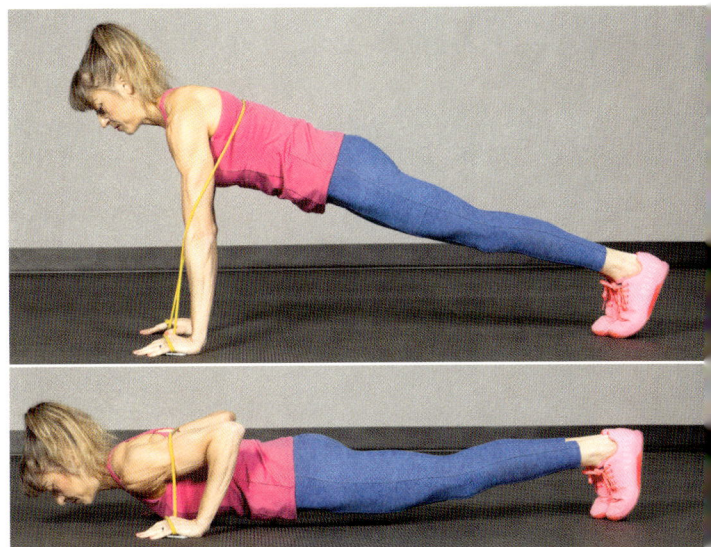

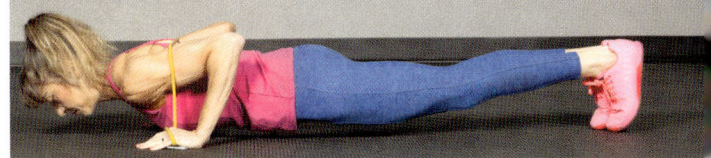

EXERCISE SWAPS: Bench press, machine chest press, cable chest press, push-up, incline push-up, Smith machine bench press, band press

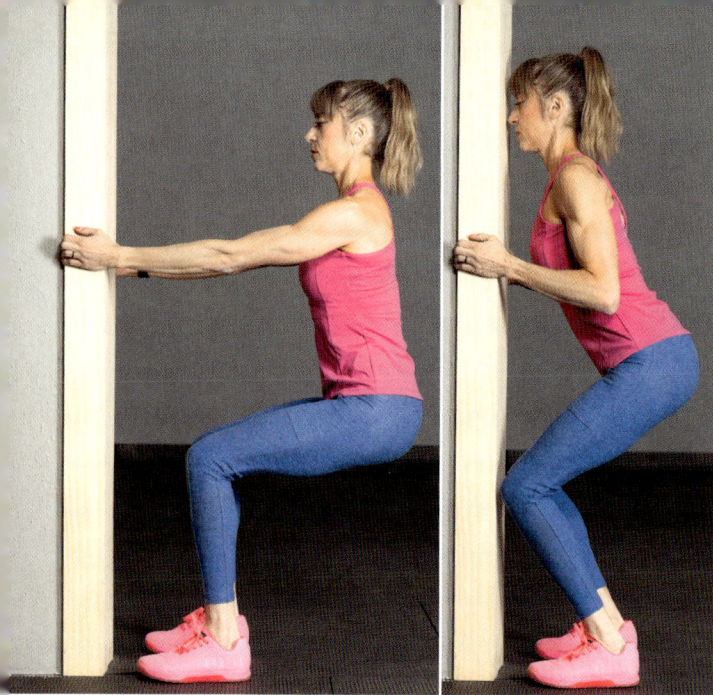

DOORWAY ROW

Hold onto a doorway or stair rail with both hands as you sink into a little squat; your hands will be at chest height or just below. Make sure to engage your lats to avoid shrugging and adjust your feet so they're about 6 inches or so from the doorway while you squat. Lean back to extend your arms to take on your weight. You can adjust the resistance by moving closer to or farther away from the door frame.

Drive your elbows down and back to pull your body toward the doorway. Do not stand up out of the squat or use your legs. Feel your back working to pull you forward. Focus on your shoulder blades moving toward your spine as you drive your elbows down and back. Do not shrug and keep your chest up nice and tall. Think wide shoulders as you row. Row in and then fully extend your arms to return to the starting position.

MODIFICATIONS: Scapular wall reps or not sinking as low in the squat are a great way to modify this movement.

EXERCISE SWAPS: Inverted row, single-arm doorway row, bent-over dumbbell rows, band row, scapular wall reps, lying scapular press, chest-supported row, mini band row

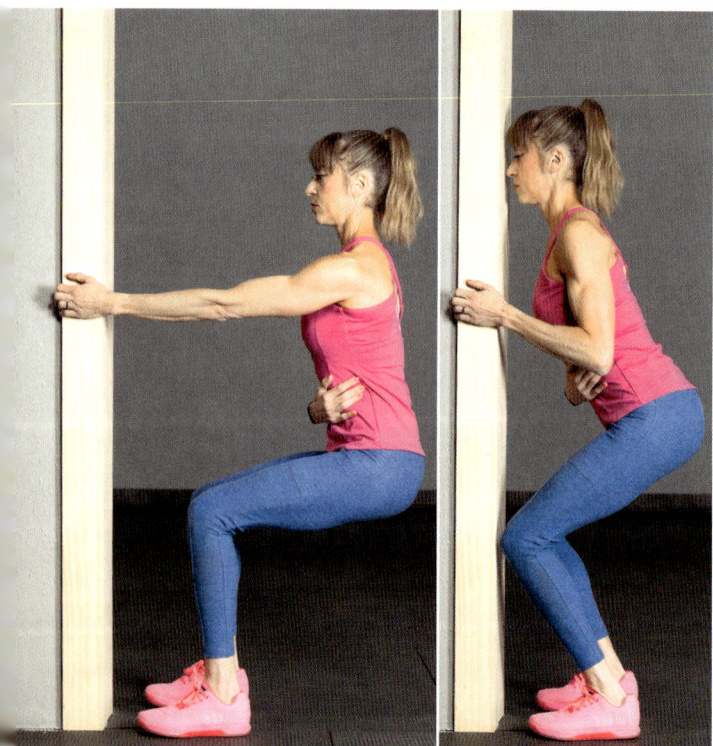

SINGLE-ARM DOORWAY ROW

Hold onto a doorway or hand rail with one hand as you sink into a little squat; your hand will be at chest height or just below. Make sure to engage your lats to avoid shrugging and adjust your feet so they're about 6 inches or so from the doorway while you squat. You can cross your free hand over your chest, but make sure you row as if you're pulling with both sides. Don't rotate or twist. Lean back to extend your arm to take on your weight. You can adjust the resistance by moving closer to or farther away from the doorframe.

Drive your elbow down and back to pull your body toward the doorway. Do not stand up out of the squat or use your legs. Feel your back working to pull you forward. Focus on your shoulder blade moving toward your spine as you drive your elbow down and back. Do not shrug and keep your chest up nice and tall. Think wide shoulders as you row. Row in and then fully extend your arm to return to the starting position.

MODIFICATIONS: Start with the two-arm doorway row or scapular wall reps.

EXERCISE SWAPS: Doorway row, scapular wall reps, lying scapular press, half-kneeling single-arm mini band row, single-arm row, single-arm band row, anti-rotational single-arm suspension trainer row

LYING SCAPULAR PRESS

Lie on your back with your knees bent and your feet flat on the ground. Bend your elbows to 90 degrees and place your arms down by your sides. Engage your abs and drive your elbows down into the ground to lift your back up, pressing your chest out. Keep your head in line with your spine as you lift, but you can just slightly tuck your chin to look forward if it helps your neck.

Focus on pressing your chest out as you pull your shoulder blades toward your spine to engage your back and shoulders. Really drive through your elbows to push up and pause; then lower back down to your back and repeat. Do not turn this into a sit-up, though. Drive off your elbows and feel your back working to press up and out!

MODIFICATIONS: Start with scapular wall reps or perform a hold based on the workout. You can also swap in a scapular push-up.

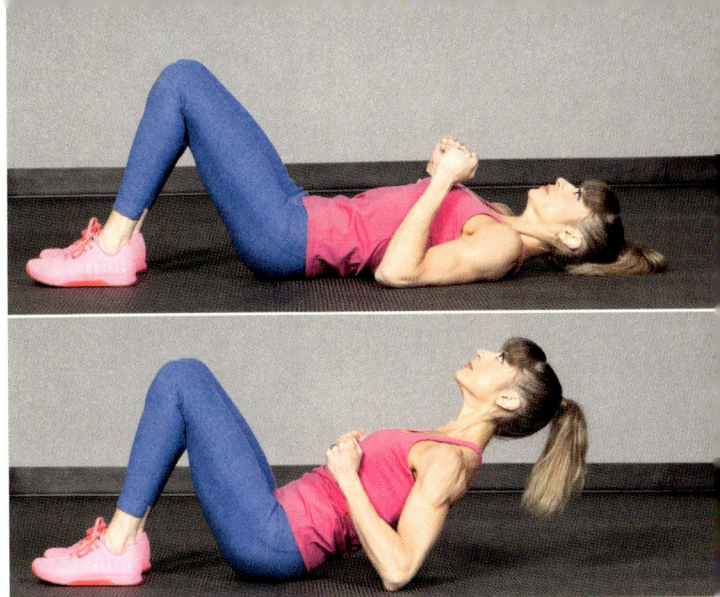

EXERCISE SWAPS: Scapular wall reps, lying scapular hold, scapular wall hold, scapular push-up, scapular wing, back shrug, bent-over row, band row, inverted row

GET-UP LUNGE

With your feet together, sit your butt back and sink into a little squat with a slight hip hinge, leaning your torso forward just enough to help you sink and sit back. You will not stand up out of this squat while performing the get-up lunges.

Keep your chest up and your back flat as you lower one knee down to the ground so that you're half-kneeling. Bring the other leg down until you're fully kneeling. Keep your chest up and your back flat, but maintain some slight hip flexion in this kneeling position without sitting back on your heels.

Return to standing one leg at a time, stepping forward with the first leg that moved to kneeling; then bring the other foot forward to just touch its toe down before reversing back into half-kneeling.

MODIFICATIONS: Kneel to a block or box or don't stay as low in the squat. You can also do the 2-way reach skater lunges or a basic squat.

EXERCISE SWAPS: Front lunge, split squat, 2-way reach skater lunge, goblet get-up lunge, barbell get-up lunge, single-leg squat

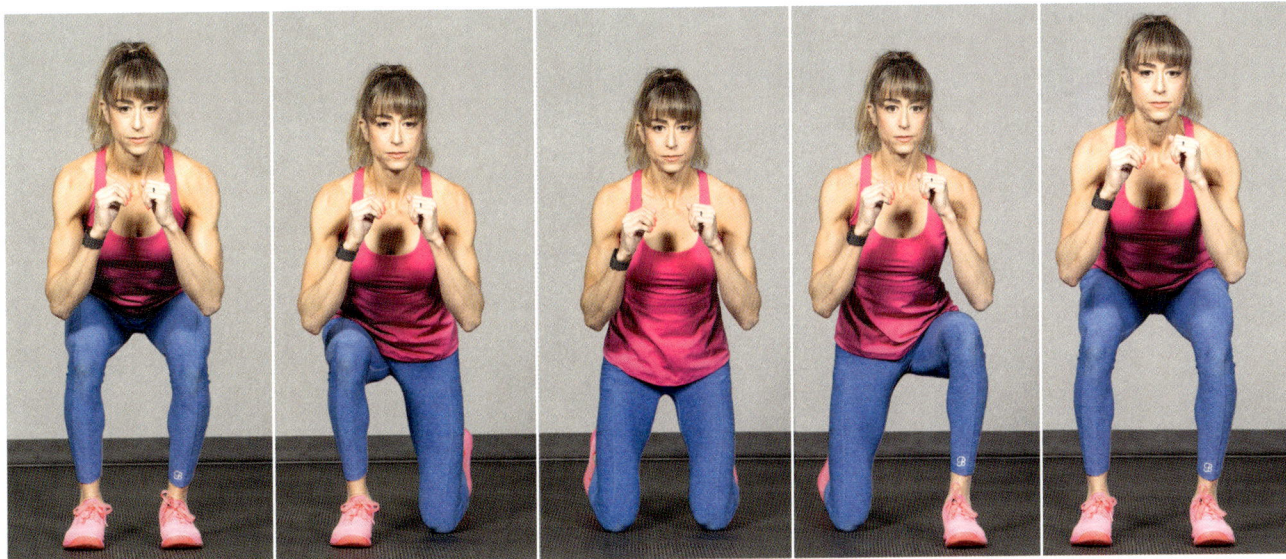

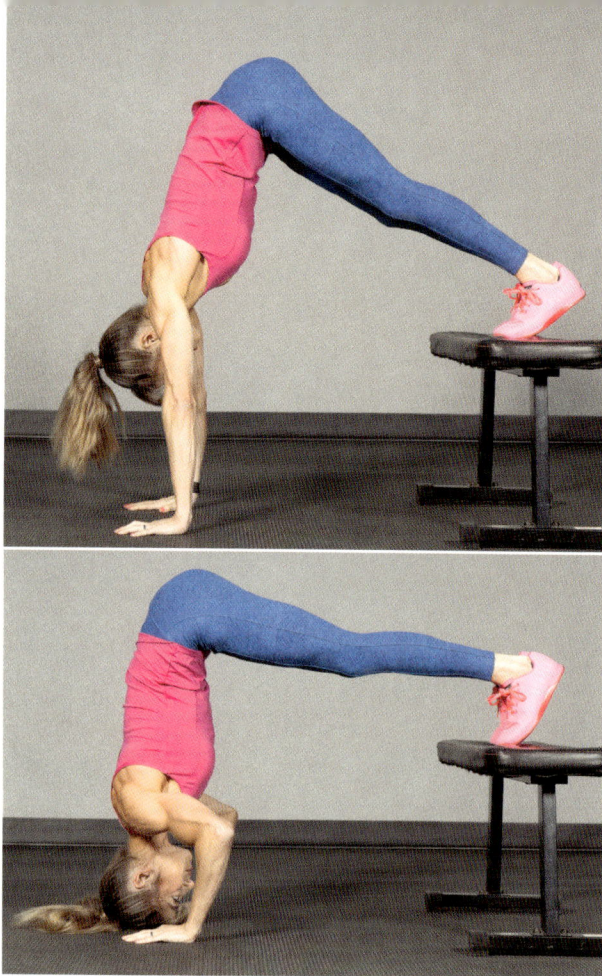

BENCH DIP

Sit on the edge of a bench, box, or chair with your hands just to the sides of your butt and turned so your fingertips hang over the edge of the support. Press through your hands to lift yourself off the bench as you walk your feet out so your butt is hovering just in front of the bench. Your legs should be straight out in front of you as you press your hands down hard into the bench to lift. Press your chest out and avoid shrugging your shoulders.

Then bend your elbows to lower your butt toward the ground. Lower as close as you can, bending your elbows to about 90 degrees. Then feel your triceps work to extend your elbows and press back up. Feel the backs of your arms and shoulders. Fully extend your arms and then repeat the dip.

This move is intensive on the shoulders, so be cautious if you've had shoulder issues in the past.

MODIFICATIONS: Bend your knees to modify the move.

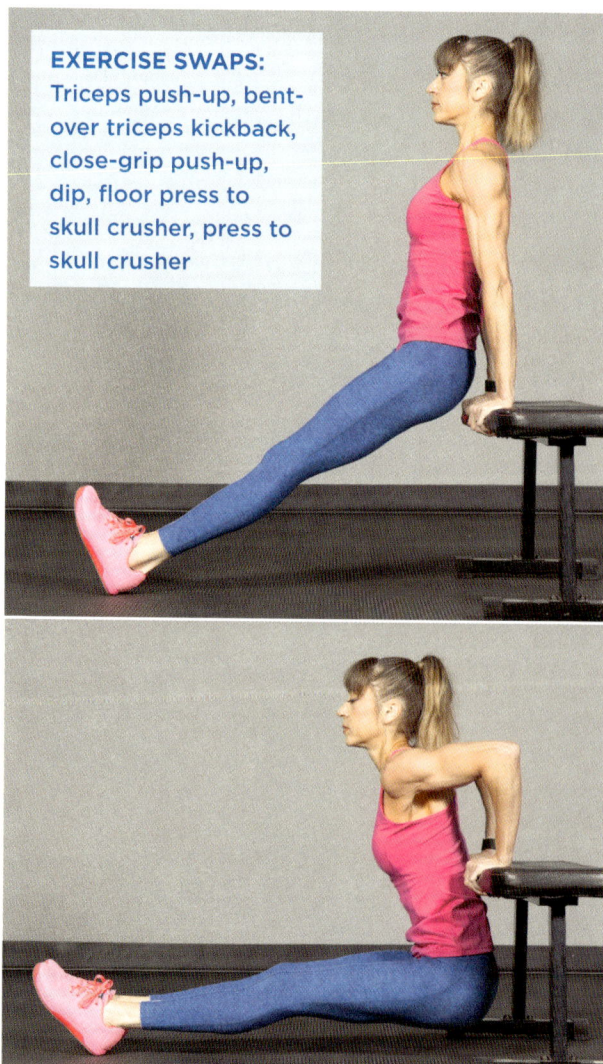

EXERCISE SWAPS: Triceps push-up, bent-over triceps kickback, close-grip push-up, dip, floor press to skull crusher, press to skull crusher

PIKE PUSH-UP

Place your feet on a bench, couch, or stair with your hands in a plank position. The higher the support, the more challenging this move will be. Walk your hands back so your butt is up in the air and your chest is facing toward the wall behind you with your arms extended. Create as straight a line as possible from your hands up to your butt.

Bend your elbows to lower your head toward the ground at about your fingertips; you will need to shift forward just slightly to bring your head to your fingertips. Lower your head to hover over or just lightly touch the ground before pressing back up. Really focus on pushing the ground away with your entire hand.

Think "vertical press" and push your butt up toward the ceiling. Do not turn this into a decline push-up.

MODIFICATIONS: Try the downward dog pike push-up or place your hands up on an incline instead of your feet to perform the move.

EXERCISE SWAPS: Downward dog pike push-up, barbell overhead press, dumbbell overhead press, landmine press, band overhead press

PLANK CLIMBER

Set up in the high plank position. Set your feet about hip-width apart or slightly wider to help you prevent rotation of your core as you climb up and down; drive back through your heels to create tension through your legs to help maintain that plank position. Make sure you aren't shrugging your shoulders as you brace your abs and squeeze your butt.

Bend one arm to place your forearm on the ground with your elbow under your shoulder. Bend the other arm to lower down into a full forearm plank. Make sure you aren't shrugging as you lower. Try to keep your hips as still as possible and do not let them sag toward the ground.

Place one hand down on the ground under your shoulder to start to push-up before placing the other hand on the ground to lift all the way. Alternate which side you lead with each rep or do a certain number of reps on one side and then switch, but make sure you lead with both sides at some point.

MODIFICATIONS: Use a bench as an incline or do this from your knees.

EXERCISE SWAPS: Bench plank climber, floor press to skull crusher, press to skull crusher, front to side raise, chest to overhead press, triceps push-up, close-grip push-up, shoulder tap push-up

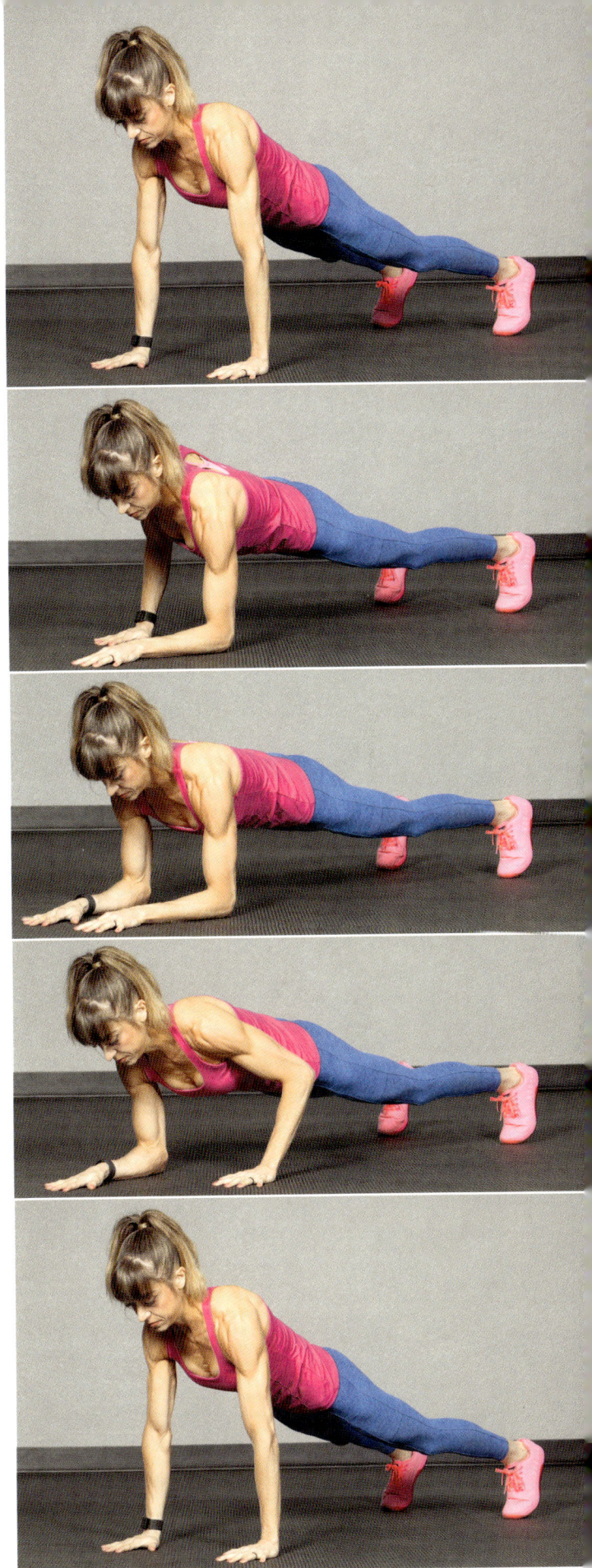

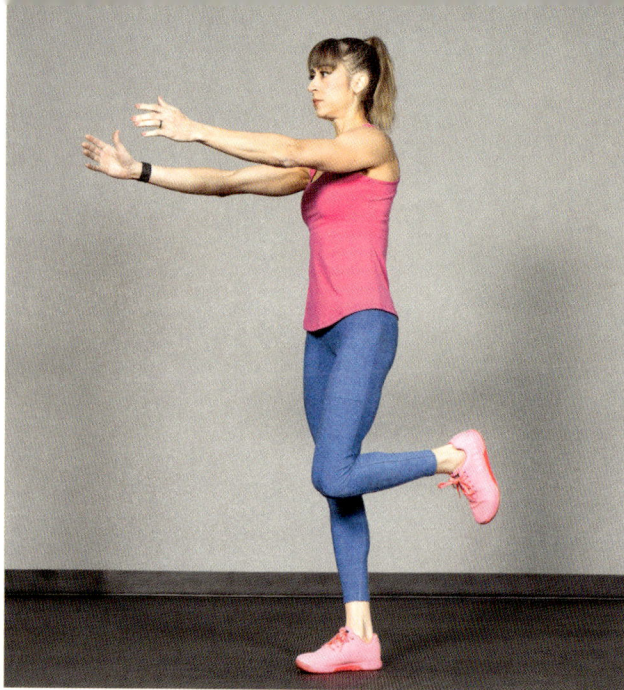

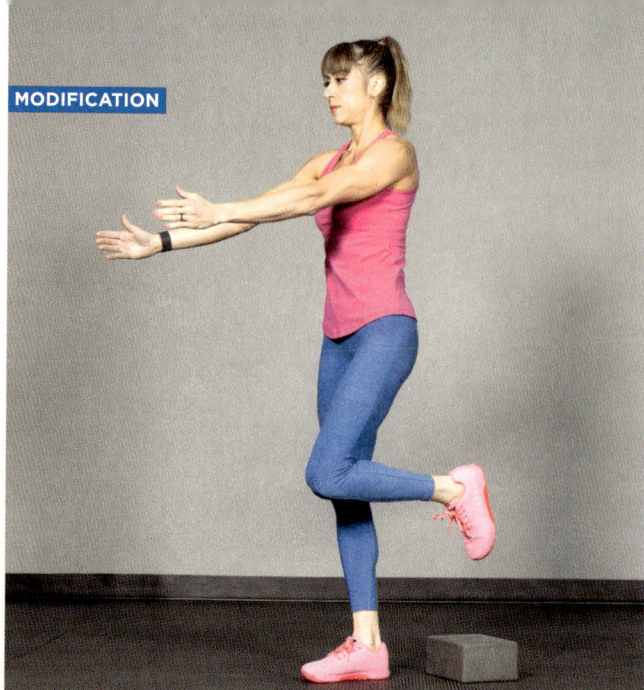

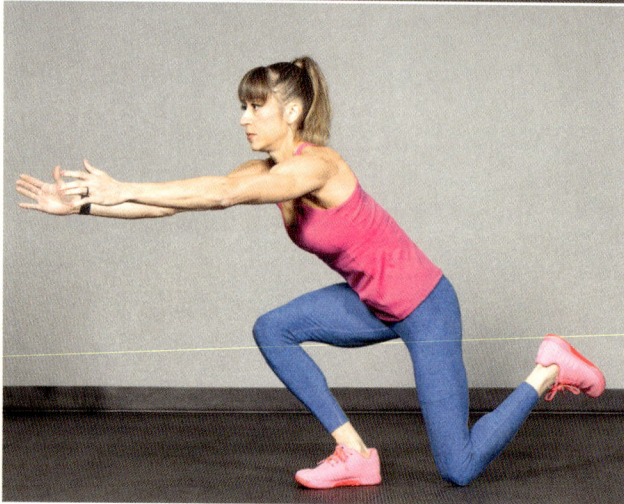

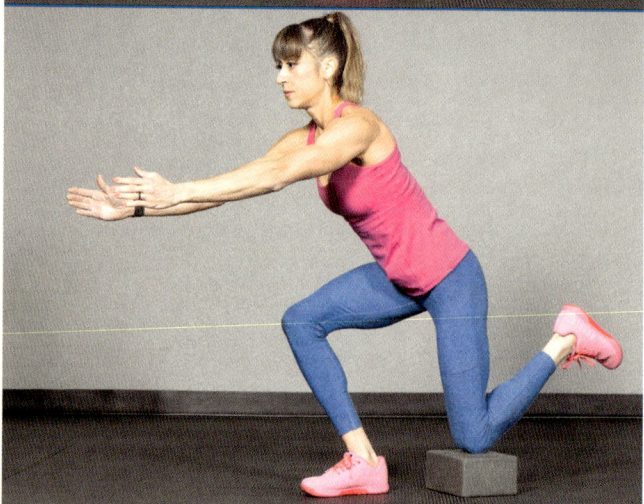

AIRBORNE LUNGE

Stand tall and shift your weight to one foot, bending the other knee to bring your heel toward your butt. You want to keep that foot pulled toward your butt so only your knee touches down when you lower. Sit your butt back to hinge at the hips as you bend your support knee to drop your back knee toward the ground. Lean forward as you hinge, but do not round over. You're leaning forward to counterbalance your weight and sit back.

Touch your knee to the ground gently without letting your raised foot touch down. Do not reach that raised leg back too far or you'll get too spread out. Your standing knee may travel over your toes. Make sure you've pushed your butt back to load your glutes while keeping the support foot, and especially your heel, firmly pressed into the ground. After lightly touching your back knee down, drive back up to standing.

Do not push off that knee or the raised foot.

You want the entire movement to be powered by your support leg. Stand tall at the top and squeeze the glute of your support leg. Try not to touch the other foot down between reps.

MODIFICATIONS: Modify the movement by holding on to a chair or suspension trainer. You can also reduce the range of motion by lowering your back knee to a block.

EXERCISE SWAPS: Suspension trainer airborne lunge, reduced ROM airborne lunge, reverse lunge, alternating slider reverse lunge, single-leg deadlift

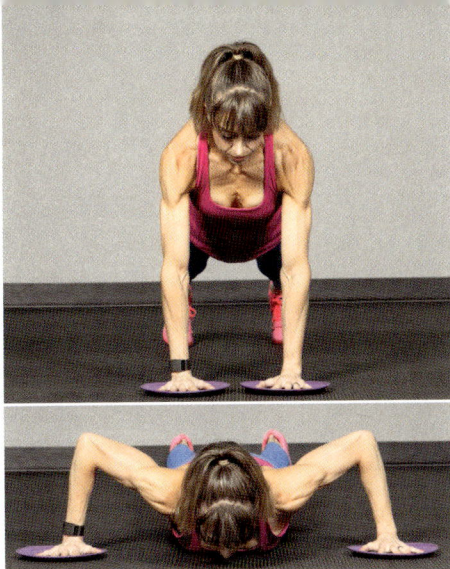

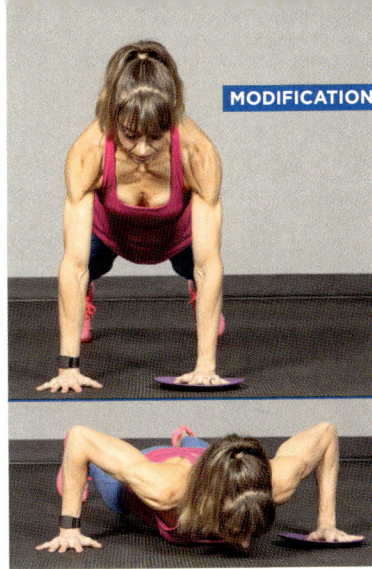

MODIFICATIONS: You can widen your feet for a more stable base or slide one hand out at a time. You can also perform this off your knees. A wide-grip push-up is also an option.

EXERCISE SWAPS: Wide-grip push-up, cable chest fly, dumbbell chest fly, pec deck, incline chest fly

FLY PUSH-UP

Set up in a push-up position with a towel or slider under each hand and your hands aligned under your chest. Place your feet about hip-width apart and drive back through your heels, creating a nice straight line from your head to your heels. Slide both hands out wide, flying your arms open so your upper arms are roughly parallel to the ground and your elbows are bent. Feel your chest stretch with this movement.

Pull with your chest muscles to bring your hands back under your chest as you straighten your arms to return to your starting position. Feel your chest working to bring your hands back in. Repeat to slide back out.

SIDE TO CURTSY LUNGE

This movement combines the side lunge with the curtsy lunge with one leg moving back and forth between the two lunges. If you lunge out to the side with your left leg, you will then step back to the center, touching only your toe down if needed, and then sink into a curtsy lunge with the left leg behind you. Your right leg will never move.

Stand tall with your feet together. Step out with one leg into the side lunge, loading that glute as you bend your knee to sit back in the hinge and sink down. Push off that leg to drive back up to standing, only tapping your toe if needed for stability before crossing that leg behind you in the curtsy lunge. Load your front glute as you cross your leg behind and lower your knee to hover over the ground. Hinge a bit to load your front glute but don't round forward.

Push off your front leg to help you come back up to standing. Without touching down—or by just tapping your toe lightly—lunge back into the side lunge to repeat the sequence.

MODIFICATIONS: Pause between each lunge and don't sink as deep. You can also break this down and just do one type of lunge. To progress, you can add dumbbells: Hold them in front of your legs to start, dropping them toward the instep of the foot of the bent knee in the side lunge. Then bring them outside your hips as you lunge back into the curtsy.

EXERCISE SWAPS: Barbell side to curtsy lunge, goblet side to curtsy lunge, side lunge, curtsy lunge

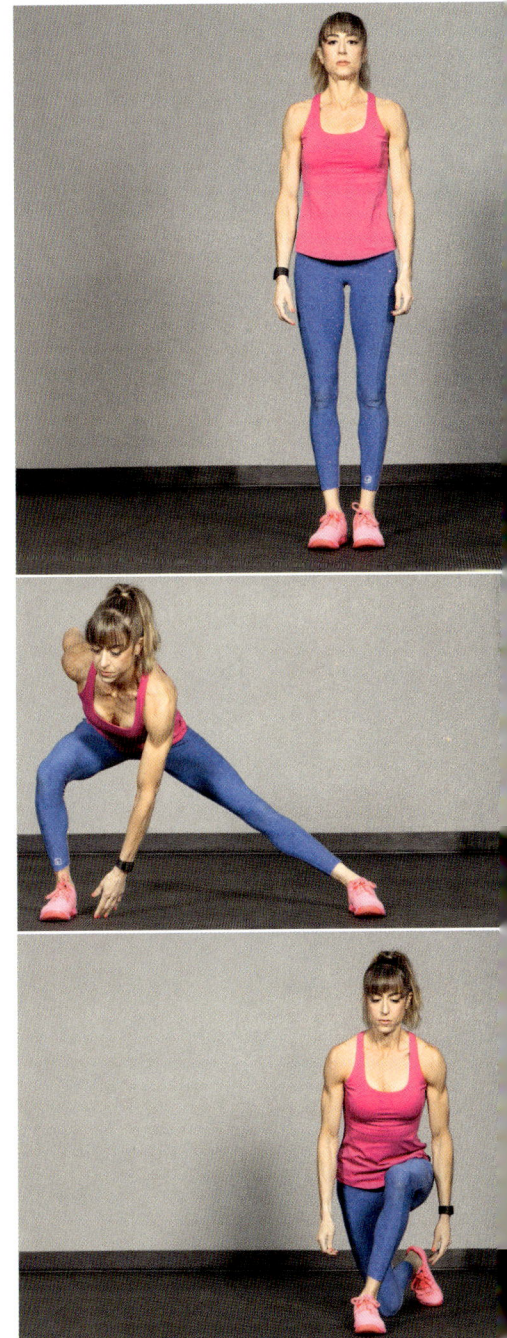

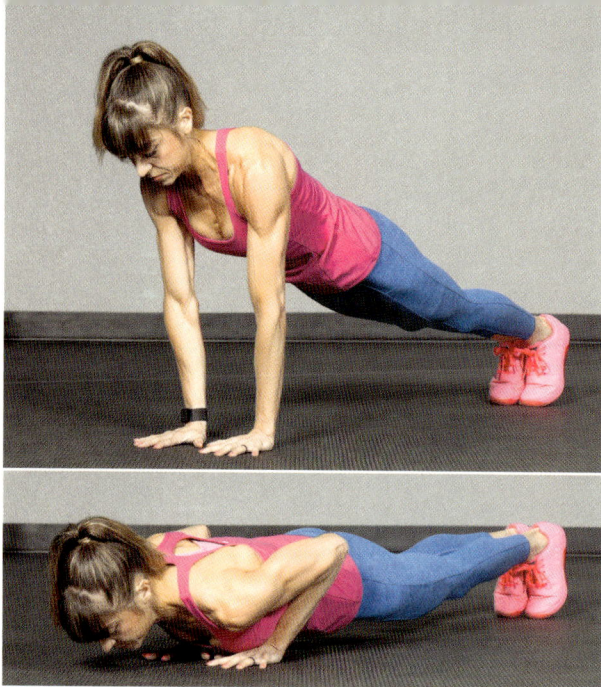

CLOSE-GRIP PUSH-UP

Set up in a high plank position but move your hands close together right under your chest. The closer your hands are together, the harder the move will be and the more your triceps will be forced to work.

Keeping your body in a nice straight line and your arms tucked to your sides, lower your chest to the ground. Your body should move as one unit without your butt going up in the air or your hips sagging. Keep tension back through your heels to maintain the plank position.

Make sure your elbows and arms stay close to your sides as you lower. Do not let them flare out, or you won't force your triceps to work as hard. Lower your chest as close to the ground as possible and then press back up.

MODIFICATIONS: Place your hands on a bench or perform the move from your knees.

EXERCISE SWAPS: Bench close-grip push-up, close-grip bench press, press to skull crusher, floor press to skull crusher, triceps push-up, bench dip, dip

LYING SIDE SLIDE

Lie on your side with a slider or towel under your bottom hand and your arm fully extended past your head. Bend your knees to help you stabilize. Place your top hand on your side so it can't assist at all.

Move to a sitting position by pulling the hand on the slider toward your shoulder while keeping your arm straight. Feel your lat working to pull your hand down as you push yourself up. Slide your hand back out to lower to the ground again.

MODIFICATIONS: Place your top hand on the ground in front of you to help you balance.

EXERCISE SWAPS: Cable single-arm lat pushdown, band single-arm lat pushdown, lat pushdown, slider ab extension, band/towel pull-down, lying W pull-down, pullover

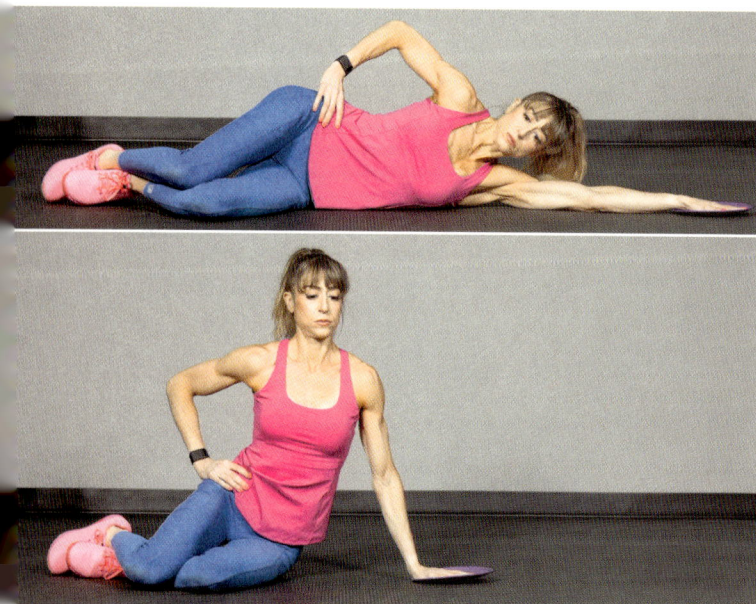

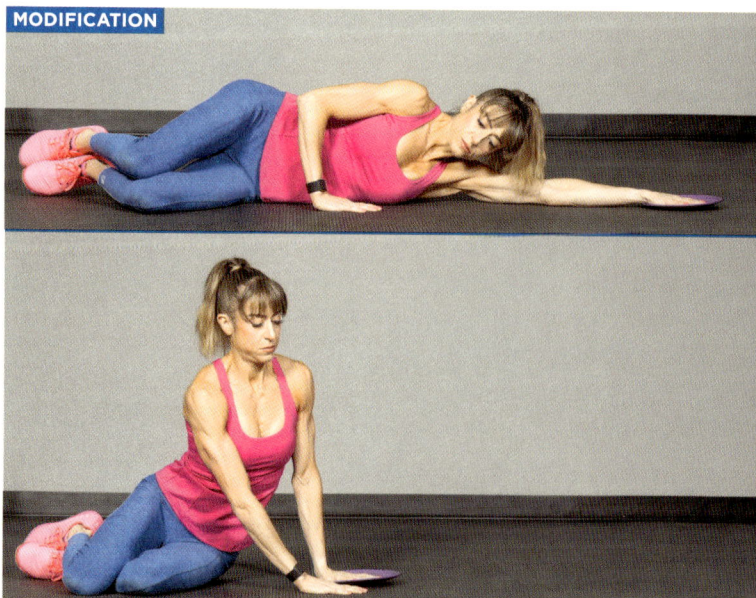

MODIFICATION

ALTERNATING SLIDER REVERSE LUNGE

Stand with each foot on a slider and your feet together. Slide one foot back as you sink into a lunge, dropping your back knee toward the ground and bending your front knee to 90 degrees. Slightly hinge at your hips to load your front glute as you keep your knee in line with your ankle. Do not round forward as you hinge.

Drive through your front foot to pull your back foot up to return to standing. Then slide the other foot back in a lunge as you bend your front knee, sinking so that your back knee hovers just off the ground. Make sure your front knee doesn't cave in as you lunge back or drive up to standing.

MODIFICATIONS: If you've had knee issues in the past, you can also perform a straighter leg lunge or not sink as deeply. The sliders reduce traction, so removing them can also help. When you feel ready to progress, hold weights down at your side.

EXERCISE SWAPS: Dumbbell reverse lunge, alternating goblet slider reverse lunge, deficit reverse lunge, alternating dumbbell slider reverse lunge, unilaterally loaded alternating slider reverse lunge, straight-leg reverse lunge

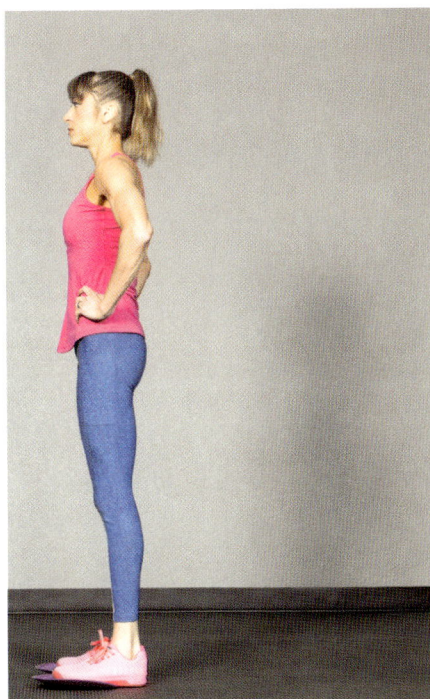

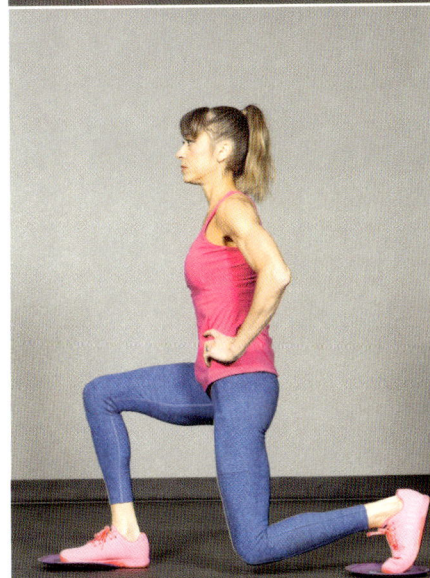

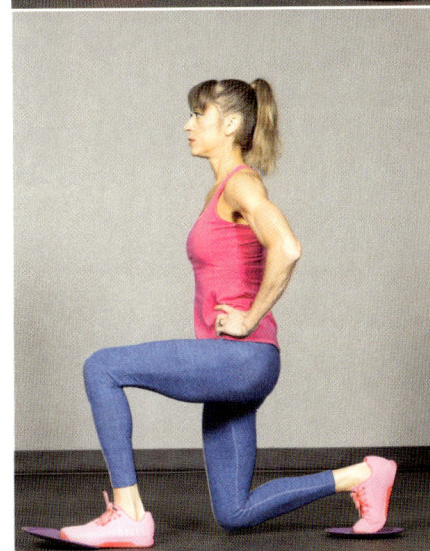

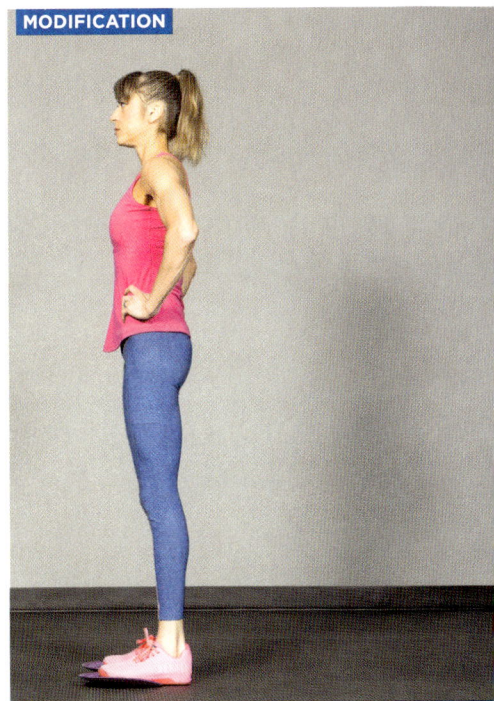

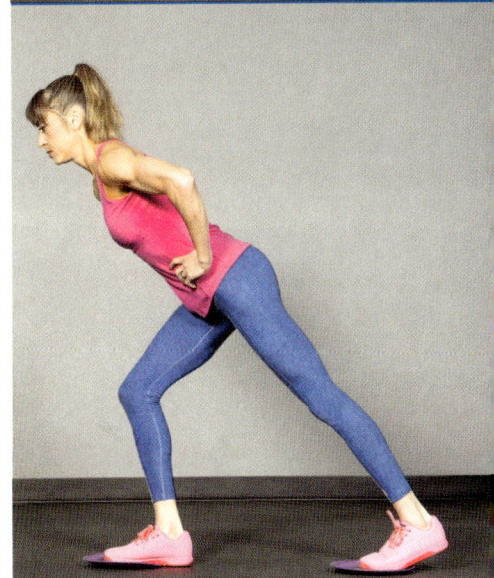

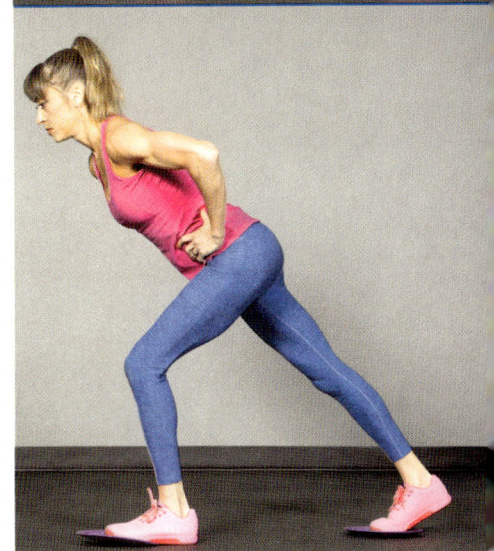

MODIFICATION

SCAPULAR WALL REPS

Bend your elbows to about 90 degrees and place them on the wall behind you with your arms in by your sides. Press off your elbows, engaging your upper back as you press your chest out. Walk your feet out from the wall, leaning back into it to apply more resistance. Do not shrug your shoulders or walk out too far.

Stand with your feet together and flex your feet, engaging your glutes and quads so you have a nice straight line from your shoulders to your heels. Pause here then relax your back into the wall before again driving off your elbows to press off the wall.

The wall and your body angle might limit how you can hold your head, but try to relax it back rather than tucking your chin. Think about lifting your chest open toward the ceiling, and don't shrug as you drive off your elbows to move your back from the wall.

MODIFICATIONS: Do not walk your feet out more than a few inches from the wall.

EXERCISE SWAPS: Lying scapular hold, lying scapular press, scapular push-up, single-arm scapular push-up, scapular wall hold, doorway row, bent-over row, band row, inverted row, chest-supported row

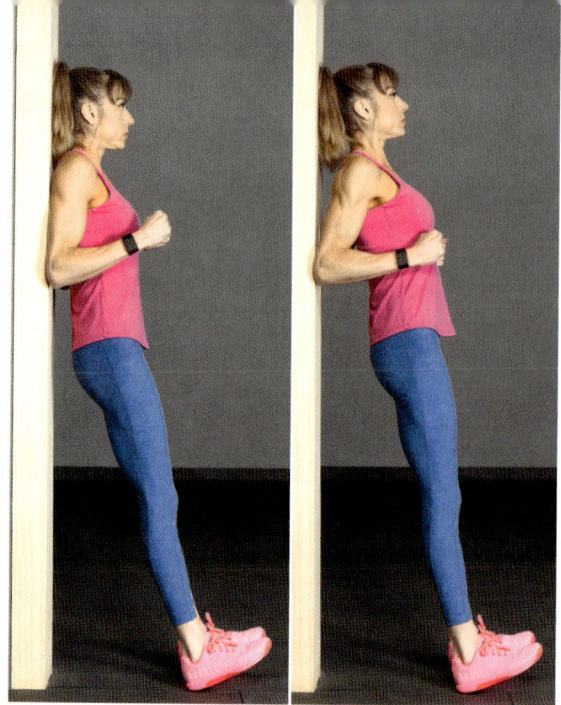

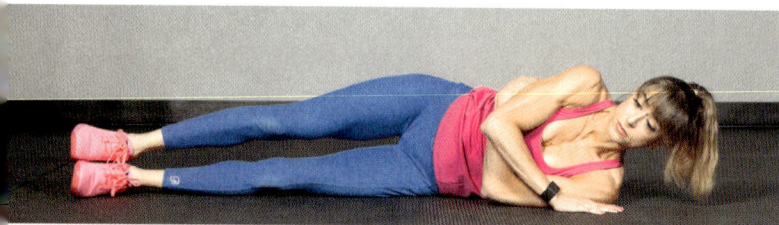

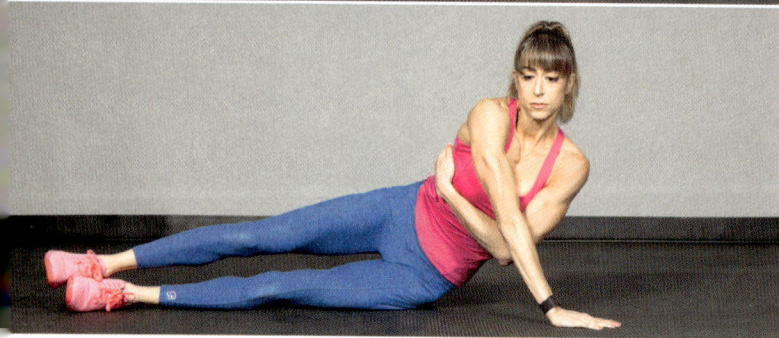

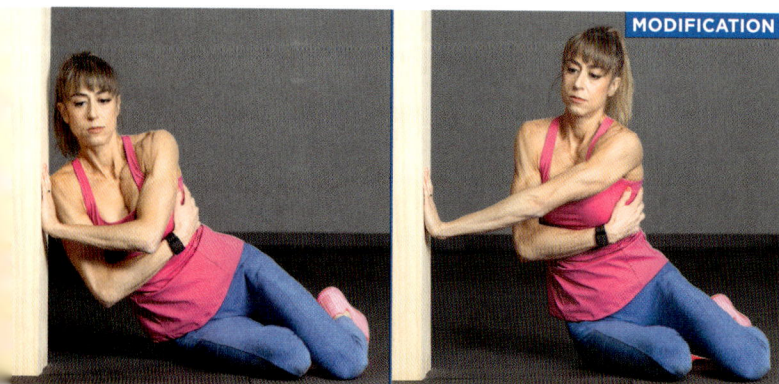

TRICEPS PUSH-UP

Lie on your side with your legs straight. Wrap your bottom arm up across your body and place your hand on your opposite shoulder or around your ribs. Place your top hand on the ground at about your shoulder or right below. The closer your hand is toward your belly button, the harder the move will be.

Push your hand into the ground, feeling your triceps work to push your upper body up. Press up until your arm is extended and then lower back to the ground. Your chest may slightly rotate toward the ground as you press, but make sure you really focus on the back of your arm working, and don't turn to face the ground. Engage your abs and don't let your legs flop around as you lift.

MODIFICATIONS: Push off a wall or bench.

MODIFICATION

EXERCISE SWAPS: Bent-over triceps kickback, triceps pushdown, bench dip, press to skull crusher, close-grip push-up, mini band triceps pushdown

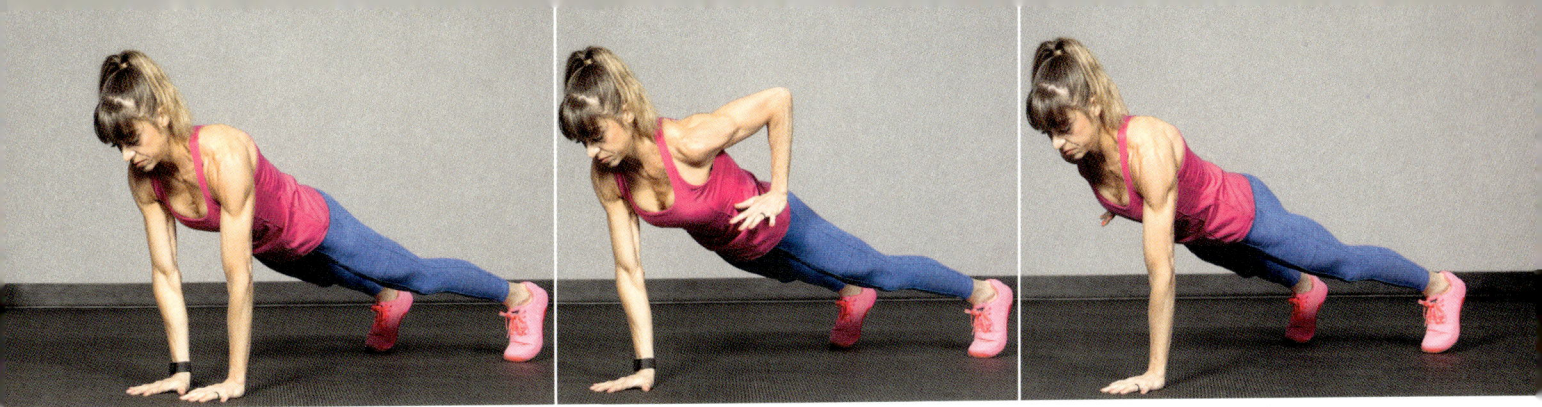

ALTERNATING-ARM PLANK ROW

Set up in a high plank position and place your hands somewhat close together under your chest. Put your feet a bit wider apart for stability.

Hold this plank position and row one hand up to your chest, driving your elbow toward the ceiling. Do not shrug as you row. Engage your lats and focus on your shoulder blade moving toward your spine as you raise your hand. Move at a controlled pace; don't rush because you're losing balance. Really fight to keep your hips and core still and prevent rotation. Lower your hand to the ground and row up on the other side. Move slowly, alternating arms.

MODIFICATIONS: Perform the row on one side only or plank from your knees or by placing your hands on a bench. To progress, set your feet closer together, but don't let your hips rotate during the row.

EXERCISE SWAPS: Renegade row, plank row, single-arm scapular push-up, scapular push-up, anti-rotational suspension trainer row, single-arm band row

ALTERNATING FRONT-ANGLED LUNGE

Stand tall with both feet together. Step forward and about 3 to 8 inches to the outside of where you would lunge if you were lunging straight ahead. Bend both knees as you step forward to sink down into a lunge. Keep your front heel down and make sure you don't turn in the direction you lunged. Both of your toes should still be pointing straight ahead with your ankle, knee, and hip of your front leg in alignment.

Drive off your front foot to push back up to standing and lunge at an angle on the other side. You should feel like your feet are wider apart than usual when you lunge. This will work your inner thighs more. Keep alternating sides, sinking as deep in the lunge as you possibly can.

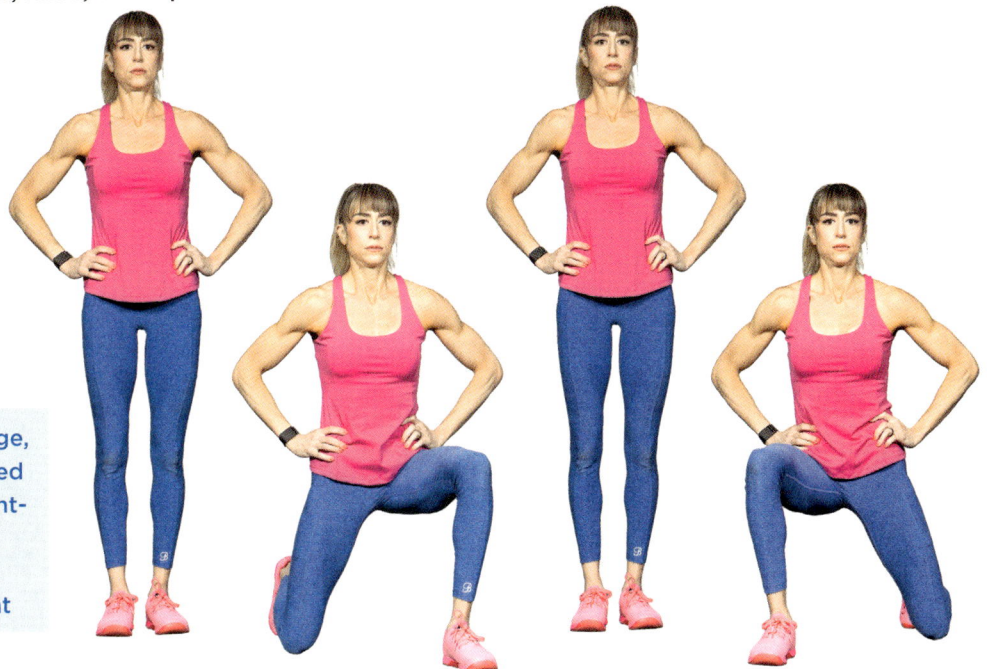

MODIFICATIONS: Keep a more vertical shin angle on your front leg to avoid overloading your quad or knee and do not lunge as deep to start. Add weights to progress the move.

EXERCISE SWAPS: Front lunge, goblet alternating front-angled lunge, barbell alternating front-angled lunge, front-angled lunge, sumo squat, Cossack squat, staggered stance squat

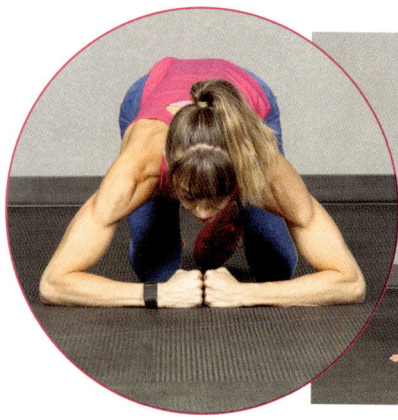

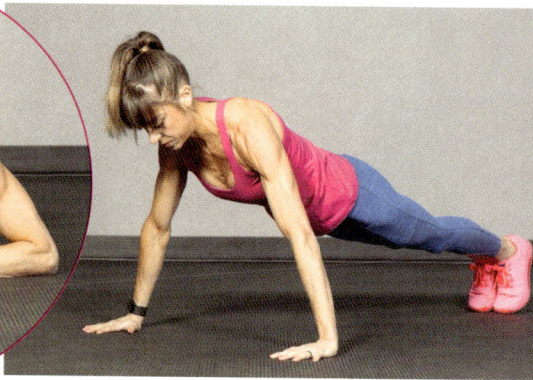

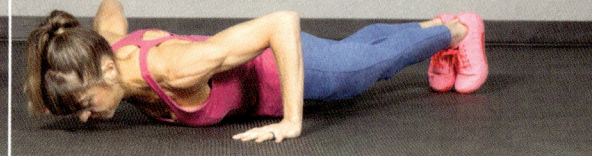

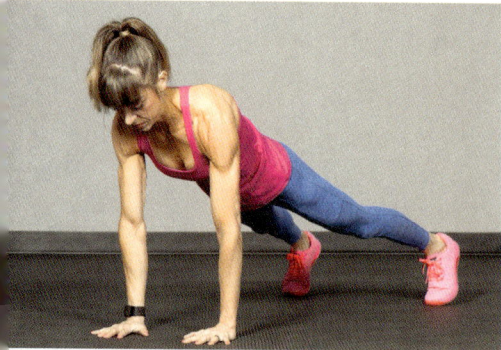

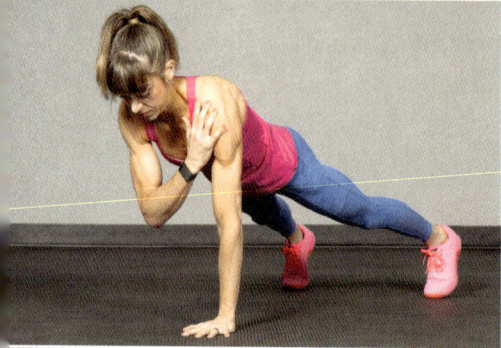

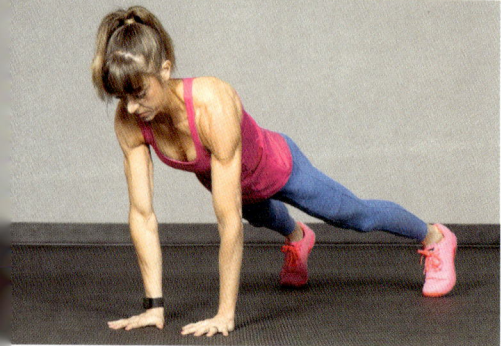

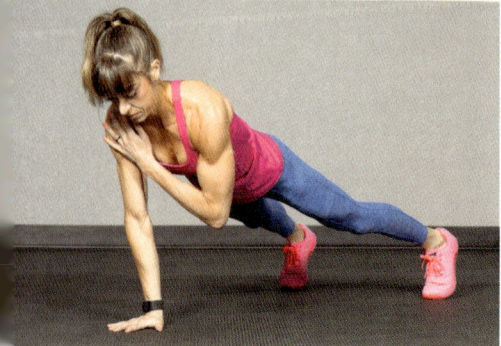

WIDE-GRIP PUSH-UP

Kneel on the ground, make your hands into fists, and place your knuckles together. Lean forward and lay your forearms on the ground. The point where your elbows are is how wide your hands should be for the push-up.

Make sure your hands are in line with your chest rather than above your shoulders as you set up in the high plank position with your feet close together and your body in a nice straight line from your head to your heels.

Press through your hands as you lower your chest to the ground. Do not let your hips sag or your butt go up in the air. Make sure your entire body moves as one unit. After you've lowered all the way down, press back up, fully straightening your arms at the top of the push-up.

MODIFICATIONS: Perform the push-up off a bench or incline or from your knees on the ground to modify.

PLANK WITH SHOULDER TAP

Set up in a high plank position and place your hands somewhat close together under your chest with your feet a bit wider apart for stability. Holding this plank position, engage your lats to support your shoulders and make sure they aren't shrugged.

Brace your abs and engage your glutes as you lift one hand up off the ground, moving it slowly to touch the opposite shoulder. Keep your hips square to the ground and do not rotate as you lift your hand. Slowly place your hand back down on the ground. Lift the other hand and tap the opposite shoulder. Try to keep your body still except for moving your hand. Do not rotate as you lift.

MODIFICATIONS: Perform the move with your hands on a bench or incline or do the plank from your knees. To progress, bring your feet closer together, but don't let your hips rotate during the shoulder tap.

SLIDER PLANK JACKS

Place a slider or towel under each foot and set up in a high plank position with your hands under your shoulders and your feet together. Your body should be in a nice straight line from your head to your heels. Keeping your core tight, slide your feet open to slightly wider than shoulder-width apart. Do not let your hips sag or your butt go up in the air as you slide your legs apart.

Quickly slide your legs back together to your starting position. Repeat, sliding your legs open and then closed again.

MODIFICATIONS: Perform the plank off a bench or slide one side out and in at a time. You can also do this without the sliders although that will not work your adductors (inner thighs) as much.

EXERCISE SWAPS: Step plank jacks, plank jacks, kneeling adductor slide, side plank adductor lift, cable adduction, glute bridge with squeeze

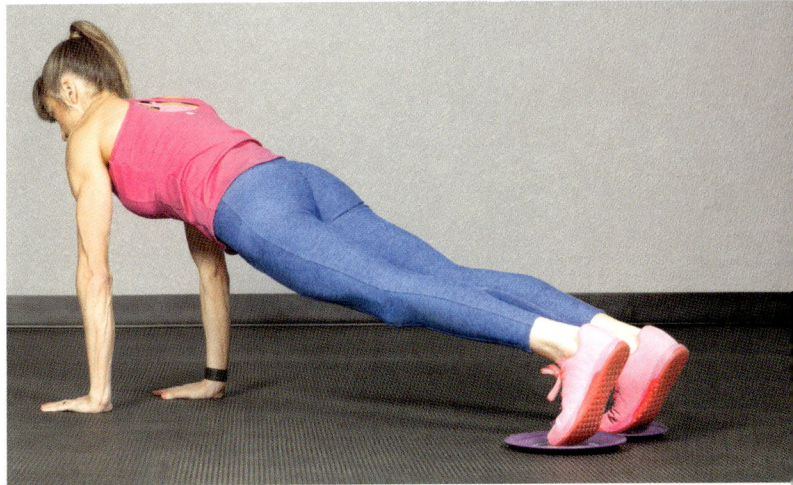

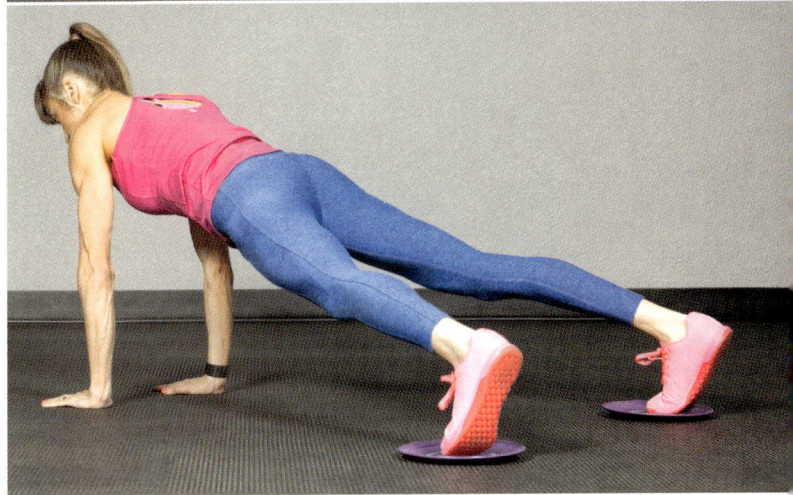

LYING KNEES

Start in a hollow body position with your hands clasped by one ear. Simultaneously swing your hands in a chopping motion toward your opposite hip as you crunch the knee of that leg toward your chest and sit up.

Return to the starting position and repeat the movement. Focus on rounding your spine to sit up as you chop and tuck your knee. Once all reps are done, switch sides.

MODIFICATIONS: Perform this move with your knees bent and feet on the ground. Tuck your knee in while your other leg stays bent with your foot on the ground. You will perform this as a crunch instead of coming to balance on your butt. Alternatively, you can raise your feet higher off the ground.

EXERCISE SWAPS: Modified lying knees, Russian twist, cable twist, band twist, side plank oblique twist, bicycle crunch, sit-thru

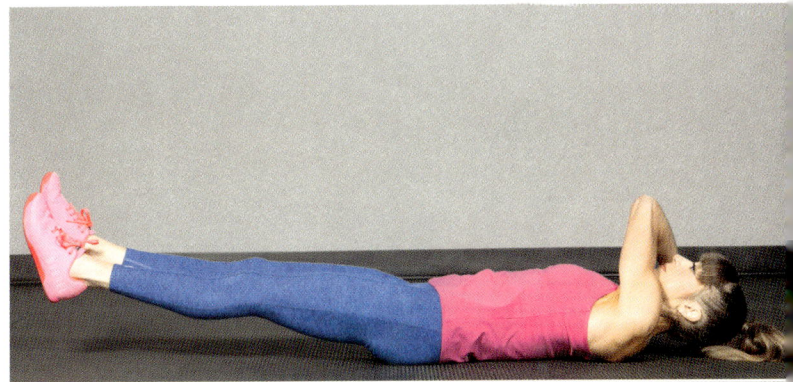

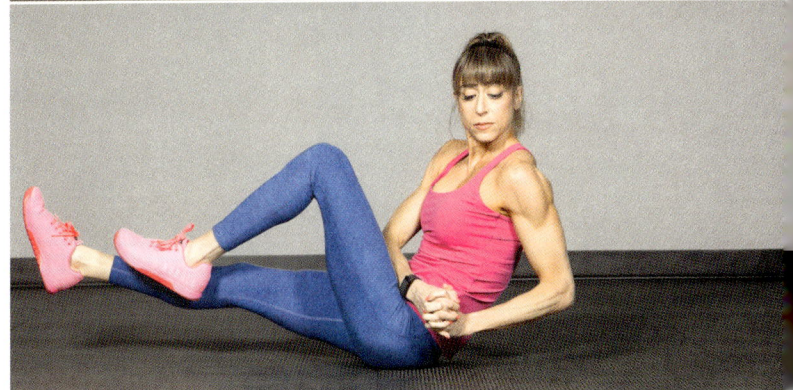

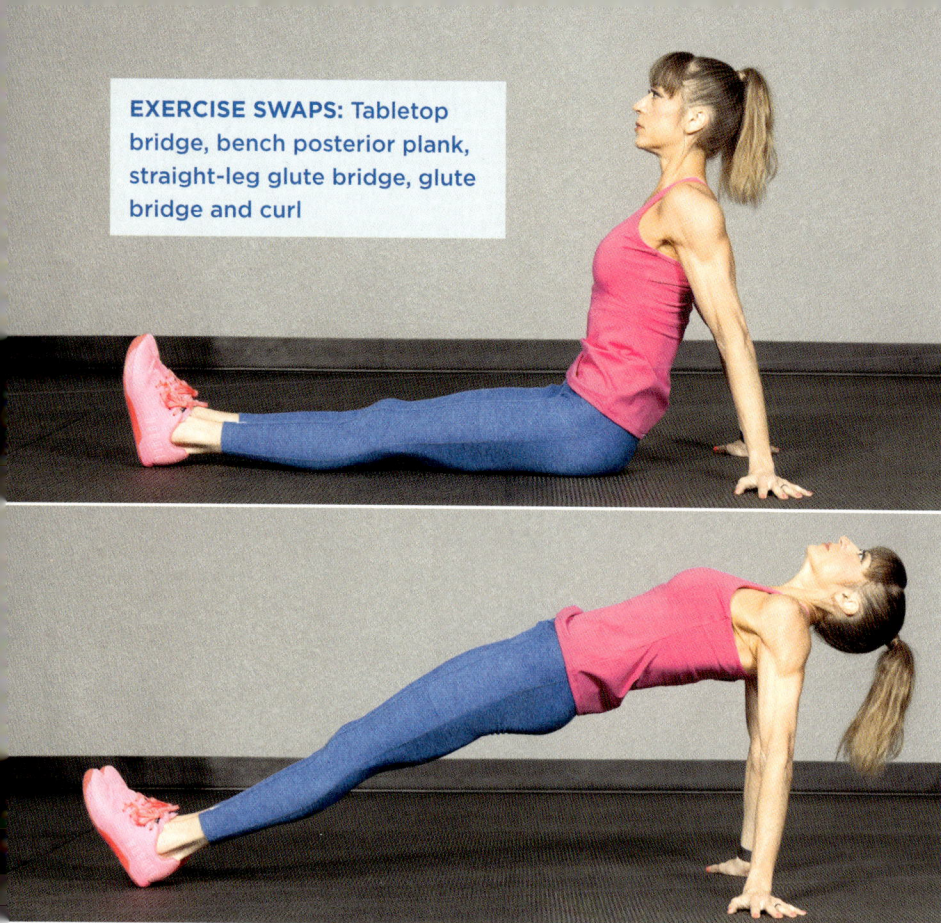

POSTERIOR PLANK

Sit on the ground with your legs extended and your hands behind you. Drive up through your heels and your hands to press your hips toward the ceiling and your chest out. Lean your head back as you bridge up.

Squeeze your butt and lift your hips up as high as you can while keeping your legs straight and your chest pressed out. Do not shrug your shoulders at the top, and make sure you don't arch your lower back. You should feel your hamstrings, upper back, and butt working. Hold at the top of the move with your body in a nice straight line; then reset and repeat.

MODIFICATIONS: Place your hands on a bench or perform a tabletop bridge.

SINGLE-LEG HIP THRUST

Sit with your upper back against a bench and your feet flat on the ground. The bench should hit just below your shoulder blades. Raise one foot off the ground and bridge up, driving through your upper back and foot on the ground.

Do not push yourself backward. Think about driving your knee toward your toe and do not let your knee cave in.

Squeeze your glute to extend your hips and pause at the top. Repeat.

MODIFICATIONS: Perform a single-leg glute bridge or 80/20 variation with one foot staggered out to assist with the hip thrust.

EXERCISE SWAPS: Weighted single-leg hip thrust, 80/20 hip thrust, single-leg glute bridge, feet-raised hip thrust

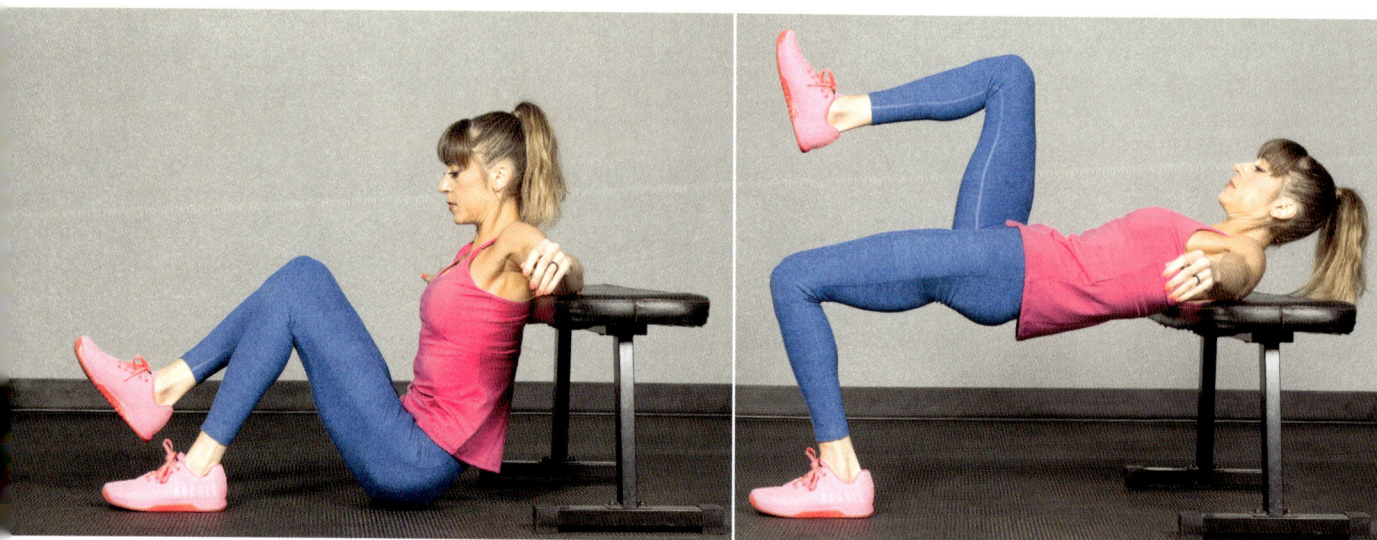

SLIDER AB EXTENSION

Place a slider or towel under each hand and set up as if you're doing a push-up from your knees. Your hands should be under your shoulders with your body in a nice straight line from your head to your knees. Brace your abs, tucking your pelvis toward your ribs and squeeze your glutes.

Slide both hands out as far as you can, keeping your arms straight, to lower your body toward the ground. Pull the sliders back under your shoulders without bending your arms to return your body to the plank position.

Do not sit your butt back or let your lower back engage as you extend your arms and pull your hands back in. You want to brace your abs and keep your body in a nice straight line the entire time. Focus on the exhale as you come back up to the plank position.

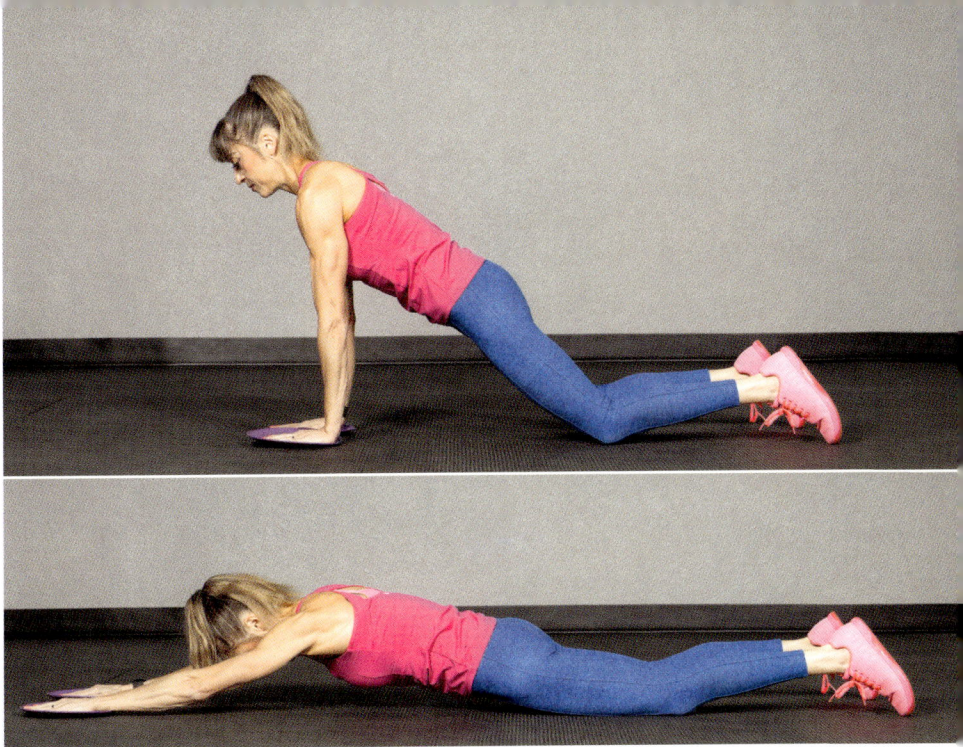

MODIFICATIONS: Do not slide out as far, and you can use a wall to stop the sliders. You also can perform an alternating single-arm variation. If you don't have sliders, you can do ab extensions using a yoga ball, suspension trainer, or ab wheel.

EXERCISE SWAPS: Ab wheel roll-out, single-arm ab extension, suspension trainer ab extension, body saw, extended plank hold, yoga ball/stability ball ab extension

STANDING QUAD KICKOUT

Balance on one foot, focusing on driving it into the ground as you engage your glute. Lift your other leg so your hip is bent to 90 degrees with your knee bent and your lower leg hanging down.

Slowly kick your lower leg out so your leg is approximately parallel to the ground. Feel your hips working to keep your hip flexed and your quads working to extend your knee. Squeeze your quad to fully extend; then bend at your knee to return to the starting position before repeating the movement. Do not lower your leg to the ground.

MODIFICATIONS: Place your hand on the wall to help you balance or perform a seated quad extension.

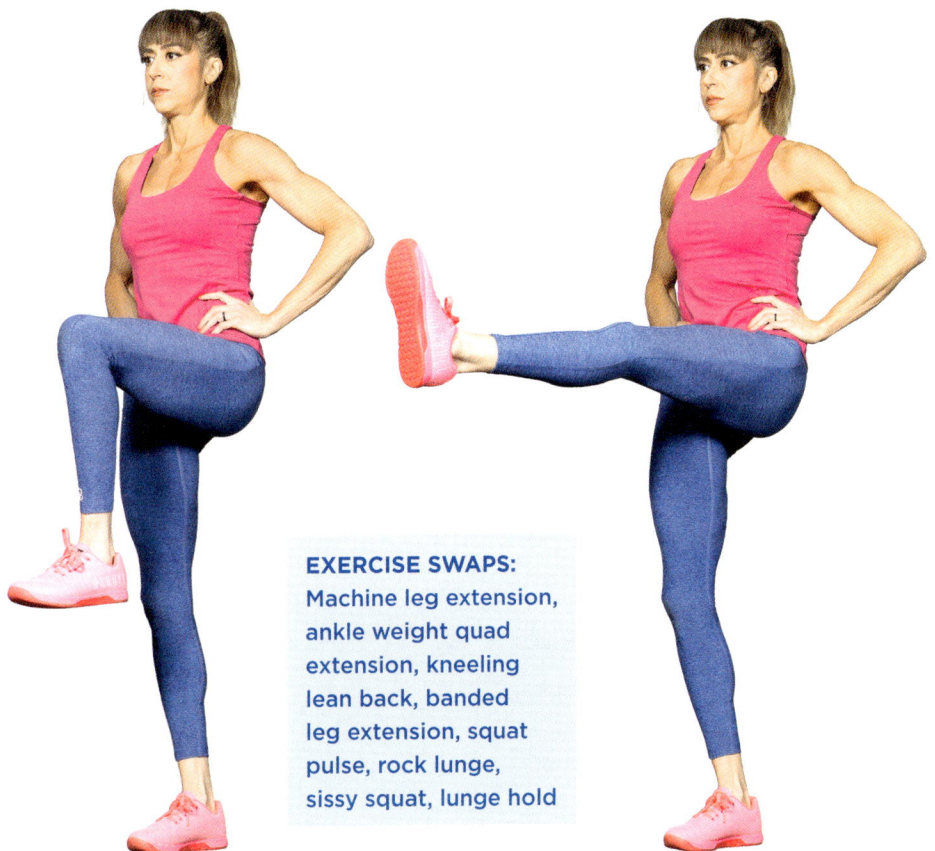

EXERCISE SWAPS: Machine leg extension, ankle weight quad extension, kneeling lean back, banded leg extension, squat pulse, rock lunge, sissy squat, lunge hold

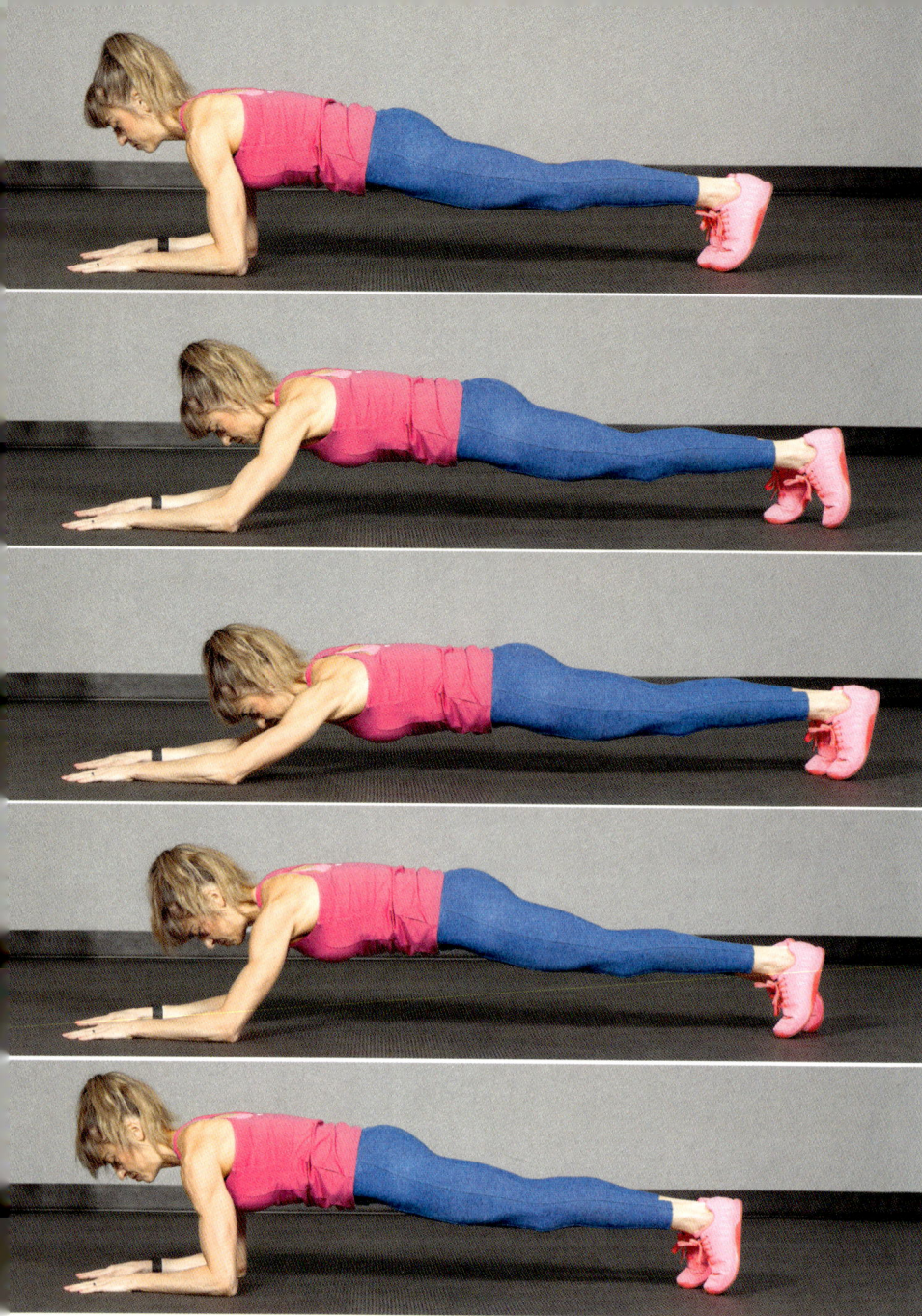

BODY SAW

Set up in a forearm plank with your feet close together. Engage your back and make sure your body is in a nice straight line to your heels.

Take small steps to walk your feet backward, without letting your hips sag toward the ground. Lengthen through your triceps and lats as you walk back as far as you can while keeping your core engaged.

Walk your feet forward until you return to the forearm plank with your elbows under your shoulders. Do not let your butt go up in the air or your hips sag.

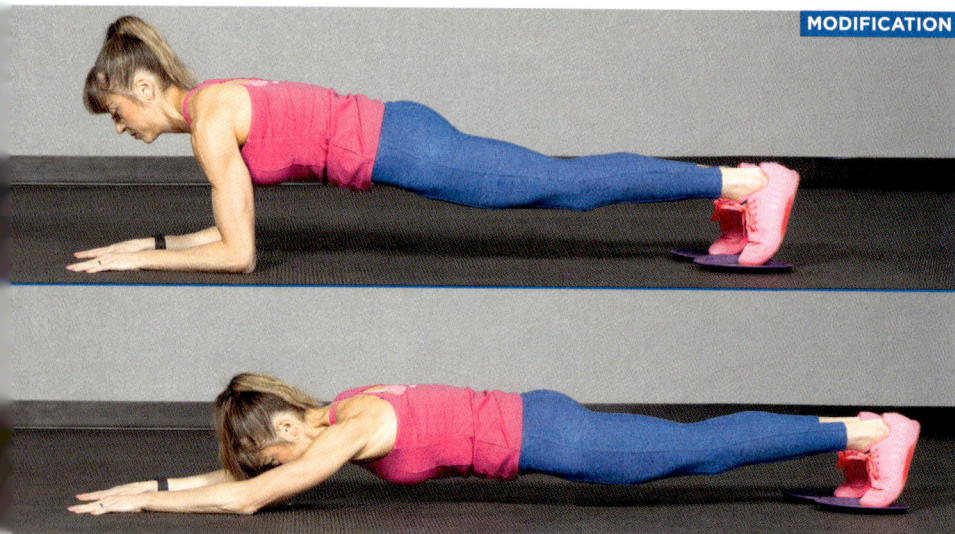

MODIFICATION

MODIFICATIONS: Perform the plank off an incline or don't walk back as far. To progress the move, place sliders or towels under your feet and slide back then engage your lats and triceps as you pull yourself back forward.

EXERCISE SWAPS: Slider ab extension, slider body saw, extended plank hold, plank rock, bench body saw

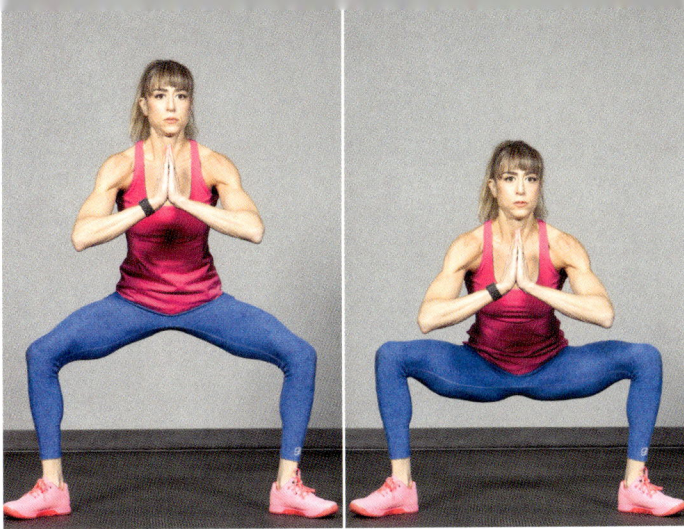

MODIFICATIONS: Hold on to a chair or suspension trainer to help you balance and don't pulse as low in the squat.

EXERCISE SWAPS: Squat pulse, kneeling adductor slide, goblet sumo squat pulse

PULSE SUMO SQUAT

Stand with your feet wider than shoulder-width apart (adjusting your stance according to your mobility). Turn your toes out to about a 45-degree angle. Make sure that your ankles, knees, and hips are in alignment as you sink into the squat. You do not want your knees caving in or bowing way open.

Squat, sitting your butt down and back as you keep your chest up. Feel your glutes pulling your knees open to keep your hips, knees, and ankles all in line. Sink to about parallel then go an inch or two lower before pulsing a few inches above parallel. Do not come more than halfway out of the squat as you pulse and make sure your feet stay firmly planted.

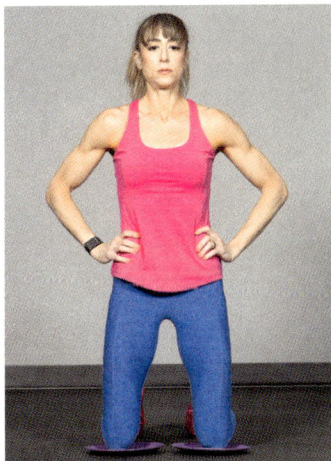

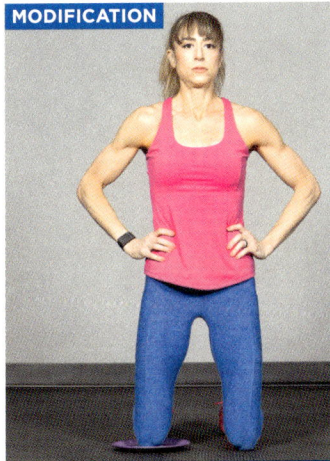

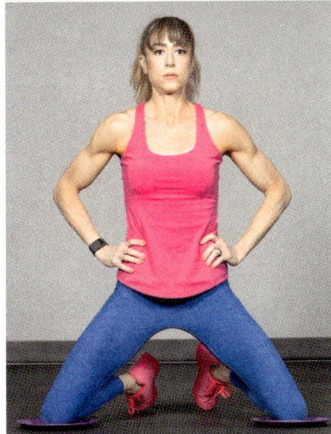

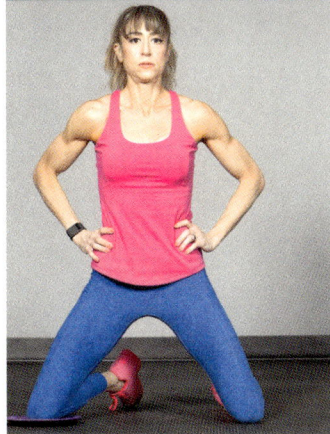

MODIFICATION

MODIFICATION

KNEELING ADDUCTOR SLIDE

Kneel on the ground with a slider or towel under each knee. Your knees should be together with your feet behind you—flex them if you need a little extra stability. Slide your knees open as far as you can with control before using your inner thighs to pull your knees back together. Do not slide out too far or you won't be able to pull the sliders back together. Do not purposefully sit back as you slide out; however, you may slightly hinge at the hips as you open up.

Drive your knees down into the sliders to maintain control and pull your knees back together.

MODIFICATIONS: Slide out one side at a time or do a side-lying adductor lift.

EXERCISE SWAPS: Cable adductions, adduction machine, side-lying adductor lift, glute bridge with squeeze, modified kneeling adductor slides, slider side lunges

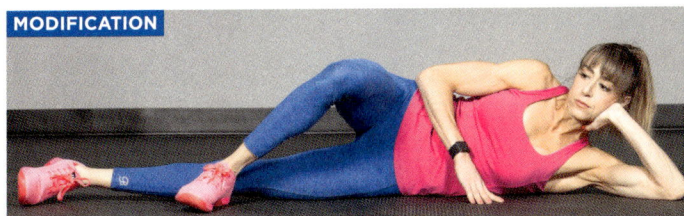

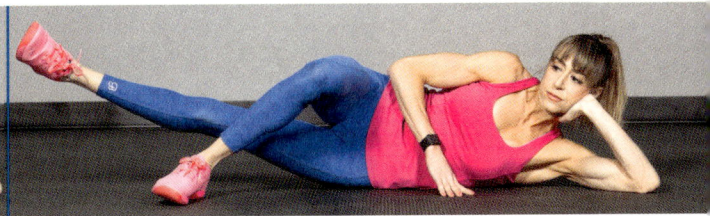

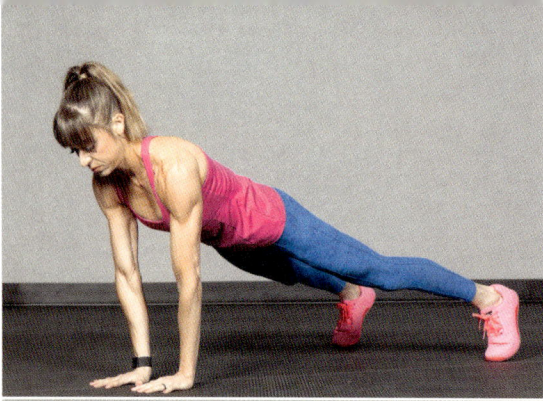

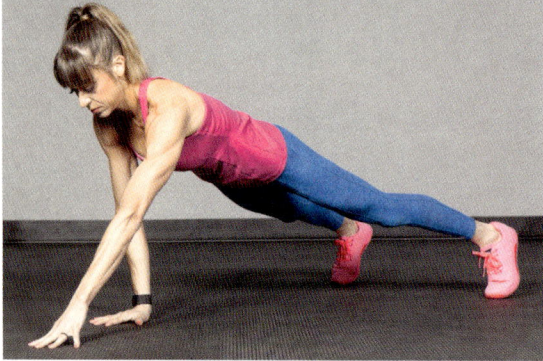

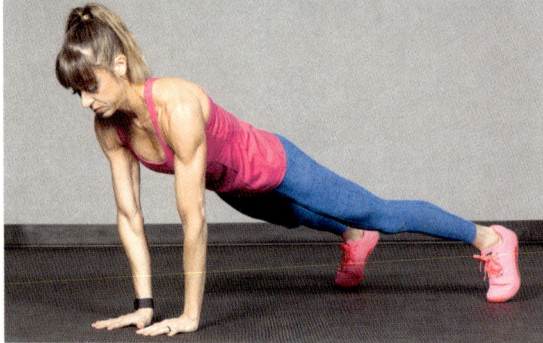

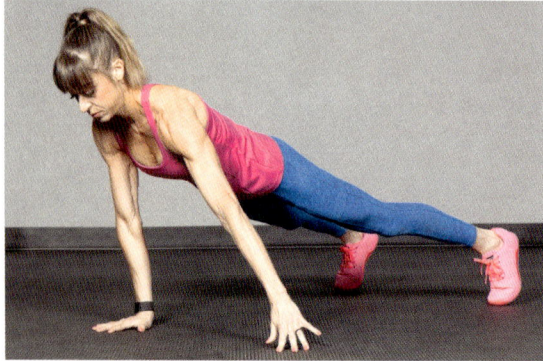

PLANK WITH TWO-WAY TAP

Set up in a high plank position with your hands somewhat close together under your chest and your feet about shoulder-width apart for stability. Brace your abs and drive back through your heels. Do not shrug your shoulders.

Reach one hand out to touch the ground beyond your head and return it to its starting position. Then reach that same hand out to the side. Return that hand to center.

Repeat the sequence with the other hand. Alternate sides, fighting the urge to rotate your hips, let them sag, or let your butt go up in the air.

MODIFICATIONS: Place your hands up on a bench or incline.

> **EXERCISE SWAPS:** Bench plank with two-way tap, plank with shoulder tap, front to side raise, chest to overhead press

T SIT-UP

Place a slider or towel under each hand and lie on your back with your arms straight out from your body at just below shoulder height. Pull your hands toward your body, keeping your arms straight to push you to sit up. Feel your back working to pull your hands in as your shoulder blades move toward your spine to power your sit-up. Make sure your shoulders aren't shrugged and that your chest is pressed out as you sit tall at the top.

Slowly round your back and extend your arms straight in line just below shoulder height to lower yourself back down. Think about lowering one vertebra at a time. Do not bend your arms as you sit up or lower. Repeat.

MODIFICATIONS: Perform a crunch variation rather than doing the full sit-up or modify to a scapular push-up or basic sit-up.

> **EXERCISE SWAPS:** Scapular push-up, alternating arm plank row, sit-up

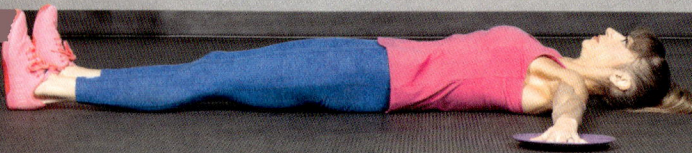

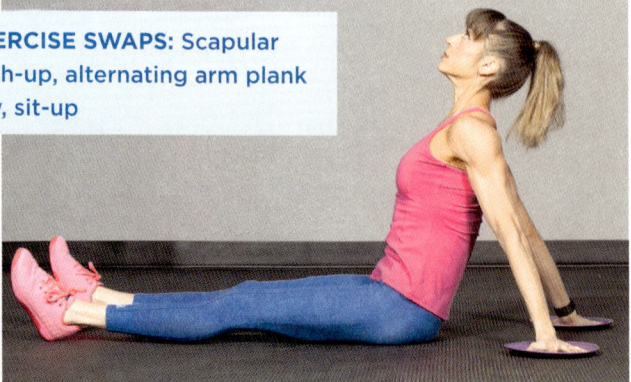

GLUTE BRIDGE TO SIT-UP

Lie on your back with your knees bent and feet flat on the ground about hip-width apart. Bend your elbows to 90 degrees and drive your upper arms into the ground. Tuck your pelvis toward your ribs and then drive through your feet, upper arms, and upper back to bridge up while squeezing your glutes.

Pause for a second before lowering your hips. Move your feet a little bit away from your butt so that you can perform the sit-up. Make sure to roll up so that you engage your abs and not your low back. Lie back down and repeat the sequence.

MODIFICATIONS: Perform a bridge to a crunch instead of a full sit-up.

EXERCISE SWAPS: Cable hip rotation, band hip rotation, glute bridge, plank with reach back and out, 3-way hip circle, bird dog plank, crunch to bridge

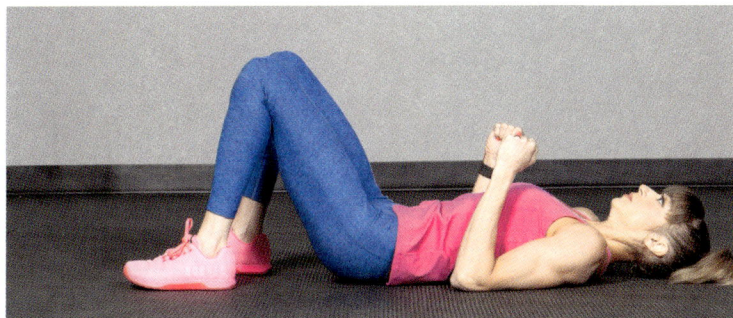

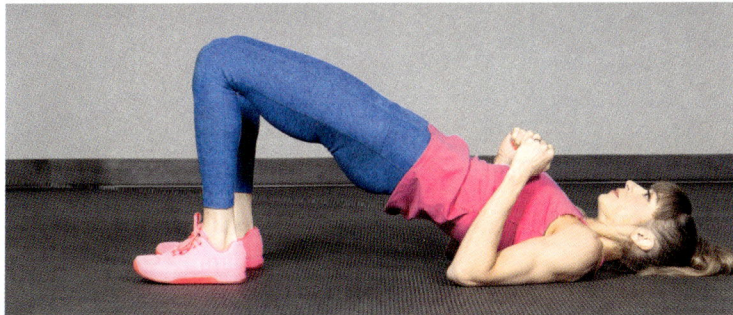

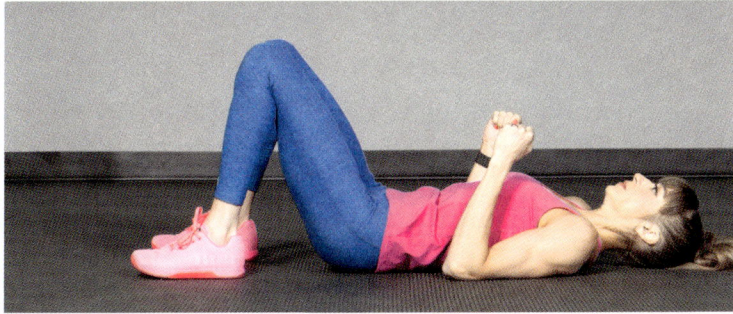

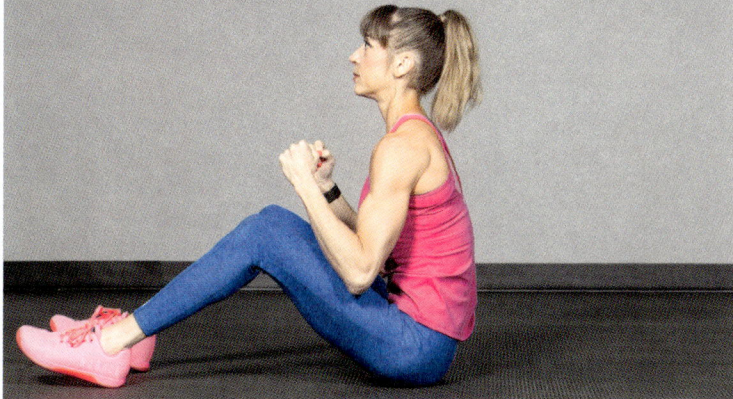

MODIFICATION

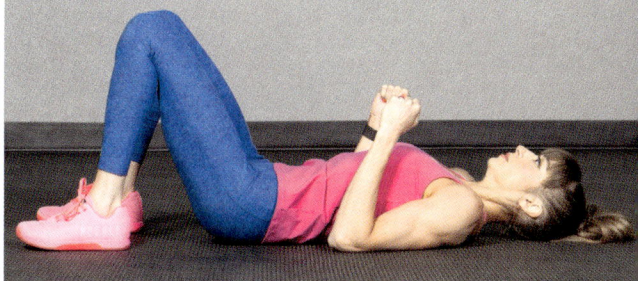

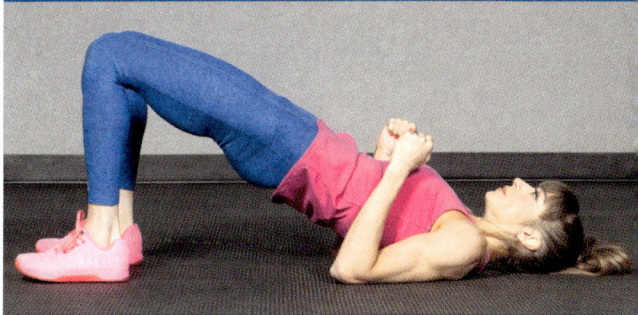

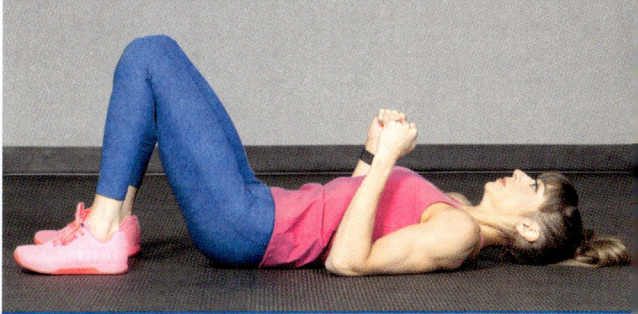

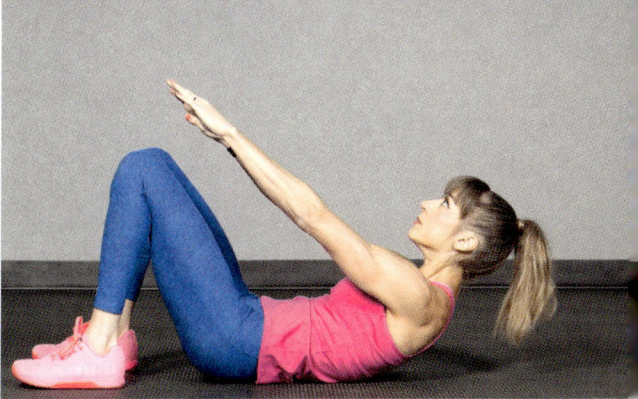

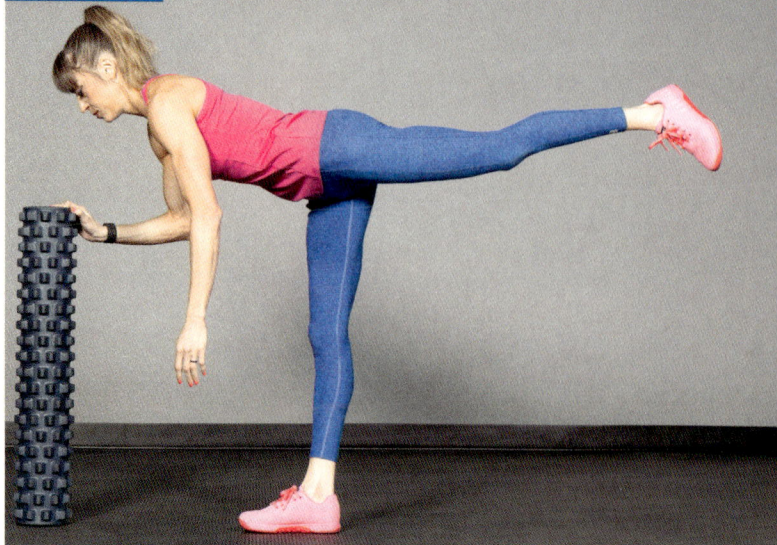

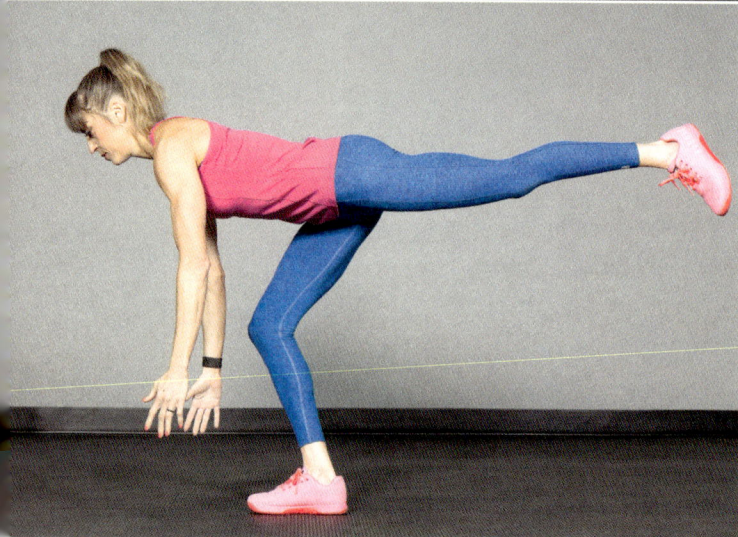

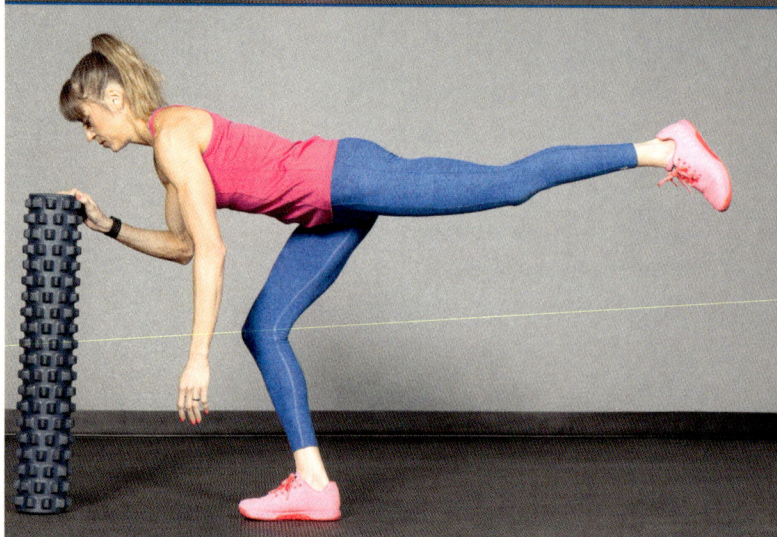

SINGLE-LEG DEADLIFT SQUAT

Balance on one foot, focusing on the two points in the ball of your foot and one point in your heel pushing down into the ground. Raise your other leg while hinging at your hips to lean your torso forward to counterbalance your leg.

Focus on leveling your pelvis so it's square to the ground as you create a straight line from your head to your raised heel. Reach your hands toward the ground or in front of your head. Straighten your support leg without locking out your knee.

Bend your knee to sink into a little squat and then straighten your leg. Do not come out of the hinge. This is a small knee bend and extend. You should feel your glute and hamstring burning through the reps.

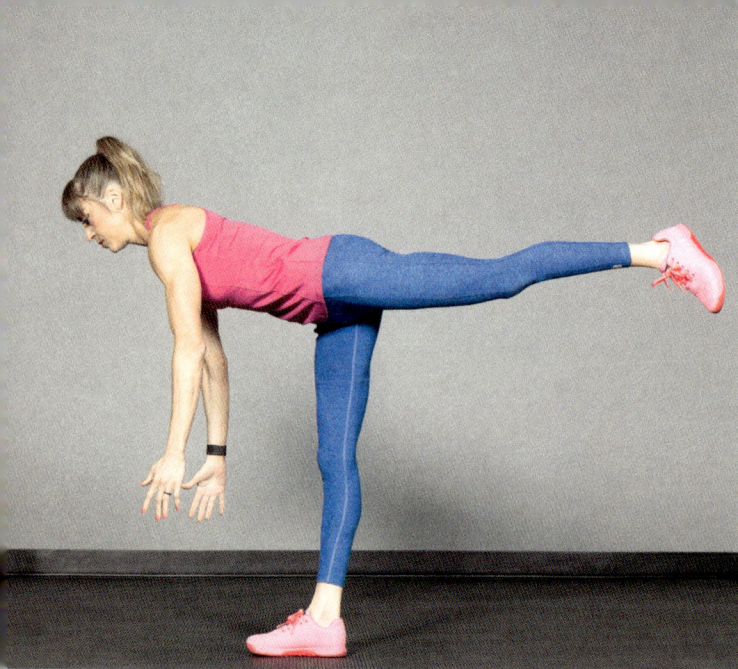

MODIFICATIONS: Place your hand on a support for stability. You can also lightly touch your back toe to the ground while staying in a hip hinge position.

EXERCISE SWAPS: Single-leg reverse hyper, single-leg deadlift hold, Romanian deadlift pulses, glute-ham hinge, straight-leg glute bridge

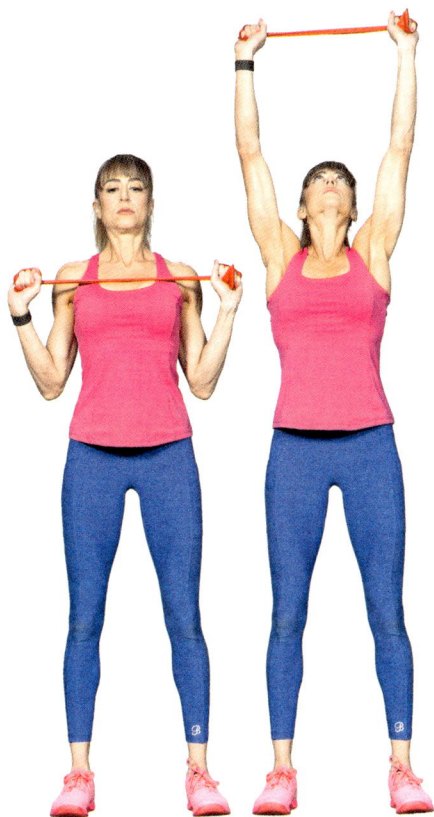

BAND/TOWEL PULL-DOWN

Hold a band or towel in both hands with your hands about shoulder-width apart. Slightly pull out on the band so that there is tension. Press your chest out and press the band overhead, keeping the band tight between your hands.

Then pull the band down toward your chest, as if pulling your chest up to the bar during a pull-up. Drive your elbows down as your shoulder blades move down and back so your back is powering the pull. Maintain tension on the band the entire time. Repeat the movement.

MODIFICATIONS: Use no band to focus on that pull-down, almost like doing a standing version of a lying W pull-down.

EXERCISE SWAPS: Lying W pull-down, pull-up, pullover, lying side slide, lat pull-down machine, band lat pull-down

SINGLE-LEG SQUAT

Stand with your back to a bench. The higher the bench, the easier the move will be. Raise one leg and sit to the bench with control. Reach your arms in front of you to help counterbalance your squat.

The more you allow yourself to sit down, the easier the move will be. If you just lightly touch the bench and come right back up, the difficulty increases. Try not to touch your other foot down each time you stand up.

MODIFICATIONS: Use a higher box or hold on to a chair or suspension trainer for support. You may also do an 80/20 or staggered stance squat. To progress, hold a weight at your chest, use a shorter box, or try a suspension trainer hand assist without sitting to a bench.

EXERCISE SWAPS: Staggered stance squat, high box single-leg squat, low box single-leg squat, pistol squat, suspension trainer single-leg squat, goblet single-leg squat, goblet squat, front squat, front lunge, step-up

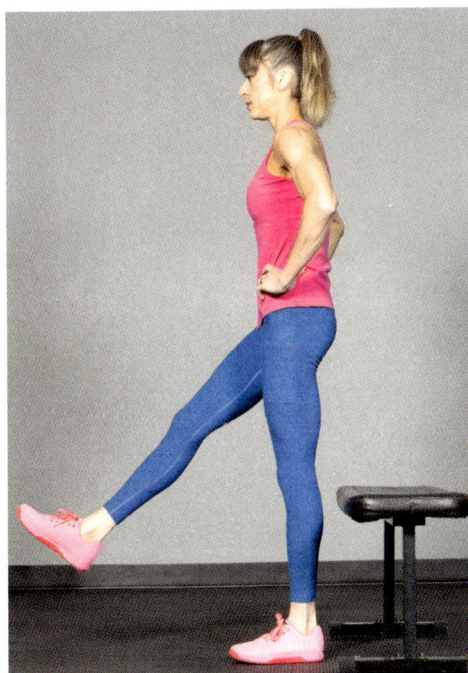

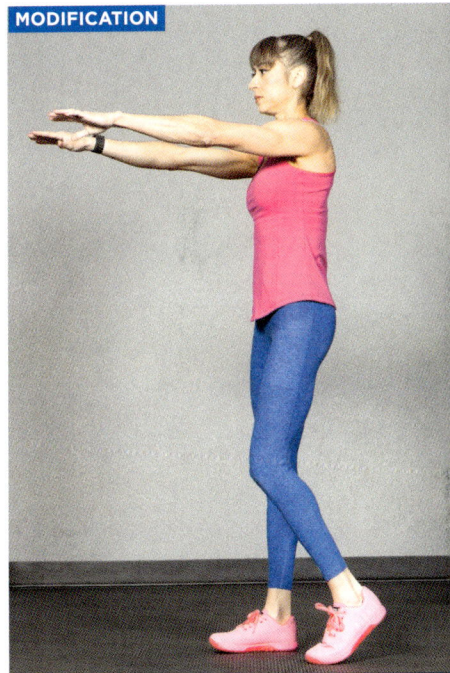

MODIFICATION

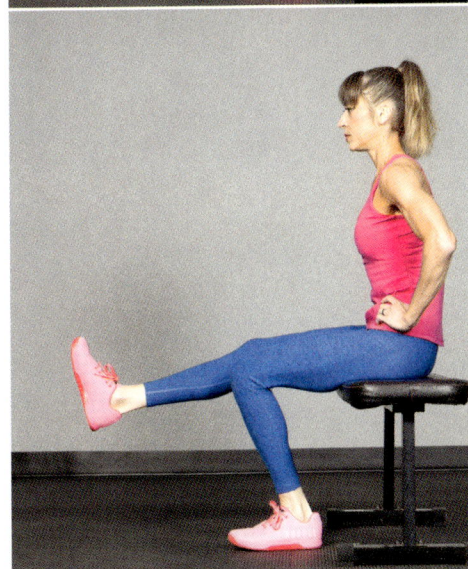

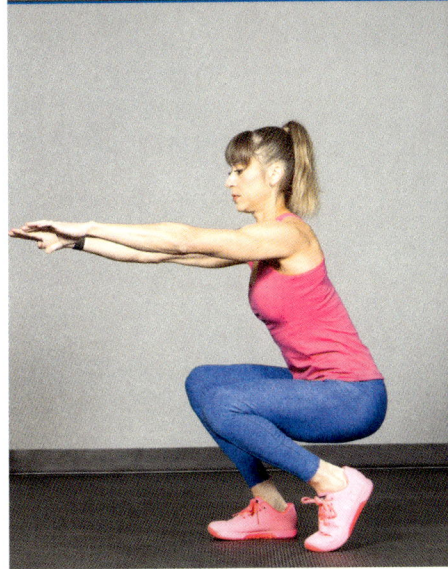

SIDE PLANK HIP DIP WITH ROTATIONAL REACH

Do a forearm side plank with your feet unstacked (your top leg in front of your bottom leg) and your elbow under your shoulder. Engage the side of your back to support your shoulder as you flex your feet to create tension down your legs. Reach your top hand up toward the ceiling.

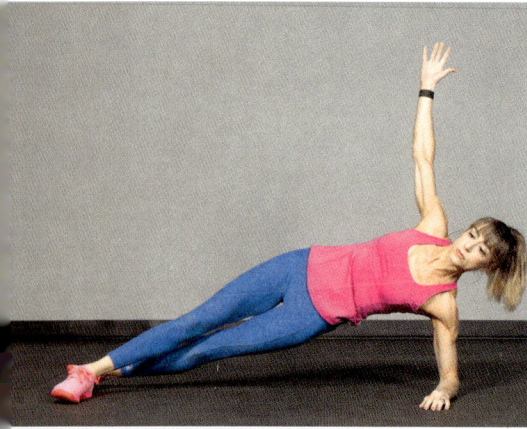

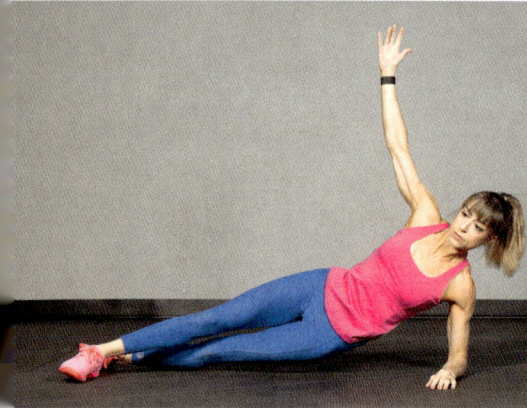

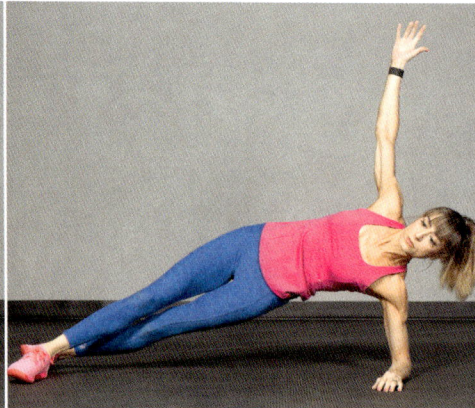

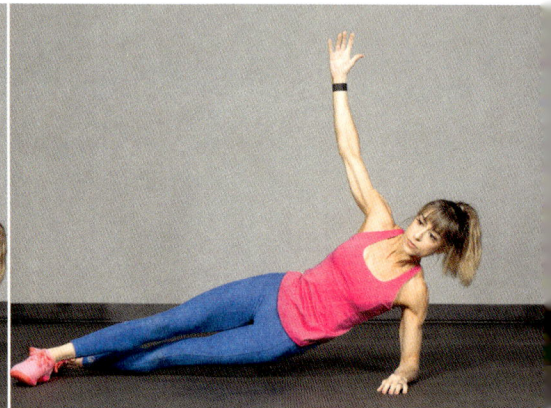

BURPEE

Stand with your feet together and then squat and place your hands on the ground while jumping your feet back into a high plank position. Perform a push-up, dropping your chest to the ground with your body moving as one unit. Push up to the plank position and jump your feet to your hands. Return to standing and jump up off the ground before repeating the movement.

MODIFICATIONS: Modify by removing the push-up or by placing your hands on a bench to do an incline plank and push-up.

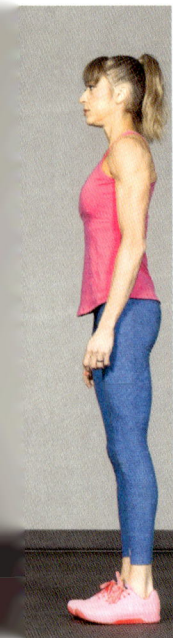

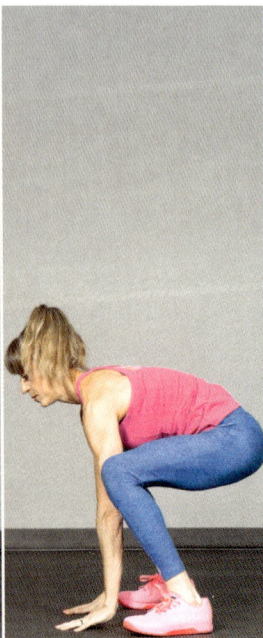

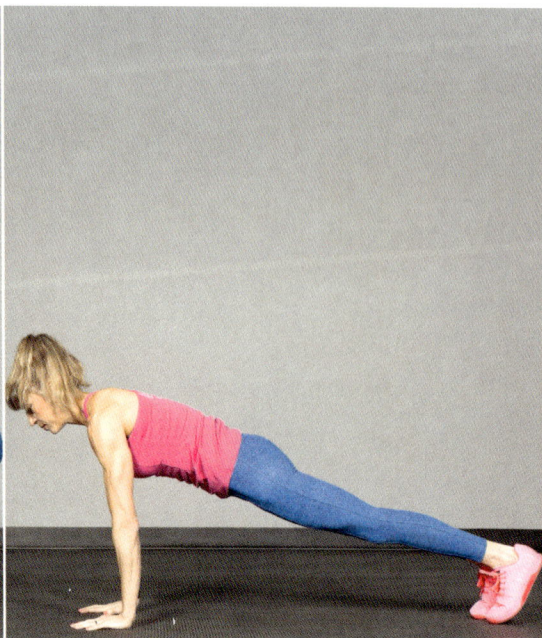

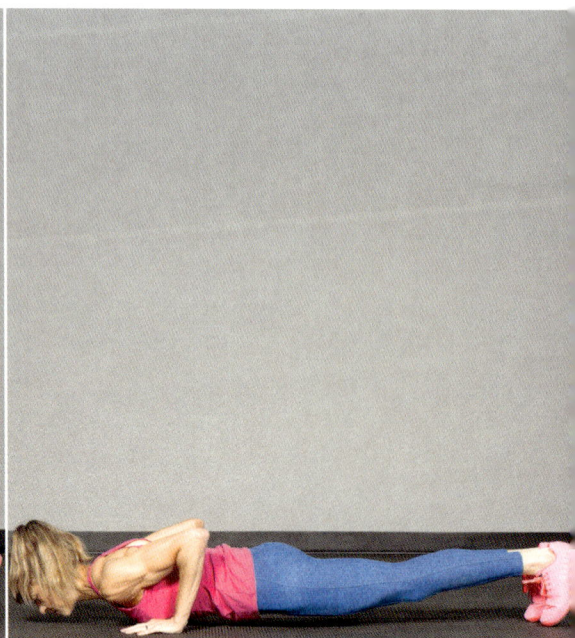

From this side plank, perform two hip dips, dropping your hip down to the ground before lifting back up into the side plank. Feel your bottom oblique and the side of your butt working. Do not let your chest rotate toward the ground and really use that bottom side to lift back up as high as you can. Do not relax on the ground when you lower.

MODIFICATIONS: Perform this move off a bench or incline to reduce the resistance on your upper body. You can also do just the rotational reach or do the hip dip movement without the reach.

After performing the two dips, reach your top hand under your body as if you're reaching for the wall behind you. As you reach under, pivot your feet as if you're moving to a front plank. Rotate back open into the side plank and repeat the hip dips.

EXERCISE SWAPS: Bench side plank hip dip with rotational reach, side plank hip dip, rotational reach plank, Russian twist, band twist, hinge and twist, side plank oblique twist

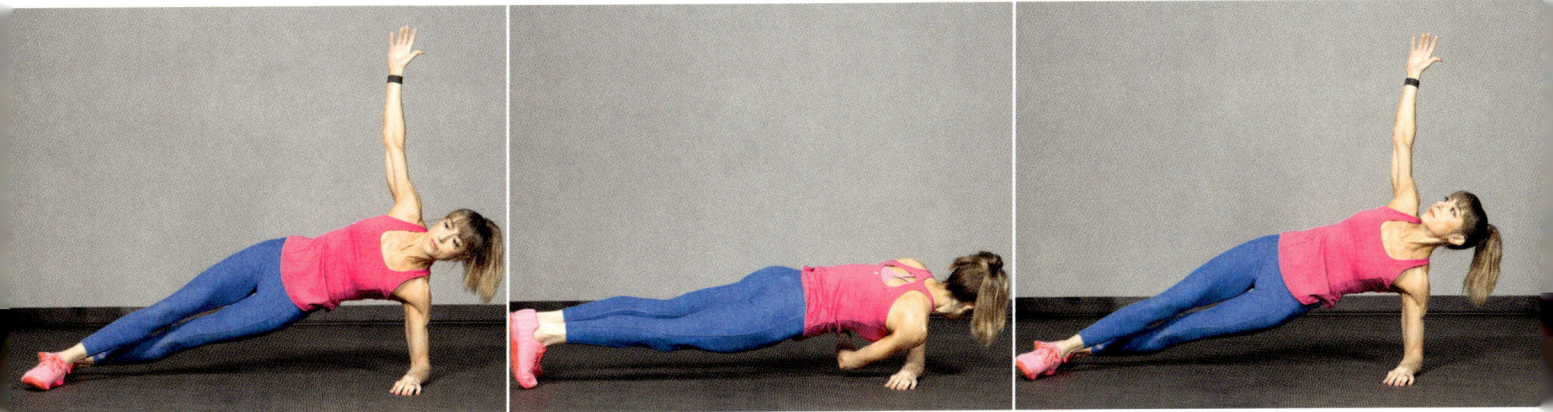

EXERCISE SWAPS: Any fun burpee variation! Squat to press, battle rope, bike sprint, sled push, rower

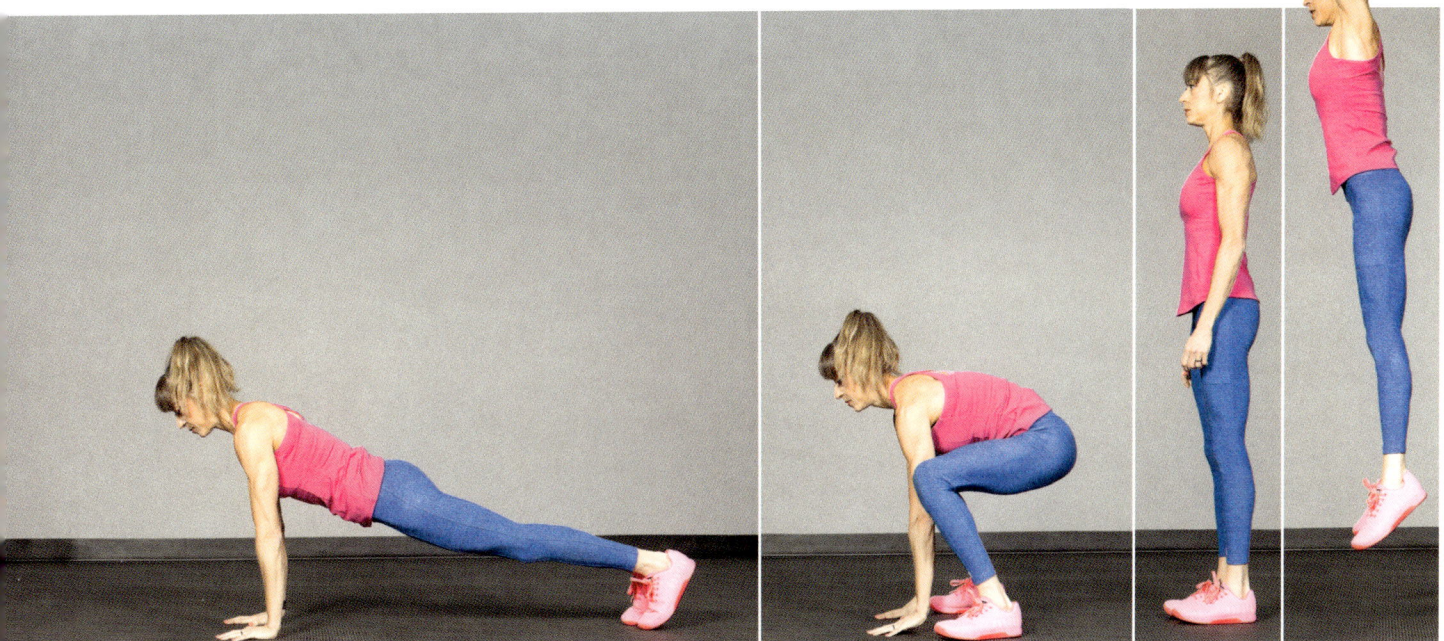

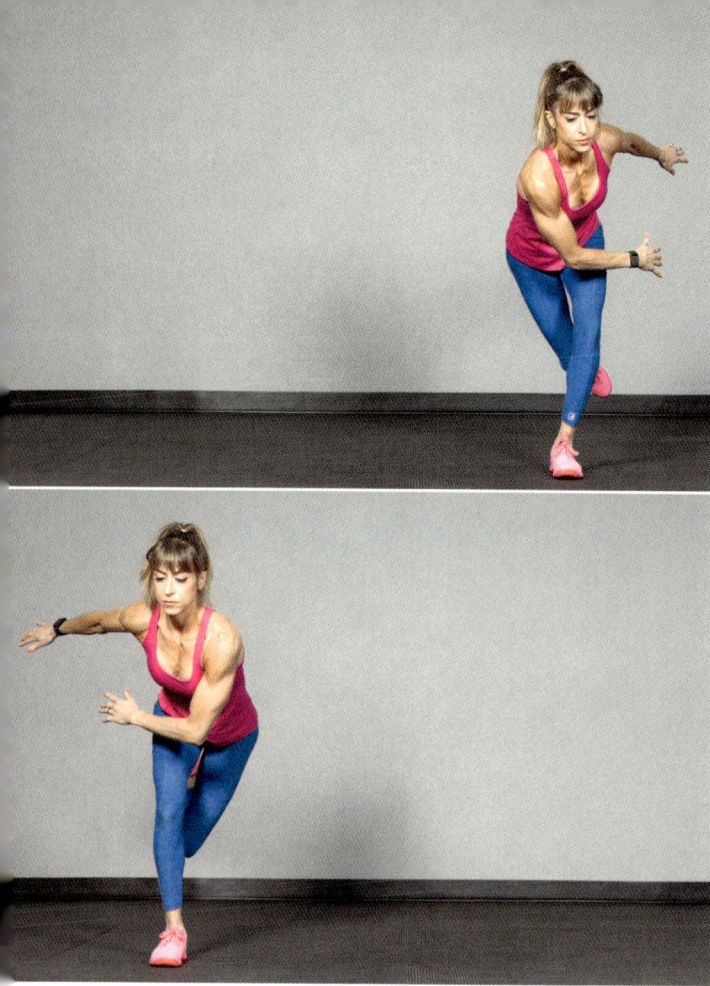

SLIDER SIDE LUNGE

Place a towel or slider under one foot and stand tall with your feet together. Bend the support leg (the one not on the slider) and sit your butt back as you slide your other foot to the side. Hinge to sit your butt back but don't round forward. Keep your support heel firmly planted on the ground. Also, make sure to slide your leg out straight to the side. Do not bend the leg on the slider.

Drive through your standing foot to pull your other foot back to your start position. Feel your inner thigh really working to slide your foot back in. Complete all reps on one side before switching.

MODIFICATIONS: Do not slide out as far to start or do the move without a slider by performing a reach and tap. To progress, go lower in the lunge, slow down the tempo, or add weight.

EXERCISE SWAPS: Cable adduction, adduction machine, side-lying adductor lift, glute bridge with squeeze, modified kneeling adductor slide, kneeling adductor slide, sumo squat

SKATER HOP

Stand to one side of the space you have available and load your weight onto your outside leg. Cross your other leg behind your support leg and sink into a little squat while swinging your arms to that side in front of you.

Load your glute and swing your arms across your body to help you power a lateral jump. Land softly on your other foot and sink into a squat on that side before pushing off to jump back to your starting position.

Feel the side of your butt really working to push and jump side to side; swing your arms outside your hip to help you launch yourself as far as possible. Try not to touch your free leg down between jumps, although you can let it swing behind.

MODIFICATIONS: Do not jump as far. If you must, touch your other leg down lightly to help with balance as you land.

EXERCISE SWAPS: Modified skater hop, alternating side lunge, side shuffle, squat with lateral leg raise, jumping jacks

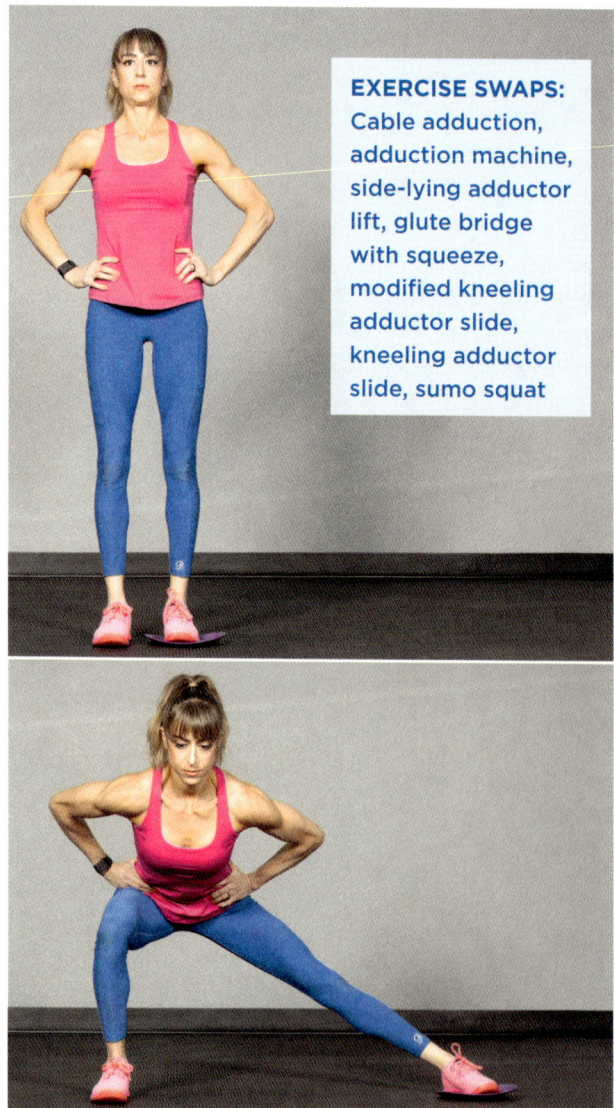

SIT-THRU

Set up on all fours. Flex your feet and press up onto your hands and the balls of your feet. Pick up one leg and bring it under your body as you pivot and lift your opposite hand to "sit through." Extend your leg in front of you as you raise your free hand toward the ceiling. Your support hand and foot are keeping you from sitting on the ground. Make sure your shoulder isn't shrugged.

Tuck your knee back under your body as you pivot back onto your hands and the balls of your feet again. Repeat the movement on the other side. Keep alternating sides, moving as quickly as you can.

MODIFICATIONS: Place your hands on a bench or incline to modify or even sit through to start without raising your hand off the ground. Check out this video for a demonstration of a regular sit-thru and the modification with a bench: https://www.youtube.com/watch?v=QYFfozU6yKk.

EXERCISE SWAPS: Russian twist, bench sit-thru, cross-body mountain climber, plank hip dip, side plank hip dip with rotational reach, side plank oblique twist, lying knees, cable twist, band twist

PLANK KNEE TUCK

Place your feet on sliders or towels and set up in a high plank position. Brace your abs and engage your back to support your shoulders.

Engage your abs to slide your feet forward to bring your knees toward your chest. Do not sit back on your heels as you tuck in or let your hands drift beyond your shoulders. Then slide your feet back out into the plank position and repeat.

You can do this using a stability ball or suspension trainer as well.

MODIFICATIONS: Slide one foot in at a time or step in instead of using the sliders. You can also modify by putting your hands on a bench or incline.

EXERCISE SWAPS: Stability ball plank knee tuck, suspension trainer plank knee tuck, step plank knee tuck, bench plank knee tuck, full body crunch, mountain climber, incline ab, hanging knee to elbow, lower body crunch

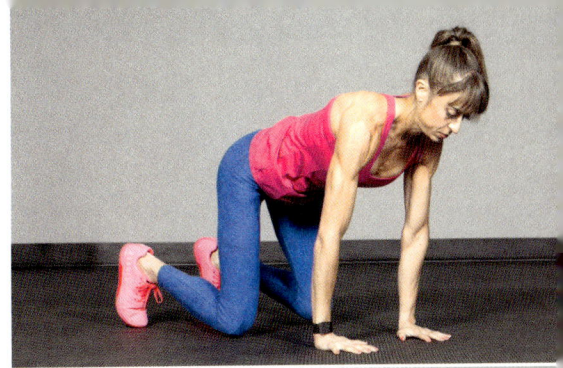

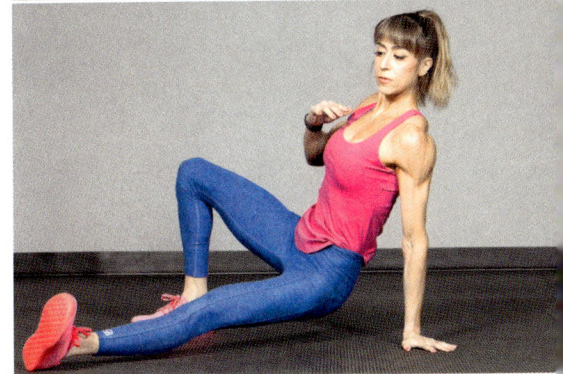

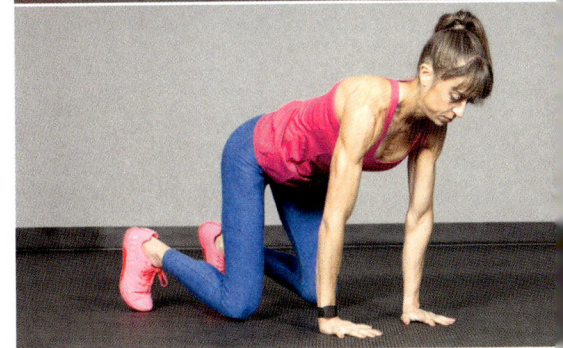

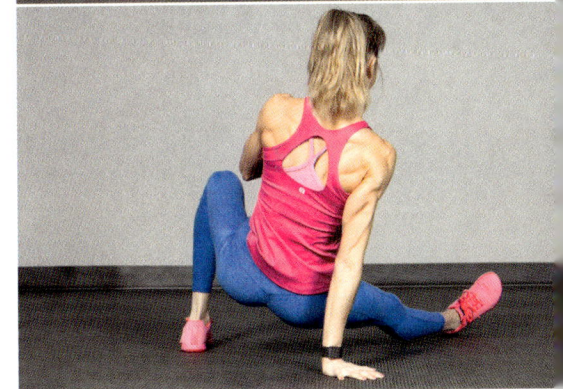

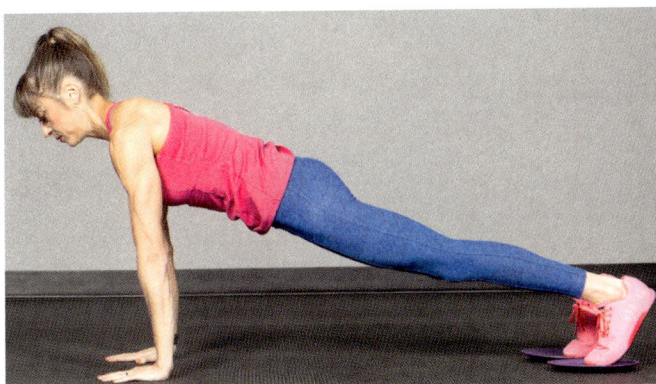

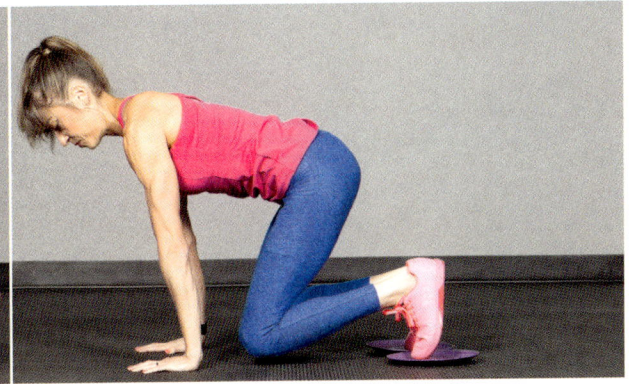

ACKNOWLEDGMENTS

> **Greatness requires the help of others.**

I was excited to write this book and share what I've learned. I thought I'd be able to do everything on my own. I'm a grinder and a very stubborn person, and I'm not good at reaching out for help. I try to bull my way through things. I'll stay up extra late and wake up extra early. I waste more hours than I should researching things and experimenting and plowing through setbacks.

I've found myself falling into this trap in the past, and I see it often with clients when they push back against "needing" the accountability, support, and guidance of coaching. We believe we can go it alone. We don't like the idea of "needing" someone else.

I think many of us can fall victim to this belief. We shy away from getting "help," seeing it as a sign of weakness or indication that we don't have the knowledge to achieve success. But I've realized how much this attitude has held me back and how much it has actually prevented me from seeing the most success I can achieve.

But really, asking for help is not in the slightest bit weak.

It's why I loved this quote from the *Arnold* documentary and love that he repeats this same idea often when giving speeches and presentations: "I always tell people that you can call me anything that you want. But don't ever, ever call me a self-made man. The only thing that was self-made was my motivation and visualization and all this stuff. There were endless amounts of people that were helping me."

We each must have drive and determination. No one can give that to us, and it's what helps us get back up when failures and setbacks happen (because they will). This is honestly what helped me countless days when I thought I just wouldn't be able to get this book finished or convey my thoughts and feelings in a way that would help.

But the more we can learn from others and stand on the shoulders of those who came before us, the more we can achieve far more than we ever thought possible.

We can't know what we don't know. We can't see the upsides to our downsides or the downsides to our upsides. We can't see the way our perspective of life colors things. Our limit to our success is ourselves.

But the more we can have that outside assistance, the further we will go to see things we can't see alone.

It isn't weakness to ask for help, to use other expertise, to have a coach, to learn from others. Asking for help is what's required to be *great*.

The more we refuse support, guidance, and coaching, the more we truly hold ourselves back.

So, I'm saying that I think I'm great and this book is great but not just because of me. I have amazing people in my life who supported me, pushed me, and challenged me, and I want to acknowledge them.

I first have to thank Ryan, my husband, my butthead, my partner in crime, who is why Redefining Strength is here today and why I had the opportunity to write this book. When I said I had a dream, he wholeheartedly supported me and worked with me to make it happen. He pushed me into the discomfortable time and time again. (And yes, I said *discomfortable*. Sometimes I make up words to get to the emotion of things, and uncomfortable things can be awkward and funny while also being uncomfortable—aka discomfortable.) He has always given me feedback and pushed me beyond my comfort zone. When filming or writing, he never hesitates to say, "Nope. Do it again." He knows I can give more. He doesn't let me settle. And honestly, I can't be thankful enough in this life to have him in my corner. (I also knew when he told me lines in this book were good that they were truly freaking magical!)

Second, my mom has always encouraged me to pursue my dreams and never let what someone else says about me hold me back from trying. Even when I was "too short" or had the lowest national ranking of my recruiting class to Boston University, she pushed me to pursue what I wanted. You miss all of the shots you don't take!

Third, my team who have helped me both indirectly and directly through their constant desire to learn and grow and help our magical community.

I have to give a special shout out to Ashley Cashdollar, who is not only a good friend but was my first true employee of Redefining Strength. Her positivity and support helped me craft what I feel is an amazing book, and she kept me going when I stared at a daunting list of exercises for the library. Her video of Kiwi and Sushi was also a gamechanger for this book!

A shout out also goes to Michelle Alley, a passionate and fabulous registered dietitian on my team. Her knowledge has helped me shape nutritional strategies to meet you where you are so you can rock those results and change not only your life but the lives of your family—allowing them to look, feel, and move their best while being their healthiest!

And butt slaps (because I'm not a hugger) of special recognition to Julia Stumpf, RD, and Brooke Harper, RD, for their extra support during this!

INDEX

ABOUT THE AUTHOR

Cori Lefkowith is the founder of Redefining Strength, an international fitness company known for its no-nonsense, educational approach to helping people get strong for life. With more than a decade of coaching experience and certifications spanning corrective exercise, performance enhancement, nutrition, menopause, pre- and postnatal fitness, and functional training, Cori has built her career on cutting through confusion and empowering individuals to take ownership of their bodies at every age.

A former Division I tennis player and state powerlifting champion, Cori's relationship with fitness has shifted dramatically over the years—from chasing perfection and battling burnout to discovering the power of sustainable, strength-driven training. Her own evolution, paired with the thousands of clients she has coached through setbacks, plateaus, life changes, and wins, led her to develop the STRONG system: a practical, adaptable framework designed to help people build habits that last and strength that carries into every part of their lives.

Since launching Redefining Strength, Cori's programs, educational videos, and daily tips have reached tens of millions worldwide. Her work has been featured in *Women's Health*, the *Guardian*, *SELF*, MindBodyGreen, Well+Good, LIVESTRONG, and more. Together with her team of coaches and dietitians, she has helped tens of thousands of clients break free from fad-diet culture, rebuild their confidence, and create results that fit real life—not the other way around.

At the heart of Cori's approach is a belief that sustainable change doesn't come from perfection, guilt, or extremes, but from taking action—especially when it's hard. Her signature phrases, including "Act as if," "Regress to progress," "Suck it up, buttercup," and "It's your choice," reflect her tough-love style and her commitment to helping people step into their strongest selves from the inside out.

Cori lives in Southern California with her husband and business partner, Ryan Heenan, and their two Bichons, Kiwi and Sushi, who monitor all workouts, coaching sessions, and writing with great enthusiasm. When she's not training, creating content, or coaching clients, she's exploring new coffee shops, filming with her pups nearby, or refining new ways to make fitness simpler and more accessible.

You can follow Cori's work at Redefining Strength, where she shares training education, programs, and practical guidance across YouTube, Instagram, Facebook, email, and her podcast.

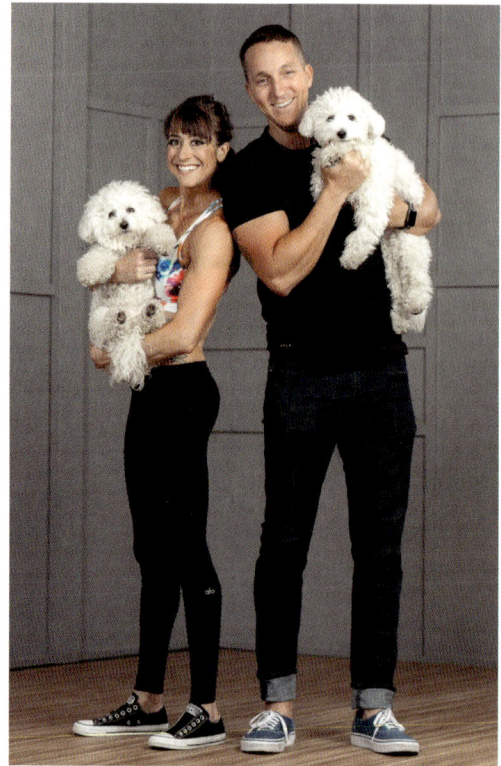